REVIEWERS

Lorraine Noll, MSN, RNC
Associate Professor
Professional Nursing Program
University of Wisconsin—Green Bay
Green Bay, Wisconsin

Fatma Youssef, DNSc, RN
Professor
School of Nursing
Marymount University
Arlington, Virginia

PREFACE

The health care system in the United States is a paradox. As a country, we spend nearly 14% of the gross domestic product on health care. Yet, only three cents of each health care dollar spent goes toward the preventive services estimated to influence over 50% of all disease, disability, and mortality in the country. Populations such as the homeless, minorities, children, elderly, uninsured, and underinsured fare poorly, although they represent more than 30% of the country's population.

The growing sense of urgency to resolve the health care crisis has turned policy makers' attention to alternative approaches that would decrease the need for institutionalized health care. Policy makers have begun looking at community-wide and community-coalition–based approaches that emphasize disease prevention, health promotion and protection, and community-based interventions. Such initiatives as President Clinton's emphasis on national health care reform (1993); legislation requiring health care reform in eight states; the PEW Health Professions Committee Reports (1991-1995) on the state of health care delivery, health professionals, and education; and the latest IOM (1994) study of the changing face of primary care have underscored the need for new approaches to solving the nation's health care problems.

As a result, the American health care system is experiencing its most dramatic transformation in history (PEW, 1995) with an emphasis on transformation of organizations and financing, health alliances, integrated networks, and public and private sector partnerships. Major transformations will not only be demanded of health care professionals but also of educational programs that prepare students to meet the demands of the changing system (PEW, 1998).

The PEW Commission (1995) indicated that health professionals of the future will need to be competent in a number of skills, including caring for the community's health, expanding access to care, coordinating care in the integrated network, practicing prevention, promoting healthy lifestyles, managing information, and participating in a racially and culturally diverse society. These competencies are all emphasized in public and community health nursing education and are needed by practicing nurses in the community.

As the nation and individual states move health care delivery toward community-oriented practice, a greater need for public and community health nurses will arise. Data indicate the long-standing existence of a shortage of nurses prepared in this area. This book is designed to assist nurses in preparing themselves for community-oriented practice by serving as a ready resource for the many questions and situations they may encounter in their practice.

The *Handbook of Public and Community Health Nursing Practice: A Health Promotion Guide* is a compilation of instruments, guides, hints, charts, graphs, and forms that provides public health and community health nurses cues that will aid in caring for clients: communities, families, and individuals. The information contained herein will also assist faculty and students in providing structure for the students' synthesis of knowledge related to all parameters of public health and community health nursing practice. In addition, researchers may find resources for application to the study of problems encountered in the community.

The cues contained in this book will assist nurses in assessing, planning, and evaluating community-oriented nursing practice. The resources in this book should not be considered exhaustive of those available to nurses but should be considered as sources that may be used as appropriate to job responsibilities or that may serve as a catalyst for searching the literature for related cues to complete the task of promoting the health of the community or population served. This work is a ready reference for the nurse to use while intervening with clients to promote their health and well being. These cues are also beneficial in evaluating client outcomes.

The *Handbook of Public and Community Health Nursing Practice: A Health Promotion Guide* is organized into four parts. The first part supplies information that nurses in the community can use daily, such as sources of HIV information; health-related, world-wide websites; resources for culturally diverse populations; and common epidemiologic rates. The second part furnishes assessment tools for a variety of client populations and settings, including community, home and industry, family, individual, and nutritional to provide an extensive assemblage of data collection instruments. The third part points to indicators of risk that help predict potential health problems, such as substance or physical abuse, depression and mental illness, and communicable disease; this part also guides the nurse's intervention. The fourth part offers teaching tools to assist the nurse in providing clients with guidance on self-examination for cancer, good nutrition, living with AIDS, caring for newborns, and other health promotion topics.

Additional resources for community health can be found on the Internet at Mosby's community health website: www.mosby.com/communityhealth/.

Handbook of Public and Community Health Nursing Practice

A Health Promotion Guide

Second Edition

MARCIA STANHOPE, RN, DSN, FAAN, C
Associate Dean and Professor
College of Nursing
University of Kentucky
Lexington, Kentucky

RUTH N. KNOLLMUELLER, RN, PhD
Clinical Associate
School of Nursing
University of Connecticut
Storrs, Connecticut

Illustrated

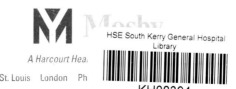

Mosby

A Harcourt Hea

St. Louis   London   Ph

Vice President, Nursing Division: Sally Schrefer
Executive Editor: June D. Thompson
Senior Developmental Editor: Linda Caldwell
Project Manager: John Rogers
Senior Production Editor: Helen Hudlin
Design: Kathi Gosche

2nd EDITION

NOTICE

Pharmacology is an ever-changing field. Standard safety precautions must be followed, but as new research and clinical experience broaden our knowledge, changes in treatment and drug therapy may become necessary or appropriate. Readers are advised to check the most current product information provided by the manufacturer of each drug to be administered to verify the recommended dose, the method and duration of administration, and contraindications. It is the responsibility of the appropriately licensed health care provider, relying on experience and knowledge of the patient, to determine dosages and the best treatment for each individual patient. Neither the publisher nor the editor assumes any liability for any injury and/or damage to persons or property arising from this publication.

Mosby, Inc., *A Harcourt Health Sciences Company,* 11830 Westline Industrial Drive, St. Louis, Missouri 63146

Printed in the United States of America

Library of Congress Cataloging-in-Publication Data

Stanhope, Marcia.
    Handbook of public and community health nursing practice : a health promotion guide / Marcia Stanhope, Ruth N. Knollmueller.—2nd ed.
        p. ; cm.
    Rev. ed. of: Public and community health nurse's consultant. c1997.
    Includes bibliographical references and index.
    ISBN 0-323-01332-5
        1. Community health nursing—Handbooks, manuals, etc.   2. Public health nursing—Handbooks, manuals, etc.   I. Knollmueller, Ruth N.   II. Stanhope, Marcia. Public and community health nurse's consultant.   III. Title.
        [DNLM: 1. Community Health Nursing—Handbooks.   2. Public Health Nursing—Handbooks. WY 49 S786p 2001]
    RT98.S783 2001
    610.73'4—dc21   00-046540

00 01 02 03 04 CL/RDC 9 8 7 6 5 4 3 2 1

We wish to thank those who have permitted their work to be shared and we acknowledge the expertise and the contributions they have made to preventing disease and promoting the health of communities, families, and individuals.

Special acknowledgment goes to Dr. Donna L. Wong for the material borrowed from the three pediatric nursing textbooks she has authored: *Whaley and Wong's Nursing Care of Infants and Children,* edition 6; *Wong and Whaley's Clinical Manual of Pediatric Nursing,* edition 5; and *Whaley and Wong's Essentials of Pediatric Nursing,* edition 5.

A special thanks to Scott Seitz and Peg Teachey for their assistance in completing this work.

Marcia Stanhope
Ruth N. Knollmueller

CONTENTS

Part One: Resource Data   1

Part Two: Assessment   71

Individual Assessment   215

Nutritional Assessment 255

Part Three: Indicators of Risk 307

Abuse 307

Mental Health   356

Accessibility Grid

	Infants	Children	Adolescents	Adults	Elderly	Men	Women	Pregnant women	Clients with special needs	Clients with mental health concerns	Clients from specific cultures and religions	Family	Community
Windshield Survey: A Micro Approach (p 71)													X
Community Assessment: A Macro Approach (p 73)													X
Community Health Assessment Model (p 76)													X
Lifespan Community Assessment—A Developmental Approach (p 79)													X
Public Health Capacity-Building (p 83)													X
Community-Oriented Health Systems (p 90)													X
Eleven Functional Health Patterns Assessment Guidelines for Communities (p 93)													X

Tool							
Assessment Survey: Housing for the Disabled (p 109)					X		
Tools for Living for the Aged and Disabled (p 115)		X			X		
Life Skills and Community Living (p 117)					X		
Family Self-Care Patterns (p 155)							X
Stages of Family Development: Health Promotion and Disease Prevention (p 160)							X
Family Health Assessment Interview (p 161)							X
Eleven Functional Health-Pattern Assessment Guidelines for Families (p 165)							X
Family Health and Functioning Assessment (p 168)							X
Suggested Areas for Assessment of Family Health-Related Lifestyle (p 170)							X
Family Career: Stages, Tasks, and Transitions (p 172)							X
Family Stage-Specific Risk Factors and Related Health Problems (p 173)							X
The Eight-Stage Family Life Cycle (p 177)							X

This grid lists all of the tools that are related to a specific client population.

Continued

Accessibility Grid—cont'd

	Infants	Children	Adolescents	Adults	Elderly	Men	Women	Pregnant women	Clients with special needs	Clients with mental health concerns	Clients from specific cultures and religions	Family	Community
Comparison of Family Life Cycle Stages of Duvall and Miller with Carter and McGoldrick (p 177)												X	
Dislocations of the Family Life Cycle by Divorce, Requiring Additional Steps to Restabilize and Proceed Developmentally (p 179)												X	
Remarried Family Formation: a Developmental Outline (p 181)												X	
Cultural Heritage Assessment Tool (p 182)											X		
Religious Beliefs that Affect Nursing Care (p 184)											X		
Cultural Characteristics Related to Healthcare of Children and Families (p 200)		X									X	X	
Genogram Form (p 212)												X	

Genogram Symbols (p 214)										X
Ecomap Form (p 215)										X
Global Assessment of Functioning (GAF) Scale (p 215)			X							
Initial Patient Assessment (p 217)			X							
Family Health and Functioning Assessment (p 219)			X							X
Short Portable Mental Status Questionnaire (SPMSQ) (p 220)			X							
Mini-Mental LLC (p 221)			X							
Mental Status Test (Mini-Mental State) and Directions (p 223)			X							
Social Assessment of the Elderly (p 252)								X		
Primary Changes of Aging (p 254)								X		
Family Nutritional Assessment Tool (p 261)										X
Nutritional Assessment of the Elderly (p 277)								X		
Recommended Nutrient Intakes for Canadians (p 284)	X				X	X	X	X		

Continued

Accessibility Grid—cont'd

	Infants	Children	Adolescents	Adults	Elderly	Men	Women	Pregnant women	Clients with special needs	Clients with mental health concerns	Clients from specific cultures and religions	Family	Community
Characteristics of Substances of Abuse (p 308)										X			
The Five Stages of Substance Abuse (p 315)										X			
Brief Drug Abuse Screening Test (B-DAST) (p 317)										X			
The CAGE Questionnaire (p 318)										X			
Selected Drugs Commonly Abused and Symptoms of Abuse (p 319)										X			
Leading Drugs Abused in the United States (p 322)										X			
Types of Child Abuse (p 322)		X											
Components of Report of Child Maltreatment (p 325)		X											

Parental Risk Factors for Child Maltreatment (p 327)											X
Methods Used to Pressure Children into Sexual Activity (p 333)			X								
Talking with Children Who Reveal Abuse (p 333)			X								X
Warning Signs of Child Abuse (p 334)			X								
Child History—Indicators of Potential or Actual Child Abuse and Neglect (p 335)			X								
Parenting Profile Assessment (p 338)											X
Definitions of Elder Abuse (p 341)					X						
Signs of Elder Mistreatment (p 342)					X						
History of Elder—Possible Indicators of Potential or Actual Elder Abuse (p 343)					X						
Abuse Assessment Screen (p 346)						X	X				X
Danger Assessment (p 347)						X	X				X
Indicators of Potential or Actual Wife Abuse from History (p 348)					X	X	X				X

Continued

Accessibility Grid—cont'd

	Infants	Children	Adolescents	Adults	Elderly	Men	Women	Pregnant women	Clients with special needs	Clients with mental health concerns	Clients from specific cultures and religions	Family	Community
Indicators of Potential or Actual Violence in a Family from Nursing History (p 351)						X	X					X	
Indicators of Potential or Actual Violence in a Family from Nursing Observation (p 354)						X	X					X	
Criteria for Possible Aggression (p 355)						X	X					X	
Behaviors Associated with Low Self-Esteem (p 356)										X			
Behavioral Characteristics of Borderline Personality Disorder (p 357)										X			
NANDA Nursing Diagnosis: Altered Family Processes (Specify) (p 358)										X		X	
Families with Disturbances in Internal Dynamics (p 359)										X		X	

Early Warning Signs of Mental Health Problems in Children and Adolescents (p 360)		X	X									
Major Depressive Disorder Subgroups (p 363)		X	X									
Behaviors Associated with Depression (p 365)												X
Illnesses Associated with Depression (p 366)												X
Differences Between Anxiety and Depression (p 368)												X
Dealing with Depression: The Nursing Process and Maslow's Hierarchy of Need (p 369)												X
Changes Symptomatic of Depression (p 372)												X
Risk Factors Related to Suicide (p 374)												X
Assessing Risk for Suicide (p 375)												X
Clues of Suicidal Risk in Adolescents (p 377)				X								X
Suicide/Self-Harm Assessment (p 378)												X
Dealing with Stress (p 380)												X

Continued

Accessibility Grid—cont'd

	Infants	Children	Adolescents	Adults	Elderly	Men	Women	Pregnant women	Clients with special needs	Clients with mental health concerns	Clients from specific cultures and religions	Family	Community
Symptoms of Stress (p 384)										X			
Strategies for Managing Stress (p 385)										X			
Family Systems Stressors-Strength Inventory (FS³I) (p 386)										X		X	
The Worry Scale (p 405)										X			
Family Crisis-Oriented Personal Evaluation Scales (F-COPES) (p 408)										X		X	
Assessment Data for Crisis Intervention (p 411)										X			
Problems Exhibited by the Crisis-Prone Person (p 413)										X			
Areas of Disordered Functioning in Anorexia Nervosa (p 413)										X			

Continued

Accessibility Grid—cont'd

	Infants	Children	Adolescents	Adults	Elderly	Men	Women	Pregnant women	Clients with special needs	Clients with mental health concerns	Clients from specific cultures and religions	Family	Community
Nurse Case Management in Rehabilitation (p 564)									X				
Access to Healthcare Services (p 575)									X				
Preserving Self: From Victim, to Client, to Disabled Person (p 588)									X				
Assessment of Equipment Needs for the Disabled Client (p 590)									X				
Physiologic Changes from Aging and Alterations in Teaching Techniques (p 606)					X								
Elderly Clients' Special Learning Needs (p 607)					X								
Teaching Guidelines for the Elderly Client with Cancer (p 608)					X								

Implications for the Toddler's Health Learning (p 613)					X							
Implications for the Preschooler's Health Learning (p 614)					X							
Implications for the School-Age Child's Health Learning (p 615)					X							
Implications for the Adolescent's Health Learning (p 616)				X								
Implications for the Young and Middle Adult's Health Learning (p 617)			X									
Implications for the Older Adult's Health Learning (p 618)		X										
Sign Language for Common Health Situations (p 619)	X											
Manual Sign Language Alphabet (p 621)	X											
Tips for Communicating with a Hearing Impaired Person (p 621)	X											
Keep It Simple—Reading Skills Rules (p 622)	X											
SMOG Testing to Check Literacy Skills (p 623)	X											

Continued

Accessibility Grid—cont'd

	Infants	Children	Adolescents	Adults	Elderly	Men	Women	Pregnant women	Clients with special needs	Clients with mental health concerns	Clients from specific cultures and religions	Family	Community
Readability Graph (p 626)									X				
Gunning Fog Index Scale (p 627)									X				
Nursing Suggestions to Encourage Language Development in Preschoolers (p 629)		X							X				
Administration and Scoring of the Preschool Readiness Experimental Screening Scale (PRESS) (p 630)		X											
The Progression and Recovery of the Alcoholic in the Disease of Alcoholism (p 633)										X			
Stages of Chemical Dependence (p 634)										X			
Substance Use Prevention (p 634)										X			

Advantages and Disadvantages of Contraceptive Methods in the Adolescent (p 636)				X			
Pelvic Muscle Exercises (p 639)			X				
Nursing Counseling for Families about Enuresis (p 640)			X				X
Blood Pressure Recommendations for Follow-up and Classifications—Adult (p 655)			X				
Vision, Hearing, and Language Screening Procedures (p 666)	X		X			X	
Major Developmental Characteristics of Hearing (p 670)	X					X	
Major Developmental Characteristics of Language and Speech (p 671)	X					X	
Landmarks of Speech, Language, and Hearing Ability During the Preschool Period (p 672)	X					X	
Nurse's Interventions for Screening Vision and Hearing of Preschoolers (p 675)	X					X	
Clues for Detecting Visual Impairment (p 676)	X				X		

Continued

Accessibility Grid—cont'd

	Infants	Children	Adolescents	Adults	Elderly	Men	Women	Pregnant women	Clients with special needs	Clients with mental health concerns	Clients from specific cultures and religions	Family	Community
Denver Eye Screening Test (p 678)		X							X				
Tuning Fork Tests (p 679)		X		X					X				
Normal Tooth Formation in the Child (p 680)		X											
Developmental Tools Used to Assess Children with Chronic Conditions (p 682)		X											
Denver Developmental Screening Test/Denver II (p 700)		X											
Cultural Awareness: The Denver Developmental Screening Tests (p 703)		X									X		
Denver II Scoring (p 704)		X											
Denver Articulation Screening Examination (p 705)		X											

Growth Measurements: Birth to 18 Years (p 710)	X	X	X									
Warning Signs that May Indicate the Presence of Childhood Cancer (p 735)		X										
Testicular Self-Examination (p 741)					X							
Breast Self-Examination (p 742)						X						
Vulvar Self-Examination (p 747)						X						
Fibrocystic Changes of the Breast (p 762)						X						
Failure to Thrive—Nonorganic (p 768)	X						X					
Clinical Manifestations of Nonorganic Failure to Thrive (p 769)	X						X					
Feeding Children with Nonorganic Failure to Thrive (p 769)	X						X					
Characteristics of Failure-to-Thrive Family (p 771)	X						X				X	
Recommended Nutritional Intake for Pregnant Adolescents (p 779)			X					X				
Recommended Nutritional Intake for Young Adults (p 780)				X								
Recommended Nutritional Intake for Elderly People (p 781)					X							

Continued

Accessibility Grid—cont'd

	Infants	Children	Adolescents	Adults	Elderly	Men	Women	Pregnant women	Clients with special needs	Clients with mental health concerns	Clients from specific cultures and religions	Family	Community
Developmental Milestones Associated with Feeding (p 782)	X	X											
Low-Gluten Diet for Children with Celiac Disease (p 809)		X							X				
Cultural and Regional Foods (p 820)											X		
Food Restrictions of Various Religions (p 825)											X		
Clinical Categories for Children with HIV Infection (p 845)		X							X				
Normal Discomforts Experienced during Pregnancy (p 858)								X					
Prenatal High Risk Factors (p 860)								X					
Risk Factors Affecting Pregnancy (p 865)								X					

Assessment Focus at First Prenatal and Return Visits (p 866)					X				
Nursing Strategies for Working with Childbearing Clients Experiencing Crisis and Grief (p 867)			X		X				
Family System Changes during the Childbearing Cycle (p 868)					X			X	
Parenting Tasks for Developmental Landmarks in Infancy (p 869)	X							X	
Normal Sleep Patterns for Infants (p 870)	X								
Visual Developmental Milestones during Infancy (p 871)	X								
Progressive Auditory Development of Infants during Infancy (p 871)	X								
Clinical Assessment of Nutritional Status (p 872)	X								
Development of Feeding Skills (p 878)	X								
Feeding for the First 12 Months of Life (p 880)	X								
Infant State-Related Behavior Chart (p 881)	X								

Continued

Accessibility Grid—cont'd

	Infants	Children	Adolescents	Adults	Elderly	Men	Women	Pregnant women	Clients with special needs	Clients with mental health concerns	Clients from specific cultures and religions	Family	Community
Common Concerns and Problems of the First Year (p 885)	X												
Infant Stimulation Guide (p 898)	X												
Tips for a Baby's Safety (p 901)	X												
Protocol for Postpartum Home Visit (p 906)	X											X	

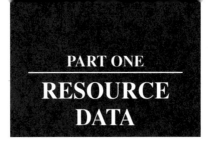

PART ONE
RESOURCE DATA

RESOURCE INFORMATION — CLIENT

Resources for reference and referral are an essential part of the nurse's repertoire. Assisting clients in seeking needed information is central to public/community health nursing practice. The following is a selected group of resources to help the nurse in working with clients, families, and communities.

Community Resources—United States

The following is a list of resources on many different health-related topics, from alcoholism to water safety. The list includes names and addresses that can be used to obtain further information. It is not by any means a complete list, but is meant to serve as a starting point. Because telephone numbers may change, please contact directory assistance for proper listings.

Acquired Immunodeficiency Syndrome (AIDS)

National AIDS Hotline
c/o American Social Health Association
PO Box 13827
Research Triangle Park, NC 27709
(800) 342-AIDS (2437) or
(800) 342-7514

Public Health Service AIDS Information Hotline
(800) 342-AIDS
(202) 245-6867 (in AK and HI only)

Advocacy

American Civil Liberties Union
125 Broad St
New York, NY 10004-2400
(212) 549-2500

Occupational Safety and Health Administration (OSHA)
US Department of Labor, Office of Public Affairs
Room N3647
200 Constitution Ave NW
Washington, DC 20210
(202) 693-1999

Alcohol and Drug Abuse

AL-ANON Family Group Headquarters, Inc
1600 Corporate Landing Pkwy
Virginia Beach, VA 23454-5617
757-563-1600
888-4AL-ANON

Alcoholics Anonymous
Call local chapters (see White Pages of phone directory)

International Commission for Prevention of Alcoholism & Drug Dependency
6830 Laurel St NW
Washington, DC 20012

MADD—Mothers Against Drunk Driving
P.O. Box 541688
Dallas, TX 75354-1688
(800) GET-MADD

National Clearinghouse for Alcohol & Drug Information, Center for Substance Abuse and Prevention
5600 Fishers Lane,
Rockville, MD 20847-2345
(301) 443-0365
800-729-6686

National Cocaine Hotline
Phoenix House
164 West 74th St
New York, NY 10023
(800) COCAINE

National Council on Alcoholism & Drug Dependence, Inc
2 West 21st St
New York, NY 10010

SADD—Students Against Driving Drunk
PO Box 800
Marlboro, MA 01752
(617) 481-3568

Alzheimer's Disease

Alzheimer's Disease Association
919 N Michigan Ave, #1100
Chicago, IL 60601
(312) 335-8700

Alzheimer's Disease Education and Referral Center (ADEAR)
PO Box 8250
Silver Springs, MD 20907-8250
(800) 438-4380

Arthritis and Collagen Disorders

American Juvenile Arthritis Organization
1314 Spring St NW
Atlanta, GA 30309
(404) 872-7100

Arthritis Foundation
1330 W Peachtree St
Atlanta, GA 30309
(404) 872-7100

National Arthritis and Musculoskeletal and Skin Diseases Information Clearinghouse
1 AMS Cr
Bethesda, MD 20892-3675

Scleroderma Research Foundation
2320 Bath St, Ste. 315
Santa Barbara, CA 93105
(800) 441-CURE

United Scleroderma
Foundation, Inc
89 Newbury St, Ste. 201
Danvers, MA 01923
(800) 722-HOPE

Asthma and Allergies

American Lung Association
1740 Broadway
New York, NY 10019
(212) 315-8700

**Asthma and Allergy
Foundation of America**
1233 20th St NW, Ste. 400
Washington, DC 20036
1 (800) ASTHMA

Bereavement

The Compassionate Friends
PO Box 3696
Oakbrook, IL 60522-3696
(650) 990-0010

SIDS Network
PO Box 520
Ledyard, CT 06339

**Survivors of Suicide (SOS):
Directory of Survivor
Groups, American
Association of Suicidology**
4201 Connecticut Ave NW,
Ste. 408
Washington, DC 20008

**Widowed Persons Service,
AARP**
601 E St NW
Washington, DC 20049
(800) 424-3410

Blindness

**American Council of the
Blind**
1155 15th St NW, Ste. 1004
Washington, DC 20005
(800) 424-8666

**American Foundation for
the Blind, Inc**
11 Penn Plaza, Ste. 300
New York, NY 10001
(212) 502-7600

Braille Institute
741 N Vermont Ave
Los Angeles, CA 90029

Guide Dogs for the Blind
PO Box 151200
San Rafael, CA 94915-1200
(800) 295-4050

The Library of Congress
National Library Service for
the Blind and Physically
Handicapped
Washington, DC 20542
(202) 707-5100

**National Association for
Visually Handicapped**
NAVH NY City
22 West 21st St
New York, NY 10010
(212) 889-3141
NAVH San Francisco
3201 Balboa St
San Francisco, CA 94121
(415) 221-3201

National Eye Institute
National Institutes of Health
Information Officer
2020 Vision Place
Bethesda, MD 20892-3655
(301) 496-5248

**National Retinitis
Pigmentosa Foundation**
1401 Mt. Royal Ave., 4th fl.
Baltimore, MD 21217
(800) 683-5555

Prevent Blindness America
500 E Remington Rd
Schaumburg, IL 60173
(800) 331-2020

Recording for the Blind, Inc
20 Roszel Rd
Princeton, NJ 08540
(609) 452-0606

Burns

National Burn Federation
3737 5th Ave
Suite 206
San Diego, CA 92103

Cancer

AMC Cancer Information
(800) 525-3777

American Association of Cancer Education
Educational Research and
Development
University of Alabama at
Birmingham
401 CHSD University St
Birmingham, AL 35294

American Cancer Society
1599 Clifford Rd NE
Atlanta, GA 30329
(800) 227-2345

American Pain Society
4700 W Lake Ave
Glenview, IL 60025
(847) 375-4715

American Society of Clinical Oncology
225 Reinekers Lane, Ste. 650
Alexandria, VA 22314
(703) 299-0150

Association of Cancer Online Resources
173 Duane St, 3rd Floor
New York, NY 10013-3334
(212) 226-5525

Association of Community Cancer Centers
11600 Nebel St, Ste. 201
Rockville, MD 20852-2557
(301) 984-9496

Association of Pediatric Oncology Nurses
4700 W Lake Ave
Glenview, IL 60025
(847) 375-4724

Encore (discussion and exercise program for women who have had breast cancer surgery)
National Board, YWCA
726 Broadway
New York, NY 10003
(212) 614-2700

Federation for Children with Special Needs
95 Berkley St
Boston, MA 02116
(800) 331-0688 (voice or
TDD)
(617) 482-2915

International Association Cancer Victors and Friends, Inc
7740 W Manchester Ave,
Ste. 110
Playa del Rey, CA 90291
(213) 822-5032

Intravenous Nurses Society
Fresh Pond Square,
10 Fawcett St
Cambridge, MA 02138
(617) 441-3009

Leukemia Society of America, Inc
733 3rd Ave
New York, NY 10017
(212) 573-8484

Make A Wish Foundation of America
2600 N Central Ave, Ste. 936
Phoenix, AZ 85004
(602) 722-9474

Make Today Count (for persons with cancer or other life-threatening illnesses)
101½ S Union St
Alexandria, VA 22314-3323
(703) 548-9674

National Association of Meal Programs (referrals)
1414 Prince St, Ste. 202
Alexandria, VA 22314
(703) 548-5558

National Lymphedema Network
Latham Square
1611 Telegraph Ave, Ste. 111
Oakland, CA 94612-2138
(800) 541-3259

National Neurofibromatosis Foundation
95 Pine St, 16th Floor
New York, NY 10015
(800) 323-7938

NIH Cancer Info Service Public Inquiries Office
Building 31, Room 10A03
31 Center Dr
Bethesda, MD 20892-2580
1 (800) Cancer
1 (800) 332-8615 (Hearing-impaired TTY)

Y-Me National Breast Cancer Organization
212 W Van Buren St
Chicago, IL 60607-3908
National hotline
(800) 221-2141
Spanish hotline
(800) 986-9505

Child Abuse

Child Help USA and Children's Defense Fund
25 E St NW
Washington, DC 20001
(800) 4ACHILD

Clearinghouse on Child Abuse and Neglect Information
330 C St NW
Washington, DC 20013
(800) 394-3366

Children

American Pediatric Society/Society for Pediatric Research
3400 Forest Dr, Ste. B-7
The Woodlands, TX 77381
(281) 419-0052

American SIDS Institute
2480 Windy Hill Rd, Ste. 380
Marietta, GA 30067
(770) 612-1030

National Tay-Sachs and Allied Disease Association
2001 Beacon St, Suite 204
Brighton, MA 02135
(800) 906-8723

Shriners Hospital Referral Line
(800) 237-5055

The Starlight Children's Foundation
5900 Wilshire Blvd,
Ste. 2530
Los Angeles, CA 90036

Diabetes

American Association of Diabetes Educators
100 W Monroe St, 4th Floor
Chicago, IL 60603-1901
(312) 424-2426

American Diabetes Association
1701 N Beauregard St
Alexandria, VA 22311
(800) DIABETES

American Diabetes Association Camp Directory
801 W Firewood Ln, Ste. 103
Anchorage, AK 99503
(800) DIABETES

Juvenile Diabetes Foundation International Hotline
120 Wall St
New York, NY 10015
(800) JDF-CURE

National Diabetes Information Clearinghouse
1 Information Way
Bethesda, MD 20892-3500

The Juvenile Diabetes Foundation
23 E 26th St
New York, NY 10010

Disabilities and Handicaps

American Stroke Association Support Groups National Center
7272 Greenville Ave
Dallas, TX 75231
(800) AHA-USA1
(888) 4 STROKE

Autism Society of America
7910 Woodmont Ave,
Ste. 300
Bethesda, MD 20814-3015

Boy Scouts of America
Scouting for the Handicapped Division
PO Box 152079
1325 Walnut Hill Ln
Irving, TX 75015-2079

Brain Injury Association, Inc
105 N Alfred St
Alexandria, VA 22314

Clearinghouse on Disability Information Office of Special Education and Rehabilitative Services
Switzer Bldg, Rm 3132
330 C St, SW
Washington, DC 20202-2524
(202) 205-8241

Disability Rights Advocates
449 15th St, Ste. 303
Oakland, CA 94612
(510) 451-8644

Farmers (services and devices for handicapped farmers)
FARM (Easter Seal Society of Iowa, Inc)
PO Box 4002
Des Moines, IA 50333

Income Tax Services for People with Disability Federal Internal Revenue Service
(for TDD users)
(800) 428-4732
(800) 382-4059 (in IN only)

Independent Living for the Handicapped
Department of Housing and Urban Development
451 7th St SW
Washington, DC 20410
(202) 401-0388
TTY: (202) 708-1455

Library of Congress
National Library Service
for the Blind and Physically
Handicapped
1291 Taylor St NW
Washington, DC 20542
(202) 707-5100

National Amputation
Foundation
38-40 Church St
Malverne, NY 11565
(516) 387-3600

National Association of the
Physically Handicapped,
Inc
754 Staeger St
Akron, OH 44306-2940
(330) 724-1994

National Association of
Retarded Citizens of the US
1010 Wayne Ave, Ste. 650
Silver Springs, MD 20910
(301) 565-3842

National Council on
Disability
1331 F St NW, Suite 1050
Washington, DC 20004-1107
(202) 272-2004
TDD: (202) 272-2074

National Easter Seal
Society
230 W Monroe St, Ste. 1800
Chicago, IL 60606
(312) 726-6200

National Foundation March
of Dimes
1275 Mamaroneck Ave
White Plains, NY 10605
(888) MODIMES

National Information
Center for Children and
Youth with Disabilities
PO Box 1492
Washington, DC 20013
(800) 695-0285

National Institute on
Disability and
Rehabilitation Research
Office of Special Education
and Rehabilitation Services
US Dept. of Education
400 Maryland Ave SW
Washington, DC 20202-0498
(800) 872-5327

National Rehabilitation
Information Center
1010 Wayne Ave, Ste 800
Silver Springs, MD 20910
(800) 346-2742 or
(301) 562-2400

United Cerebral Palsy
Association
16602 C Street NW, Ste. 700
Washington, DC 20036
(800) 872-5827

Down Syndrome

National Association for
Down's Syndrome
PO Box 4542
Oak Brook, IL 60522
(630) 325-9112

National Down Syndrome
Society Hotline
666 Broadway
New York, NY 10012
(800) 221-4602

Elderly

Administration on Aging
330 Independence Ave SW
Cohen Bldg, Room 4760
Washington, DC 20201
(202) 619-0556

American Academy of Physical Medicine and Rehabilitation
122 S Michigan Ave,
Ste. 1300
Chicago, IL 60603-6107
(312) 922-9366

American Association for Geriatric Psychiatry
PO Box 376A
Greenbelt, MD 20768
(301) 220-0952

American Association for International Aging
1133 20th St NW, Ste. 333
Washington, DC 20036
(202) 822-8893

American Association of Homes and Services for the Aging
901 E Street NW, Ste. 500
Washington, DC 20004

American Association of Retired Persons (AARP)
601 E St NW
Washington, DC 20049
(202) 434-2277

American Bar Association
Commission on Legal Problems of the Elderly
1800 M St NW
Washington, DC 20036
(202) 331-2297

American College of Nursing Home Administrators
4650 East-West Freeway
Washington, DC 20014

American Congress of Rehabilitation Medicine
5700 Old Orchard Rd
Skokie, IL 60077
(708) 966-0095

American Federation for Aging Research (AFAR)
1414 Avenue of the Americas
18th Floor
New York, NY 10019
(212) 752-AFAR
FAX: (212) 832-2298

American Geriatric Society
770 Lexington Ave, Ste. 400
New York, NY 10021
(212) 308-1414

American Lung Association
1740 Broadway
New York, NY 10019-4373
(212) 315-8700

American Parkinson's Disease Association
1250 Hylan Boulevard,
Ste. 4B
Staten Island, NY 10305-1946
(800) 223-2732 or
(718) 981-8001

American Society for Geriatric Dentistry
211 E Chicago Ave
17th Floor
Chicago, IL 60611
(312) 440-2500 (×2660)

American Society for Parenteral and Enteral Nutrition
8630 Fenton St, Ste. 412
Silver Springs, MD 20910-3805
(301) 587-6315

American Society on Aging
833 Market St, Ste. 511
San Francisco, CA 94103-1824
(415) 882-2910

**Association for Gerontology
in Higher Education**
1001 Connecticut Ave NW,
Ste. 410
Washington, DC 20036-5504
(202) 429-9277

**Association of Hospital-
Based Nursing Facilities**
3500 Masons Hill Business
Park
Ste. 501A
Huntington Valley, PA 19006
(215) 657-9992

**Association of Humanistic
Gerontology**
1711 Solano Ave
Berkeley, CA 94707

Children of Aging Parents
1609 Woodbourne Rd,
Ste. 302-A
Levittown, PA 19057
(215) 945-6900

**Commission on Legal
Problems of the Elderly**
1800 M St NW
Washington, DC 20036
(202) 331-2297

**Concern in Care of the
Aging**
(See American Association of
Homes and Services for the
Aging)

**Consultant Dietitians in
Healthcare Facilities**
PO Box 60
Armada, MI 48005
(313) 784-9766

**Consumer Product Safety
Commission**
5401 Westbound Ave
Washington, DC 20207
(301) 492-6580

**Department of Veterans
Affairs**
Veterans Health
Administration
Nursing Service Program
(118c)
810 Vermont Ave NW
Washington, DC 20420
(202) 299-4000

**Design for Aging/
Architecture for Health**
American Institute of
Architects
1735 New York Ave NW
Washington, DC 20006
(202) 626-7361

**Directory of Aging
Resources**
Business Publishers
951 Pershing Dr
Silver Springs, MD 20910-
4464
Updated periodically. Cost
approx $100
(800) BPI-6737
FAX: (301) 585-9075

Family Caregiver Alliance
425 Bush St, Ste. 500
San Francisco, CA 94108

Federal Council on Aging
330 Independence Ave SW
Room 4280 HHS-N
Washington, DC 20201

**Foundation for Hospice and
Home Care**
519 C St NE
Washington, DC 20002
(202) 547-6586

Gerontological Nutritionists
4103 44th St
Sacramento, CA 95820
(916) 451-7149

Gerontological Society of America
1275 K St NW, Ste. 350
Washington, DC 20005-4006
(202) 842-1275

Gray Panthers
1424 16th St NW, Ste. 602
Washington, DC 20036
(202) 387-3111

House Select Committee on Aging
House Office Bldg.
Annex 1, Room 712
Washington, DC 20515

Huntington's Disease Society of America
140 W 22nd St
New York, NY 10011-2420
(212) 242-1968

Institute for Retired Professionals
New School of Social Research
60 W 12th St
New York, NY 10011

International Federation on Aging
Secretariat—Canada
380 St. Antoine St W,
Ste. 3200
Montreal, Quebec H24 3X7
(514) 987-8191
FAX: (514) 987-1948

International Senior Citizens Association
537 S Commonwealth Ave,
Ste. 4
Los Angeles, CA 90020
(213) 380-0135

Lighthouse National Center for Vision and Aging
800 Second Ave
New York, NY 10017
(212) 808-0077

Managed Care and Aging Network
American Society on Aging
833 Market St, Ste. 511
San Francisco, CA 94103-1824

Managed Care: An AARP Guide
American Association of Retired Persons
611 E St NW
Washington, DC 20049

Mental Disorders of the Aging
Research Branch DCR
Room 11 C-03
5600 Fishers Ln
Rockville, MD 20857

National Alliance of Senior Citizens
2525 Wilson Blvd
Arlington, VA 22201

National Asian-Pacific Center on Aging
Melbourne Tower
1511 Third Ave, Ste. 914
Seattle, WA 98101
(206) 624-1221

National Association for Hispanic Elderly
3325 Wilshire Blvd, Ste. 800
Los Angeles, CA 90010-1724
(213) 487-1922

National Association for Home Care
519 C St NE
Washington, DC 20002-5809
(202) 547-7424

**National Association for
Senior Living Industries**
184 Duke of Gloucester St
Annapolis, MD 21401-2523
(410) 263-0991

**National Association of
Area Agencies on Aging**
1112 16th St NW, Ste. 100
Washington, DC 20036
(202) 296-8130

**National Association of
Directors of Nursing
Administration in Long-
Term Care (NADONA-
LTC)**
10999 Reed Hartman Hwy,
Ste. 229
Cincinnati, OH 45242
(800) 222-0539

**National Association of
Meal Programs**
206 E St NE
Washington, DC 20002
(202) 547-6157

**National Association of
Nutrition and Aging
Services Programs**
2675 44th St SW, Ste. 305
Grand Rapids, MI 49509
(616) 531-9909 or
(800) 999-6262

**National Association of
Rehabilitation Facilities**
1730 N Lynn St, Ste. 502
Arlington, VA 22209
(703) 525-1191

**National Association of
Spanish Speaking Elderly**
2025 I St NW, Ste. 219
Washington, DC 20006

**National Association of
State Units on Aging**
2033 K St NW, Ste. 304
Washington, DC 20006
(202) 785-0707

**National Caucus and
Center on Black Aged**
1424 K St NW, Ste. 500
Washington, DC 20005
(202) 637-8400

**National Citizens Coalition
for Nursing Home Reform**
1224 M St NW, Ste. 301
Washington, DC 20005
(202) 393-2018

**National Clearinghouse on
Technology and Aging**
College of Health and Human
Services
Ohio University
Athens, OH 45701
(614) 593-2133
FAX: (614) 593-0555

**National Committee for
Prevention of Elder Abuse**
(see National Institute on
Aging)

**National Conference on
Geriatric Nurse
Practitioners**
PO Box 270101
Fort Collins, CO 80527-0101
(303) 493-7793

**National Council of Senior
Citizens**
1311 F St NW
Washington, DC 20004-1171
(202) 347-8800
FAX: (202) 624-9595

National Council on the Aging
(Includes National Institute of Senior Citizens and National Institute on Adult Day Care)
409 3rd St SW, Ste. 200
Washington, DC 20024
(202) 479-1200

National Gerontological Nursing Association
c/o Mosby
7250 Parkway Dr, Ste. 510
Hanover, MD 21076
(800) 723-0560

National Hospice Organization (NHO)
1901 N Moore St, Ste. 901
Arlington, VA 22202
(703) 243-5900

National Indian Council on Aging
6400 Uptown Blvd NE, Ste. 510W
Albuquerque, NM 87110
(505) 242-9505

National Institute on Aging
Public Information Office
Federal Bldg. 31-C, Room 5C27
9000 Rockville Pike
Bethesda, MD 20892

National Meals on Wheels Foundation
1133 20th St NW, Ste. 321
Washington, DC 20036
(202) 463-6039

National Osteoporosis Foundation
1150 17th St NW, Ste. 500
Washington, DC 20036
(202) 223-2226

National Policy Center on Housing and Living Arrangements for Older Americans
University of Michigan
2000 Bonisteel Blvd
Ann Arbor, MI 48109

National Senior Citizens Law Center
1815 H St NW, Ste. 700
Washington, DC 20006
(202) 887-5280

National Stroke Association
8480 E Orchard Rd, Ste. 1000
Englewood, CO 80111-5015
(303) 771-1700

Older Women's League (OWL)
666 11th St NW, Ste. 700
Washington, DC 20001
(202) 783-6686

Senate Special Committee on Aging
Dirksen Senate Office Bldg
Room 623
Washington, DC 20510

Senior Care Centers of America, Inc
26 E Second St, A-1
Moorestown, NJ 08057
(609) 778-0624

Social Security Administration
6401 Security Blvd.
Baltimore, MD 21235
1 (800) 772-1213
1 (800) 325-0778 (TTY)

Video Respite™
Innovative Caregiving Resources
PO Box 17332
Salt Lake City, UT 84117
(801) 272-9446

Epilepsy

Epilepsy Foundation of America
4351 Garden City Dr
Landover, MD 20785
(800) 332-1000

Family Planning/Pregnancy

AAA Pregnancy Hotline
(800) 560-0717

American Society of Human Genetics
Administrative Office
9650 Rockville Bldg
Bethesda, MD 20814-3898
(301) 571-1825

International Childbirth Education Association, Inc
PO Box 20048
Minneapolis, MN 55420-0048

La Leche League International, Inc
1400 W Meacham Rd
Schaumburg, IL 60173-4048
(847) 517-7730

National Abortion Federation
1755 Massachusetts Ave NW, Ste. 600
Washington, DC 20036
(800) 772-9100 (hotline);
(202) 667-5881

National Abstinence Clearinghouse
801 East 41st St
Sioux Falls, SD 57105
(888) 577-2966

National Maternal and Child Health Clearinghouse
2072 Chain Bridge Rd
Vienna, VA 22182
(888) 434-4MCH

Office of Population Affairs Clearinghouse
PO Box 30686
Bethesda, MD 20824-0686
(301) 654-6190

Planned Parenthood Federation of America, Inc
810 7th Ave
New York, NY 10019
(212) 541-7800

Pregnancy Crisis Center
(pregnancy crisis hotline)
(800) 344-7211

Food (See also Nutrition)

Food and Drug Administration
Office of Consumer Affairs
5600 Fishers Ln, Rm 16-05
Rockville, MD 20857
(888) FDA-INFO

Food and Nutrition Information Center
National Agricultural Library Building
10301 Baltimore Ave
Beltsville, MD 20705
(301) 504-5755

Gastrointestinal Disorders

Crohn's and Colitis Foundation of America
386 Park Ave S, 17th Floor
New York, NY 10016-8804
(800) 932-2423

National Digestive Diseases Education and Information Clearinghouse
2 International Way
Bethesda, MD 20892-3570
(301) 654-3810

United Ostomy Association
19772 MacArthur Blvd,
Ste. 200
Irvine, CA 92612-2405
(949) 660-8624

General Public Information

Consumer Information Center US General Services Administration
Consumer Information
Room G-142
1800 F Street NW
Washington, DC 20405

Food and Drug Administration
Office of Consumer Affairs
HFE-88
5600 Fishers Ln
Rockville, MD 20857
(301) 827-5006

US Department of Health and Human Services Public Health Service
Agency for Healthcare
Research and Quality
2101 E Jefferson St, Ste. 501
Rockville, MD 20852
(800) 952-7664

US Department of Labor Occupational Safety and Health Administration (OSHA)
Office of Public Affairs
Room N3647
200 Constitution Ave NW
Washington, DC 20210
(202) 693-1999

Health

American Alliance for Health, Physical Education, Recreation, and Dance
1900 Association Dr
Reston, VA 20191
(800) 213-7193

American Council on Exercise
5820 Oberlin Dr, Ste. 102
San Diego, CA 92121-3787
(858) 535-8227

American Health Care Association, Inc
23123 State Rd 7, Ste. 330
Boca Raton, FL 33428
(800) 535-2681

American Health Foundation
320 E 43rd St
New York, NY 10018

American Holistic Nurses' Association
PO Box 2130
Flagstaff, AZ 86003-2130
(800) 278-AHNA

American Hospital Association Center for Health Promotion
1 N Franklin
Chicago, IL 60606
(800) 424-4301

American Nurses' Association
600 Maryland Ave SW,
Ste. 100 W
Washington, DC 20024
(800) 274-4ANA

American Public Health Association
810 I St NE, Ste. 500
Washington, DC 20002-4267
(202) 682-0100

Center for Health
Promotion and Education
Centers for Disease Control
and Prevention
1600 Clifton Rd
Atlanta, GA 30333
(800) 711-3435

Citizens Council on Health
Care
1954 University Ave W,
Ste. 8
St. Paul, MN 55104

Clearinghouse on Health
Indexes
National Center for Health
Statistics,
Division of Epidemiology
and Health Promotion
6525 Belcrest Rd
Hyattsville, MD 20782-2003
(301) 436-7035

Healthy America, National
Coalition for Health
Promotion and Disease
Prevention
1015 15th St NW, Ste. 424
Washington, DC 20005

International Council on
Health, Physical Education
and Recreation
1201 16th St NW
Room 417
Washington, DC 20036

National Council on Health
Care Services
1200 15th St NW, Ste. 601
Washington, DC 20005

National Health Council
1730 M St NW, Ste. 500
Washington, DC 20036
(202) 785-3910

National Health
Information Clearinghouse
PO Box 1133
Washington, DC 20013-1133
(800) 336-4797
(703) 522-2590 (in VA only)

National Indian Health
Board, Inc
1602 S Parker Rd, Ste. 200
Denver, CO 80231

National Institutes of Health
9000 Rockville Pike
Bethesda, MD 20892
(301) 496-4000

National League of Nursing
61 Broadway
New York, NY 10006
(212) 363-5555
(800) 669-1656

National Wellness Institute
1300 College Court
PO Box 827
Stevens Point, WI 54481-
0827
(715) 342-2969

US Department of Health
and Human Services
Office of Disease Prevention
and Health Promotion
Washington, DC 20201
(301) 468-3028

Health—Dental

American Dental
Association
211 E Chicago Ave
Chicago, IL 60611
(312) 440-2800

Health—Eyes

American Optometric
Association
243 N Lindbergh Blvd
St Louis, MO 63141
(314) 991-4100

Health—Mental

National Clearinghouse for Mental Health Information
National Institute of Mental Health
5600 Fishers Ln
Room 7C-02
Rockville, MD 20857
(301) 443-4513

Hearing and Speech

Alexander Graham Bell Association for the Deaf and Hard of Hearing
3417 Volta Pl NW
Washington, DC 20007-2778
(202) 337-5220
TTY: (202) 337-5221

American Speech, Language, and Hearing Association
10801 Rockville Pike
Rockville, MD 20852
(800) 321-ASHA or
(800) 498-2071

AT&T Communications
Reston, VA
(473) 473-7373

Better Hearing Institute
515 King St
Alexandria, VA 22314
(800) EAR-WELL

International Hearing Society
1680 Middlebelt Rd
Livonia, MI 47154-3367

National Center for Stuttering
(800) 221-2483

National Hearing Aid Helpline
(800) 521-5247

Self-Help for Hard of Hearing People
7910 Woodmont Ave, Ste. 200
Bethesda, MD 20814
(301) 657-2248
TTY: (301) 657-2249

Telecommunications for the Deaf
8630 Fenton St, Ste. 604
Silver Springs, MD 20910-3803
TTY: (301) 589-3006
(800) 733-7258

Heart

American Heart Association
7272 Greenville Ave
Dallas, TX 75231
(800) AHA-USA1

Council on Arteriosclerosis of the American Heart Association
7320 Greenville Ave
Dallas, TX 75231

High Blood Pressure Information Center
National Institutes of Health
9000 Rockville Pike
Bethesda, MD 20892
(301) 496-1809

Mended Hearts, Inc
7272 Greenville Ave
Dallas, TX 75231-4596
(800) AHA-USA1

National Heart, Lung, and Blood Institute
National Institutes of Health
Bethesda, MD 20892

Hospital Care

Association for the Care of Children in Hospitals
3615 Wisconsin Ave NW
Washington, DC 20016

Hill-Burton Hospital Free Care
(800) 638-0742
(800) 492-0359 (in MD only)

Incontinence

National Association for Continence
PO Box 8310
Spartanburg, SC 29305-8310

The Simon Foundation for Continence
PO Box 835
Wilmette, IL 60091
(800) 23-SIMON

Kidney Disease

American Kidney Fund
6110 Executive Blvd,
Ste. 1010
Rockville, MD 20052
(800) 638-8299

National Kidney Foundation
30 E 33rd St
Room 1100
New York, NY 10016
(800) 622-9010

Lung

American Lung Association
1740 Broadway
New York, NY 10019
(212) 315-8700

Asthma and Allergy Foundation of America
1233 20th St SW, Ste. 402
Washington, DC 20036
(800) 7ASTHMA

National Asthma Center
National Jewish Hospital and
Research Center
(800) 222-5864
(303) 398-1477 (in CO only)

National Jewish Center for Immunology and Respiratory Medicine
1400 Jackson St
Denver, CO 80206
(303) 388-4461
(800) 222-LUNG

Medicare/Medicaid

DHHS Inspector General's Office Fraud Hotline
(800) HHS-TIPS
330 Independence Ave, SW
Washington, DC 20201

Neuromuscular Diseases

American Parkinson Disease Association, Inc
1250 Hylan Blvd, Ste. 4B
Staten Island, NY 10305-1946
(800) 223-2732
(718) 981-8001

Amyotrophic Lateral Sclerosis Association
27001 Agourard, Ste. 150
Calabasas Hills, CA 91301-5104
(800) 782-4747

Huntington's Disease Society of America, Inc
158 29th St, 7th Floor
New York, NY 10001-5300
(800) 345-HDSA

Muscular Dystrophy Association, USA
3300 E Sunrise Dr
Tucson, AZ 85718
(800) 572-1717

Myasthenia Gravis Foundation of America
123 W Madison St, Ste. 800
Chicago, IL 60602
(800) 541-5454

**National Multiple Sclerosis
Society**
753 Third Ave
New York, NY 10017
(800) FIGHTMS

**National Parkinson
Foundation**
1501 NW 9th Ave
Bob Hope Rd.
Miami, FL 33136
(800) 327-4545

**Parkinson's Disease
Foundation, Inc**
710 W 168th St
New York, NY 10032-9982
(800) 457-6676

Nutrition (See also Food)
**American Dietetic
Association (ADA)**
216 W Jackson Blvd
Chicago, IL 60606-6995
(312) 899-0040
(800) 877-1600

**Center for Nutrition Policy
and Promotion**
1120 20th St NW, Ste. 200
Washington, DC 20036
(202) 418-2312

**Consumer Information
Center**
Pueblo, CO 81009
(719) 948-4000

Osteoporosis
**National Osteoporosis
Foundation**
1232 22nd St NW
Washington, DC 20037-1292
(202) 223-2226

Organ Donors
**Organ Donation, Dept. of
Health and Human Services**
Health Resources and Service
Administration
5600 Fishers Ln
Parklawn Bldg., Rm 13A-19
Rockville, MD 20857
(301) 443-7577

TransWeb
1327 Jones Dr, Ste. 105
Ann Arbor, MI 48105
(734) 998-7314

Personal Care/Ostomy Resources
**About Faces Permanent
Cosmetics**
1001 Bridgeway Blvd,
Ste. 432
Sausalito, CA 94965
(415) 331-0663

**Blanchard Ostomy
Products**
1510 Raymond Ave
Glendale, CA 91201
(818) 242-6789

Cymed Ostomy Co
1336-A Channing Way
Berkeley, CA 94702
(800) 582-0707

**Marlen Manufacturing &
Development Co**
5150 Richmond Rd
Bedford, OH 44146-1331
(216) 292-7060

Nu-Hope Laboratories, Inc
PO Box 331150
Pacoima, CA 91333-1150
(800) 899-5017

Ostomy USA
PO Box 859
Tallevast, FL 34270-0859
(800) 846-5994

United Ostomy Association, Inc
(800) 826-0826

VPI, A Cook Group Company
127 S Main St,
PO Box 266
Spencer, IN 47460-0266
(800) 843-4851
(812) 829-4891

Pain

Agency for Health Care Policy and Research (for acute pain)
(800) 358-9295

American Academy of Head, Facial, and Neck Pain and TMJ Orthopedics
(800) 322-7651

American Academy of Orofacial Pain
10 Joplin Ct
Lafayette, CA 94549-1913
(510) 945-9298
FAX: (510) 945-9299

American Academy of Pain Management
13947 Mono Way, #A
Sonora, CA 95370
(209) 533-9744
FAX: (209) 533-9750

American Academy of Pain Medicine
4700 W Lake Ave
Glenview, IL 60025-1485
(847) 375-4731
FAX: (847) 375-4777

American Association for the Study of Headache
19 Mantua Rd
Mount Royal, NJ 08061
(609) 423-0258

The American Back Pain Association
PO Box 135
Pasadena, MD 21222-0135
(410) 255-3633
FAX: (410) 255-7338

American Back Society
27647 E 14th St, Ste. 401
Oakland, CA 94601
(510) 536-9929

American Board of Anesthesiology
(205) 522-9857

American Cancer Society
(800) ACS-2345

American Chronic Pain Association
PO Box 850
Rocklin, CA 95677-0850
(916) 632-0922
FAX: (916) 632-3208

American College of Osteopathic Pain Management and Sclerotherapy
107 Maple Ave
Silverside Heights
Wilmington, DE 19809
(302) 792-9280
FAX: (302) 792-9283

American Council for Headache Education
19 Mantua Rd
Mount Royal, NJ 08061
(609) 423-0258

American Pain Society
4700 W Lake Ave
Glenville, IL 60025-1485
(847) 375-4715
FAX: (847) 375-4777

American Society of Clinical Oncology
(312) 644-0878

American Society of Law, Medicine, and Ethics
765 Commonwealth Ave
16th Floor
Boston, MA 02215
(617) 262-4990
FAX: (617) 437-7596

American Society of Pain Management Nurses
7794 Grow Dr
Pensacola, FL 32514
(888) 34-ASPMN (342-7766)
(850) 473-0233 (in FL)
FAX: (850) 484-8762

American Society of Regional Anesthesia
PO Box 11086
Richmond, VA 23230-1086
(804) 282-0010
FAX: (804) 282-0090

Arachnoiditis Information Network
(314) 394-5741

Arizona Cancer Pain Coalition
(603) 285-3000

Arthritis Foundation
1330 W Peachtree St
Atlanta, CA 30309
(404) 872-7100

Arthritis Society of Canada National Office
(416) 967-1414

Back Pain Association of America
(410) 255-3633

Carpal Tunnel Syndrome/Association for Repetitive Motion Syndromes
PO Box 514
Santa Rosa, CA 95402
(707) 571-0597

Children's Hospice International
(703) 684-0330

Collaborating Center for Cancer Pain, Research and Education Pain Service
Memorial Sloan-Kettering Hospital
1275 York Ave
New York, NY 10021

Committee on Pain Therapy
American Society of Anesthesiologists
(708) 825-5586

Endometriosis Association
(800) 992-3636

Fibromyalgia Network
PO Box 31750
Tucson, AZ 85751-1750
(590) 290-5508

Greater Philadelphia Pain Society
(610) 664-0809

Hospice Association of America
(202) 547-7424

Institute for the Advancement of Health
(212) 832-8282

International Association for the Study of Pain
909 NE 43rd St, Ste. 306
Seattle, WA 98105-6020
(206) 547-6409
FAX: (206) 547-5004

International Pain Foundation
(206) 547-2157

Interstitial Cystitis Association (ICA)
PO Box 1553
Madison Square Station
New York, NY 10159
(212) 979-6057

Mayday Pain Resource Center
(626) 301-8345

National Alliance of Statewide Cancer Pain Initiatives
(608) 265-4013

National Association for Breast Cancer
9 E 37th St, 10th Floor
New York, NY 10016
(212) 889-0606

National Cancer Institute
Bldg. 31, Rm. 10A03
31 Center Drive
Bethesda, MD 20892-2580
(800) 4-CANCER or
(301) 496-5583
(800) 332-8615 (TTY)

National Center for Medical Rehabilitation Research (National Institute of Child Health and Human Development)
(301) 402-2242

National Chronic Pain Outreach Association
PO Box 274
Millboro, VA 24460
(540) 997-5004

National Coalition for Cancer Research
(202) 544-1880

National Committee on the Treatment of Intractable Pain
1333 New Hampshire Ave
NW, Ste. 600
Washington, DC 20036
(202) 452-4836

National Headache Foundation
428 W St. James Pl
Chicago, IL 60614
(800) 843-2256

National Hospice Organization
(800) 658-8898

The Neuropathy Association
60 E 42nd St, Ste. 942
New York, NY 10165
(212) 692-0662

Oncology Nurses Society
(412) 921-7373

Pain Institute
(810) 827-7790

Patient Advocates for Advanced Cancer Treatment
1143 Parmelee NW
Grand Rapids, MI 49504
(616) 453-1477

Pennsylvania Department of Health
Cancer Control Program
(800) 537-4063

Reflex Sympathetic Dystrophy Syndrome Association
116 Haddon Ave, Ste. D
Haddonfield, NJ 08803
(215) 955-5444 or
(609) 795-8845

Roxane Pain Institute
(800) 335-9100 or
(614) 276-4000

**Sickle Cell Disease
Association of America**
200 Corporate Pointe,
Ste. 495
Calver City, CA 90230-7633
(800) 421-8453 or
(310) 216-6363

**Society for Pain Practice
Management**
11111 Nall, #202
Leawood, KS 66211
(913) 491-6451
FAX: (913) 491-6453

**Stanford University Pain
Management Service**
(415) 723-6238

**The Resource Center for
State Cancer Pain
Initiatives**
(608) 265-4013

TMJ Association Ltd
PO Box 26771
Milwaukee, WI 53226-0770
(414) 259-3223

**Trigeminal Neuralgia
Association**
PO Box 340
Barnegat Light, NJ 08006
(609) 361-1014
FAX: (609) 361-0982

**Triumph Over Pain
Foundation**
1341 W Folterton Pkwy,
Ste. 120
Chicago, IL 60614
(773) 327-5198

**University of
Vermont–Vermont
Rehabilitation Engineering
Center for Lower Back
Pain**
(800) 527-7320 or
(802) 656-4582

**US Department of Health
and Human Services,
National Institute of Dental
and Craniofacial Research,
Intramural Research
Division, Pain Research
Center**
9000 Rockville Pike
Bethesda, MD 20892
(301) 496-4261

Vulvar Pain Foundation
PO Office Drawer 177
Graham, NC 27255
(910) 226-0704

VZV Research Foundation
40 E 72nd, #4B
New York, NY 10021
(212) 472-7148

**Wisconsin Cancer Pain
Initiative**
(608) 262-0978

Personal Care
Resources\Cosmetics

Beautiful Shapes by Olga
(breast prostheses,
mastectomy accessories)
2753 Nostrand Ave
Brooklyn, NY 11210
(877) OLGABRA

**Cancer Information Center
National Cancer Institute**
Building 31, Room 10A03
31 Center Dr, MSC 2580
Bethesda, MD 20892-2580
(800) 4-CANCER

Designs for Comfort, Inc
(a combination cap and hair
piece called the *Headliner* as
an alternative to wigs)
PO Box 671044
Marietta, GA 30066
(800) 443-9226

**Holly Cosmetics/Medical
Image Products**
(corrective cosmetics)
3014 Springcrest Dr
Louisville, KY 40241
(800) 222-3964

Intimacies by Alice
(for women who have had
breast surgery)
3 Hudson Watch Dr
Ossining, NY 10562
(914) 923-2010

Jodee
(mastectomy products)
3100 N 29th Ave
Hollywood, FL 33020
(954) 926-1900

**Worldwide Home Health
Center, Inc**
(a distributor for healthcare
products and services)
926 E Tallmadge Ave
Akron, OH 44310
(800) 223-5938 (in OH)
(800) 621-5938

Poison/Toxic Substances

Poison Control Branch
Food and Drug
Administration
5600 Fishers Ln
Parklawn Building,
Rm 15B-23
Rockville, MD 20857
(301) 443-6260

**Toxic Substances Control
Act Hotline**
(800) 424-9065
(202) 554-1404 (in
Washington, DC area only)

**US Environmental
Protection Agency**
Natural Pesticide
Telecommunication
(800) 858-7378

Pregnancy (See Family Planning/Pregnancy)

Product Safety

**Consumer Product Safety
Commission**
Washington, DC 20207-0001
(800) 638-CPSC
(800) 638-8270 (TDD)

Rape

**National Center for Injury
Prevention and Control**
Mailstop K60
4770 Buford Hwy NE
Atlanta, GA 30341-3724
(770) 448-4410

Rehabilitation

**National Rehabilitation
Information Center**
1010 Wayne Ave, Ste. 800
Silver Springs, MD 20910
(800) 346-2742

**Rehabilitation
International**
25 E 21st St
New York, NY 10010
(212) 420-1500

Rehabilitation Services Administration
Department of Education,
Office of Special Education
and Rehabilitative Services
400 Maryland Ave SW
Washington, DC 20202
(800) USA LEARN

Society for the Rehabilitation of the Facially Disfigured
550 1st Ave
New York, NY 10016
(212) 340-5400

Safety

Clearinghouse for Occupational Safety and Health Information
Information Resources
Branch
4676 Columbia Pkwy
Cincinnati, OH 45226
(800) 356-4674

HUD User (Housing)
PO Box 6091
Rockville, MD 20849
(800) 245-2691

Medic Alert Foundation International
PO Box 19008
Turlock, CA 95381-1009

National Highway Traffic Safety Administration
US Department of
Transportation
400 7th St SW
Washington, DC 20590
(800) 327-4236

National Injury Information Clearinghouse
US Consumer Products
Safety Commission
Washington, DC 20207

Sexually Transmitted Diseases

Centers for Disease Control and Prevention
1600 Clifton Rd
Atlanta, GA 30333
(800) 311-3435

Sexuality Information and Education Council of the US
130 W 42nd St, Ste. 350
New York, NY 10036-7802
(212) 819-9770

Smoking

Office on Smoking and Health
Centers for Disease Control
and Prevention
Mail Stop K50
4770 Buford Hwy NE
Atlanta, GA 30341-3724
(770) 488-5705

Spinal Cord Injury

National Spinal Cord Injury Association
8701 Georgia Ave, Ste. 500
Silver Springs, MD 20910
(800) 962-9629

National Spinal Cord Injury Foundation
369 Elliot St
Newton Upper Falls, MA
02169

National Spinal Cord Injury Hotline
(800) 526-3456

Paralyzed Veterans of America
7315 Wisconsin Ave,
Ste. 301-W
Washington, DC 20014

Spina Bifida

Spina Bifida Information and Referral
(800) 621-3141

Surgery

National Second Surgical Opinion Program Hotline
(800) 638-6833

Community Resources—Canada

Aboriginal Nurses Association of Canada
12 Stirling Ave, 3rd Floor
Ottawa, ON K1Y 1P8
(613) 724-4677
FAX: (613) 724-4718

Al-Anon Family Groups (Canada)
9 Antares Dr, Ste. 245
Nepean, ON K2E-7V5
(613) 723-8484
FAX: (613) 723-0151

Alcoholics Anonymous
234 Eglinton Ave E, Ste. 202
Toronto, ON M4P 1K5
(416) 487-5591
FAX: (416) 487-5855

Allergy/Asthma Information Association
130 Bridgeland Ave
Ste. 424
Toronto, ON M6A 1Z4
(416) 783-8944
FAX: (416) 783-7538

Allergy Foundation of Canada
PO Box 1904
Saskatoon, SK S7K 3S5
(306) 373-7591

Alzheimer Society of Canada
20 Eglinton Ave W, Ste. 1200
Toronto, ON M4R 1K8
(416) 488-8772
FAX: (416) 488-3778

Amyotrophic Lateral Sclerosis Society of Canada
265 Yorkland Blvd, Ste. 300
Toronto, ON M2J 1S5
(416) 497-2267
FAX: (416) 497-1256

Aplastic Anemia Family Association of Canada
22 Aikinhead Rd
Etobicoke, ON M9R 2Z3
(416) 235-0468
FAX: (416) 864-9929

Arthritis Society
393 University St, Ste. 1700
Toronto, ON M5G 1E6
(416) 979-7228
FAX: (416) 979-8366

Asthma Society of Canada
130 Bridgeland Ave, Ste. 425
North York, ON M6A 1Z4
(416) 787-4050
FAX: (416) 787-5807

Bulimia Anorexia Nervosa Association
300 Cabana Rd E
Windsor, ON N9G 1A3
(519) 969-2112
FAX: (519) 969-0227

Canada Safety Council
1020 Thomas Spratt Pl
Ottawa, ON K1G 5L5
(613) 739-1535
FAX: (613) 739-1566

**Canadian AIDS
Hotline/AIDS
Clearinghouse**
(613) 725-3769 (Ottawa)
(416) 392-AIDS (Toronto)

Canadian AIDS Society
130 Albert St, Ste. 900
Ottawa, ON K1P 5G4
(613) 230-3580
FAX: (613) 563-4998

**Canadian Association for
Community Care**
1 Nicholas St, Suite 520
Ottawa, ON K1N 7B7
(613) 241-7510
FAX: (613) 241-5923

**Canadian Association for
Community Living**
Kinsmen Building
4700 Keele St
Downsview, ON M3J 1P3
(416) 661-9611
FAX: (416) 661-5701

**Canadian Association for
Health, Physical Education
and Recreation**
1600 James Naismith Dr
Gloucester, ON K1B 5N4
(613) 748-5622
FAX: (613) 748-5737

**Canadian Association for
School Health**
2835 Country Woods Dr
Surrey, BC V4P 9P9
(604) 535-7664
FAX: (604) 531-6454

**Canadian Association on
Gerontology**
824 Meath St, Ste. 100
Ottawa, ON K1Z 6E8
(613) 728-9347
FAX: (613) 728-8913

**Canadian Association of
Occupational Therapists**
CTTC Building
1125 Colonel By Drive,
Ste. 3400
Ottawa, ON K1S 5R1
(613) 523-CAOT or
(800) 434-CAOT
FAX: (613) 523-2552

**Canadian Association of
Optometrists**
234 Argyle Ave
Ottawa, ON K2P 1B9
(613) 235-7924
FAX: (613) 235-2025

**Canadian Association of
Practical Nurses and
Nursing Assistants**
10403 172 St, Ste. 230
Edmonton, AB T5S 159
(780) 484-8886
FAX: (780) 484-9069

**Canadian Association of
Social Workers**
383 Parkdale Ave, Ste. 402
Ottawa, ON K1Y 4R4
(613) 729-6668
FAX: (613) 729-9608

**Canadian Association of
Speech-Language
Pathologists and
Audiologists**
130 Albert St, Ste. 2006
Ottawa, ON K1P 5G4
(613) 567-9968
FAX: (613) 567-2859

**Canadian Association of
the Deaf**
251 Bank St, Suite 203
Ottawa, ON K2P 1X3
(613) 565-2882 (TTY)
FAX: (613) 565-1207

Canadian Breast Cancer Foundation
790 Bay St, Suite 1000
Toronto, ON M5G 1N8
(800) 387-9816 or
(416) 596-6773
FAX: (416) 596-7857

Canadian Cancer Society
10 Alcorn Ave, Suite 200
Toronto, ON M4V 3B1
(416) 961-7223
FAX: (416) 961-4189

Canadian Cardiovascular Society
222 Queen St, Suite 1403
Ottawa, ON K1P 5V9
(613) 569-3407
FAX: (613) 569-6574

Canadian Centre for Occupational Health and Safety
250 Main St E
Hamilton, ON L8N 1H6
(800) 668-4284 or
(905) 572-2981
FAX: (905) 572-2206

Canadian Centre on Substance Abuse
75 Albert St, Suite 300
Ottawa, ON K1P 5E7
(613) 235-4048
FAX: (613) 235-8101

Canadian Child Care Federation
383 Parkdale Ave, Suite 201
Ottawa, ON K1Y 4R4
(613) 729-5289
FAX: (613) 729-3159

Canadian Chiropractic Association
1396 Eglinton Ave W
Toronto, ON M6C 2E4
(416) 781-5656
FAX: (416) 781-7344

Canadian Coalition for the Prevention of Developmental Disabilities
c/o Canadian Institute of
Child Health
885 Meadowlands Dr,
Suite 512
Ottawa, ON K2C 3N2
(613) 224-4144
FAX: (613) 224-4145

Canadian Coalition on Medication Use and Seniors
112 Eddy St, Suite 100
Hull, QC J8X 2W5
(819) 770-3131
FAX: (819) 770-5833

Canadian Coalition on Organ Donor Awareness
Canada's Research-Based
Pharmaceutical Companies
1111 Prince of Wales Dr
Suite 302
Ottawa, ON K2C 3T2
(613) 727-1380
FAX: (613) 727-1407

Canadian Council of the Blind
396 Cooper St, Suite 200
Ottawa, ON K2P 2H7
(613) 567-0311
FAX: (613) 567-2728

Canadian Council on Social Development
441 MacLaren St, 4th Floor
Ottawa, ON K2P 2H3
(613) 236-8977
FAX: (613) 236-2750

Canadian Council for Tobacco Control
170 Laurier Ave W,
Suite 1000
Ottawa, ON K1P 5V5
(613) 567-3050
FAX: (613) 567-2730

Canadian Cultural Society of the Deaf, Inc
11337 61st Ave, Suite 144
Edmonton, AB T6H 1M3
(780) 436-2599 (TTY/TDD)
FAX: (780) 430-9489

Canadian Cystic Fibrosis Foundation
2221 Yonge St, Suite 601
Toronto, ON M4S 2B4
(416) 485-9149
FAX: (416) 485-0960

Canadian Deaf-Blind and Rubella Association
350 Brant Ave
Owen Sound, ON N4K 2G9
Brantford, ON N3T 3J5
(519) 754-0729
FAX: (519) 754-5400

Canadian Dental Association
1815 Alta Vista Dr
Ottawa, ON K1G 3Y6
(613) 523-1770
FAX: (613) 523-7736

Canadian Diabetes Association
15 Toronto St, Suite 800
Toronto, ON M5C 2E3
(416) 363-3373
FAX: (416) 363-3393

Dietitians of Canada
480 University Ave
Suite 604
Toronto, ON M5G 1V2
(416) 596-0857
FAX: (416) 596-0603

Canadian Down Syndrome Society
14th St NW, Suite 811
Calgary, AB T2N 2A4
(403) 270-8500
FAX: (403) 270-8291

Canadian Fire Safety Association
2175 Sheppard Ave E
Suite 310
Willowdale, ON M2J 1W8
(416) 492-9417
FAX: (416) 491-1670

Canadian Guidance and Counselling Association
116 Albert St, Suite 702
Ottawa, ON K1P 5G3
(613) 237-1099
FAX: (613) 237-9786

Canadian Hard of Hearing Association
2435 Holly Ln, Suite 205
Ottawa, ON K1V 7P2
(613) 526-1584
(613) 526-2692 (TTY/TDD)
FAX: (613) 526-4718

Canadian Healthcare Association
17 York St, Ste. 100
Ottawa, ON K1N 9J6
(613) 241-8005
FAX: (613) 241-5055

Canadian Hearing Society
271 Spadina Rd
Toronto, ON M5R 2V3
(416) 964-9595
(416) 964-0023 (TTY/TDD)
FAX: (416) 928-2523

Canadian Hemophilia Society
625 President Kennedy
Suite 1210
Montreal, Quebec H3A 1K2
(514) 848-0503
FAX: (514) 848-9661

Canadian Institute for Health Information
377 Dalhousie St, Suite 200
Ottawa, ON K1N 9N8
(613) 241-7860
FAX: (613) 241-8120

Canadian Institute of Child Health
384 Bank St, Suite 300
Ottawa, ON K2P 1Y4
(613) 230-8838
FAX: (613) 230-6654

Canadian Institute of Stress
PO Box 665
Station "U"
Toronto, ON M8Z 5Y9
(416) 236-4218

Canadian Liver Foundation
365 Bloor St E, Suite 200
Toronto, ON M4W 3L4
(416) 964-1953
FAX: (416) 964-0024

Canadian Medical Association
1867 Alta Vista Dr
Ottawa, ON K1G 3Y6
(613) 731-9331
FAX: (613) 731-9013

Canadian Medic Alert Foundation
250 Ferrand Dr, Suite 301
Toronto, ON M3C 3G8
(800) 668-1507 or
(416) 696-0267
FAX: (416) 696-0156

Canadian Mental Health Association
111 Simcoe St. N
Oshawa, ON L1G 4S4
(905) 436-8760
FAX: (905) 436-1569

Canadian National Institute for the Blind
1929 Bayview Ave
Toronto, ON M4G 3E8
(416) 480-7580
FAX: (416) 480-7677

Canadian Nurses Association
50 Driveway
Ottawa, ON K2P 1E2
(613) 237-2133
FAX: (613) 237-3520

Canadian Orthopaedic Association
1440 St. Catherine St W
Suite 320
Montreal, PQ H3G 1R8
(514) 874-9003
FAX: (514) 874-0464

Canadian Osteopathic Association
575 Waterloo St
London, ON N6B 2R2
(519) 439-5521
FAX: (519) 439-2616

Canadian Paediatric Society
2204 Walkley Rd
Ottawa, ON K1G 4G8
(613) 526-9397
FAX: (613) 526-3332

Canadian Paraplegic Association
1101 Prince of Wales Dr
Suite 230
Ottawa, ON K2C 3W7
(800) 720-4933
(613) 723-1033
FAX: (613) 723-1060

Canadian Psychiatric Association
441 MacLaren St, Suite 260
Ottawa, ON K2P 2H3
(613) 234-2815
FAX: (613) 234-9857

Canadian Psychological Association
151 Slater St, Suite 205
Ottawa, ON K1P 5H3
(613) 237-2144
FAX: (613) 237-1674

Canadian Public Health Association
1565 Carling Ave, Suite 400
Ottawa, ON K1Z 8R1
(613) 725-3769
FAX: (613) 725-9826

Canadian Red Cross Society
909 Fairfield Rd
Victoria, BC V8V 3A3
(604) 382-2043
FAX: (604) 382-3420

Canadian Society for International Health
1 Nicholas St, Suite 1105
Ottawa, ON K1N 7B7
(613) 241-5785
FAX: (613) 241-3845

Canadian Society for the Prevention of Cruelty to Children
PO Box 700
356 1st St
Midland, ON L4R 4P4
(705) 526-5647
FAX: (705) 526-0214

Canadians for Health Research
PO Box 126
Westmount, PQ H3Z 2T1
(514) 398-7478
FAX: (514) 398-8361

Catholic Health Association of Canada
1247 Kilborn Pl
Ottawa, ON K1H 6K9
(613) 731-7148
FAX: (613) 731-7797

Centre for Health Promotion
University of Toronto
Banting Institute
100 College St, Suite 207
Toronto, ON M5G 1L5
(416) 978-1809
FAX: (416) 971-1365

Council of Canadians with Disabilities
294 Portage Ave, Suite 926
Winnipeg, MB R3C 0B9
(204) 947-0303
FAX: (204) 942-4625

Council on Drug Abuse
16 Scarlett Rd
Toronto, ON M6N 4K1
(416) 763-1491
FAX: (416) 767-5343

DAWN Canada (DisAbled Women's Network)
PO Box 22003
Brandon, MB R7A 6Y9
Tel./FAX: (204) 726-1406

Dying With Dignity: Canadian Society Concerned With the Quality of Dying
55 Eglinton Ave E, Suite 705
Toronto, ON M4P 1G8
(416) 486-3998
FAX: (416) 489-9010

Epilepsy Canada
1470 Peel St, Suite 745
Montreal, QC H3A 1T1
(514) 845-7855
FAX: (514) 845-7866

Family Service Canada
383 Parkdale
Ottawa, ON K1Y 4R4
(613) 722-9006
FAX: (613) 722-8610

Heart and Stroke Foundation of Canada
222 Queen St, Suite 1402
Ottawa, ON K1P 5V9
(613) 569-4361
FAX: (613) 569-3278

International Social Service Canada
151 Slater St, Suite 714
Ottawa, ON K1P 5H3
(613) 236-6161
FAX: (613) 233-7306

Juvenile Diabetes Foundation Canada
7100 Woodbine Ave,
Suite 311
Markham, ON L3R 5J2
(877) 287-3533 or
(905) 944-8700
FAX: (905) 944-0800

Kidney Foundation of Canada
5165 Sherbrooke St W
Montreal, QC H4A 1T6
(514) 369-4806
FAX: (514) 369-2472

La Leche League Canada
PO Box 29
18C Industrial Dr
Chesterville, ON K0C 1H0
(613) 448-1842
FAX: (613) 448-1845

Learning Disabilities Association of Canada
323 Chapel St, Suite 200
Ottawa, ON K1N 7Z2
(613) 238-5721
FAX: (613) 235-5391

Lung Association— National Office
1900 City Park Dr, Suite 508
Gloucester, ON K1J 1A3
(613) 747-6776
FAX: (613) 747-7430

Lupus Canada
Box 64034
5512 4th St NW
Calgary, AB T2K 6J1
(800) 661-1468
Tel./FAX: (403) 274-5599

Migraine Association of Canada
365 Bloor St E, Suite 1912
Toronto, ON M4W 3L4
(800) 663-3557 or
(416) 920-4916
FAX: (416) 920-3677

Multiple Sclerosis Society of Canada
250 Bloor St E
Suite 1000
Toronto, ON M4W 3P9
(416) 922-6065
FAX: (416) 922-7538

Muscular Dystrophy Association of Canada
2345 Yonge St, Suite 900
Toronto, ON M4P 2E5
(416) 488-0030
FAX: (416) 488-7523

National Anti-Poverty Organization
325 Dalhousie St, Suite 440
Ottawa, ON K1N 7G2
(613) 789-0096
FAX: (613) 789-0141

National Cancer Institute of Canada
10 Alcorn Ave, Suite 200
Toronto, ON M4V 3B1
(416) 961-7223
FAX: (416) 961-4189

National Eating Disorder Information Centre
CW 1-211
200 Elizabeth St
Toronto, ON M5G 2C4
(416) 340-4156
FAX: (416) 340-4736

National Institute of Nutrition
265 Carling Ave, Suite 302
Ottawa, ON K1S 2E1
(613) 235-3355
FAX: (613) 235-7032

**North American Chronic
Pain Association of Canada**
150 Central Park Dr, Suite 105
Brampton, ON L6T 2T9
(905) 793-5230
FAX: (905) 793-8781

**One Parent Families
Association of Canada**
1099 Kingston Rd, Suite 222
Pickering, ON L1V 1B5
(905) 831-7098
FAX: (905) 831-2580

**Osteoporosis Society of
Canada**
33 Laird Dr
Toronto, ON M4G 3S9
(416) 696-2663
FAX: (416) 696-2673

**Parkinson Foundation of
Canada**
4211 Yonge St, Suite 316
Toronto, ON M2P 2A9
(416) 227-9700
FAX: (416) 227-9600

**Planned Parenthood
Federation of Canada**
1 Nicholas St, Suite 430
Ottawa, ON K1N 7B7
(613) 241-4474
FAX: (613) 241-7550

**PRIDE (Parent Resources
Institute for Drug
Education) Canada**
University of Saskatchewan
College of Pharmacy
Saskatoon, SK S7N 5C9
(800) 667-3747 or
(306) 975-3755

**Schizophrenia Society of
Canada**
75 The Donway W, Suite 814
Don Mills, ON M3C 2E9
(800) 809-4673 or
(416) 445-8204
FAX: (416) 445-2270

**Sleep/Wake Disorders
Canada**
3089 Bathurst St, Suite 304
Toronto, ON M6A 2A4
(800) 387-9253 or
(416) 787-5374
FAX: (416) 787-4431

**Smoking and Health Action
Foundation**
720 Spadina Ave, Suite 221
Toronto, ON M5S 2T9
(416) 928-2900
FAX: (416) 928-1860

**Spina Bifida Association of
Canada**
388 Donald St, Suite 220
Winnipeg, MB R3B 2J4
(800) 565-9488 or
(204) 925-3650
FAX: (204) 925-3654

**Stay Alert . . . Stay Safe
Organization**
2180 Yonge St, 17th Floor
Toronto, ON M4P 2V8
(416) 480-8225
FAX: (416) 480-8556

**Tourette Syndrome
Foundation of Canada**
194 Jarvis St, Suite 206
Toronto, ON M5B 2B7
(416) 861-8398
FAX: (416) 861-2472

Turner's Syndrome Society
814 Glencairn Ave
Toronto, ON M6B 2A3
(800) 465-6744 or
(416) 781-2086
FAX: (416) 781-7245

United Way Canada
56 Sparks St, Suite 404
Ottawa, ON K1P 5A9
(613) 236-7041
FAX: (613) 236-3087

Victorian Order of Nurses
for Canada
5 Blackburn Ave
Ottawa, ON K1N 8A2
(613) 233-5694
FAX: (613) 230-4376

YMCA Canada
42 Charles St E, 6th Floor
Toronto, ON M4Y 1T4
(416) 967-9622
FAX: (416) 967-9618

RESOURCE INFORMATION—NURSE
PROFESSIONAL RESOURCES

Professional resources serve to assist the nurse in defining scope of practice and in assessing health risks for individual clients and the community. New nurses to the specialty will want to be oriented to their practice, and the nurse manager can use a standard procedure for providing this orientation. The following is a selected group of resources that will provide direction for this.

ANA Standards of Public Health Nursing Practice

Public health nursing is the practice of promoting and protecting the health of populations using knowledge from nursing, social, and public health sciences (American Public Health Association, Public Health Nursing Section 1996). Public health nursing is population-focused, community-oriented nursing practice. The goal of public health nursing is the prevention of disease and disability for all people through the creation of conditions in which people can be healthy.

STANDARDS OF CARE
Standard I. Assessment
The public health nurse assesses the health status of populations using data, community resources identification, input from the population, and professional judgment.

Standard II. Diagnosis
The public health nurse analyzes collected assessment data and part-

From American Nurses' Association: *Scope and standards of public health nursing practice,* Washington DC, 1999, The Association. Reprinted with the permission of ANA.

ners with the people to attach meaning to those data and determine opportunities and needs.

Standard III. Outcomes Identification

The public health nurse participates with other community partners to identify expected outcomes in the populations and their health status.

Standard IV. Planning

The public health nurse promotes and supports the development of programs, policies, and services that provide interventions that improve the health status of populations.

Standard V. Assurance: Action Component of the Nursing Process for Public Health Nursing

The public health nurse assures access and availability of programs, policies, resources, and services to the population.

Standard VI. Evaluation

The public health nurse evaluates the health status of the population.

STANDARDS OF PROFESSIONAL PERFORMANCE
Standard I. Quality of Care

The public health nurse systematically evaluates the availability, accessibility, acceptability, quality, and effectiveness of nursing practice for the population.

Standard II. Performance Appraisal

The public health nurse evaluates his or her own nursing practice in relation to professional practice standards and relevant statutes and regulations.

Standard III. Education

The public health nurse acquires and maintains current knowledge and competency in public health nursing practice.

Standard IV. Collegiality

The public health nurse establishes collegial partnerships while interacting with healthcare practitioners and others, and contributes to the professional development of peers, colleagues, and others.

Standard V. Ethics

The public health nurse applies ethical standards in advocating for health and social policy, and delivery of public health programs to promote and preserve the health of the population.

Standard VI. Collaboration

The public health nurse collaborates with the representatives of the population and other health and human service professionals and organizations in providing for and promoting the health of the population.

Standard VII. Research

The public health nurse uses research findings in practice.

Standard VIII. Resource Utilization

The public health nurse considers safety, effectiveness, and cost in the planning and delivery of public health services when using available resources, to ensure the maximum possible health benefit to the population.

ANA Scope and Standards of Home Health Nursing Practice

Home health nursing refers to the practice of nursing applied to a client with a health condition in the client's place of residence. Clients and their designated caregivers are the focus of home health nursing practice. The goal of care is to initiate, manage, and evaluate the resources needed to promote the client's optimal level of well-being and function. Nursing activities necessary to achieve this goal may warrant preventive, maintenance, and restorative emphases to prevent potential problems from developing.

Home health nursing is a specialized area of nursing practice with its roots firmly placed in community health nursing.

STANDARDS OF CARE
Standard I. Assessment

The home health nurse collects client health data.

Standard II. Diagnosis

The home health nurse analyzes the assessment data in determining diagnoses.

From American Nurses' Association: *Scope and standards of home health nursing practice,* Washington DC, 1999, The Association. Reprinted with the permission of ANA.

Standard III. Outcome Identification

The home health nurse identifies expected outcomes to the client and the client's environment.

Standard IV. Planning

The home health nurse develops a plan of care that prescribes intervention to attain expected outcomes.

Standard V. Implementation

The home health nurse implements the interventions identified in the plan of care.

Standard VI. Evaluation

The home health nurse evaluates the client's progress toward attainment of outcomes.

STANDARDS OF PROFESSIONAL PERFORMANCE
Standard I. Quality of Care

The home health nurse systematically evaluates the quality and effectiveness of nursing practice.

Standard II. Performance Appraisal

The home health nurse evaluates his or her own nursing practice in relation to professional practice standards, scientific evidence, and relevant statutes and regulations.

Standard III. Education

The home health nurse acquires and maintains current knowledge and competency in nursing practice.

Standard IV. Collegiality

The home health nurse interacts with and contributes to the professional development of peers and other health care practitioners as colleagues.

Standard V. Ethics

The home health nurse's decisions and actions on behalf of clients are determined in an ethical manner.

Standard VI. Collaboration

The home health nurse collaborates with the client, family, and other health care practitioners in providing client care.

Standard VII. Research

The home health nurse uses research findings in practice.

Standard VIII. Resource Utilization

The home health nurse assists the client or family in becoming informed consumers about the risks, benefits, and cost of planning and delivering client care.

ANA Scope and Standards of Parish Nursing

Parish nurse is the most common title given to a registered professional nurse who serves as a member of the ministry staff of a faith community to promote health as wholeness of the faith community, its family and individual members, and the community it serves through the independent practice of nursing as defined by the nurse practice act in the jurisdiction in which he or she practices and the standards of practice set forth in this document.

STANDARDS OF CARE
Standard I. Assessment

The parish nurse collects health data.

Standard II. Diagnosis

The parish nurse analyzes collected data about the client to determine the diagnosis.

Standard III. Outcome Identification

The parish nurse, with the client, identifies expected outcomes specific to the client's desired health outcomes.

Standard IV. Planning

The parish nurse assists the client in developing a plan for health promotion and other interventions that empowers the client to achieve desired health outcomes. The plan identifies the self-care activities to be done by the client, the interdependence with other systems, the interventions to be performed by the parish nurse, and the collaboration with and referral to other healthcare professionals and providers on the basis of the expected outcomes.

From American Nurses' Association: *Scope and standards of parish nursing,* Washington DC, 1998, American Nurses' Publishing. Reprinted with the permission of the ANA.

Standard V. Implementation

The parish nurse assists the client in implementing the interventions identified in the health promotion plan.

Standard VI. Evaluation

The parish nurse continually evaluates client responses to interventions in order to determine the progress made toward desired outcomes.

STANDARDS OF PROFESSIONAL PERFORMANCE
Standard I. Quality of Care

The parish nurse systematically participates in evaluation of the quality and effectiveness of his or her parish nursing practice.

Standard II. Performance Appraisal

The parish nurse evaluates his or her own nursing practice in relation to professional standards, relevant statutes, and regulations.

Standard III. Education

The parish nurse acquires and maintains current knowledge in nursing practice and health promotion.

Standard IV. Collegiality

The parish nurse contributes to the professional development of peers, colleagues, and other health ministers.

Standard V. Ethics

The parish nurse's decisions and actions reflect and are guided by client, personal, and professional ethical considerations.

Standard VI. Collaboration

The parish nurse collaborates with the client system, other health ministers, healthcare providers, and community agencies in promoting client health.

Standard VII. Research

The parish nurse uses research findings in practice.

Standard VIII. Resource Utilization

The parish nurse considers the effectiveness measures of appropriateness, accessibility, acceptability, and affordability of resources in the development and implementation of health promotion programs for clients.

ANA Scope and Standards of Forensic Nursing Practice

Forensics nursing is multidimensional and includes the responsibilities, functions, roles, and skills that involve a specific body of knowledge. Characteristics unique to forensic nursing practice may include but are not limited to:

- Assessment, diagnosis, identification, planning, implementation of interventions and human responses to individuals of all ages, including but not limited to victims of sexual assault, physical assault, homicide, child abuse, and spousal abuse
- Identifying injuries and deaths with forensic implications
- Collecting evidential material required by law enforcement or medical examiners
- The scientific investigation of death
- Provisions of care in uncontrolled or unpredictable environments and providing continuity of care from the emergency department to the court of law
- Crisis intervention for unique patient populations
- Expert witness testimony
- Recording the medical-legal documentation to be used in a court of law
- Interacting with grieving families
- Thoroughly reviewing and analyzing medical records
- Consulting with other agencies whenever forensic interests interact

STANDARDS OF CARE
Standard I. Assessment

The forensic nurse shall provide an accurate assessment, based upon data collected, of the physical and/or psychological issues of the client as related to forensic nursing and/or forensic pathology.

Standard II. Diagnosis

The forensic nurse shall analyze the assessment data to determine a diagnosis pertaining to forensic issues in nursing.

Standard III. Outcomes Identification

The forensic nurse will identify expected individual outcomes based on the forensic diagnoses of the client.

Standard IV. Planning

The forensic nurse develops a comprehensive plan of action for the forensic client appropriate to forensic interventions to attain expected outcomes.

Standard V. Implementation

The forensic nurse implements a plan of action based on forensic issues derived from assessment data, nursing diagnoses, and medical diagnoses, when applicable and scientific knowledge.

Standard VI. Evaluation

The forensic nurse evaluates and modifies the plan of action to achieve expected outcomes.

STANDARDS OF PROFESSIONAL PERFORMANCE
Standard I. Quality of Care

The forensic nurse systematically evaluates the quality and effectiveness of forensic nursing practice.

Standard II. Performance Appraisal

The forensic nurse evaluates his or her own forensic nursing practice in relation to professional practice standards and relevant statutes and regulations.

Standard III. Education

The forensic nurse acquires and maintains current knowledge in forensic nursing practice.

Standard IV. Collegiality

The forensic nurse contributes to the professional development of peers, colleagues, and others.

Standard V. Ethics

The forensic nurse's decisions and actions are determined in an ethical manner.

Standard VI. Collaboration

The forensic nurse collaborates with the forensic client, family members, significant others, and multidisciplinary team members.

Standard VII. Research

The forensic nurse recognizes, values, and utilizes research as a method to further forensic nursing practice.

Standard VIII. Resource Utilization

The forensic nurse considers factors related to safety, effectiveness, and cost in planning and delivering forensic services.

ANA Scope and Standards of Nursing Practice in Correctional Facilities

NURSING PRACTICE IN CORRECTIONAL FACILITIES

The major thrust of nursing care in correctional settings is the provision of primary care services for the population. Primary health services in this field include screening activities, providing direct healthcare services, analyzing individual health behaviors, teaching, counseling, and assisting individuals in assuming responsibility for their own health to the best of their ability, knowledge, and circumstances.

STANDARDS OF CARE
Standard I. Assessment

The nurse collects client health data.

Standard II. Diagnosis

The nurse analyzes the assessment data in determining diagnoses.

Standard III. Outcome Identification

The nurse identifies expected outcomes individualized to the client.

Standard IV. Planning

The nurse develops a care plan that prescribes interventions to attain expected outcomes.

From American Nurses' Association: *Scope and standards of nursing practice in correctional facilities,* Washington, DC, 1995, American Nurses Publishing. Reprinted with the permission of the ANA.

Standard V. Implementation

The nurse implements the interventions identified in the care plan.

Standard VI. Evaluation

The nurse evaluates the client's progress toward attainment of outcomes.

STANDARDS OF PROFESSIONAL PERFORMANCE
Standard I. Quality of Care

The nurse systematically evaluates the quality and effectiveness of nursing practice.

Standard II. Performance Appraisal

The nurse evaluates his or her own nursing practice in relation to professional practice standards and relevant statutes and regulations.

Standard III. Education

The nurse acquires and maintains current knowledge in nursing practice.

Standard IV. Collegiality

The nurse contributes to the professional development of peers, colleagues, and others.

Standard V. Ethics

The nurse's decisions and actions on behalf of clients are determined in an ethical manner.

Standard VI. Collaboration

The nurse collaborates with the client, significant others, other criminal justice system personnel, and healthcare providers in providing client care.

Standard VII. Research

The nurse uses research findings in practice.

Standard VIII. Resource Utilization

The nurse considers factors related to safety, effectiveness, and cost in planning and delivering client care.

ANA Scope and Standards of College Health Nursing Practice

College health nursing services vary in size and scope. They range from a staff of one nurse who addresses the needs of the campus community, to complex nursing services that are a part of a comprehensive ambulatory care agency with a full interdisciplinary team. The client population served by college health nurses is also varied. Students, faculty, staff and, occasionally, families, friends, or campus visitors, may be served.

The college health nurse is a licensed professional nurse prepared as a generalist at the baccalaureate nursing level. It is noted, however, that advanced practice nurses educated at the master's degree or higher level also practice in college health.

STANDARDS OF CARE
Standard I. Assessment
The college health nurse collects client data.

Standard II. Diagnosis
The college health nurse analyzes the assessment data in determining diagnosis.

Standard III. Outcome Identification
The college health nurse identifies the expected outcomes individualized to the client or group of clients.

Standard IV. Planning
The college health nurse develops a plan of care that prescribes interventions to attain expected outcomes.

Standard V. Implementation
The college health nurse implements the interventions identified in the plan of care.

Standard VI. Evaluation
The college health nurse evaluates the client's progress toward attainment of outcomes.

From American Nurses' Association: *Scope and standards of college health nursing practice,* Washington, DC, 1997, American Nurses Publishing. Reprinted with the permission of the ANA.

STANDARDS OF PROFESSIONAL PERFORMANCE
Standard I. Quality of Care

The college nurse systematically evaluates the quality and effectiveness of college health nursing practice and the college health program.

Standard II. Performance Appraisal

The college health nurse evaluates his or her own nursing practice in relation to professional practice standards and relevant statutes and regulations.

Standard III. Education

The college health nurse acquires and maintains current knowledge in nursing practice and the diverse health issues affecting college students.

Standard IV. Collegiality

The college health nurse contributes to the professional development of peers, colleagues, and others.

Standard V. Ethics

The college health nurse's decisions and actions on behalf of clients are determined in an ethical manner.

Standard VI. Collaboration

The college health nurse collaborates with the client, significant others, other members of the campus community and healthcare providers in providing client care and college health activities.

Standard VII. Research

The college health nurse contributes to nursing and college health through innovations in theory and practice and through participation in research, and uses research findings in practice.

Standard VIII. Resource Utilization

The college health nurse considers factors related to safety, effectiveness, and cost in planning and delivering client care.

Standard IX. Organization of Nursing Services

Nursing services provided in college health settings are planned and organized to meet existing needs and identify future needs of the client. These services are administered by a professional registered nurse with education and experience commensurate with his or her responsibilities.

Standard X. Community Health Systems

The college health nurse participates with other members of the community in assessing, identifying outcomes, planning, implementing, and evaluating college health services and community health services.

Standard XI. Health Promotion, Health Protection, and Disease Prevention

The college health nurse provides active health promotion, health protection, and disease prevention services for individuals and groups.

NASN Standards of Professional School Nursing Practice

The *Standards of Professional School Nursing Practice* delineates the professional responsibilities of all school nurses engaged in clinical practice. The use of this and other documents could serve as a basis for:

- Quality improvement systems
- Databases
- Regulatory systems
- Healthcare reimbursement and financing methodologies
- Development and evaluation of nursing service delivery systems and organizational structures
- Certification activities
- Position descriptions and performance appraisals
- Agency policies, procedures, and protocols
- Educational offerings

Standards, as well as practice guidelines, must be evaluated on a regular basis. School nurses are invited to provide feedback to the Standards Task Force regarding the utility, effectiveness, and comprehensiveness of these standards.

STANDARDS OF CARE
Standard I. Assessment

The school nurse collects client data.

From National Association of School Nurses: *Standards of professional school nursing practice,* Scarborough, Maine, 1998, National Association of School Nurses.

Standard II. Diagnosis

The school nurse analyzes the assessment data in determining nursing diagnoses.

Standard III. Outcome Identification

The school nurse identifies expected outcomes individualized to the client.

Standard IV. Planning

The school nurse develops a plan of care/action that specifies interventions to attain expected outcomes.

Standard V. Implementation

The school nurse implements the interventions identified in the plan of care/action.

Standard VI. Evaluation

The school nurse evaluates the client's progress toward attainment of outcomes.

STANDARDS OF PROFESSIONAL PERFORMANCE
Standard I. Quality of Care

The school nurse systematically evaluates the quality and effectiveness of school nursing practice.

Standard II. Performance Appraisal

The school nurse evaluates his or her own nursing practice in relation to professional practice standards and relevant statutes, regulations, and policies.

Standard III. Education

The school nurse acquires and maintains current knowledge and competency in school nursing practice.

Standard IV. Collegiality

The school nurse interacts with and contributes to the professional development of peers and school personnel as colleagues.

Standard V. Ethics

The school nurse's decisions and actions on behalf of clients are determined in an ethical manner.

Standard VI. Collaboration

The school nurse collaborates with the student, family, school staff, community, and other providers in providing student care.

Standard VII. Research

The school nurse promotes use of research findings in school nursing practice.

Standard VIII. Resource Utilization

The school nurse considers factors related to safety, effectiveness, and cost when planning and delivering care.

Standard IX. Communication

The school nurse uses effective written, verbal, and nonverbal communication skills.

Standard X. Program Management

The school nurse manages school health services.

Standard XI. Health Education

The school nurse assists students, families, the school staff, and community to achieve optimal levels of wellness through appropriately designed and delivered health education.

AOHN Standards of Occupational and Environmental Health Nursing

Occupational and environmental health nursing is the specialty practice that provides for and delivers health and safety services to employees, employee populations, and community groups. The practice focuses on promotion and restoration of health, prevention of illness and injury, and protection from occupational and environmental hazards. Occupational and environmental health nurses make independent nursing judgements in providing healthcare services within this autonomous specialty.

The nurse is key to the coordination of a holistic, multidisciplinary approach to delivery of safe, quality, and comprehensive occupational health and safety services, which include:

From American Association of Occupational Health Nurses: *Standards of occupational and environmental health nursing,* Atlanta, 1999, American Association of Occupational Health Nurses.

- Clinical and primary care, including assessment, diagnosis, management, and documentation of occupational and nonoccupational illness and injury
- Case management for occupational and nonoccupational illnesses and injuries
- Health hazard assessment and surveillance of employee populations, workplaces, and community groups
- Investigation, monitoring, and analysis of illness and injury episodes and trends as well as methods to promote and protect employee health and safety
- Compliance with laws, regulations, and standards governing health and safety for employees and the environment
- Management and administration of occupational and environmental health services
- Health promotion and disease prevention strategies using primary, secondary, and tertiary principles
- Counseling, health education, and training programs using adult learning approaches
- Research related to occupational and environmental health

Standard I. Assessment

The occupational and environmental health nurse systematically assesses the health status of the individual client or population and the environment.

Standard II. Diagnosis

The occupational and environmental health nurse analyzes assessment data to formulate diagnoses.

Standard III. Outcome Identification

The occupational and environmental health nurse identifies outcomes specific to the client.

Standard IV. Planning

The occupational and environmental health nurse develops a goal-directed plan that is comprehensive and formulates interventions to attain expected outcomes.

Standard V. Implementation

The occupational and environmental health nurse implements interventions to attain desired outcomes identified in the plan.

Standard VI. Evaluation

The occupational and environmental health nurse systematically and continuously evaluates responses to interventions and progress toward achievement of desired outcomes.

Standard VII. Resource Management

The occupational and environmental health nurse secures and manages the resources that support an occupational health and safety program.

Standard VIII. Professional Development

The occupational and environmental health nurse assumes accountability for professional development to enhance professional growth and maintain competency.

Standard IX. Collaboration

The occupational and environmental health nurse collaborates with employees, management, other healthcare providers, professionals, and community representatives.

Standard X. Research

The occupational and environmental health nurse uses research findings in practice and contributes to the scientific base in occupational and environmental health nursing to improve practice and advance the profession.

Standard XI. Ethics

The occupational and environmental health nurse uses an ethical framework as a guide for decision making in practice.

EXPECTED OUTCOMES IN OCCUPATIONAL AND ENVIRONMENTAL HEALTH PRACTICE

Examples of expected outcomes that occupational and environmental health nurses may identify include:

- Improvement in health status of the employee/workforce
- Reduction in morbidity and mortality
- Increase in knowledge of associated risk factors
- Elimination or reduction in risk or hazards related to the work environment, work processes, and work practices
- Improved employee health and safety through initiation, improvement, or utilization of prevention and control strategies

- Increased knowledge related to health promotion, preventive health, and therapeutic strategies
- Reduction in healthcare costs/premiums
- Identification and utilization of appropriate community and personal resources
- Use of appropriate resources to enhance coping skills
- Ability to meet job requirements

Guidelines for Public Health Nursing

Definition

Public health nursing is the practice of promoting and protecting the health of populations using knowledge from nursing, social, and public health sciences.

Nursing combines critical thinking and creative problem solving with the process of assessment, planning, intervention, and evaluation to achieve health outcomes.

1. Assessment is the collection and analysis of relevant data to evaluate health status and to identify problems, opportunities, needs, and assets.
2. Planning requires collaborative goal setting and mapping strategies to achieve those goals.
3. Intervention involves carrying out a plan of care in partnership with the client based on priority of need.
4. Evaluation entails determining the effectiveness of the interventions and changing the plan as indicated.

The practice of nursing and the core public health functions are both forms of analytical thinking and the scientific process.

A mix of skills that are critical to public health nursing:

- Epidemiology
- Skills to impact change organization
- Measurement of health status and organizational change
- How people connect to organizations
- Environmental health
- Policy
- Negotiation, collaboration, communication, advocacy
- Data analysis, statistics

From Association of State and Territorial Directors of Nursing: *Public health nursing: a partner for healthy populations,* Washington, DC, 2000, American Nurses Association.

- Health economics
- Interdisciplinary teams
- Program evaluation
- Coalition building
- Population-based principles, interventions
- Politics of health
- How to build on differences, diversity
- Quality improvement approach

Tenets of Public Health Nursing

The following guidelines explain public health nursing:

- The process of population-based assessment, policy development, and assurance is systematic and comprehensive.
- In all processes partnerships with representatives of the people are essential.
- Primary prevention is given priority.
- Creating healthy environmental, social, and economic conditions in which people live guides selection of intervention strategies.
- The practice incorporates an obligation to actively reach out to all who might benefit from an intervention or service.
- The dominant concern is for the greater good of all of the people or the population as a whole.
- The wise stewardship and allocation of the available resources is supported in order to gain the maximum population health benefit from the use of those resources.
- The health of the people is most effectively promoted and protected through collaboration with members of other professions and organizations.

Orientation of New Nurse to Public Health Core Functions Guide

CORE FUNCTIONS OF PUBLIC HEALTH

Assessment–encompasses all the activities involved in the concept of community diagnosis, such as surveillance, identifying needs, analyzing the causes of problems, collecting and interpreting data, case finding, monitoring and forecasting trends, research, and evaluation of outcomes.

From Association of State and Territorial Directors of Nursing: *Public health nursing: a partner for healthy populations,* Washington, DC, 2000, American Nurses Association.

Policy development–occurs as the result of interactions among many public and private organizations and individuals. It is the process by which decisions about problems are made, goals and the proper means for reaching them are chosen, conflicting views about solutions are handled, and resources are allocated.

Assurance–provides services necessary to reach agreed upon goals, either by encouraging private sector action, by requiring it, or by providing services directly. The assurance function in public health involves stimulating the implementation of legislative mandates as well as maintaining statutory responsibilities.

ESSENTIAL PUBLIC HEALTH SERVICES

Monitor health status to identify community health problems

Diagnose and investigate health problems and health hazards in the community

Inform, educate, and empower people about health issues

Mobilize community partnerships to identify and solve health problems

Develop policies and plans that support individual and community health efforts

Enforce laws and regulations that protect health and ensure safety

Link people to needed personal health services and assure the provision of healthcare when otherwise unavailable

Assure a competent public health and personal healthcare workforce

Evaluate effectiveness, accessibility, and quality of personal and population-based health services

Research for new insights and innovative solutions to health problems

EXAMPLES OF NURSING ACTIVITIES FOR EACH ESSENTIAL SERVICE

1. Monitor health status to identify community health problems.

Public health nurses:
    Participate in community assessment.
    Identify sub-populations at risk for disease or disability.
    Collect information on interventions to special populations.
    Define and evaluate effective strategies and programs.
    Identify potential environmental hazards.

2. Diagnose and investigate health problems and health hazards in the community.

Public health nurses:

Understand and identify determinants of health and disease.

Apply knowledge about environmental influences on health.

Recognize multiple causes of or factors in health and illness.

Participate in case identification and treatment of persons with communicable disease.

3. Inform, educate, and empower people about health issues.

Public health nurses:

Develop health and educational plans for individuals and families in multiple settings.

Develop and implement community-based health education.

Provide regular reports on the health status of special populations in clinic settings, community settings, and groups.

Advocate for and with underserved and disadvantaged populations.

Assure health planning that includes primary prevention and early intervention strategies.

Identify health population behaviors and maintain successful intervention strategies through reinforcement and continual funding.

4. Mobilize community partnerships to identify and solve health problems.

Public health nurses:

Interact regularly with many providers and services within each community.

Convene groups and providers who share common concerns and interests in special populations.

Provide leadership to prioritize community problems and development of interventions.

Explain the significance of health issues to the public and participate in developing plans of action.

5. Develop policies and plans that support individual and community health efforts.

Public health nurses:

Participate in community and family decision-making.

Provide information and advocate for the interests of special groups in program development.

Develop programs and services to meet the needs of high-risk populations as well as members of the broader community.

Participate in disaster planning and mobilization of community resources in emergencies.

Advocate for appropriate funding for services.

6. Enforce laws and regulations that protect health and ensure safety.

Public health nurses:

Regulate and support safe care and treatment for dependent populations such as children and the frail elderly.

Implement ordinances and laws that protect the environment.

Establish procedures and processes that ensure competent implementation of treatment schedules for diseases critical to public health.

Participate in the development of local regulation that protects communities and the environment from potential hazards and pollution.

7. Link people to needed personal health services and assure the provision of health care when otherwise unavailable.

Public health nurses:

Provide clinical preventive services to certain high-risk populations.

Establish programs and services to meet special needs.

Recommend clinical care and other services to clients and their families in clinics, homes, and the community.

Provide referrals through community links to needed care.

Participate in community provider coalitions and meetings to educate others and to identify service centers for community populations.

Provide clinical surveillance and identification of communicable disease.

8. Ensure a competent public health and personal health care workforce

Public health nurses:

Participate in continuing education and preparation to assure competence.

Define and support proper delegation to unlicensed assistive personnel in community settings.

Establish standards for performance.

Maintain patient record systems and community documents.

Establish and maintain procedures and protocols for patient care.

Participate in quality assurance activities, such as record audits, agency evaluations, and clinical guidelines.

9. Evaluate effectiveness, accessibility, and quality of personal and population-based health services.

Public health nurses:

Collect data and information on community interventions.

Identify unserved and underserved populations in communities.

Review and analyze data on the health status of communities.

Participate with communities in assessing services and outcomes of care.

Identify and define enhanced services required to manage health status of complex populations and special risk groups.

10. Research for new insights and innovative solutions to health problems.

Public health nurses:

Implement nontraditional interventions and approaches to effect change in special populations.

Participate in the collection of information and data to improve the surveillance and understanding of special problems.

Develop collegial relationships with academic institutions to explore new interventions.

Participate in early identification of factors detrimental to the community's health.

Formulate and use investigative tools to identify and affect care delivery and program planning.

Building Capacity of the Public Health Nursing Workforce: A Focus on Competency

The transition from a predominantly personal health and clinical-based practice to a population health practice can be facilitated by:

1. Identifying current models of population health using the core public health functions and essential health services as a framework.
2. Collaborating with local schools of public health and schools of nursing to design population health educational programs.
3. Participating in the national network of public health professionals engaged in developing the competencies for the future public health workforce.
4. Developing educational training programs based on the competencies outlined in the documents described in this manual.

From Association of State and Territorial Directors of Nursing: *Public health nursing: a partner for healthy populations,* Washington, DC, 2000, American Nurses Association.

CLINICAL RESOURCES

Industry Inspection List for OSHA

Use this list as a guide for making plant inspections. Details on requirements are found in the OSHA *General Industry Standards.* Keep records of what you see and the action taken!

Walking—working surfaces
Slippery
Damaged
Clear
Openings
Egress
Electrical
Disconnects
Defective
Exposed
Controls
Housekeeping/general plant environment
Clean
Debris
Ventilation
Sanitation
Vehicles
Authorized use
Defective
Rules and regulations
Adequate safeguards
Charging areas
Preventive maintenance and
   tag-out procedure
Cranes and hoisting equipment
Defective
Capacity
Controls
Authorized use

Material handling and storage
Hazardous material
Proper use
Identification
Containment
Proper location
Hazardous materials
Chemicals
Powered tools
Defective
Guards
Use
Storage
Personal protective equipment
Eye protection
Hearing protection
Body protection
Emergency equipment
Sanitation and storage
Fire hazards
Flammable materials
Access
Areas identified
Storage
Compressed air and gases
Storage
Secured
Use

From Occupational Safety and Health Administration: US Department of Labor, online http://www.osha-slc.gov.2000.

Machinery and equipment
Defective
Lock-out
Use
Guarding
Controls
Safety devices
Pinch points

Fumes
Noise
Dusts
Safe job procedures
Job safety analysis conducted
Proper training
Job procedures

Laboratory Values of Clinical Importance

$$\text{mmol/L} = \frac{\text{mg/dL} \times 10}{\text{atomic weight}}$$

$$\text{mg/dL} = \frac{\text{mmol/L} \times \text{atomic weight}}{10}$$

Body Fluids and Other Mass Data

Body fluid, total volume: 50% (in obese) to 70% (lean) body weight
    Intracellular: 30-40% body weight
    Extracellular: 20-30% body weight
Blood:
    Total volume:
      Male: 69 mL/kg body weight
      Female: 65 mL/kg body weight
    Plasma volume:
      Male: 39 mL/kg body weight
      Female: 40 mL/kg body weight
    RBC volume:
      Male: 30 mL/kg body weight (1.15-1.21 L/m^2 body surface area)
      Female: 25 mL/kg body weight (0.95-1.00 L/m^2 body surface area)

$$\text{Body surface area (m}^2) = \frac{(\text{wt in kg})^{0.425} \times (\text{ht in cm})^{0.725}}{139.315}$$

From Harrison: *Principles of internal medicine,* ed 13, New York, 1995, McGraw-Hill.

CSF

Glucose: 2.2-3.9 mmol/L (40-70 mg/dL)
Total protein: 0.2-0.5 g/L (20-50 mg/dL)
CSF pressure: 50-180 mm H_2O
Leukocytes:
    Total: <5 per mL
    Differential:
        Lymphocytes: 60-70%
        Monocytes: 30-50%
        Neutrophils: None

Chemical Constituents of Blood

Albumin, serum: 35-55 g/L (3.5-5.5 g/dL)
Aldolase: 0-100 nkat/L (0-6 U/L)
Aminotransferases, serum:
    Aspartate (AST, SGOT): 0-0.58 μkat/L (0-35 U/L)
    Alanine (ALT, SGPT): 0-0.58 μkat/L (0-35 U/L)
Ammonia, as NH_3 plasma: 6-47 μmol/L (10-80 μg/dL)
Amylase, serum: 0.8-3.2 μkat/L (60-180 U/L)
Arterial blood gases:
    [HCO_3]: 21-28 mmol/L (21-30 mEq/L)
    P_{CO_2}: 4.7-5.9 kPa (35-45 mm Hg)
    pH: 7.38-7.44
    P_{O_2}: 11-13 kPa (80-100 mm Hg)
Bilirubin, total, serum (Malloy-Evelyn): 5.1-17 μmol/L
    (0.3-1.0 mg/dL)
    Direct, serum: 1.7-5.1 μmol/L (0.1-0.3 mg/dL)
    Indirect, serum: 3.4-12 μmol/L (0.2-0.7 mg/dL)
Calcium, ionized: 1.1-1.4 mmol/L (4.5-5.6 mg/dL)
Calcium, plasma: 2.2-2.6 mmol/L (9-10.5 mg/dL)
Carbon dioxide content, plasma (sea level): 21-30 mmol/L (21-30
    mEq/L)
Carbon dioxide tension (P_{CO_2}), arterial blood (sea level): 4.7-6.0 kPa
    (35-45 mm Hg)
Chloride, serum: 98-106 mmol/L (98-106 mEq/L)
Cholesterol, plasma: <5.20 mmol/L (<200 mg/dL)
Complement, serum:
    C3: 0.55-1.20 g/L (55-120 mg/dL)
    C4: 0.20-0.50 g/L (20-50 mg/dL)
Creatine kinase, serum (total):
    Male: 0.42-1.50 μkat/L (25-90 U/L)
    Female: 0.17-1.17 μkat/L (10-70 U/L)

Creatinine, serum: <133 μmol/L (<1.5 mg/dL)

Digoxin, serum:
   Therapeutic level: 0.6-2.8 nmol/L (0.5-2.2 ng/mL)
   Toxic level: >3.1 nmol/L (>2.4 ng/mL)

Ethanol, plasma:
   Behavioral changes: >4.3 mmol/L (>20 mg/dL)
   Legal intoxication: >17 mmol/L (>80 mg/dL)
   Coma and death: >65 mmol/L (>300 mg/dL)

Ferritin, plasma:
   Male: 15-400 μg/L (15-400 ng/mL)
   Female: 10-200 μg/L (10-200 ng/mL)

Glucose (fasting), plasma:
   Normal: 4.2-6.4 mmol/L (75-115 mg/dL)
   Diabetes mellitus: >7.8 mmol/L (>140 mg/dL) (on more than one occasion)

Glucose, 2-hour postprandial, plasma:
   Normal: <7.8 mmol/L (<140 mg/dL)
   Impaired glucose tolerance: 7.8-11.1 mmol/L (140-200 mg/dL)
   Diabetes mellitus: >11.1 mmol/L (>200 mg/dL) (on more than one occasion)

Hemoglobin, blood (sea level):
   Males: 140-180 g/L (14-18 g/dL)
   Females: 120-160 g/L (12-16 g/dL)
   Hemoglobin A_{1c}: Up to 6% of total hemoglobin

Immunoglobins, serum:
   IgA: 0.9-3.2 g/L (90-325 mg/dL)
   IgD: 0-0.08 g/L (0-8 mg/dL)
   IgE: <0.00025 g/L (<0.025 mg/dL)
   IgG: 8.0-15.0 g/L (800-1500 mg/dL)
   IgM: 0.45-1.5 g/L (45-150 mg/dL)

Iron, serum: 9.0-27 μmol/L (50-150 μg/dL)

Iron-binding capacity, serum: 45-66 μmol/L (250-370 μg/dL)
   Saturation: 20-45%

Lactate dehydrogenase, serum:
   1.7-3.2 μkat/L (100-190 U/L)

Lipoproteins, plasma (desirable):
   LDL cholesterol: <3.36-4.14 mmol/L (<130 mg/dL)
   HDL cholesterol: >1.8 mmol/L (>70 mg/dL)

Magnesium, serum: 0.8-1.2 mmol/L (2-3 mg/dL)

Osmolality, plasma: 285-295 mosmol/kg of serum water

Phenytoin, plasma:
   Therapeutic range: 40-80 μmol/L (10-20 mg/L)
   Toxic level: >120 μmol/L (>30 mg/L)

Phosphatase, acid, serum: 0.90 nkat/L (0-5.5 U/L)
Phosphatase, alkaline, serum: 0.5-2.0 μkat/L (30-120 U/L)
Phosphorus, inorg., serum: 1.0-1.4 mmol/L (3-4.5 mg/dL)
Potassium, serum: 3.5-5.0 mmol/L
Proteins, total, serum: 55-80 g/L (5.5-8.0 g/dL)
Protein fractions, serum:
   Albumin: 35-55 g/L (3.5-5.0 g/dL) (50-60%)
   Globulin: 20-35 g/L (2.0-3.5 g/dL) (40-50%)
   Alpha$_1$: 2-4 g/L (0.2-0.4 g/dL) (4.2-7.2%)
   Alpha$_2$: 5-9 g/L (0.5-0.9 g/dL) (6.8-12%)
   Beta: 6-11 g/L (0.6-1.1 g/dL) (9.3-15%)
   Gamma: 7-17 g/L (0.7-1.7 g/dL) (13-23%)
Sodium, serum: 136-145 mmol/L (136-145 mEq/L)
Triglycerides, plasma: <1.8 mmol/L (<160 mg/dL)
Urea nitrogen, serum: 3.6-7.1 mmol/L (10-20 mg/dL)
Uric acid, serum:
   Male: 150-480 μmol/L (2.5-8.0 mg/dL)
   Female: 90-360 μmol/L (1.5-6.0 mg/dL)

Function Tests

Circulation

Cardiac output (Fick): 2.5-3.6 L/m^2 body surface area per min.
Ejection fraction, stroke volume/end-diastolic volume (SV/EDV):
   Normal range: 0.55-0.78, average 0.67
Pulmonary vascular resistance: 2-12 kPa·s/L (20-120 [dyn·s]/cm^5)
Systemic vascular resistance: 77-150 (dyn·s)/cm^5
   (770-1500 [kPa·s]/L)

Gastrointestinal

D-Xylose absorption test: After an overnight fast, 25 g xylose is given
   PO in aqueous solution; urine collected for the following 5 hours
   should contain 33-53 mmol (5-8 g) (or >20% of ingested dose);
   serum xylose should be 1.7-2.7 mmol/L (25-40 mg per 100 mL) 1
   hour after the oral dose.
Gastric juice:
   Volume:
      24 hours: 2-3 L
      Nocturnal: 600-700 mL
      Basal, fasting: 30-70 mL/h
   pH: 1.6-1.8

Acid output:
  Basal:
    Male: (mean ± 1 SD): 0.8 ± 0.6 μmol/sec (3.0 ± 2.0 mEq/h)
    Female: (mean ± 1 SD): 0.6 ± 0.5 μmol/sec (2.0 ± 1.8 mEq/h)
  Maximal (after subcutaneous histamine acid phosphate
    0.004 mg/kg and preceded by 50 mg promethazine; or after beta-zole 1.7 mg/kg or pentagastrin 6 μg/kg):
    Male: 6.4 ± 1.4 μmol/s (23 ± 5 mEq/h)
    Female: 4.4 ± 1.4 μmol/s (16 ± 5 mEq/h)
Secretin test (pancreatic exocrine function: 1 U/kg body weight, IV):
  Volume (pancreatic juice): >2.0 mL/kg in 80 min.
  Bicarbonate concentration: >80 mmol/L
  Bicarbonate output: >10 mmol in 30 min.

Metabolic and endocrine
Adrenal steroids, plasma:
  Cortisol:
  8 AM 140-690 nmol/L (5-25 μg/dL)
  4 PM 80-330 nmol/L (3-12 μg/dL)
Adrenal steroids, urinary excretion:
  Aldosterone: 14-53 nmol/day (5-19 μg/day)
  Cortisol, free: 55-275 nmol/day (20-100 μg/day)
  17-Hydroxycorticosteroids: 5.5-28 μmol/d (2-10 mg/day)
  17-Ketosteroids:
    Male: 20-69 μmol/day (6-20 mg/day)
    Female: 20-59 μmol/day (6-17 mg/day)
Estradiol:
  Male: <180 pmol/L (<50 pg/mL)
  Female: 70-220 pmol/L (20-60 pg/mL), higher at ovulation
Progesterone:
  Male: prepubertal, preovulatory, and postmenopausal female: <6 nmol/L (2 ng/mL)
  Females, luteal, peak: 6-60 nmol/L (2-20 ng/mL)
Testosterone:
  Male: 10-35 nmol/L (3-10 ng/mL)
  Female: <3.5 nmol/L (<1 ng/mL)
  Prepubertal boys and girls: 0.17-0.7 nmol/L (0.05-0.2 ng/mL)
Thyroid function tests:
  Radioactive iodine uptake, 24 hours: 5-30% (range varies in different areas owing to variations in iodine intake)
  Resin T_3 uptake: 25-35% (varies among laboratories)

Thyroid-stimulating hormone (TSH): 0.4-5 mU/L (0.4-5 μU/mL)
Thyroxine (T_4), serum radioimmunoassay: 64-154 nmol/L
  (5-12 μg/dL)
Triiodothyronine (T_3), plasma: 1.1-2.9 nmol/L (70-190 ng/dL)

Renal
Clearances (corrected to 1.72 m^2 body surface area):
  Insulin clearance (mean ± 1 SD):
    Male: 2.1 ± 0.4 mL/sec (124 ± 25.8 mL/min)
    Female: 2.0 ± 0.2 mL/sec (119 ± 12.8 mL/min)
  Endogenous creatinine clearance: 1.5-2.2 mL/sec (91-130 mL/min)
Concentration and dilution test:
  Specific gravity of urine:
    After 12-hour fluid restriction: 1.025 or more
    After 12-hour deliberate water intake: 1.003 or less

Hematologic Examinations
(See also "Chemical Constituents of Blood")
Carboxyhemoglobin:
  Nonsmoker: 0-2.3%
  Smoker: 2.1-4.2%
Haptoglobin, serum: 0.5-2.2 g/L (50-220 mg/dL)
Hematocrit
  Male: 0.42-0.52
  Female: 0.37-0.48
Hemoglobin, adults:
  Females: 7.4-9.9 mmol/L (12-16 g/dL)
  Males: 8.1-11.2 mmol/L (13-18 g/dL)
Leukocytes, total, adults: 4.3-10.8 × 10^9/L (4.3-10.8 × 10^3/mm^3)

Differential count	Approx. % of total
Neutrophils	45-74
Bands	0-4
Lymphocytes	16-45
Monocytes	4-10
Eosinophils	0-7
Basophils	0-2

Platelets and coagulation parameters:
  Fibrinogen: 2-4 g/L (200-400 mg/dL)
  Fibrin split products: <10 mg/L (<10 μg/mL)
  Platelets: 130,000-400,000/mm^3

Sedimentation rate:
  Westergren, <50 years of age:
    Male: 0-15 mm/hr
    Female: 0-20 mm/hr
  Westergren, >50 years of age:
    Male: 0-20 mm/hr
    Female: 0-30 mm/hr

Urine

Creatinine: 8.8-14 mmol/d (1.0-1.6 g/day)
Protein: <0.15 g/d (<150 mg/day)
Potassium: 25-100 mmol/day (varies with intake)
Sodium: 100-260 mmol/day (varies with intake)

Common Epidemiologic Rates

General Mortality Rates

Crude mortality rate
$$\frac{\text{Number of deaths occurring during 1 year}}{\text{Midyear population}} \times 100,000$$

Cause-specific mortality rate
$$\frac{\text{Number of deaths from a stated cause during 1 year}}{\text{Midyear population}} \times 100,000$$

Case-fatality rate
$$\frac{\text{Number of deaths from a specific disease}}{\text{Number of cases of the same disease}} \times 100$$

Proportional mortality ratio
$$\frac{\text{Number of deaths from a specific cause within a given time period}}{\text{Total deaths in the same time period}} \times 100$$

Age-specific mortality rate
$$\frac{\text{Number of persons in a specific age group dying during 1 year}}{\text{Midyear population of the specific age group}} \times 100,000$$

Maternal and Infant Indices

Crude birth rate
$$\frac{\text{Number of live births during 1 year}}{\text{Midyear population}} \times 1000$$

General fertility rate
$$\frac{\text{Number of live births during 1 year}}{\text{Number of females aged 15-44 at midyear}} \times 1000$$

From Harkness GA: *Epidemiology in nursing practice,* St Louis, 1995, Mosby.

Maternal mortality rate	$\dfrac{\text{Number of deaths from puerperal causes during 1 year}}{\text{Number of live births during same year}} \times 100{,}000$
Infant mortality rate	$\dfrac{\text{Number of deaths of children under 1 year of age during 1 year}}{\text{Number of live births during same year}} \times 1000$
Perinatal mortality rate	$\dfrac{\text{Number of fetal deaths plus infant deaths under 7 days of age during 1 year}}{\text{Number of live births plus fetal deaths during same year}} \times 1000$
Neonatal mortality rate	$\dfrac{\text{Number of deaths of children under 28 days of age during 1 year}}{\text{Number of live births during same year}} \times 1000$
Fetal mortality rate	$\dfrac{\text{Number of fetal deaths during 1 year}}{\text{Number of live births plus fetal deaths during same year}} \times 1000$

Handwashing Technique

1. Use a sink with warm running water, soap, and paper towels.
2. Push wristwatch and long uniform sleeves up above wrists. Remove jewelry, except a plain band, from fingers and arms.
3. Keep fingernails short and filed.
4. Inspect the surface of the hands and fingers for breaks or cuts in the skin and cuticles. Report such lesions when caring for highly susceptible clients.
5. Stand in front of the sink, keeping hands and uniform away from the sink surface. (If hands touch the sink during handwashing, repeat the process.) Use a sink where it is comfortable to reach the faucet.
6. Turn on the water. Turn on hand-operated faucets by covering the faucet with a paper towel.
7. Avoid splashing water against your uniform or clothes.
8. Regulate flow of water so the temperature is warm.
9. Wet hands and lower arms thoroughly under running water. Keep the hands and forearms lower than the elbows during washing.

Modified from Potter PA, Perry AG: *Fundamentals of nursing: concepts, process, and practice,* ed 4, St Louis, 1998, Mosby.

10. Apply 1 mL of regular or 3 mL of antiseptic liquid soap to the hands, lathering thoroughly. If bar soap is used, hold it throughout the lathering period. Soap granules and leaflet preparations may be used.

11. Wash the hands, using plenty of lather and friction for at least 10 to 15 seconds. Interlace the fingers and rub the palms and back of hands with a circular motion at least 5 times each.

12. If areas underlying fingernails are soiled, clean them with fingernails of the other hand and additional soap or a clean orangewood stick. Do not tear or cut the skin under or around the nail.

13. Rinse hands and wrists thoroughly, keeping hands down and elbows up.

14. Repeat steps 10 through 12 but extend the actual period of washing for 1-, 2-, and 3-minute hand washings.

15. Dry the hands thoroughly from the fingers up to the wrists and forearms.

16. Discard paper towel in proper receptacle.

17. To turn off a hand faucet, use a clean, dry paper towel.

Remember to treat the inside of your "black bag" as clean. Always wash hands before removing supplies and equipment from bag or putting clean supplies in the bag. Carry soap and paper towels in outside packets of your bag or at inner top.

REPORTABLE DISEASES

The Centers for Disease Control and Prevention requires states, agencies, and health providers to provide information about specific diseases. Furthermore, states and localities also often have such requirements related to specific disease states within communities. Following is a listing of the national reportable diseases and an example of one state's reportable diseases. Users may obtain updated information from their state's health department.

National Reportable Diseases

Acquired immunodeficiency syndrome (AIDS)
Anthrax
Botulism
Brucellosis
Chancroid
Chlamydia trachomatis, genital infections
Cholera
Coccidioidomycosis

Cryptosporidiosis
Cyclosporiasis
Diphtheria
Ehrlichiosis, human granulo-
    cytic
Ehrlichiosis, human monocytic
Encephalitis, California
    serogroup viral
Encephalitis, Eastern equine
Encephalitis, St. Louis
Encephalitis, Western equine
Escherichia coli O157:H7
Gonorrhea
Haemophilus influenzae, inva-
    sive disease
Hansen's disease (leprosy)
Hantavirus pulmonary syn-
    drome
Hemolytic uremic syndrome,
    post-diarrheal
Hepatitis A
Hepatitis B
Hepatitis, C/non-A, non-B
HIV infection, adult (≥13
    years)
HIV infection, pediatric (<13
    years)
Legionellosis
Listeriosis
Lyme disease
Malaria

Measles
Meningococcal disease
Mumps
Pertussis
Plague
Poliomyelitis, paralytic
Psittacosis
Q fever
Rabies, animal
Rabies, human
Rocky Mountain spotted fever
Rubella
Rubella, congenital syndrome
Salmonellosis
Shigellosis
Streptococcal disease, invasive,
    Group A
Streptococcus pneumoniae,
    drug-resistant
Streptococcal toxic-shock syn-
    drome
Syphilis
Syphilis, congenital
Tetanus
Toxic-shock syndrome
Trichinosis
Tuberculosis
Tularemia
Typhoid fever
Varicella (deaths only)
Yellow fever

From CDC Centers for Disease Control and Prevention. Available at: http://www.cdc.gov/eps/dphsi/infdis.htm, Feb 2000.

State and Local Reportable Diseases

Category I

Report immediately by telephone to the Department of Health Services and to your patient's local health department the occurrence or suspicion of any of the diseases listed below. Also mail a communicable disease report within 24 hours.

Animal bite
Anthrax
Botulism (other than infant botulism
Campylobacteriosis
Cholera
Diphtheria
Encephalitis
Gonococcal infections (all suspected or confirmed antibiotic-resistant strains)
Hepatitis (viral)
Measles
Meningitis (and other invasive disease caused by *Haemophilus influenzae* type B)
Meningitis caused by *Neisseria meningitidis*
Meningococcemia

Pertussis (whooping cough)
Plague
Poliomyelitis
Rabies (human)
Rubella (including congenital rubella syndrome)
Salmonellosis
Shigellosis
Syphilis (primary, secondary, congenital, or early latent)
Trichinosis
Tuberculosis*
Typhoid fever
Yellow fever
Yersiniosis
A suspected epidemic of any disease

*Report directly to the local health department or to the Tuberculosis Control Program.

Category II

Complete and mail a Communicable Disease Report within 7 days of diagnosis.

Acquired immunodeficiency syndrome (AIDS)
Amebiasis
Botulism
Brucellosis
Chancroid
Chlamydia infections
Cryptococcosis
Ehrlichiosis (human)

Giardiasis
Gonococcal infections (other than antibiotic-resistant strains)
Granuloma inguinale
Herpes simplex infections (genital)
Histoplasmosis

Human immunodeficiency virus (HIV) infection
Kaposi's sarcoma
Kawasaki syndrome
Legionellosis
Leprosy
Leptospirosis
Lyme disease
Lymphogranuloma venereum
Malaria
Mumps
Mycobacterium avium-intracellulare infection
Pneumocystis carinii pneumonia
Positive tuberculin skin tests (in children 6 years of age or less)

Psittacosis
Q fever
Reye's syndrome
Rocky Mountain spotted fever
Syphilis (all stages other than those listed previously)
Tetanus
Toxic-shock syndrome
Toxoplasmosis
Tularemia
Typhus
Varicella (chickenpox—adult)

Report the number of cases of chickenpox on a weekly basis.

Category III

Reporting required within 3 months:

Asbestosis
Coal worker's pneumoconiosis

Mesothelioma
Silicosis

Current Status of HIV Reporting as of December 7, 1998

Name-based reporting:	Non-name-based reporting:	Reporting not required:
Alabama	Georgia	Alaska
Arizona	Illinois	California
Arkansas	Kansas	Connecticut-1
Colorado	Kentucky	Delaware
Florida	Maine	Hawaii
Idaho	Maryland-4	Massachusetts-6
Indiana	Montana	New York-6
Iowa	New Hampshire	Pennsylvania
Louisiana	Oregon-3	Puerto Rico
Michigan	Rhode Island	Vermont
Minnesota	Texas-2	Washington-6
Mississippi	Virgin Islands-6	District of Columbia

(Continued)

Current Status of HIV Reporting as of December 7, 1998— cont'd

Name-based reporting:	Non-name-based reporting:	Reporting not required:
Missouri		
Nebraska		
Nevada		
New Jersey		
New Mexico		
North Carolina		
North Dakota		
Ohio		
Oklahoma		
South Carolina		
South Dakota		
Tennessee		
Utah		
Virginia		
West Virginia		
Wisconsin		
Wyoming		

1 Requires named reports of HIV infection in children <13 years of age. Reports of HIV infection not required for adults/adolescents 13 and older.

2 Uses unique identifier system for HIV reporting. Requires named reporting of HIV infection in children <13 years of age.

3 Requires named reporting only for HIV infection in children <6 years of age and in limited other circumstances.

4 Uses unique identifier system for HIV reporting for person 13 years of age and older. Requires named reporting of symptomatic HIV infection and AIDS.

5 Requires named reporting of symptomatic HIV infection and AIDS.

6 Name-based reporting passed by law, rule or regulation in 1998, but not yet implemented.

7 Maryland and Texas conduct HIV case surveillance using a 12 digit unique identifier (UI) and attempt to conduct follow-up activities to fill gaps in the information received. Providers, hospitals, and labs in the other states in this column send health departments individual-level HIV data using a variety of non-name-based identifiers, such as initials, a date of birth, or a test number. These states generally do not conduct any follow-up activities on this HIV case information and have not evaluated the usefulness or completeness of their HIV reporting systems.

States in *italics* offer only confidential and not anonymous HIV testing. All other U.S. states and territories offer anonymous testing.

Courtesy of the AIDS Action Council.

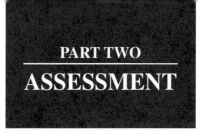

PART TWO

ASSESSMENT

COMMUNITY ASSESSMENT

Caring for the community has been an important part of practice for the public and community health nurse. In order to be knowledgeable about relevant care to individuals and family members, it is essential to know the community where they live, to identify resources that may participate in care, and to learn about deficits that might be strengthened through public and community health nursing practice.

Windshield Survey: A Micro Approach

This tool is designed to assist the nurse traveling around the community in identifying objective data that will help define the community, trends, stability, and changes which can affect the health of the population.

Boundaries

To what extent do the identified boundaries of the catchment reflect the boundaries (such as a river or a different terrain), constructed (such as a highway or railroad) or economic (such as a difference in real estate or the presence of industrial or commercial units along with residential ones)? Does the neighborhood have an identity or a name? Is it displayed? Are there unofficial names? Are there subcommunities within the area?

Housing and zoning

How old are the houses? What style are they and of what materials are they constructed? Are all the neighborhood houses similar? If not, how would you characterize the differences? Are there single or multifamily homes? What size are the lots? Are there signs of disrepair (such as broken doors, steps, or windows)? Are there vacant houses?

Modified from Mizrahi TM. School of Social Work, Richmond, VA, Virginia Commonwealth University, September, 1992.

Signs of decay

Is the neighborhood on the way up or down? Is it "alive"? How would you decide? Is there trash, abandoned cars, boarded-up buildings, rubble, dilapidated sheds, rubble-filled vacant lots, poor drainage, disease vector harborage, or the like?

Parks and recreational areas

Are there parks and recreational areas in the neighborhood? Is the open space public or private? Who uses it?

"Commons"

What are the neighborhood hangouts? For what groups, and at what hours (e.g., school year, candy store, bar, restaurant, park)? Does the "commons" have a sense of territoriality, or is it open to strangers?

Stores

What supermarkets or neighborhood stores are available? How do residents travel to the store? Are there drug stores, laundries, or dry cleaners?

Transportation

How do people get in and out of the neighborhood? What is the condition of the streets? Is there a major highway near the neighborhood? Whom does it serve? Is public transportation available?

Service centers

Are there social agencies, clinics, recreation centers, or schools? Are there doctors, dentists, or other healthcare providers? Is there a hospital in the area?

Street people

If you are traveling during the day, who is on the streets (women, children, teenagers, community health nurses, collection agents, salesmen, etc.)? How are they dressed? What animals do you see (strays, pets, watchdogs, or livestock)?

Protective services

Is there evidence of police and fire protection in the area?

Race

Of what ethnicity are the residents (black, white, Asian)? How are the different racial groups residentially located? Is the area integrated?

Ethnicity

Are there indicies of ethnicity—food stores, restaurants, churches, private schools, language information other than in English?

Religion

What churches and church-operated schools are in the neighborhood? How many are there?

Socioeconomic

How would you categorize the residents: I, upper class; II, upper-middle class; III, middle class; IV, working class; V, lower class? On what do you base this judgment?

Health and morbidity

Are there evidences of acute or chronic diseases or conditions, of accidents, communicable diseases, alcoholism, drug abuse, or mental illness? On what do you base this judgment?

Politics

Do you see any political campaign posters? Is there a party headquarters? Is there any evidence of a predominant party affiliation?

Community Assessment: A Macro Approach

The following questions have been designed to assist personnel in analyzing the data collected relative to the communities. The list is not exhaustive but is designed to stimulate thinking as providers residing within their communities begin to determine health needs. Analysis of the data is one step of the nursing process. The data analysis may best be done by those most familiar with the community, in preference to analysis performed by those less familiar with the community (that is, the state agency).

1. Identify the boundaries of this community.
    a. People
    b. Place
    c. Social interaction and/or common goals, interests, or characteristics

Adapted from Community Health Faculty, Undergraduate Program, University of Maryland School of Nursing: *Community assessment tool,* Baltimore, 1975, University of Maryland School of Nursing. In Smith CM, Maurer FA: *Community health nursing: theory and practice,* ed 2, Philadelphia, 2000, WB Saunders.

2. Identify the suprasystem and explain the importance of looking at the suprasystem during a community assessment.
3. Identify the goals of this community.
4. Describe the community's physical and psychosocial characteristics.
   a. Physical characteristics
      (1) How long has the community existed?
      (2) Obtain demographic data about the community's members (age, race, sex, ethnicity, housing, density of population).
      (3) Identify physical features of the community that influence behavior.
   b. Psychosocial characteristics
      (1) Religion
      (2) Socioeconomic class
      (3) Education
      (4) Occupation
      (5) Marital status
5. Which external influences (inputs) from the environment (suprasystem) are resources? Which are demands?

	Resources	Demands
Money:		
Facilities:		
Human services:		
Formal		
Informal		
Health information:		
Legislation:		
Values of suprasystem		
(i.e., what external values		
affect this community?):		

6. Internal functions (throughputs): Identify resources and demands within the community that influence its level of health.
   a. Economy
      (1) Formal and informal human services: What formal and informal human services are available within the community (resources)?
      (2) Money: What is the budget? How is revenue generated from within the community?
      (3) Facilities, equipment, goods: What healthcare facilities are available within the community? What does the community produce? What equipment/supplies does it have to produce its goods?
      (4) Education: How are members educated/socialized to function productively?
      (5) Analysis of economy subsystem functioning: What is the ratio of resources to demands?
      (6) How accessible, adequate, and appropriate are the services, facilities, finances, and education in this community?
   b. Polity: Describe the political system within the community used to attain community goals.
      (1) What is the basic organizational structure?
      (2) Who are the formal and informal leaders?

    (3) What is the pattern of decision making? How have decisions been made in the past?

    (4) What methods of social control are used?

    (5) Analysis of the polity subsystem: What is the ratio of demands to resources?

  c. Communication: Describe the communication within the community that fosters a sense of belonging and provides identity and support to its members.

    (1) Nonverbal communication: What is the "personality"/emotional tone of the community? How do people talk about their community? What clubs and organizations are present?

    (2) Verbal communication: What is the pattern of communication? Who communicates with whom? Is it vertical or horizontal? How is communication achieved? What is the form of communication? When does the communication occur?

    (3) Analysis of communication subsystem: How well does the community communicate a sense of identity or belonging to its members? How adequate is the communication?

  d. Values: Identify the ideas, attitudes, and beliefs of community members that serve as general guides to behavior.

    (1) Traditions: What traditions are upheld?

    (2) Subgroups: What subgroups or cliques are obvious in this community?

    (3) Environment: Describe the environment, and explain how it reflects values.

    (4) Health:

      (a) What types of health facilities are used? How often?

      (b) What are people's attitudes about health and healthcare professionals?

      (c) What priority do community members place on health?

    (5) Homogeneity vs. heterogeneity: Is the community homogeneous or heterogeneous in its beliefs and values?

    (6) Analysis of values subsystem: How well does the community provide guidelines for the behavior of its members?

7. Health behavior and health status (outputs):

  a. People factors:

    (1) Describe the general trends regarding size of community.

    (2) What are the trends in mortality and morbidity?

      (a) What is the mortality rate?

      (b) What are the major causes of death?

      (c) What major diseases/illnesses are present?

      (d) Who are the vulnerable groups? What are the risky behaviors?

      (e) What presymptomatic illness or problems might be expected?

      (f) What is the level of social functioning in this community?

      (g) What types of disabilities and/or impairments are present or might be found in this community?

  b. Environmental factors:

    (1) Physical environmental factors: What is the quality of the physical environment (air, water, housing, work or home environment)?

(2) Social environmental factors: What is the emotional tone and stability of the population?

8. Describe feedback from the environment about the community's functioning.
9. Make inferences about the level of health of this community.
   a. What are some actual health problems or needs?
   b. What are some potential health problems or needs?
   c. How well is the community working to meet its health needs? What is its proposed action to meet its health needs?
   d. How has the community solved similar problems in the past?
   e. What are the strengths of the community?
10. Identify one actual or potential health need for which you, as a nurse, could plan an intervention.

Community Health Assessment Model

Definition of community: A locality-based entity—composed of systems of formal organizations reflecting societal institutions, informal groups, and aggregates, which are interdependent—whose function (expressed intent) is to meet a wide range of collective needs.

Definition of community health: The meeting of collective needs through identifying problems and managing interactions within the community and between the community and the larger society. This requires commitment, self-other awareness and clarity of situational definitions, articulateness, effective communication, conflict containment and accommodation, participation, management of relations with the larger society, and machinery for facilitating participant interaction and decision making.

COMMUNITY HEALTH ASSESSMENT GUIDE CATEGORIES

A. Community
   1. Place
      a. Geopolitical boundaries of community
      b. Local or folk name for community
      c. Size in square miles/areas/blocks/census tracts
      d. Transportation avenues
      e. Physical environment

From Stanhope M, Lancaster J: *Community and public health nursing,* ed 5, St Louis, 2000, Mosby.

2. People
- **a.** Number and density of population
- **b.** Demographic structure of populations
- **c.** Informal groups
- **d.** Formal groups
- **e.** Linking structures

3. Function
- **a.** Production–distribution–consumption of goods and services
- **b.** Socialization of new members
- **c.** Maintenance of social control
- **d.** Adapting to ongoing and unexpected change
- **e.** Provision of mutual aid

B. Community health

1. Status
- **a.** Vital statistics
- **b.** Disease incidence and prevalence for leading causes of mortality and morbidity
- **c.** Health risk profiles
- **d.** Functional ability levels

2. Structure
- **a.** Health facilities
- **b.** Health-related planning groups
- **c.** Health manpower
- **d.** Health resource utilization patterns

3. Process
- **a.** Commitment
- **b.** Self-other awareness and clarity of situational definitions
- **c.** Articulateness
- **d.** Effective communication
- **e.** Conflict containment and accommodation
- **f.** Participation
- **g.** Management of relations with larger society
- **h.** Machinery for facilitating participant interaction and decision making

DATABASE

This form provides a structured method for recording data. The name of the community and the assessment category and/or subcategory are noted at the top of the page. These categories correspond to those of the assessment guide. The data are collected and the source of the information and the data are recorded. Data are often entered using the SOAP format. An example of the COHR Database form is depicted on the next page.

DATABASE

Name of community _____

Assessment category _____ Subcategory _____

Date	Data Source	Data*

*Note with an asterisk the themes identified and meanings given.

COMMUNITY HEALTH NURSING DIAGNOSIS OF THE PROBLEM

Headings of columns for the Community Health Diagnosis List are Date, Number, Diagnosis/Concern, and Supportive Data (title of appropriate section of database and capsule summary of relevant data).

COMMUNITY CAPABILITY LIST

Heading of columns for this list are Date, Number, Capability, Supportive Data (title of appropriate section of database and capsule summary of relevant data).

PROBLEM ANALYSIS

Problems come from the Community Health Nursing Diagnosis. A line labeled Problem/Statement is included at the top of the form below Name of Community. Heading of columns are Problem Correlates, Relationship of Correlates of Problem, and Data Supportive to Relationships (refer to appropriate sections of database and relevant research findings in current literature).

PROBLEM PRIORITIZATION

Headings of columns are Criteria, Criteria Weights (1-10), Problem, Problem Rating (1-10), Rationale for Rating, Problem Ranking/ (Weight × Rate).

Goals and Objectives

This form includes a line labeled Problem/Concern as well as lines for Goal Statement at the top under Name of Community.

Plan

A line labeled Objective Number and Statement is included under Name of Community. Column headings are Date, Intervener Activities/ Means, Value (1-10), and Activity/Means Selected for Implementation.

Progress Notes

A line labeled Goal is included under Name of Community. Column headings are Date, Narrative Assessment Plan (NAP), and Budget and Time. A footnote to the second column explains the NAP procedure: Record both objective and subjective data. Interpret these data in terms of (1) whether the objectives were achieved and (2) whether the intervener activities utilized were effective. The plan is dependent on the assessment and may include both new (or revised) objectives and activities.

Lifespan Community Assessment: A Developmental Approach

Suggested use

The lifespan perspective of human development has the potential for providing a comprehensive model for community health nursing practice. The community can be viewed from this lifespan perspective. The nurse can observe the dynamic relations between a developing community and its changing context. The sources of data and data collection methods that are appropriate for this type of assessment are similar to those used in other community analyses. What is important is the concept of time. The nurse should gather information over several points of time to offer a true feel for the life and health of a community.

Community assessment instrument

I. Population
- A. Total population
- B. Age distribution
    1. List by age groups of 5 years (0-4, 5-9, etc.).
    2. Give actual numbers and percentages for each group.
- C. Sex distribution (Actual numbers and percentages)
- D. Race distribution (As above)
- E. Ethnicity (As above)
- F. Religion
    1. As above
    2. Separate "other," separating persons in nonmajor denominations from actual nonbelievers.
- G. Education (As above)
- H. Socioeconomic status
    1. Incomes of families. (As above, in increments of $10,000 until $40,000 and above.)
    2. Categories of occupations
    3. Unemployment levels

II. Environment
- A. Geography
    1. Topography
    2. Location
    3. Boundaries
- B. Climate
- C. Sanitation
    1. Water supply source
    2. Sewage disposal
    3. Trash and garbage
- D. Protection
    1. Fire. Describe services
    2. Police. Describe services
- E. Housing.
    1. Ownership. Give numbers and percentages; describe
    2. Rental (As above)

From McCool, Susman: Life span perspective of community health, *Public Health Nurs* 7(1), 1990.

F. Pollution-safety hazards
    1. Air
    2. Water
    3. Land

III. Organization
  A. Government
    1. Type
    2. Leaders
  B. History. Include major changes (such as shifts in industry, highway development, urban renewal, regionalization).
  C. Economics. List primary sources of government and private income.
  D. Recreation
    1. Parks (public and private)
    2. Entertainment
      a. Theaters
      b. Museums
      c. Amateur/professional sporting teams
    3. Social organizations
  E. Education. Levels, types, and number of schools.
  F. Religion
    1. Churches (Number and size)
    2. Religious organizations
  G. Power structure
    1. Community leaders
    2. Decision makers

IV. Technology/business
  A. Leading industries
    1. Name
    2. Type
    3. Number of employees
  B. Utilities
    1. Energy sources (such as electricity, oil, gas, coal, solar)
    2. Telephone services
  C. Transportation
    1. Highways
    2. Train
    3. Bus
    4. Air
  D. Business organizations
  E. Basic services
    1. Food (Sources, major stores)
    2. Clothing (As above)

V. Communication
- A. Newspapers
  1. Name
  2. Publication schedule
  3. Circulation
- B. Radio stations
  1. Name
  2. Format style and content
  3. Frequencies
- C. Television
  1. Name
  2. Commercial/public
- D. Informal networking

VI. Health
- A. Vital statistics
  1. Live births
  2. Mortality
     a. Leading causes of death, including number and rate.
     b. Neonatal, infant, and maternal deaths, including number and rate.
  3. Morbidity. Chronic diseases, number and rate.
- B. Hospitals
  1. Name
  2. Ownership
  3. Number of beds
  4. Types of service
  5. Average length of stay
- C. Nursing homes
  1. Name
  2. Ownership
  3. Bed capacity/number of beds
  4. Services offered
- D. Ambulatory services/clinics
  1. Name
  2. Public/private ownership
  3. Services offered
- E. Mental health facilities
  1. Name
  2. Ownership
  3. Number of beds
  4. Services offered
- F. Emergency services
  1. Name
  2. Ownership

      3. Personnel involved

      4. Availability

  G. Social/health services

      1. Occupational

      2. School

      3. Voluntary agencies

      4. Comprehensive health centers/clinics

      5. Prepaid group health plans

      6. Health councils

      7. Social service agencies

  H. Healthcare personnel

      1. Physicians

      2. Registered nurses

      3. Dentists

      4. Social workers

      5. Chiropractors

      6. Others

Data-Gathering Sources and Strategies

The table on pp. 84-87 provides a list of sources of information that may be helpful in completing the community assessment. This list is not exhaustive. Others may be added as appropriate to a specific community. The nurse may use maps, aerial photos, community photos, government reports, newspaper articles, census data, local books, health department vital statistics, agency annual reports, participant observation, windshield survey, key informant interviews (government, school, church, healthcare system), citizen and consumer interviews, community forums of interested persons, diaries, checklists, community self-surveys, and sketch maps as strategies to collect data for each of the components of the categories described.

Public Health Capacity-Building

Public Health Practices

Assessment practices

  1. **Assess the health needs of the community** by establishing a systematic needs assessment process that periodically

From Turnock B: *Public health: what it is and how it works,* Gaithersburg, MD, 1997, Aspen.

Data gathering sources and strategies

Categories/components	History	Boundaries	Resources	Technology	Norms and values	Roles and positions	Power structures
Family	Ethnic origin Traditions Extended family	Migration patterns Strength Land and home use Community interaction	Census data Income Education Home Recreation	Nutrition Shelter Hygiene Health Education	Diary Family stories Celebrations Family functions	Family assessment Individual interview Observation	Family influence in community Family involvement in groups
Education	Growth of schools Curricula trends Reports Diary Survey	School districts School sites Number of schools Survey administrators	Board of education Census data Annual reports Interviews with parents, teachers, school nurses	PTO/PTA Teachers Administrators Student surveys Windshield survey	Interviews Budget Active PTO Type of curriculum Attendance Absenteeism	Number of elected and appointed positions Policies on relationships	Key figures Tenure policy PTO influence
Government	Historical society Newspaper columns Reports Books Library Key informants Observation	Maps Aerial photographs Census tracts Population density Voting districts	Key informants Tax structure Budget Population trends Trained personnel Eligible voters	Government structure Government departments Services offered Tax networks Government planning office	Citizen attendance Elected party Expansion laws	Sketch map List of office holders Government duties Services offered	Key figures Stability of office Number of community factions

Economy Family finances Industrial finances Community finances	Changes in median household and per capita incomes Welfare records Population trends Past/present industry	Intra/interstate use of products Geographic distribution of labor force Local/national financing	Census data Land use Number in labor force Banks Unemployment rate	City planner interviews City commissioner interviews Plant facilities and equipment State welfare records	Stability Windshield survey Employee interviews "Good worker" standard Income adequacy	Job descriptions Employer and employee surveys	Formal leaders Informal leaders Windshield survey Unions
Religion	Library Historical society Church libraries Newspaper archives	Types of churches Number of churches Population served Number of participants Geographic distribution of members	Budgets Size of congregation National affiliations	Organizational structures Number of new members Religious practices of church and citizens	Rituals Church size Programs of church Citizen commitment Social changes Intergroup activities	Windshield survey Lay participation in church Religious leaders' behaviors	Turnover of leaders Stability of leaders Lay leaders
Recreation and safety	Trends Popular support Key personalities	Area served Facilities Types of activities Schedules	City planner Fire, police departments Water department Sewage treatment plants	Professional or volunteer workers Equipment	Traditional vs. new practices Personnel interviews Organized or informal services	Stability Turnover Key informants	Personal interviews Organizational structure
Social issues	Library Historical society Ethnic origins Trends in distribution	Geography Social structure Types of people moving in and out	Census data Income Land use Number in educational levels Occupations		Citizen interviews Citizen participation with groups Subcultures	Sketch map of citizen associations and communications	Informal leaders Styles Ranking of classes

Continued

Data gathering sources and strategies—cont'd

Categories/ components	History	Boundaries	Resources	Technology	Norms and values	Roles and positions	Power structures
Communication networks and transportation	Growth trends Library Chamber of commerce	Population and housing census data Transportation authorities State highway departments TV and newspaper	Number of TV/ radio stations and newspapers Local airports and bus terminals Telephone services	Media sources Transportation sources	Windshield survey Resident interviews Community survey Types of news	Sketch map Use of transportation Public attention to media	Censorship Community opinion Types of editorials Transportation service distribution Participant observation Key informants Employee interview Consumer interview
Health and illness	Statistical trends Health planning agency reports Agency annual reports Census data Health department vital statistics Epidemics	Number of like agencies Health planning agency Agency service area Location of services	Phone directory Community resource book Annual reports Budgets Services offered	Treatment patterns Preventive services Diagnostic aids	Folk vs. scientific medicine Self-care activities Cost of care Quality of life	Key leaders Job descriptions Practice laws and patterns	

Agriculture	Maps Aerial photos Census data Chamber of commerce	Distribution size	Census data Crops Income Laborers State agricultural department	Individual Family farms Coop farms Machines Farm labor	Farm support Prices Federal subsidy	Windshield survey Personal interviews	Citizen interviews Community participation by farmers
Industry	Department of labor and statistics Chamber of commerce Census data	Organizational charts Policies Size and number of plants	Census data Union records Employee support services	Small industry White collar vs. blue collar industry Large firms	Employee demographics Policies Work space and size Support services Recreation facilities Company social activities	Job descriptions Organizational structure Types of jobs	Key informants Influential members serving community Commitment to community

provides information on the health status/needs of the community.

2. **Investigate the occurrence of adverse health effects and health hazards in the community** by conducting timely investigations that identify the magnitude of health problems, duration, trends, location, and populations at risk.

3. **Analyze the determinants of identified health needs** in order to identify etiologic and contributing factors that place certain segments of the population at risk for adverse health outcomes.

Policy development practices

4. **Advocate for public health, build constituencies, and identify resources in the community** by generating supportive and collaborative relationships with public and private agencies and constituent groups for the effective planning, implementation, and management of public health activities.

5. **Set priorities among health needs** based on the size and seriousness of the problems, the acceptability, economic feasibility, and effectiveness of interventions.

6. **Develop plans and policies to address priority health needs** by establishing goals and objectives to be achieved through a systematic course of action that focuses on local community needs and equitable distribution of resources and involves the participation of constituents and other related governmental agencies.

Assurance practices

7. **Manage resources and develop organizational structure** through the acquisition, allocation, and control of human, physical, and fiscal resources; maximize the operational functions of the local public health system through coordination of community agencies' efforts and avoidance of duplication of services.

8. **Implement programs** and other arrangements ensuring or providing direct services for priority health needs identified in the community by taking actions that translate plans and policies into services.

9. **Evaluate programs and provide quality assurance** in accordance with applicable professional and regulatory standards to ensure that programs are consistent with plans and policies; provide feedback on inadequacies and changes needed to redirect programs and resources.

10. Inform and educate the public on public health issues of concern in the community, promoting an awareness about public health services availability and health education initiatives that contribute to individual and collective changes in health knowledge, attitudes, and practices toward a healthier community.

Performance Measure—Local Health Department
Assessment practices
Assess
1. Reviews health status and needs of entire jurisdiction
2. Includes community input and participation
3. Includes mortality and morbidity information from vital records
4. Includes information from behavioral risk factor surveys

Investigate
5. Monitors all outbreak and adverse health effects

Analyze
6. For determinants of health problems
7. For population groups at risk
8. For adequacy of existing health resources

Policy development practices
Advocate
9. Meets with health-related organizations
10. Reports on issues disseminated to the community
11. Regularly informs media
12. Publicly reviews mission and role

Prioritize
13. Based on consequences of health problems
14. Based on acceptability, economic feasibility, and effectiveness of interventions

Plan
15. Community health action plan addresses priority health needs
16. Incorporates public participation
17. Agency strategic plan is linked to community health action plan

Assurance practices

Manage
18. Organizational self-assessment completed
19. Job descriptions and minimum qualifications updated
20. Strategy for securing funding in place

Implement
21. Mandated programs are addressed
22. Agency providing or ensuring services for each priority health need

Evaluate
23. Compliance with professional and regulatory standards
24. Program goals and objectives monitored
25. Program changes made on basis of evaluation and quality assurance activities

Inform and educate
26. Public information and education

Community-Oriented Health Systems

The building blocks of regional systems are their component primary care systems (Figure 2-1). To be fully effective and efficient, local primary care systems should be organized into community health networks that:

- Are community based
- Ensure collaborative relationships between local or regional providers
- Provide integration of the full range of services, with an emphasis on early intervention, disease prevention, and primary care, to residents of the community served
- Provide health promotion services, including community outreach and incentives for the appropriate utilization of such services targeted to meet special community health needs as identified by regular assessments of community health status
- Demonstrate accountability to the community by, at a minimum, including public health and other community leaders in the governing

From Rohrer JE: *Planning for community-oriented health systems,* Washington, DC, 1996, American Public Health Association.

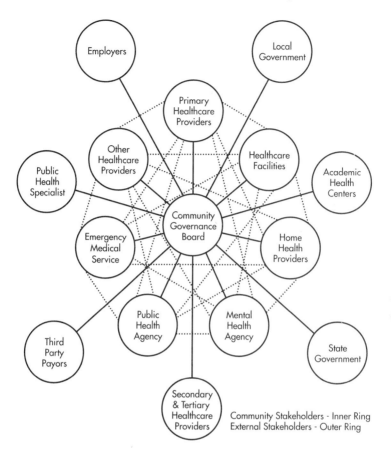

Figure 2-1 The community-based health network. *Adapted from Merchant J, Rohrer J, Walkner L, et al:* Provision of comprehensive health care to rural Iowans in the 21st century, *PEW and Robert Wood Johnson Public Report, 1994, Ames, Iowa, University of Iowa.*

board and providing regular reports on health outcomes, costs, timeliness of service, and other measures of quality

- Secure geographic accessibility to all individuals residing in the area served, without social, cultural, communication, or other barriers to healthcare
- Incorporate continuing health education and health professional training with an emphasis on community-based primary and preventive healthcare
- Incorporate methods for evaluation of health outcomes addressing identified community health needs

Principles for Successful System Development

Developing a primary care system out of the fragmented components present in most communities is a difficult task. Those who have done it successfully suggest that following certain principles will increase the chances for success:

1. State at the outset that the purpose of planning is to create a shared vision of how the local system can function.

2. Expand participation beyond healthcare providers to include the larger community. All relevant constituencies should be represented so that the planning group will be perceived as having legitimacy. An effective chairperson is needed who is neutral and respected and possesses group process skills. Without local leadership, community system development efforts cannot succeed.

3. Take advantage of internal problems and external threats in a constructive way. For example, financial insolvency of the local hospital or encroachments on the local market from external provider groups can motivate communities to take planning more seriously.

4. Use a road map for the process. Participants will be reassured and more productive when they understand the sequence of activities. However, the group may not be prepared to think about major system changes when it begins planning under these circumstances. It may be better just to focus on needs assessment and developing a shared vision. The group must be ready for more advanced topics before they are raised, since it can easily balk or even disband.

5. Rethink the appropriate scope of local health services. The planning group may assume that the historical service mix is reasonable for the future unless challenged to reconsider.

6. Analyze the health system. All major strengths and weaknesses should be identified to the extent possible. These may include quality of care, local service needs, leadership, financial performance, teamwork, consumer satisfaction, and utilization patterns. Amundson recommends that an outside consultant be used, particularly for the needs assessment.

7. Provide briefings to the steering committee on key topics.

8. Use effective group process methods. Experience in conducting meetings, communication, team building, and conflict management can all be helpful.

9. Commit resources. Communities that are unwilling to invest in a planning process are unlikely to change. Some local organi-

zation may be required to put up cash. However, if start-up funds are available from elsewhere, investment of time and energy may be a sufficient commitment from board members.

10. Continue the planning process. Evaluation of the impact of implemented plans is necessary; the planning group will need to make changes each year.

11. Take advantage of assistance from larger provider organizations. Sometimes a large hospital system will see primary care system development as being to its advantage. Empowering a community group to serve as a governing board may lead to constructive changes that could never have been forced on the community. For example, when a regional hospital has a management contract with a small hospital that is failing, it may seek to disengage to avoid losses while fearing a backlash from the local physicians, on whom it depends for referrals. Consequently, the regional hospital may choose to subsidize a planning effort without controlling the outcome, in the belief that the result will be goodwill and, possibly, rational restructuring to emphasize primary care.

Eleven Functional Health Patterns Assessment Guidelines for Communities

Communities develop health patterns. In some practice settings the community is the primary client. In other cases an individual client or a family may have, or be predisposed to, certain problems that require an assessment of certain community patterns. The following are guidelines for a comprehensive community assessment, but selected patterns can also be assessed, depending on the focus of care delivery:

1. *Health-perception–health-management pattern*
   History (community representatives):
   a. In general, what is the health/wellness level of the population on a scale of 1 to 5, with 5 being high? Any major health problems?
   b. Any strong cultural patterns influencing health practices?
   c. Do people feel that they have access to health services?
   d. Is there demand for any particular health services or prevention programs?
   e. Do people feel that fire, police, safety programs are sufficient?

From Gordon M: *Manual of nursing diagnosis: 1993-1994,* St Louis, 1993, Mosby.

Examination (community records):

a. Morbidity, mortality, disability rates (by age group, if appropriate)?

b. Accident rates (by district, if appropriate)?

c. Currently operating health facilities (types)?

d. Ongoing health promotion–prevention programs; utilization rates?

e. Ratio of health professionals to population?

f. Laws regarding drinking age?

g. Arrest statistics for drug use/drunk driving by age group?

2. *Nutritional-metabolic pattern*

History (community representatives):

a. In general, do most people seem well nourished? Children? Elderly?

b. Food supplement programs? Food stamps: rate of use?

c. Is cost of foods reasonable in this area relative to income?

d. Are stores accessible for most? "Meals on Wheels" available?

e. Water supply and quality? Testing services (if most have own wells)? (If appropriate: water usage cost? Any drought restrictions?)

f. Any concern that community growth will exceed good water supply?

g. Are heating/cooling costs manageable for most? Programs?

Examination:

a. General appearance (nutrition, teeth, clothing appropriate for climate)? Children? Adults? Elderly?

b. Food purchases (observations at food store checkout counters)?

c. "Junk" food (machines in schools, etc.)?

3. *Elimination pattern*

History (community representatives):

a. Major kinds of wastes (industrial, sewage, etc.)? Disposal systems? Recycling programs? Any problems perceived by community?

b. Pest control? Food service inspection (restaurants, street vendors, etc.)?

Examination:

a. Communicable-disease statistics?

b. Air pollution statistics?

4. *Activity-exercise pattern*

History (community representatives):

a. How do people find the transportation here? To work? For recreation? To healthcare?

b. Do people (senior, others) have/use community centers? Recreation facilities for children? Adults? Seniors?

c. Is housing adequate (availability, cost)? Public housing?

Examination:

a. Recreation/cultural programs?

b. Aids for the disabled?

c. Residential centers, nursing homes, rehabilitation facilities relative to population needs?

d. External maintenance of homes, yards, apartment houses?

e. General activity level (e.g., bustling, quiet)?

5. *Sleep-rest pattern*

History (community representatives):

a. Generally quiet at night in most neighborhoods?

b. Usual business hours? Are industries 'round-the-clock?

Examination:

a. Activity/noise levels in business district? Residential?

6. *Cognitive-perceptual pattern*

History (community representatives):

a. Do most groups speak English? Bilingual?

b. Educational level of population?

c. Schools seen as good/need improving? Adult education desired/available?

d. Types of problems that require community decisions? Decision-making process? What is best way to get things done/changed here?

Examination:

a. School facilities? Dropout rate?

b. Community government structure; decision-making lines?

7. *Self-perception–self-concept pattern*

History (community representatives):

a. Good community to live in? Going up in status, down, or about the same?

b. Old community? Fairly new?

c. Does any age group predominate?

d. People's mood, in general: enjoying life, stressed, feeling "down"?

e. People generally have the kinds of abilities needed in this community?

f. Community/neighborhood functions? Parades?

Examination:

a. Racial, ethnic mix (if appropriate)?

b. Socioeconomic level?

c. General observations of mood?

8. *Role-relationship pattern*

History (community representatives):

 a. Do people seem to get along well together here? Places where people tend to go to socialize?

 b. Do people feel that they are heard by the government? High/low participation in meetings?

 c. Enough work/jobs for everybody? Are wages good/fair? Do people seem to like the kind of work available (happy in their jobs/job stress)?

 d. Any problems with riots, violence in the neighborhoods? Family violence? Problems with child/spouse/elder abuse?

 e. Does community get along with adjacent communities? Do people collaborate on any community projects?

 f. Do neighbors seem to support each other?

 g. Community get-togethers?

Examination:

 a. Observation of interactions (generally or at specific meetings)?

 b. Statistics on interpersonal violence?

 c. Statistics on employment, income/poverty?

 d. Divorce rate?

9. *Sexuality-reproductive pattern*

History (community representatives):

 a. Average family size?

 b. Do people feel there are any problems with pornography, prostitution, or other?

 c. Do people want/support sex education in schools/community?

Examination:

 a. Family sizes and types of households?

 b. Male/female ratio?

 c. Average maternal age? Maternal mortality rate? Infant mortality rate?

 d. Teen pregnancy rate?

 e. Abortion rate?

 f. Sexual violence statistics?

 g. Laws/regulations regarding information on birth control?

10. *Coping–stress-tolerance pattern*

History (community representatives):

 a. Any groups that seem to be under stress?

 b. Need/availability of phone help lines? Support groups (health-related, other)?

Examination:

 a. Statistics on delinquency, drug abuse, alcoholism, suicide, psychiatric illness?

 b. Unemployment rate by race/ethnic group/sex?

11. *Value-belief pattern*

History (community representatives):

a. Community values: what seem to be the top four things that people living here see as important in their lives? (Note health-related values, priorities.)

b. Do people tend to get involved in causes/local fund-raising campaigns? (Note if any are health-related.)

c. Are there religious groups in the community? Churches available?

d. Do people tend to tolerate/not tolerate differences or socially deviant behavior?

Examination:

a. Zoning/conservation laws?

b. Scan of community government health committee reports (goals, priorities)?

c. Health budget relative to total budget?

ENVIRONMENTAL ASSESSMENT: HOME AND INDUSTRY

Assessment of the environment where individuals and families live and work is an integral aspect of community health nursing practice. These tools will assist the nurse in establishing a baseline for evaluating that environment and for teaching and planning appropriate interventions.

Building Accessibility Checklist

The following checklist can be used as a guide to comply with the American National Standards Institute (ANSI) and Uniform Federal Accessibility Standards (UFAS) for making buildings accessible to the physically handicapped. The following checklist is based on both the ANSI standards and UFAS. In some areas where UFAS differs from ANSI, both specifications are included. This is done particularly in the use of technical terms.

Adapted from Uniform Accessibility Standards, available online: http://www.access-board.gov/ufas/ufas.htm; Americans with Disabilities, Information Center, available online: http://www.ada-infonet.org; Occupational Safety and Health Administration, available online: http://www.osha-slc.gov.

Type of building or project
1. A new construction?
2. An addition?
3. An alteration?
4. A historic preservation building?
5. A leased building?
6. A housing or dwelling unit?

Building site, exterior, route
1. Does the grading of the building site allow the approaches to the building to be substantially level?
2. Is there parking within 200 feet of the building entrance?
3. Is any of the parking reserved for the handicapped?
4. Are any parking spaces open on one side to allow easy access for wheelchairs and for people who use braces to get in and out of the automobile?
5. Are the parking spaces on level ground?
6. Are there ramps or level spaces to allow people to enter the building without crossing a curb?
7. How many accessible parking spaces are there?
8. Is there an accessible route connecting buildings, facilities, other architectural elements and spaces on the same site?
9. Is there an accessible route within the site from transportation stops, accessible parking spaces, passenger loading zones, and public streets and sidewalks?
10. Are ground and floor surfaces free of protruding objects and otherwise accessible?

Walkways
1. Are walks at least 48 inches wide?
2. Is the gradient not greater than a 1-foot rise in 20 feet (5%)?
3. Are walks without interruption (i.e., steps or abrupt changes in level)?
4. If the walks cross a driveway, parking lot or other walks, do they blend into a common, level surface?
5. On elevated walks, is there at least a 5 × 5 foot platform if a door swings out onto the platform or 3 × 5 foot platform if the door swings in?
6. Do walks have nonslip or slip-resistant surfaces?

Buildings: ramps
1. Do ramps have a slope no greater than a 1-foot rise in 12 feet (8.33%)?

2. If ramps are steeper than a 5% gradient rise (a rise of 6 inches) or have a horizontal projection of more than 72 inches, are handrails provided?

3. If there are handrails, are they at least 32 inches above the ramp surface?

4. Are there handrails on both sides?

5. Are the ramp surfaces smooth?

6. Is the clear width of the ramp at least 36 inches (3 feet)?

7. Do the handrails extend 1 foot beyond the top and bottom of the ramp?

8. Are the ramp surfaces nonslip or slip-resistant?

9. Do ramps have a level 6-foot clearance at the bottom?

10. Do ramps with a gradient steeper than 5% have level spaces (a minimum of 3 feet in length) at 30-foot intervals?

11. Are these level rest areas at least 5 feet wide (to provide for turns)?

12. Is the cross slope 1:50 or less?

13. Are edges protected to preclude slipping off?

14. Will water accumulate on an outdoor ramp or the approach to it?

Buildings: entrances and exits

1. Is at least one entrance to the building accessible to people in wheelchairs?

2. Is at least one entrance accessible to wheelchairs on a level that would make the elevators accessible?

3. Is the accessible entrance on an accessible route?

4. Is the service entrance the only accessible entrance?

Buildings: doors and doorways

1. Do doors have a clear opening at least 32 inches wide?

2. Can doors be opened in a single effort? Can handles, pulls, latches, locks be grasped and operated with one hand?

3. Is the floor of the doorway level within 5 feet from the door in the direction it swings?

4. Does this level space extend 1 foot beyond each side of the door?

5. Does it extend 3 feet in the direction opposite to the door swing?

6. Do thresholds exceed ½ inch (¾ inches for exterior sliding doors)?

7. Is the speed of door closers at least 3 seconds?

8. Does the door require more than 5 pounds of pressure to open?

9. Where there are hinged or pivoted doors in a series, are they at least 48 inches wide plus the width of the swinging inward door path?

Buildings: stairs and steps

1. Do the steps avoid protruding lips and abrupt nosings at the edge of each step?
2. Do stairs have handrails at least 32 inches above step level?
3. Will water accumulate on outdoor stairs and approaches?
4. Are tread heights and risers uniform?
5. How many accessible stairs and sets of stairs are there?
6. Do stairs have handrails on both sides that extend at least 12 inches beyond the top and at least 19 inches from the bottom step?
7. Do steps have risers 7 inches or less?

Buildings: floors

1. Do floors have nonslip or slip-resistant surface?
2. Are floors on each story at a common level or connected by a ramp?
3. Is carpet (or carpet tile) securely attached?
4. Do grates have a maximum opening of ½ inch?

Buildings: restrooms

1. How many toilets for either sex are there on each floor with facilities for the physically handicapped?
2. Can physically handicapped persons, particularly those in wheelchairs, enter the restroom?
3. Do toilet rooms have turning space 60 × 60 inches to allow traffic of individuals in wheelchairs?
4. Do toilet rooms have at least one toilet stall that:
   - Is 3 feet wide?
   - Is at least 4 feet, 8 inches deep?
   - Has a door that is 32 inches wide and swings out?
   - Has a handrail on each side, 33 inches high and parallel to floor, 1½ inches in diameter, with 1½ inches clearance between rail and wall, fastened securely to wall at the ends and center?
   - Has a toilet seat of 17-19 inches from stand?
5. Do toilet rooms have wash basins with narrow aprons, which when mounted at standard height are no greater than 34 inches at the top, and which have a clearance underneath of 29 inches?
6. Are drainpipes and hot water pipes covered or insulated?
7. Is one mirror as low as possible and no higher than 40 inches above the floor?
8. Is one shelf at a height within range and reach of a person in a wheelchair and no lower than 15 inches above the floor?
9. Do toilet rooms for men have wall-mounted urinals with the opening of the basin 19 inches (17 inches under UFAS standards)

from the floor, or have floor-mounted urinals that are level with the main floor of the toilet rooms?

10. Are flush controls automatic or hand-operated? Are they 44 inches or less from the floor?

11. Do toilet rooms have controls, coat hooks, towel racks, and towel dispensers mounted no lower than 15 inches from the floor and otherwise within reach?

12. Are disposal units mounted no higher than 40 inches from the floor?

13. Are towel racks, towel dispensers, and other appropriate disposal units located to the side rather than above the basins?

14. Is there a shower or bathtub with an accessible seat, grab bars, controls, and proper spacing?

Buildings: water fountains

1. How many drinking fountains for use by physically handicapped persons are there on each floor?

2. Can persons in wheelchairs wheel up to fountain?

3. Do water fountains have up-front spouts and controls?

4. Are they hand-operated?

5. If coolers are wall-mounted, are they hand-operated? Are basins 36 inches or less from the floor?

Buildings: public telephones

1. How many public telephones in each bank of phones are accessible to the physically handicapped?

2. Is the height of the dial 48 inches or less from the floor?

3. Is the coin slot located 48 inches or less from floor?

4. Is there a clear space of at least 30 × 40 inches to allow forward or parallel approach?

5. Are these telephones equipped for persons with hearing disabilities? Are those telephones identified as such?

6. Are telephone books (if provided) 48 inches or less from the floor?

7. Are push-button controls (if available) provided?

Buildings: elevators/lifts

1. If in more than a one-story building, how many elevators are available for the physically handicapped?

2. Can physically handicapped persons, particularly those in wheelchairs, enter the elevator?

3. Are outside call buttons centered 48 inches (42 inches under UFAS standards) or less from the floor? Do they have visual signals?

4. Are control buttons inside at least ¾ inches raised? Are they located 48 inches or less from floor?

5. Are the buttons labeled with raised or indented letters beside them?
6. Are they touch-sensitive and easy to push?
7. Is the elevator cab at least 5 × 5 feet?
8. Are visual and audible signals provided at each elevator group to indicate which car is answering the call?
9. Do jambs of each elevator have raised floor designations on both sides?
10. Does the elevator door remain open at least 3 seconds?
11. Can a person in a wheelchair facing the rear see floor numbers, either by mirror or floor identification at rear of car?
12. Are floors announced orally by recorded devices for the benefit of the blind?
13. Are there platform lifts with operable controls, adequate clearances, and appropriate surfaces?

Building: controls

1. Are light switches no more than 48 inches above the floor?
2. Are controls for heating, cooling, and ventilation no more than 48 inches above the floor?
3. Are controls for fire alarms and other warning devices no more than 48 inches from floor?
4. Are other frequently used controls, such as drapery pulls, no more than 48 inches from floor?
5. Is the force needed to operate the controls no more than 5 pounds?
6. Is there clear space to allow a forward or parallel approach by a person in a wheelchair?

Building: identification

1. Are raised or recessed letters or numbers used to identify rooms or offices?
2. Is identification placed on wall, either to right or left of door?
3. Is identification at a height between 4 feet, 6 inches and 5 feet, 6 inches (measured from floor)?
4. Are doors that might prove dangerous to a blind person if he or she were to enter or exit through them made quickly identifiable to the touch?

Buildings: warning signals/alarms

1. Are audible warning signals accompanied by simultaneous visual signals for the benefit of those with hearing and sight disabilities? Are they set at a level not to exceed 120 decibels (dB)?
2. Are visual alarms flashing at less than 5 Hertz (Hz)?

Buildings: hazards, tactile warnings, protruding objects

1. When hazards such as open manhole covers, panels and excavation exits are present, are barricades placed on all open sides at least 8 feet from the hazard? Are warning devices installed?
2. Are there low-hanging door closers that remain within opening of doorways which might protrude dangerously or are more than 2 inches into regular corridors or traffic ways?
3. Are there low-hanging signs, ceiling lights, fixtures, or similar objects that protrude more than 4 inches into regular corridors or traffic ways?
4. Is lighting on ramps adequate?
5. Are exit signs easily identifiable to all disabled persons?
6. Are there tactile warnings on doors to hazardous areas?
7. Are there at least 80 inches of clear head room in walls, halls, corridors, aisles, passageways, and circulation spaces?

The following items are not contained in the ANSI standards, but are included in the UFAS document.

Dwelling units

1. How many units are accessible?
2. How many units are adaptable?
3. Has consumer information about adaptability been provided to the owner or occupant of the dwelling?
4. Has consumer information been provided to the parties who will be responsible for making adaptations?
5. Does the kitchen have at least 40-inch clearances for cabinets, countertops, appliances and walls (in U-shaped kitchens: 60 inches)?
6. Is there at least 30 × 48 inches of clear floor space in the kitchen?
7. Are all controls in the kitchen within reach of a person in a wheelchair?
8. In the kitchen is there at least one 30-inch work surface not more than 34 inches above the ground and at least 2 inches thick?
9. Is the maximum height of the sink 34 inches? Is the sink and counter width a maximum of 30 inches?
10. Are ranges and cooktops and their controls insulated or otherwise protected to prevent burns, abrasions, or shocks?
11. Is there a maximum 48-inch height for at least one shelf of all cabinets and storage shelves above work counters?
12. Are ovens self-cleaning with controls on front panels?

13. Are refrigerator and freezers side-by-side or over-and-under types?
14. Are dishwater racks accessible from the front of the machine?
15. Are laundry facilities on an accessible route? Are the controls within reach?

Food service areas (restaurant or cafeteria)

1. Is at least 5% of all fixed seating or tables 27 inches high, 30 inches wide, and 19 inches deep for knee clearance? Is the tabletop 28-34 inches from the floor?
2. Are there accessible aisles?
3. Where there are mezzanine levels, loggias, or raised platforms, are the same services and decorative character provided on accessible routes?
4. Do food service lines have a minimum clear width of 35 inches?
5. Are tray slides mounted no higher than 34 inches?
6. Are vending machines within reach and easily operable by persons in wheelchairs?
7. Are tableware, dishes, condiments, foods, and beverages displayed and dispensed within reach of a person in a wheelchair, bearing in mind width, turning space, and clearances?

Healthcare

1. Is there an accessible entrance to the facility that is protected from the weather by canopy or roof overhang?
2. Does the accessible entrance have an accessible passenger loading zone?
3. Do patient rooms have adequate clear floor and turning space as well as an accessible toilet?

Libraries

1. Is at least 5% (minimum of 1 seating area) of fixed seating, tables, and study carrels accessible in terms of having seating and work surfaces and allowing passage and use by persons in wheelchairs?
2. Is there at least one lane (including any traffic control, security gate, or turnstile) at each checkout area that is accessible?
3. Is the clear aisle space at card catalogs, magazine displays, and reference stacks at least 35 inches?
4. Is the clear aisle width in the stacks 42 inches if possible (36 inches minimum)?
5. Are all public areas accessible?

Self-Assessment of Environmental Health

Primary prevention

Occupational

1. Do I work with substances that my employer, my doctor, official agencies, or I consider potentially hazardous to my health? Frequency? Duration?
2. Am I asked to use safety/personal protective devices while I work? Why? When? Where? Who else?
3. Do I use the safety/personal protective devices my employer requires me to use while performing my job? If not, why not? If yes, when? Where? With whom?
4. Do I notice any patterns of illness in my working peers or family members? What specifically? Does anyone consider this a problem? Family? Company?
5. In describing my workplace, is/are there clutter, vapors, liquids, dust, fumes, heat, or vibration?
6. Do I feel that my work or workplace presents physical dangers such as falls, slips, or falling objects?

Home

1. What hobbies do I or family members participate in while in our home? What products are used? Are warning or special use labels present on any of these products?
2. Do we undergo regular checkups with our primary healthcare provider or doctor? Frequency? Has our healthcare provider advised us to change any personal or environmental factors present within our lives? If so, what?
3. Are all family members up to date on their immunization status?
4. What cleaning, home-maintenance, or home-repair products are used or stored within our home? Do package directions indicate proper use and storage? How are they used and stored? Does this comply with directions?
5. What type of insulation is used in my home? Are there known health hazards with this type of home insulation?
6. What type of heating is used in my home? Are there health hazards associated with this type of heating?
7. What source of water is used for my home (ground, surface, reclaimed, desalinated, or rain)? Are there any problems known to be

From Bomar P: *Nurses and family health promotion,* ed 2, Philadelphia, 1996, WB Saunders.

associated with this water resource? Is water purified, filtered, and/or chlorinated prior to entering my home?

Recreational

1. List all playtime activities. List frequency and duration of the activity.
2. Are there any known dangers associated with these recreational activities?
3. Are there any substances or chemicals required to perform the recreational pastime? If so, what? Are directions for use and storage present? Do we/I follow them precisely?
4. Is safety equipment recommended for the recreational activity? If so, is it used? If recommended and not used, why not?

Environmental

1. Draw a map of known greenbelts, industries, dumps, housing patterns, and bodies of water.
2. Is my community targeted as a "high-risk" area for any toxic waste or radiation? If so, where? Do family members have any contact with resources from this area?
3. Are environmental problems suspected within my immediate neighborhood? If yes, what?
4. List your immediate concern when you think of environmental problems within your community.

Personal

1. Do I or other family members smoke?
2. How much alcohol consumption occurs during one week for each family member? Has alcohol ever been a problem in daily life (i.e., driving, business, school)?
3. Do I or other family members use recreational/illicit drugs? If so, which ones and how frequently?
4. How many sexual partners do individuals within the family encounter within a month? A year? Can you/they describe "safe sex" practices? Do they/you use safe sex practices?

Do any of the above risk factors combine to increase the risk of disease (e.g., tobacco smoking and asbestos mining)?

Secondary prevention

Occupational

1. Have I experienced any changes in my health, possibly related to my job, that caused me or my family to worry during the last week, month, or year?

2. Describe a typical work week.
   a. Do I feel better on the first day of my work week or the last day?
   b. Is there any change between the way I feel on weekends and during the work week?
   c. Are my coworkers showing signs of illness? If so, what signs?
   d. How much sick leave have I used this quarter? How many sick-leave days are spent in bed due to illness or poor health? How many days are spent off work and not in bed? When did I last see a doctor during a sick-leave period? What information did the doctor give me about my illness?
   e. Do I think I need to see a physician or healthcare provider soon? If so, who? Why?
   f. During the performance of my work, am I at risk for physical injury or disease?

Home

1. If I work or play at home, have I become exposed to substances that cause detectable illness?
2. Are there any illnesses that have been experienced within the home by more than one family member? If yes, what disease or symptoms? Is there any pattern of association common to all members?
3. Are family members acutely or chronically ill? If so, what diseases or conditions? Are they transmittable? Are they detectable through screening tests (e.g., tuberculosis)?

Recreational

1. Have I experienced any injuries related to my playtime activities in recent months or years? If so, what? Do these injuries indicate a need to seek screening for disease or chronic injury (e.g., neurologic compromise due to falls or moving vehicle accidents)?
2. Do any recreational activities aggravate preexisting diseases or injuries?

Environmental

1. Is my community or neighborhood targeted for any screening for disease or disability?
2. Do any environmental conditions exist (historical or current) that would alarm health officials or family members and indicate need for screening for disease? If so, what conditions? What exposures (e.g., radiation, infectious disease, etc.)?

Personal

1. Are family members at high risk for AIDS or other sexually transmitted diseases (homosexual men, IV drug abusers, multiple sex partners, sexual partners of the aforementioned)? Do I have single or multiple sex partners? Do I or my partners practice safe sex? Is HIV screening and treatment available within my community? Am I or is a family member in a risk group that indicates the need for screening and early diagnosis?

2. Do I or family members have habits that may put me or them at risk for diseases (e.g., IV drug abuse, illicit substance abuse, alcohol abuse)? Are they wishing screening and treatment? What services are available for screening and treatment within our community? What is the cost for screening and treatment?

3. Is a family member a smoker with recent unexplained weight loss? When was last physical examination? When was last chest x-ray?

4. Is there any personal history of exposure that might indicate a need for periodic screening (e.g., radiation exposure)?

5. Is there any endemic disease I should be regularly tested for due to lifestyle or location (e.g., tuberculosis)?

Do any of the above risk factors combine to increase the risk for disease (e.g., tobacco smoking, asbestos mining)?

Tertiary prevention
Occupational
1. Do I feel better or worse when I am in my normal work environment? Which circumstances or activities make me feel worse? Which make me feel better?

2. Does my condition require that my employer accommodate the activities and circumstances that make me feel better? Are the accommodations made? Do the accommodations impose hardship on coworkers?

3. Can adjustments of the environment or equipment be made to allow me to work? Is retraining (habilitation) feasible? Do I or my family wish me to change jobs or retrain?

Home
1. How does the illness affect my role within the family and the completion of my tasks within the home?

2. Can adjustments of the environment or equipment be made so that I may better complete my activities within the home?

3. Do any home chores or activities exacerbate my illness or condition? If so, which ones? Can they be modified?

Recreational

1. Are my recreational activities limited due to illness or disability? If so, which ones? Can they be altered to accommodate the conditions without causing an increase in symptoms or exacerbation of illness?
2. Do any recreational activities worsen my condition? If so, which ones? Have they been altered or avoided to diminish physical or mental stress?

Environmental

1. Do environmental conditions exist within my community or home that exacerbate my condition (e.g., smog)? If so, are they alterable? If so, how?
2. Describe the climatic and general environmental conditions that potentiate your wellness. Can they be achieved within your current locale? If not, why not? If so, how?

Personal

1. Do my habits worsen my illness or conditions (e.g., smoking and emphysema)?
2. Is there a personal behavior I can enact that will facilitate recovery or rehabilitation? If so, what? If so, what lifestyle changes or resources will be needed? If so, are the resources available, accessible, or acceptable?

Do any of the above risk factors combine to increase the risk for disease (e.g., tobacco smoking and asbestos mining)?

HOME

Assessment Survey: Housing for the Disabled

Access considerations

Outdoors

Parking and distance from entrance
Location of mailbox
Storage of vehicle and access to home from the storage area
Access to home: width of doors; ability to turn key, open and close doors; need for ramps, handrails
Lighting in entrances
Community buildings used regularly; access to these buildings

From Hoeman S: *Rehabilitation nursing: process and application,* ed 2, St Louis, 1996, Mosby.

Access to private or public transportation: distance from home, cost, assistance required, ability to operate own vehicle safely

Parking areas marked for handicapped; adequate space to maneuver

Width, height of incline of ramps, sidewalks

Indoors: general

Thresholds, floor obstructions, steps inside home

Arrangement of furniture and ability to use

Location of telephone

Ability to raise/lower windows

Floor coverings: slippery, scatter rugs; can a wheelchair be maneuvered?

Location of all rooms; ability to maneuver a wheelchair or assistive device

Location of fuse box

Ability to control heat

Width of walkways, doorways, halls: space to maneuver

Access to outlets; ability to change light bulbs

Type of furniture and ability to use safely

Elevator: threshold, timing of door, adapted for hearing and visual impairments

Indoors: kitchen

Access to stove, sink, cupboards, storage, work space, refrigerator, contents, other appliances

Countertop and sink height; opening under sink for wheelchair access

Ability to operate faucets, use microwave, reach knobs on stove

Convenient arrangement of appliances

Indoors: bathroom

Height of sink and toilet, shower/tub, and location of faucets

Space for maneuvering wheelchair or assistive device

Threshold for shower

Ability to use facilities safely

Presence and location of grab bars, securely anchored

Indoors: bedroom

Height of bed

Access to closet, ability to reach rods, storage area

Firmness of mattress

Ability to transfer in and out of bed safely; adequate space around bed

Arrangement of furniture: space to maneuver

Safety considerations
General

House number clearly visible and readable for quick identification during an emergency

Locks secure; deadbolts; ability to use

Ability to see and talk to visitor at the door without being seen

Steps, porch, front door lighted and protected from the weather

Nonslip doormat

Ability to use telephone, emergency response system

Ability to control water temperature

Wiring, outlet covers for children

Smoke detectors: type, location, access

Lighting in rooms, hallways; access to control lights inside and outside the home

Ability to respond to a fire emergency: fire exits/access, use of stairs instead of elevator, use of fire extinguisher, fire drills

Use of oxygen: precautions and appropriate signs in the home

Access to telephone, radio, television while in bed

Use of space heaters: type, location

Location of knobs on stove, safety around stove, cleanliness of stove; ability to use good judgment when cooking

Ability to dispose of infectious materials safely

Safe play area

Ability to transport food from kitchen to table

Ventilation in all rooms

Pest-free method of trash storage

Assessment of Immediate Living Environment

Home evaluation checklist

Name _____ Date _____
Address _____
Diagnosis _____

Mobility status
    ❑ ambulatory, no device   ❑ walker
    ❑ cane   ❑ wheelchair

Adapted from Occupational/Physical Therapy Home Evaluation Form, Ralph K. Davies Medical Center, San Francisco and Occupational Therapy Home Evaluating Form, Alta Bates Hospital, Albany, California, 1993. In Pedretti L, Occupational therapy: practice skills for physical dysfunction, *ed 4, St. Louis, 1996, Mosby.* Continued

Assessment of Immediate Living Environment—cont'd

Exterior

Home located on ☐ level surface ☐ hill

Type of house ☐ owns house ☐ mobile home
☐ apartment ☐ board and care

Number of floors ☐ one story ☐ split level ☐ two story

Driveway surface ☐ inclined ☐ level ☐ smooth ☐ rough
Is the DRIVEWAY negotiable? ☐ yes ☐ no
Is the GARAGE accessible? ☐ yes ☐ no

Entrance

Accessible entrances ☐ front ☐ side ☐ back

Steps number _____ height of each _____ width _____ depth _____

Are there HANDRAILS? ☐ yes ☐ no

If yes, where are they located? ☐ left ☐ right

HANDRAIL height from step surface? _____

If no, how much room is available for HANDRAILS? _____

Are landings negotiable? ☐ yes ☐ no

Briefly describe any problems with LANDINGS: _____

_____

Ramps ☐ yes ☐ no ☐ front ☐ back
height _____ width _____ length _____

Are there HANDRAILS? ☐ yes ☐ no

If yes, where are they located? ☐ left ☐ right height ___

If no ramp, how much room is available for one? _____

Porch
width _____ length _____
Level at threshold? ☐ yes ☐ no

Door
width _____
threshold height _____ Negotiable? ☐ yes ☐ no
☐ swing in ☐ swing out ☐ sliding

Interior

Living room
Is furniture arranged for easy maneuverability? ☐ yes ☐ no
Is frequently used furniture accessible? ☐ yes ☐ no
Type of floor covering: _____
Comments_____

Hallways
Can wheelchair or walking aide be maneuvered in hallway? ☐ yes ☐ no
hall width _____ door width _____ Sharp turns? ☐ yes ☐ no
Steps? ☐ yes ☐ no
number _____
Are there HANDRAILS? ☐ yes ☐ no
If yes, where are they located? ☐ left ☐ right height _____

Bedroom
☐ single ☐ shared
Is there room for a W/C? ☐ yes ☐ no
Door:
width _____ threshold height _____ Negotiable? ☐ yes ☐ no
☐ swing in ☐ swing out

Bed:

◻ twin   ◻ double   ◻ queen   ◻ king   ◻ hospital bed

Overall height _____   Accessible?   ◻ yes   ◻ no

Would hospital bed fit into room if needed?   ◻ yes   ◻ no

Clothing:

Are drawers accessible?   ◻ yes   ◻ no   ◻ on right   ◻ on left

Is closet accessible?   ◻ yes   ◻ no   ◻ on right   ◻ on left

Comments: _____

Bathroom

Door:

width _____   threshold height _____   Negotiable? ◻ yes   ◻ no

Tub:

height, floor-rim _____   height, tub bottom rim _____

tub width inside _____   glass doors?   ◻ yes   ◻ no

width of tub doors _____   overhead shower?   ◻ yes   ◻ no

is tub accessible?   ◻ yes   ◻ no

Stall Shower: ◻ yes   ◻ no

door width _____   height of bottom rim   _____

Accessible?   ◻ yes   ◻ no

Sink:

height _____ faucet type _____   ◻ open   ◻ closed

Accessible?   ◻ yes   ◻ no

Toilet:

height from floor _____   location of toilet paper _____

distance from toilet to side wall   **L**...........

R...........

Grab bars: ◻ yes   ◻ no

Location _____

Comments: _____

Kitchen

Door:

width _____

threshold height _____   Negotiable?   ◻ yes   ◻ no

Stove:

height _____

Location of controls   ◻ front   ◻ back

Is stove accessible for use?   ◻ yes   ◻ no

Oven:

Height from floor to door hinge & door handle _____

Location of oven _____

Sink:

Will W/C fit underneath?   ◻ yes   ◻ no

Type of faucets _____

Cupboards:

Accessible from W/C?   ◻ yes   ◻ no

Refrigerator:

hinges on   ◻ left   ◻ right

Accessible from W/C?   ◻ yes   ◻ no

Switches/Outlets

Accessible?   ◻ yes   ◻ no

Kitchen table

height from floor _____

Accessible?   ◻ yes   ◻

Comments: _____

Continued

Assessment of Immediate Living Environment—cont'd

Laundry

Door: width   _____

          threshold height _____   Negotiable?   ❑ yes   ❑ no

Steps: ❑ yes   ❑ no

          number _____   height _____   width _____

          Are there HANDRAILS?   ❑ yes   ❑ no

          If yes, where are they located?   ❑ left   ❑ right   height _____

Washer:

          ❑ topload   ❑ front load

          Accessible?   ❑ yes   ❑ no

Dryer:

          ❑ topload   ❑ front load

          Accessible?   ❑ yes   ❑ no

Safety

Throw rugs

          ❑ yes   ❑ no

          Location _____

Phone

          Accessible?   ❑ yes   ❑ no

          Location _____

Emergency phone numbers

          ❑ yes   ❑ no

          Location _____

Mailbox

          Accessible?   ❑ yes   ❑ no

          Location _____

Thermostat

          Accessible?   ❑ yes   ❑ no

          Location _____

Electric Outlets/switches

          Accessible?   ❑ yes   ❑ no

Imperfect floor?

          ❑ yes   ❑ no

          Location _____

Sharp-edged furniture?

          ❑ yes   ❑ no

          Location _____

Insulated hot water pipes   ❑ yes   ❑ no

          Location _____

Cluttered areas?

          ❑ yes   ❑ no

          Location _____

Fire extinguisher?

          ❑ yes   ❑ no

          Location _____

Equipment present: _____

_____

_____

Problem list: _____

_____

_____

_____

Recommendations for modifications: _____

_____

_____

_____

_____

Equipment recommendations: _____

_____

_____

Tools for Living for the Aged and Disabled

The following items are suggested for use in the home to assist the elderly and disabled in self-help.

Location/activity	Equipment
Kitchen	
Meal preparation	Pots and pans with large-diameter handles
	Extended faucets for finger or wrist force
	Lazy Susans and Ferris wheel–type holders for cans and spices in cabinet
	Side-by-side refrigerator
	Microwave and crock pots
	Electric can opener
	Lid removers
	Rocker knives
	Containers to hold food in small packages
	Label packages
	Provide Braille labels for visually impaired
Eating	Rocker knife for single-hand function
	Scoop dish with plate guard
	Electric self-feeder
	Utensils with built-up handles
	Long straws
	Mugs
	ADL/Universal cuff, C-clip holder

From Pedretti L: *Occupational therapy: practice skills for physical dysfunction,* ed 4, St Louis, 1996, Mosby.   *Continued*

Tools for Living for the Aged and Disabled—cont'd

Location/activity	Equipment
Doors	Lever-type action doorknob
	Vertical bar door openers to push with hand, foot, wheelchair footrest
	Electric power doors
Floors	Nonskid linoleum
	Easy-to-clean floors
Stairs	Small chairlift
	Small elevator
Walls	Waist-level electrical outlet bars
Bathroom	
Bathing,	Grab bars for tubs, showers, toilets
toileting	Elevated toilet seat
	Bathtub bench
	Nonskid mats
	Long-handled sponge
	Suction nail
	Soap-on-a-rope
	Wash mitt
	Raised-faucet letters for visually impaired
	Digital readout temperature faucets
Hygiene—other	
Hair	Long-handled brush or comb
	C-clip holder
	Built-up handles
Brushing teeth	Built-up handle toothbrush
	Suction denture brush
	Electric toothbrush
Shaving	Electric shaver
	Electric razor
	Shaving cream dispenser with handle
Bedroom	Ceiling poles near bed to help get in/out of bed
	Bedrails
	Pressure mattress
	Dynamic rocking bed
	Electric bed
	Bedside light and appliance control
Communication	Large button telephones
	Amplified receivers
	Ringing light for hearing impaired
	Remote-controlled TV, recorders, stereos
	Low-mounted telephone
	Telephone shoulder rest
	Automatic dialer
	Portable telephone
	Dialing stick

Location/activity	Equipment
Dressing	Button loops
	Velcro closures for buttons, shoes, bra
	Long shoe horn
	Slip-in shoes
	Dressing stick
	Stocking aid
	Trouser pull
	Leg lifter
	Zipper pull
Mobility	Canes and walkers
	Large handgrips on above
	Large rubber tips on above
	Cut canes so that when the tip is on the floor, the arm is slightly flexed
	Have wheelchair seats fitted to client
	Adjust wheelchair arm and footrests
	Three-wheeled power chair
	Van with lift or ramp
	Wheelchair drive controls (hand, breath, chin)
Security	System to monitor client activity in home (such as Lifecall)
	Small transmitter for wrist or neck attached to security
Recreation	Talking books
	Page turners
	Keys attached to tape recorders for ease of turning on
	Stationary cycle for ambulatory clients
	Taped ministries from church
	Elevated gardens for wheelchair clients

Life Skills and Community Living

Safe and accessible housing, transportation, vocational rehabilitation, disability management in the workplace, educational programs, adaptive equipment to facilitate community living, support services and advocacy groups, and community resources are essential for the maximum functioning of the disabled person. These are issues to consider.

From McCourt A, editor: *The specialty of rehabilitation nursing: a core curriculum,* ed 3, Skokie, IL, 1993, The Rehabilitation Nursing Foundation of the Association of Rehabilitation Nurses.

I. Housing: selection and assessment
   A. Factors and alternatives to consider in selecting housing
      1. Be aware that many alternatives are available depending on the client's functional ability, support systems, needs, and goals
      2. Secure an appropriately adapted residence; if necessary, make adaptations
         a. Build access ramp(s)
         b. Widen doors
         c. Modify the kitchen and bathroom so that all facilities and appliances are easily accessible
         d. Make parking available
      3. Consider moving client into congregate housing with or without attendant services
      4. Encourage client to join an independent living program that allows people with disabilities to remain in their own dwellings while offering, but not managing, provision of support services
         a. Support services related to activities of daily living (ADLs)
            (1) Training in communication techniques
            (2) Communal meals
            (3) Training in homemaking skills
            (4) Supervision of and guidance in transportation skills
            (5) Recreational opportunities
            (6) Emergency procedures
            (7) Housing options
         b. Support services related to personal health management
            (1) Training in communication techniques
            (2) Counseling regarding sexuality and family relationships
            (3) Management of attendants
         c. Support services related to counseling assistance
            (1) Advocacy services
            (2) Peer counseling
            (3) Consumer and legal information
            (4) Personal business management
      5. Be aware of laws governing housing availability and accessibility
         a. The Housing Act of 1959: Provided funding for mortgage loans to developers to build housing for the elderly and the handicapped

    b. The Architectural Barriers Act of 1968: Mandated physical accessibility to any federally-funded building being constructed

    c. The Rehabilitation Act of 1973: Prohibited discrimination against the disabled when they rented or purchased federally subsidized property

    d. The Housing and Community Development Act of 1974: Subsidized rent payments to low-income families

    e. The Rehabilitation, Comprehensive Services, and Developmental Disabilities Amendment of 1978: Issued grants for housing

    f. The Americans With Disabilities Act of 1990: Established new laws governing physical access to the community, which need to be evaluated in relation to access to services and ways to implement them in communities in order to ensure access

6. Consider alternative housing situations for clients who are unable to remain in their previous residence

    a. Independent living programs

    b. Residential living—an arrangement in which a group of people with disabilities live in the same building or geographic area and share support services—can involve several challenges

       (1) Finding accessible housing

       (2) Securing attendant assistance

       (3) Providing accessible transportation

       (4) Obtaining rent subsidies

    c. Extended-care facilities such as subacute rehabilitation, neurobehavioral programs, skilled care facilities

B. Factors to consider in assessing a home

1. Availability of occupational therapy, physical therapy, and nursing evaluations to assist in determining safety, access, interventions, and the patient's ability to function in his or her own environment

2. Definition of the type of living quarters; design of the building

3. Lighting of the residence and its entrance, heating, running water, electrical outlets, and toilet facilities

4. Access to the residence and the need for wider doors, assistance with door opening, and handrails; bathroom and kitchen modifications

5. Assistive devices needed to facilitate mobility and safe participation in community environments

6. Availability of support systems to assist with mobility

7. Patient's level of independence regarding transfers, homemaking skills, personal care, food procurement and preparation, and household maintenance

8. Availability and adequacy of communications devices

9. Clutter in the environment—for example, scatter rugs, cords, carpets, toys, animals that might pose safety risks

10. Presence and accessibility of an elevator, availability of adaptive equipment such as Braille buttons, an elevator bell to indicate floor for visually impaired; automatic door timing for opening and closing

11. Furniture—arrangement, functionality, client's ability to use it safely, the need for adaptive equipment such as chair with a seat lift

12. Type of floor surface and ability to maneuver assistive device(s) on it

13. Storage of a vehicle and access to residence from the storage area

14. Ability to hear the telephone, fire alarms, doorbells, and availability of required adaptive equipment

II. Transportation

  A. Legislative mandates for public transportation systems and buildings—designed to guarantee all persons two basic rights

    1. Equal access to public transportation

    2. Completion of required modifications of airplanes, terminals, buses, subways, and public railroad systems

      a. Space to accommodate wheelchairs

      b. Wider doors and aisles, shorter or tiered steps

      c. Ramp or lift systems, elevators

  B. Issues related to modifications for vehicles for people with disabilities

    1. Hand controls, lifts, seating, and transfer mechanisms

    2. Funding for vehicle modification

    3. Travel programs and clubs for the disabled

  C. Adapted driver education and evaluation procedures

  D. Considerations regarding public transportation for those with disabilities

    1. Transportation services should be contacted prior to use to ensure that assistive services and accommodations are available

a. The Chamber of Commerce in many cities can provide booklets with information regarding community accessibility

b. The US Department of Transportation has information regarding highways and airports

2. It is vital that people with disabilities have access to the workplace, medical services, shopping, support services, recreational facilities, churches, public buildings, banks, clinics, post offices, grocery stores, and clothing stores, among other places to increase independence in self-care and community participation

3. Other transportation factors to be considered for people with disabilities

a. Distance from residence to public transportation

b. Cost of both public transportation and privately owned, specially adapted vehicles

c. Availability of assistance

d. Amount of assistance required

III. Vocational rehabilitation

A. Federal law mandates that each state have a public agency that provides vocational rehabilitation (Office of Vocational Rehabilitation [OVR])

B. Funding is provided for various aspects of vocational rehabilitation to facilitate a return to competitive work or supported employment

1. Vehicle and home modifications

2. Work-hardening programs, assessment of work capacities

3. Assessment of training facilities, equipment, and transportation

4. Determination of each individual's vocational limitations

5. Identification of vocational interests, previous work experience, and current abilities

6. Assessment of the job market

7. Employer education and development

8. Matching the disabled person's functional, cognitive, and emotional abilities with job placement options

a. Job training

b. Job modification

c. Job placement

C. Supported employment integrates people with disabilities into work settings

1. History
   a. Rehabilitation Act Amendments of 1986: Describe the content of supported employment programs
   b. Traditional vocational rehabilitation programs have served individuals with disabilities primarily in sheltered environments
2. Foci of supported employment settings
   a. Providing services to the severely disabled is a priority
   b. Workers are paid
   c. Work settings are integrated—persons with disabilities work in settings with able-bodied workers
   d. Ongoing support is provided
      (1) Supervision
      (2) Job adaptations
      (3) Personal care
      (4) Money management
      (5) Social skills
      (6) Transportation

IV. Disability management programs in the workplace
   A. Emphasize early identification of disabled workers and focus on prevention of work-related injuries
   B. Identify conditions in the work environment that result in worker disability
   C. Provide evaluations to identify the medical, social, and psychological assistance that would enable the worker to return to work
   D. Provide case management services in the form of job analysis, job modifications, and job placement
   E. Monitor services to address problems that arise after job placement occurs
   F. Motivate businesses to develop these programs owing to the cost of worker disabilities and subsequent healthcare costs
   G. Develop work-hardening programs
   H. May result in favorable outcomes
      1. Lower workers' compensation costs
      2. Reduced absenteeism
      3. Reduced costs of rehabilitation services
      4. Reduced medical costs
      5. Employee retention

V. Educational program considerations

A. Availability of institutions offering programs for the disabled such as residential schools for hearing-impaired, blind, or head-injured persons
B. Special services offered for the disabled to facilitate access to educational services
  1. Services related to the learning process
     a. Adaptation of educational materials such as talking books, Braille books, textbook recordings, cognitive software, computer-assisted learning programs
     b. Equipment such as reading machines, audiology services, communication augmentation devices, voice-activated computers
     c. Tutors, interpreters, or note-takers
  2. Other access issues—access to
     a. Classrooms, including parking
     b. Cafeteria, library, bookstore, dorms, chapel
     c. Social activities
     d. Entertainment, recreation, or sports activities
     e. Adapted bathrooms and shower facilities
C. Availability of support services
  1. Financial assistance
  2. Attendant services for students residing on campus
  3. Healthcare services
  4. Career planning and placement services
  5. Accessibility of programs for persons with disabilities
  6. Programs that take into consideration each individual's functional and cognitive abilities
  7. Vocational or guidance counseling
D. Adapted driver evaluation and education—modification of existing driver education program within the school system or referral to a rehabilitation facility for adapted driver training (e.g., a teenager with a spinal cord injury who has never driven)
VI. Adaptive equipment to facilitate community reintegration—considerations
  A. Devices for ADLs and mobility
    1. Specific type needed for physical mobility, such as a wheelchair, walker, crutches, commode, braces, scooter, or sliding board
    2. Adaptive equipment needed for independent functioning (personal hygiene, dressing, cooking)
      a. Need for and availability of amplification systems,

assistive listening devices, telecommunication devices, vibrator for alarm clock, visual alert systems, telephone amplifiers

b. Provision of round-the-clock relay services by telephone companies that is mandated by the Americans with Disabilities Act of 1990 (effective as of June 26, 1993) for individuals who have telecommunication devices for the deaf (TDDs) so they can communicate with those who do not

c. Communication boards, speech synthesizers

d. Hearing-ear dogs for the hearing-impaired, guide dogs for the visually impaired, independence dogs

3. Devices needed to prevent medical sequelae after a disability—for example, a wheelchair cushion or equipment for self-catheterization

B. Funding needed for equipment or devices

C. Availability of vendor and repair contracts

D. Client and family education regarding use, repair, and replacement of equipment

VII. Support and advocacy groups

A. Associations established and composed of individuals with disabilities such as the National Head Injury Foundation or the Paralyzed Veterans of America

B. Self-help organizations that assist the disabled by providing a variety of services, such as the Easter Seal Society or Variety Clubs

1. Offer mutual assistance

2. Assist with development of coping strategies

3. Foster abilities and skills to combat isolation and alienation

4. Develop information networks and counseling

C. National Institute on Disability and Rehabilitation Research

1. Oversees comprehensive rehabilitation service programs under the supervision and auspices of the US Department of Education

2. Participates in research and data collection, provides research grants

3. Emphasizes community reentry

Home Environment Assessment Guide

	Okay (y/n)	Plan to improve	
Basic Structure			
Intact roof			
Solid floors and stairs			
Functioning toilet (or outhouse)			
Source of fresh water			
Wheelchair ramp			
Temperature Control			
Fan/air conditioner			
Proper use of heating pads			
Proper hot water heater temperature			
Adequate heat/insulation			
Nutrition			
Kitchen condition/food storage			
Evidence of alcohol use			
Pests			
Fire Prevention and Response			
Use of kerosene heaters			
Use of open gas burners on stove for heat			
Smoking in bed			
Use of oxygen			
Dangerous electrical wiring			
Smoke alarms			
Exit plans in case of fire			
Self-Injury/Violence Prevention			
Locks			
Method of calling for help			
Proximity of neighbors			
Surrounding criminal activity			
Emergency phone numbers by telephone			
Loaded guns/knives			
Household toxins			
Water/bathtub			
Power tools			
Medication Management			
Duplicate medicines, outdated drugs, pill box			
Correct labeling			
Storage safety, accessibility, refrigeration			
Caregiver familiarity			
Wandering Control (for confused patients)			
Doortap latches, special locks			
Fenced yards with hidden latches			
Identification bracelets			
Electronic wandering alarms			

Use for:
— client
X clinician

Client's signature ____

Clinician's signature ____

Date ____

RESIDENCE

Adapted from Yoshikawa TAT, Cobbs EL, Brummel-Smith K: *Ambulatory geriatric care,* St Louis, 1993, Mosby, p 162. In Ebersole P, Hess P: *Toward healthy aging: human needs and nursing response,* ed 5, St Louis, 1998, Mosby.

INDUSTRY

Occupational/Environmental Health History

Occupational/Environmental Health History— Adapted to Neuman's Systems Model
Identifying data: medical record #:
Name:
Address:
Telephone:
Social Security #:
Sex (circle): Male   Female
Age: ____ Date of Birth: _____

Stressors perceived by the client:
I. Chief complaint:
This statement is to be in the patient's own words. It should reflect the reason why the client is currently seeking healthcare information or services.

Key questions:
1. Describe the health problem or injury you are currently experiencing.
2. Does any other member of your family experience this problem? Any co-worker? Any acquaintance?
3. Do you smoke (packs per day, length of time in years)? Use chewing tobacco? Consume alcohol (how much)?
4. Do you smoke while on the job? At home? Do your co-workers smoke while on the job? Do your family members smoke while you are in the room?
5. Have you missed work within the past 6 weeks? When did these symptoms begin? Have you been forced to stay in bed since the onset of this problem? Are you distressed by this level of disability?
6. Have you ever worked at a job or hobby that caused you to have this problem before? If so, describe the pattern of illness or difficulty. Have you ever found yourself short of breath, lightheaded, dizzy, with a cough, or wheezing while at work or after work? At the beginning of a work week? At the end of a work week? During the weekend?

From Bomar P, editor: *Nurses and family health promotion: concepts, assessment, and interventions,* ed 2, Philadelphia, 1996, WB Saunders.

7. Have you ever changed jobs, homes, or hobbies due to a health condition?

8. Have you ever experienced musculoskeletal difficulties, such as back pain, fractures, or muscle strain, related to work, home, or play?

9. Name the chemicals and compounds you work with and the frequency of contact with each.

10. Describe your neighborhood. Map out the location of industrial areas, waste disposal sites, water sources, and waste disposal.

11. Are there any community environmental problems that have evolved in recent time? Toxic spills, sewage breakage, smog changes, NIOSH/OSHA investigations pertinent to your condition?

12. Do you use pesticides, cleaning solutions, glues, solvents, heavy metals, or poisons within the home?

13. Type of heating and cooling within the home (electric, natural gas, other) and its impact on the (temporal) illness pattern.

II. Lifestyle patterns:

Note changes in previously stated patterns. It's important to note changes within the physical living environment, occupational setting (of client or other family members), and recreational environment.

Power and authority: Who makes decisions for the family? Is there a struggle for power within the family unit? Does this illness evidence possibly impact on power distribution within family?

Allocation of role and division of labor: Are roles perceived as appropriate by the client? Do the roles meet the client's needs? How are family chores and responsibilities divided among family members? Does the client perceive that this issue will affect the distribution of labor in any particular fashion?

Financial resources: Note the income and major outflow stressors. Will this illness cause any change within the home (physical) environment or location? Will this stressor cause perceived changes within the occupational and recreational spheres?

Spiritual beliefs: What are the spiritual beliefs of this family? Do such beliefs have bearing on the physical environment?

Activities of daily living: Include information about dietary habits, transportation method and patterns, housekeeping patterns and products, care of ill and infirm family members, sleep and rest patterns. Does the client perceive any of these areas to be of major concern?

Process characteristics: Note atmosphere within the home, methods of communication, developmental tasks, and use of extended family network. How does the family process information from the physical environment? How does the family or individual respond to adverse conditions within the occupational, recreational, or general environment? Are they able to act when the physical environment appears dangerous? When given advice about issues within their physical environment, are they able to process the information and make changes that diminish stressors?

Coping patterns: What makes the symptom or problem diminish or go away? Temporal sequence—map out the correlation of symptoms with work time, play time, home time, and recreational habits of the patient and individuals within the family.

Availability of resources: What resources are available from personal, local government, or national government assets to treat this environmental stressor? Is the family able to act independently on advice to use services within the healthcare system or general community, or must a professional assist? Is this stressor occupationally induced or exacerbated? If so, what resources are available through the employer to deal with this stressor?

Client goals and perceived assets: What does the client perceive as his or her sphere of influence on this problem? Health beliefs and attitudes—observable wellness activities, fatalism, use of emergency department or clinics. Does the client show evidence of a primary provider of healthcare services or use of informal nonprofessional network of healthcare providers?

Stressors as perceived by the caregiver:

List the major problems or stressors as perceived by the provider.

Do these observations differ from the client's perceptions? If so, how so?

How have previous problems or stressors paralleled this situation? How did the client treat the problem? What was the outcome?

What resources does the client possess? What resources are missing? What available resources need augmentation?

What do you perceive the client expects from the healthcare provider? What role will you play in the illness and recovery?

Impressions:
1. Intrapersonal factors
   a. Physical factors
   b. Psychosociocultural
   c. Developmental
2. Interpersonal factors—summarize the resources of immediate and extended family, work environment, and recreational environment.
3. Extrapersonal factors—summarize community resources, occupational, and federal and state programs that may facilitate resolution of this problem.
4. Problem statement—use nursing diagnosis to formulate your problem statement. Note target dates for reassessment, and state changes in stressors, intra-, inter-, and extrapersonal stressors when reassessing a problem.

Taking an Exposure History

This section provides two examples of environmental and occupational history-taking forms that could be used by nurses in a variety of practice settings. The first form, *Comprehensive Occupational and Environmental History,* was created for a faculty development workshop on Environmental and Occupational Health offered by the University of Maryland at Baltimore (June 1993); the second, *Occupational and Environmental Health History Form,* is reprinted with permission from Alyce B. Tarcher's *Principles and Practice of Environmental Medicine* (Plenum Publishing Co, 1992). Both forms enable nurses and other healthcare professionals to assess individual risk and the need for prevention, to diagnose and treat occupational and environmental illnesses, and to develop a sensitivity to the environmental conditions in a community that may contribute to ill health. Taking an exposure history also provides an opportunity for nurses to enhance their relationship with patients by learning more about an individual's workplace, home, and community environments.

Comprehensive Occupational and Environmental History

Work history

1. List your current and past longest held jobs, including the military:

Company	Dates employed	Job title	Known exposure
_____	_____	_____	_____
_____	_____	_____	_____
_____	_____	_____	_____

2. Do you work full-time? NO ____ YES ____ How many hours per week? ____

3. Do you work part-time? NO ____ YES ____ How many hours per week? ____

4. Please describe any health problems or injuries that you have experienced in connection with your present or past jobs:

5. Have you ever had to change jobs due to health problems or injuries? NO ____ YES ____
If so, describe:

Did any of your coworkers experience similar problems?

6. In what type of business do you currently work?

7. Describe your work (what do you actually do?):

8. Have you had any current or past exposure (through breathing or touching) to any of the following?

___ acids	___ beryllium
___ alcohols	___ cadmium
___ alkalies	___ carbon
___ ammonia	tetrachloride
___ arsenic	___ chlorinated
___ asbestos	napthalenes
___ benzene	___ chloroform

From Pope A, Snyder M, Mood L, editors: *Nursing, health and the environment*, Washington, D.C., 1995, Institute of Medicine, National Academy Press.

___ chloroprene

___ chromates

___ coal dust

___ cold (severe)

___ dichlorobenzene

___ ethylene dibromide

___ ethylene dichloride

___ fiberglass

___ halothane

___ heat (severe)

___ isocyanates

___ ketones

___ lead

___ manganese

___ mercury

___ methylene chloride

___ nickel

___ noise (loud)

___ PBBs

___ PCBs

___ perchloroethylene

___ pesticides

___ phenol

___ phosgene

___ radiation

___ rock dust

___ silica powder

___ solvents

___ styrene

___ toluene

___ TDI or MDI

___ trichloroethylene

___ trinitrotoluene (TNT)

___ vibration

___ vinyl chloride

___ welding fumes

___ x-rays

___ talc

9. Did you receive any safety training about these agents?
NO ___ YES ___
Explain:

10. Are you involved in any work processes, such as grinding, welding, soldering, or polishing, that create dust, mists, or fumes?
NO ___ YES ___ (If yes, describe)

11. Did you use any of the following personal protective equipment when exposed?

___ boots

___ coveralls

___ earplugs/muffs

___ glasses/goggles

___ gloves

___ respirator

___ safety shoes

___ shield

___ sleeves

___ welding mask

12. Is your work environment generally clean? If not, describe:

13. What ventilation systems are used in your workplace?

14. Do they seem to work? Are you aware of any chemical odors in your environment? (If so, explain)

15. Where do you eat, smoke, and take your breaks when you are on the job?

16. Do you use a uniform or have clothing that you wear only to work?

17. How is your work clothing laundered (at home, by employer, other)?

18. How often do you wash your hands at work and how do you wash them (running water, special soaps, other)?

19. Do you shower before leaving the worksite?

20. Do you have any physical symptoms associated with work? If yes, describe:

21. Are other workers similarly affected?

Home exposures

1. Which of the following do you have in your home?

   __ air conditioner   __ woodstove
   __ air purifier   __ central heating (gas)
   __ electric stove   __ central heating (oil)
   __ fireplace

2. In approximately what year was your home built?

3. Have there been any recent renovations? If yes, describe:

4. Have you recently installed new carpet, bought new furniture, or refinished existing furniture? If yes, explain:

5. Do you use pesticides around your home or garden? If yes, describe:

6. What household cleaners do you use? (List most common and any new products you use.)

7. List all hobbies done at your home:

   Are any of the agents listed earlier for work exposures encountered in hobbies or recreational activities?

   Is any special protective equipment or ventilation used during hobbies? If so, explain:

8. What are the occupations of other household members?

9. Do other household members have contact with any form of chemicals at work or during leisure activities? If so, explain:

10. Is anyone else in your home environment having symptoms similar to yours? If yes, explain briefly:

Community exposures

1. Are any of the following located in your community?

   ___ industrial plant   ___ toxic spill
   ___ landfill   ___ waste site
   ___ major source of   ___ other (specify: _____)
       air pollution

2. What is your source of drinking water?
   ___ private well   ___ other (specify: _____)
   ___ public water source

3. Are neighbors experiencing any health problems similar to yours? If yes, explain:

Occupational exposure

1. Describe any health problems or injuries related to present or past jobs.

2. Have you or your co-workers had health problems or injuries?

3. Do you believe you have health problems related to your present or past work?

4. Have you been absent from work because of a work-related illness or injury? If so, describe:

5. Have you worked with a substance that caused a skin rash? What was the substance? Describe your reaction:

6. Have you had trouble with breathing, coughing, or wheezing while at work? If so, describe:

7. Do you have any allergies? If so, describe:

8. Have you had difficulty conceiving a child?

9. Do you have any children who were born with abnormalities?

10. Do you smoke or have you ever smoked cigarettes, cigars, or pipes? For how long and how many per day?

11. Do you smoke on the job?

12. Have you ever worked at a job or hobby in which you came into direct contact with any of the following substances through breathing, touching, or direct exposure? If so, please place a checkmark beside the substance.

___ acids
___ alcohols (industrial)
___ alkalis
___ ammonia
___ arsenic
___ asbestos
___ benzene
___ beryllium
___ cadmium
___ carbon tetrachloride
___ chlorinated napthalenes
___ chloroform
___ chloroprene
___ chromates
___ coal dust
___ cold (severe)
___ dichlorobenzene
___ ethylene dibromide
___ ethylene dichloride
___ fiberglass
___ halothane
___ heat (severe)
___ isocyanates
___ ketones
___ lead

___ manganese
___ mercury
___ methylene chloride
___ nickel
___ noise (loud)
___ PBBs
___ PCBs
___ perchloroethylene
___ pesticides
___ phenols
___ phosgene
___ radiation
___ rock dust
___ silica powder
___ solvents
___ styrene
___ talc
___ toluene
___ TDI or MDI
___ trichloroethylene
___ trinitrotoluene (TNT)
___ vibration
___ vinyl chloride
___ welding fumes
___ x-rays

If you have answered "yes" to any of the above, please describe your exposure on a separate sheet of paper.

Environmental exposure

1. Do you live in the central city or in a rural, urban, or suburban area?

2. Have you ever changed your residence or home because of a health problem? If so, describe:

3. Do you live in the immediate vicinity of a refinery, smelter, factory, battery recycling plant, hazardous waste site, or other potential pollution source?

4. Do you (and your child) live in or regularly visit a building with peeling or chipped lead paint (such as those built before 1960)? Has there been recent, ongoing, or planned renovation or remodeling of this structure(s)?

5. Do any members of your household have contact with dusts or chemicals in the workplace that are then brought into the home?

6. Do you have a hobby that you do at home? If so, describe:

7. Do you fumigate your home or use pesticides in and around your home and on a pet? Do you use mothballs?

8. What cleaning agents and solvents are used in your home?

9. Is there evidence of mold in your home?

10. Which of the following do you use in your home?

___ air conditioner   ___ humidifier
___ electric stove   ___ wood stove
___ air purifier   ___ gas stove
___ fireplace   ___ unvented kerosene or gas heater

11. What is your source of drinking water?

___ community water system   ___ bottled water
___ private well

Key occupational and environmental health questions to be asked with all histories

1. What are your current and past longest-held jobs?

Occupational and environmental health history form

I. Identification

Name _____   Soc. Sec. # _____

Address _____   Sex: M ___ F ___

Telephone: home _____ work _____ Zip _____   Birthdate _____

II. Occupational history   Fill in the table below listing all jobs at which you have worked, including short-term, seasonal, and part-time employment. Start with your present job and go back to the first. Use additional paper if necessary.

Workplace (employer's name and address or city)	Dates worked		Type of industry (describe)	Your job duties (describe)	Health hazards in workplace (gases, dust, metals, solvents, radiation, infectious agents, etc.)	Protective equipment used (describe)	Health problems related to work (describe)
	From	To					

2. Have you been exposed to any radiation or chemical liquids, dusts, mists, or fumes?

3. Is there any relationship between current symptoms and activities at work or at home?

Agency for Toxic Substances and Disease Registry 1993 Priority List of Rank-Ordered Top 10 Hazardous Substances

Hazardous agents	Sources	Exposure pathways	Systems affected
Lead	Storage batteries Manufacture of paint, enamel, ink, glass, rubber, ceramics, chemicals	Ingestion Inhalation	Hematologic Renal Neuromuscular GI CNS
Arsenic	Manufacture of pigments, glass, pharmaceuticals, insecticides, fungicides, rodenticides Tanning	Ingestion Inhalation	Neuromuscular Skin GI
Metallic mercury	Electronics Paints Metal and textile production Chemical manufacturing Pharmaceutical production	Inhalation Percutaneous and GI absorption	Pulmonary CNS Renal
Benzene	Manufacture of organic chemicals, detergents, pesticides, solvents, paint removers	Inhalation Percutaneous absorption	CNS Hematopoietic
Vinyl chloride	Production of polyvinyl chloride and other plastics	Inhalation Ingestion	Hepatic Neurologic Pulmonary

NOTE: *CNS,* central nervous system; *GI,* gastrointestinal.

From Pope A, Snyder M, Mood L, editors, *Nursing, health and the environment,* Washington, DC, 1995, Institute of Medicine, National Academy Press.

Hazardous agents	Sources	Exposure pathways	Systems affected
Vinyl chloride —cont'd	Chlorinated compounds Used as a refrigerant		
Cadmium	Electroplating Solder	Inhalation	Pulmonary Renal
Polychlorinated biphenyls	Formerly used in electrical equipment	Inhalation Ingestion	Skin Eyes Hepatic
Benzo(a)pyrene*	Emissions from refuse burning and autos Used as laboratory reagent Found in charcoal-grilled meats and cigarette smoke	Inhalation Ingestion Percutaneous absorption	Pulmonary Skin Eyes
Chloroform	Aerosol propellants Fluorinated resins produced during chlorination of water Used as a refrigerant	Inhalation Percutaneous absorption Ingestion	CNS Renal Hepatic Mucous membrane Cardiac
Benzo(b)-fluoranthene	Cigarette smoke	Inhalation	Pulmonary

*BAP is a probable human carcinogen.

Selected Work-Related Health Risks

Diseases, disorders, and conditions associated with various agents, industries, or occupations: infections, malignant neoplasms, and hematological, cardiovascular, pulmonary, neurological, and miscellaneous disorders

Diseases, disorders, and conditions	Industry or occupation	Agent
Infections		
Anthrax	Shepherds, farmers, butchers, handlers of imported hides or fibers, veterinarians, veterinarian pathologists, weavers	*Bacillus anthracis*

From Tarcher AB, editor: *Principles and practice of environmental medicine,* New York, 1992, Plenum Publishing.   *Continued*

Selected Work-Related Health Risks—cont'd

Diseases, disorders, and conditions	Industry or occupation	Agent
Infections—cont'd		
Brucellosis	Farmers, shepherds, veterinarians, medical lab and slaughterhouse workers	*Brucella abortus, B. suis*
Plague	Shepherds, farmers, ranchers, hunters, field geologists	*Yersinia pestis*
Hepatitis A	Day-care centers, orphanage and mental retardation institution staff, medical personnel	Hepatitis A virus
Hepatitis B	Nurses and aides, anesthesiologists, orphanage and mental institution staff, medical lab workers, general dentists, oral surgeons, physicians	Hepatitis B virus
Hepatitis C (formerly included in non-A, non-B)	Same as hepatitis A and B	Hepatitis C virus
Ornithosis	Psittacine bird breeders, pet shop and zoo workers, poultry producers, veterinarians	*Chlamydia psittaci*
Rabies	Veterinarians, game wardens, lab workers, farmers, ranchers, trappers	Rabies virus
Rubella	Medical personnel	Rubella virus
Tetanus	Farmers, ranchers	*Clostridium tetani*
Tuberculosis (pulmonary)	Physicians, medical personnel, medical lab workers	*Mycobacterium tuberculosis*
Tuberculosis (silicotuberculosis)	Quarrymen, sandblasters, silica processors, miners, foundry workers, ceramic industry workers	Silicon dixoide (silica) *M. tuberculosis*
Tularemia	Hunters, fur handlers, sheep industry workers, cooks, veterinarians, ranchers, veterinarian pathologists	*Francisella tularensis*

Diseases, disorders, and conditions	Industry or occupation	Agent
Malignant neoplasms		
Bladder	Rubber and dye workers	Benzidine, 1- and 2-naphthyl-amine, auramine, magenta, 4-aminobi-phenyl, 4-nitrophenyl
Bone	Dial painters, radium chemists and processors	Radium
Kidney and other urinary tract organs	Coke oven workers	Coke oven emissions
Liver	Vinyl chloride polymeriza-tion industry workers	Vinyl chloride monomer
Liver hemangio-sarcoma	Vintners	Arsenical pesticides
Lung, bronchial, tracheal	Asbestos industry workers, asbestos users	Asbestos
	Topside coke oven workers	Coke oven emis-sions
	Uranium and fluorspar miners	Radon daughters
	Chromium producers, pro-cessors, users	Chromates
	Smelters	Arsenic
	Mustard gas formulators	Mustard gas
	Ion-exchange resin makers, chemists	Bis(chloro-ethyl)-ether, chloro-methyl, methyl ether
Nasal cavity	Woodworkers, furniture makers	Hardwood dusts
	Boot and shoe industry workers	Unknown
	Radium chemists and pro-cessors, dial painters	Radium
	Chromium producers, pro-cessors, users	Chromates
	Nickel smelting and refin-ing workers	Nickel Asbestos
Peritoneal, pleural mesothelioma	Asbestos industry workers, asbestos users	Asbestos

Continued

Selected Work-Related Health Risks—cont'd

Diseases, disorders, and conditions	Industry or occupation	Agent
Malignant neoplasms—cont'd		
Scrotal	Automatic lathe operators, metalworkers	Mineral, cutting oils
	Coke oven workers, petroleum refiners, tar distillers	Soots and tars, tar distillates
Hematologic disorders		
Agranulocytosis or neutropenia	Workers exposed to benzene	Benzene
	Explosives manufacturing and pesticide industry workers	Phosphorus
	Pesticide, pigment, pharmaceutical industry workers	Inorganic arsenic
Anemia (aplastic)	Explosives manufacturing	TNT
	Workers exposed to benzene	Benzene
	Radiologists, radium chemists, dial painters	Ionizing radiation
Anemia (hemolytic, nonautoimmune)	Whitewashing and leather industry workers	Copper sulfate
	Electrolytic processes, arsenical ore smelting	Arsines
	Plastics industry workers	Trimellitic anhydride
	Dye, celluloid, and resin industry workers	Naphthalene
Leukemia (acute lymphoid)	Rubber industry workers	Unknown
	Radiologists	Ionizing radiation
Leukemia (acute myeloid)	Workers exposed to benzene	Benzene
	Radiologists	Ionizing radiation
Leukemia (erythroleukemia)	Workers exposed to benzene	Benzene
Methemoglobinemia	Explosives manufacturing, dye industry workers	Aromatic amino and nitro compounds (e.g., aniline, TNT, nitroglycerin)
Cardiovascular disorders		
Angina	Auto mechanics, foundry workers, wood finishers, traffic control, driving in heavy traffic	Carbon monoxide

Diseases, disorders, and conditions	Industry or occupation	Agent
Arrhythmias	Metal cleaning, solvent use, refrigerator maintenance	Solvents, fluorocarbons
Raynaud's phenomenon	Lumberjacks, chain sawyers, grinders, chippers	Whole-body or segmental vibration
(Secondary)	Vinyl chloride polymerization industry workers	Vinyl chloride monomer
Pulmonary disorders		
Alveolitis (extrinsic, allergic)	Farmers (farmer's lung, bagassosis), bird breeders (bird-breeder's lung), cook handlers (suberosis), brewery and distillery workers (maltworker's lung); mushroom workers (mushroom worker's lung); maple bark disease, cheese makers (cheese maker's, cheese-washer's lung) coffee workers (coffee-worker's lung), fish meal workers (fish-meal–worker's lung), furriers (furrier's lung); logging and sawmill workers (sequoiosis); woodworkers (woodworker's lung); mill workers (miller's lung)	Various agents
Asbestosis	Asbestos industry workers, asbestos users	Asbestos
Asthma (extrinsic)	Jewelry, alloy, catalyst makers	Platinum
	Polyurethane, adhesive, paint workers	Isocyanates
	Alloy, catalyst, refinery workers	Chromium, cobalt
	Solderers	Aluminum soldering flux
	Plastic, dye, insecticide makers	Phthalic anhydride
	Foam workers, latex makers, biologists	Formaldehyde
	Printing industry	Gum arabic
	Nickel platers	Nickel sulfate

Continued

Selected Work-Related Health Risks—cont'd

Diseases, disorders, and conditions	Industry or occupation	Agent
Pulmonary disorders—cont'd		
Asthma (extrinsic)	Bakers	Flour
	Plastics industry workers	Trimellitic anhydride
	Woodworkers, furniture makers	Red cedar, wood dusts
	Detergent formulators	Bacillus-derived exoenzymes
	Animal handlers	Animal dander
Beryllium disease (chronic)	Beryllium alloy, ceramic, cathode-ray tube, nuclear reactor workers	Beryllium
Bronchitis, pneumonitis, pulmonary edema (acute)	Refrigeration, fertilizer, oil-refining industry workers	Ammonia
	Alkali, beach industry workers	Chlorine
	Silo fillers, arc welders, nitric acid workers	Nitrogen oxides
	Paper, refrigeration, oil-refining industry workers	Sulfur dioxide
	Cadmium smelters, processors	Cadmium
	Plastics industry workers	Trimellitic anhydride
Byssinosis	Cotton industry workers	Cotton, flax, hemp, cotton-synthetic dusts
Pneumoconiosis	Coal miners, bauxite workers	Coal dust, bauxite fumes
Silicosis	Mining, metal, and ceramic industry workers, quarrymen, sand blasters, silica processors	Silica
Talcosis	Talc processors	Talc
Neurologic disorders		
Cerebellar ataxia	Chemical industry	Toluene
	Electrolytic chlorine production workers, battery manufacturing workers, fungicide formulators	Organic mercury
Encephalitis (toxic)	Battery, smelter, foundry workers	Lead
	Electrolytic chlorine production workers, battery manufacturing workers, fungicide formulators	Organic, inorganic mercury

Diseases, disorders, and conditions	Industry or occupation	Agent
Neuropathy (toxic and inflammatory)	Pesticide, pigment, pharmaceutical industry workers	Arsenic, arsenic compounds
	Furniture refinishers, degreasers	Hexane
	Plastic-coated-fabric workers	Methyl butyl ketone
	Explosives industry workers	TNT
	Rayon manufacturing workers	Carbon disulfide
	Plastics, hydraulics, coke industry workers	Tri-*o*-cresyl phosphate
	Battery, smelter, foundry workers	Inorganic lead
	Dentists, chloralkali workers	Inorganic mercury
	Chloralkali, fungicide, battery workers	Organic mercury
	Plastics, paper manufacturing workers	Acrylamide
Parkinson's disease (secondary)	Manganese processors, battery manufacturing workers, welders	Manganese
	Internal combustion engine industry workers	Carbon monoxide
Miscellaneous		
Abdominal pain	Battery manufacturing workers, enamelers, smelters, painters, ceramics workers, plumbers, welders	Lead
Cataract	Microwave, radar technicians	Microwaves
	Explosives industry workers	TNT
	Radiologists	Ionizing radiation
	Blacksmiths, glass blowers, bakers	Infrared radiation
	Moth repellent formulators, fumigators	Naphthalene
	Explosives, dye, herbicide, pesticide industry workers	Dinitrophenol, dinitro-*o*-cresol

Continued

Selected Work-Related Health Risks—cont'd

Diseases, disorders, and conditions	Industry or occupation	Agent
Miscellaneous—cont'd		
Dermatitis (contact, allergic)	Adhesives, sealants, and plastics industry workers; leather tanning workers, poultry dressing workers, fish packing workers, boat building and repair workers, electroplating workers, metal cleaning workers, machining, housekeeping	Irritants (cutting oils, solvents, phenols, acids, alkalis, detergents, fibrous glass), allergens (nickel, epoxy resins, chromates, formaldehyde, dyes, rubber products)
Headache	Firefighters, foundry workers, wood finishers, dry cleaners, traffic control workers, driving in heavy traffic	Carbon monoxide, solvents
Hepatitis (toxic)	Solvent users, dry cleaners, plastics industry workers	Carbon tetrachloride, chloroform, tetrachlorethane, trichloroethylene
	Explosives and dye industry workers	Phosphorus, TNT
	Fire and waterproofing additive formulators	Chloronaphthalene
	Plastics formulators	4,4-methylenedianiline
	Fumigators, gasoline and fire-extinguisher formulators	Ethylene dibromide
	Disinfectant, fumigant, synthetic resin formulators	Cresol
Inner ear damage	Various	Excessive noise
Infertility (male)	Formulators	Kepone
	Producers, formulators, applicators	1,2-dibromo-3-chloropropane
Psychosis (acute)	Gasoline, seed, and fungicide workers; wood preservation, rayon manufacturing	Lead (especially organic), mercury, carbon disulfide.

Diseases, disorders, and conditions	Industry or occupation	Agent
Renal failure (acute, chronic)	Battery manufacturing, plumbers, solderers	Inorganic lead
	Electrolytic processes, arsenical ore smelting	Arsine
	Battery manufacturing, jewelers, dentists	Inorganic mercury
	Fluorocarbon, fire-extinguisher formulators	Carbon tetra-chloride
	Antifreeze manufacturing	Ethylene glycol

Selected Job Categories, Exposures, and Associated Work-Related Diseases and Conditions

Job categories	Exposures	Work-related diseases and conditions
Agricultural workers	Pesticides, infectious agents, gases, sunlight	Pesticide poisoning, farmer's lung, skin cancer
Anesthetists	Anesthetic gases	Reproductive effects, cancer
Animal handlers	Infectious agents, allergens	Asthma
Automobile workers	Asbestos, plastics, lead, solvents	Asbestosis, dermatitis
Bakers	Flour	Asthma
Battery makers	Lead, arsenic	Lead poisoning, cancer
Butchers	Vinyl plastic fumes	Meat wrapper's asthma
Caisson workers	Pressurized work environments	Nitrogen narcosis (Caisson disease, the bends)
Carpenters	Wood dust, wood preservatives, adhesives	Nasopharyngeal cancer, dermatitis
Cement workers	Cement dust, metals	Dermatitis, bronchitis
Ceramics workers	Talc, clays	Pneumoconiosis
Demolition workers	Asbestos, wood dust	Asbestosis
Drug manufacturers	Hormones, nitroglycerin, etc.	Reproductive effects

From Tarcher AB, editor: *Principles and practice of environmental medicine.* 1992, New York, Plenum Publishing.   *Continued*

Selected Job Categories, Exposures, and Associated Work-Related Diseases and Conditions—cont'd

Job categories	Exposures	Work-related diseases and conditions
Dry cleaners	Solvents	Liver disease, dermatitis
Dye workers	Dyestuffs, metals, solvents	Bladder cancer, dermatitis
Embalmers	Formaldehyde, infectious agents	Dermatitis
Felt makers	Mercury, polycyclic hydrocarbons	Mercuralism
Foundry workers	Silica, molten metals	Silicosis
Glass workers	Heat, solvents, metal powders	Cataracts
Hospital workers	Infectious agents, cleansers, radiation	Infections, accidents
Insulators	Asbestos, fibrous glass	Asbestosis, lung cancer, mesothelioma
Jackhammer operators	Vibration	Raynaud's phenomenon
Lathe operators	Metal dusts, cutting oils	Lung disease, cancer
Laundry workers	Bleaches, soaps, alkalis	Dermatitis
Lead burners	Lead	Lead poisoning
Miners (coal, hard rock, metals, etc.)	Talc, radiation, metals, coal dust, silica	Pneumoconiosis, lung cancer
Natural gas workers	Polycyclic hydrocarbons	Lung cancer
Nuclear workers	Radiation, plutonium	Metal poisoning, cancer
Office workers	Poor lighting, poorly designed equipment	Joint problems, eye problems
Painters	Paints, solvents, spackling compounds	Neurologic problems
Paper makers	Acids, alkalis, solvents, metals	Lung disorders, dermatitis
Petroleum workers	Polycyclic hydrocarbons, catalysts, zeolites	Cancer, pneumoconiosis
Plumbers	Lead, solvents, asbestos	Lead poisoning
Railroad workers	Creosote, sunlight, oils, solvents	Cancer, dermatitis
Seamen	Sunlight, asbestos	Cancer, accidents
Smelter workers	Metals, heat, sulfur dioxide, arsenic	Cancer
Steel workers	Heat, metals, silica	Cataracts, heat stroke
Stone cutters	Silica	Silicosis

Job categories	Exposures	Work-related diseases and conditions
Textile workers	Cotton dust, fabrics, fin-ishers, dyes, carbon disulfide	Byssinosis, dermatitis, psychosis
Varnish makers	Solvents, waxes	Dermatitis
Vineyard workers	Arsenic, pesticides	Cancer, dermatitis
Welders	Fumes, nonionizing radiation	Lead poisoning, cata-racts

A Model Assessment Guide for Nursing in Industry

Components	Questions to ask
The company	
Historic development	How, why, and by whom was the company founded?
Organization chart	What is the formal order of the system and to whom are the health providers respon-sible?
Company policies	Is there a policy manual? Are the workers aware of existence of the manual?
Length of the work week	How many days a week does the industry operate?
Length of the work time	Are there several shifts? How many breaks? Is there paid vacation?
Sick leave	Is there a clear policy? Do the workers know it?
Safety and fire provisions	Is management aware of situations or sub-stances in the plant that represent a po-tential danger? Are there organized fire drills? (The *Federal Register* is the source of information for federal stan-dards and serves as a helpful guide.)
Support services (benefits)	
Insurance programs	Is there a system for health insurance and life insurance, and is it compulsory? Does the company pay all or part? Who fills out the necessary forms?
Retirement program	Are the benefits realistic?
Educational support	Can the workers further their education? Will the company help financially?

Adapted from Serafini P: Nursing assessment in industry: a model, *Am J Public Health* 66(8):755-760, 1976. In Anderson E, McFarlane J: *Community as partner: theory and practice in nursing,* ed 2, Philadelphia, 1996, Lippincott. *Continued*

A Model Assessment Guide for Nursing in Industry—cont'd

Components	Questions to ask
Support services (benefits)—cont'd	
Safety committee	If there is no committee, do certain people routinely handle emergencies? The Red Cross First Aid Course through programmed instruction is excellent (for information, consult your local Red Cross).
Recreation committee	Do the workers have any communication with or interest in each other outside the work setting?
Employee relations	Are there problems in employee relations? (This is difficult information to obtain, but it is important to get a sense of employees generally feelings about management and vice versa.)
The plant	
General physical setting	What is the overall appearance?
The construction	What is the size and general condition of buildings and grounds?
Parking facilities and public transportation stops	How far do workers have to walk to get inside?
Entrances and exits	How many people must use them? How accessible are they?
Physical environment	What conditions exist in the physical environment? (Comment on heating, air-conditioning, lighting, glare, drafts, etc.)
Communication facilities	Are there bulletin boards and newsletters?
Housekeeping	Is the physical setting maintained adequately?
Interior decoration	Are the surroundings conducive to work? Are they pleasing?
Work areas	
Space	Are workers isolated or crowded?
Heights: workplace and supply areas	Is there a chance of workers falling or being injured by falling objects? (Falls and falling objects are dangerous and costly to industry.)
Stimulation	Is the worker too bored to pay attention?
Safety signs and markings	Are dangerous areas well marked?
Standing and sitting facilities	Are chairs safe and comfortable? Are there platforms to stand on, especially for wet processes?

Components	Questions to ask
Safety equipment	Do the workers make use of hard hats, safety glasses, face masks, radiation badges, etc.? Do they know the safety devices that the OSHA regulations require? to get a drink of water when they want to?
Nonwork areas	
Lockers	If the work is dirty, workers should be able to change clothes. Are they accidentally carrying toxic substances home on their clothes?
Hand-washing facilities	If facilities and supplies are available, do workers know how and when to wash their hands?
Restrooms	How accessible are restrooms and what condition are they in?
Drinking water	Can workers leave their jobs long enough to get a drink of water when they want to?
Recreation and rest facilities	Can a worker who is not feeling well lie down? Do workers feel free to use the facilities?
Telephones	Can a worker receive or make a call? Does a working mother have to stay home for a call because she can't be reached at work?
Ashtrays	Are people allowed to smoke in designated areas? Are they safe areas?
The working population*	
General characteristics	(Be as accurate as possible, but estimate when necessary.)
Total number of employees	(Usually, if an employer has 500 or more employees, full-time nursing services are necessary.)
General appearance	Are there records of heights, weights, cleanliness, and so forth? Ask to see them.
Age and sex distribution	What are the proportions of the different groups? (Certain screening programs are specific for young adults, whereas others are more for the elderly. Some programs are more for women, and others are more for men.) Is there any difference between day and evening shift populations? Are the problems of the minority sex unattended?
Race distribution	Does one race predominate? How does this compare with the general community?
Socioeconomic distribution	Are there great differences in worker salaries? (This can sometimes cause problems.)

---

*Include worker and management, but separate data for comparison.   *Continued*

A Model Assessment Guide for Nursing in Industry—cont'd

Components	Questions to ask

The working population—cont'd

General characteristics—cont'd

Components	Questions to ask
Religious distribution	Does one religion predominate? Are religious holidays observed?
Ethnic distribution	Is there a language barrier?
Marital status	What proportion of the workers are widowed, single, or divorced? (These groups often have different needs.)
Education background	Can all teaching be done at approximately the same level?
Lifestyles practiced	Is there disapproval of certain lifestyles?
Types of employment offered	
Background necessary	What education level is required? Skilled versus unskilled?
Work demands on physical condition	What level of strength is needed? Is the work sedentary or active?
Work status	How many employees work full-time? Part-time? Is there overtime?
Absenteeism	Is there a record kept? By whom? Why?
causes	What are the five most common reasons for absence?
Length	What are the patterns of absences? (Absenteeism is costly to the employer. There is some difference between one 10-day absence and 10 one-day absences by the same person.)
Physically handicapped	Does the company have a policy about hiring the handicapped?
Number employed	Where do they work? What do they do?
Extent of handicaps	Are they specially trained? Are they in a special program? Do they use prosthetic devices?
Personnel taking medication	What medication does each of these employees take? Where does each person work?
Personnel with chronic illness	At what stage of illness is the employee? Where does the employee work? Will he or she be able to continue at this job?

The industrial process: What does the company produce and how?

Components	Questions to ask
Equipment used	Is the equipment portable or fixed? Light or heavy?
General description of placement	Ask to have each piece of large equipment marked on a scale map.
Type of equipment	Fans, blowers, fast moving, wet, or dry?

Components	Questions to ask

The industrial process: What does the company produce and how?—cont'd

Nature of the operation	Ask for a brief description of each stage of the process so that you can compare the needs and abilities of the worker with the needs of the job.
Raw materials used	What are they and how dangerous are they? Are they properly stored? (Check the *Federal Register* for guidelines on storage.)
Nature of the final product	Can the workers take pride in the final product, or do they just "make parts"?
Description of the jobs	Who does what? Where? (Label the map.)
Waste products produced	What is the system for waste disposal? Are the pollution-control devices in place and functioning?
Exposure to toxic substances	To which toxins are the workers exposed? What is the extent of exposure? (Include physical and emotional hazards. Remember that chronic effects of industrial exposure are subtle; a person often gets used to having mild symptoms and won't report them. The *Federal Register* contains specifications for exposure to toxins, and some states issue state standards.)

The health program*

Existing policies	Are there informal, unwritten policies?
Objectives of the program	Are they clear?
Preemployment physicals	Are they required? Are they paid for by the company? Is the information used to hire?
First-aid facilities	What is available? What is not available?
Standing orders	Is there a company physician who is responsible for first aid or emergency policy? (If so, work closely with him or her in planning nursing services.)
Job descriptions for health personnel	Are they in writing? (If there are no guidelines to be followed, write some.)
Existing facilities and resources:	Sometimes an industry that denies having a health program has more of a system than it realizes.
Trained personnel	Who responds in an emergency?
Space	Where is the sick worker taken? Where is the emergency equipment kept?
Supplies	What are they? Where are they kept? (Make a list and describe the condition of each item.)

*Outline what is actually in existence as well as what employees perceive to be in existence.

Continued

A Model Assessment Guide for Nursing in Industry—cont'd

Components	Questions to ask
The health program—cont'd	
Existing facilities and resources—cont'd	
Records and reports	What exists? (OSHA requires that employers keep three types of records: a log of occupational injuries and illnesses, a supplemental record of certain illnesses or injuries, and an annual summary [forms 100, 101, and 102 are provided under the act]. Good records provide data for good planning.)
Services rendered in the past year:	Describe as specifically as possible.
Care needed	Chronic or acute? Why?
Screening done	Where? By whom? Why?
Referrals made	By whom? To whom? Why?
Counseling done	Formal or informal? (Often informal counseling goes unnoticed.)
Health education	What individual or group education was offered by the company?
Accidents in the past year	During working hours? After hours? (Include those that occur after work hours; some may be directly or indirectly work related.)
Reasons why employees sought health care	What are the five major reasons?
Stressors	
As identified by employees	What pressures are felt on the job?
As identified by health providers	What problems do they perceive?

FAMILY ASSESSMENT

Family assessment is a central part of public health and community health nursing practice. These tools will serve as cues to assist the nurse in making key observations about how families live, work, and play together. It is essential to understand the structure and function of the family and the roles that each individual plays in order for the nurse to be effective in disease prevention and health promotion activities.

Family Self-Care Patterns

The following tool suggests a method for identifying family health goals and monitoring progress toward these goals.

Designed for (family name): _____

Family form: _____

Family members:

Name	Sex	Position in family	Birth-date	Occupation (if employed)
_____	_____	_____	_____	_____
_____	_____	_____	_____	_____
_____	_____	_____	_____	_____
_____	_____	_____	_____	_____
_____	_____	_____	_____	_____

Home address: _____

Home telephone number: _____

Work telephone number: _____

Cultural background: _____

Spiritual-religious orientation: _____

Major formal roles of family members: _____
_____
_____
_____
_____

Community affiliations of family: _____
_____
_____
_____
_____
_____

Communication patterns (verbal and nonverbal, including expression of caring and affection):

Family decision-making patterns:

From Pender NL: *Health promotion in nursing practice,* ed 3, Norwalk, Conn, 1996, Appleton & Lange.

Family values with highest rank:

1. _____
2. _____
3. _____
4. _____
5. _____

Rank order of health as a value (if not listed above): _____

Value conflicts in family (if any):

Goals important to family:	Mutual goal or specific to dyad (d) or triad (t)
_____	_____
_____	_____
_____	_____
_____	_____

Family strengths:

Major sources of stress for family and perceived ability to deal with stressors:

Current or recent family developmental or situational transitions:

Family concerns or challenges:

Family self-care patterns

Current health protecting or preventive behaviors (e.g., immunization, self-examination, periodic screening or examination by health professionals, avoidance of toxic exposure, use of seat belts):

Current health-promoting behaviors (lifestyle review):
  Nutritional practices:

  Physical-recreational activities:

  Sleep-relaxation patterns:

  Stress management:

  Family sense of purpose:

  Family actualization efforts:

  Relationships in family and with others:

  Environmental control:

Information-seeking patterns of family in relation to health promotion:

Use of health-promotion facilities or services by family:

Other behaviors:

Consistency among family values, goals, and health actions:

Family health goals

Target health goal

Goals	Family priority (1 = most important)

Areas for improvement in family health

Target health goal

Area of change (see categories under family self-care patterns)	Specific behavior change	Family priority (1 = most desirable)	Approaches selected to facilitate family change

Evaluation of progress toward change in family lifestyle

Two weeks:

One month:

Three months:

Six months:

One year:

Stages of Family Development: Health Promotion and Disease Prevention

The following table presents nursing roles for families in various stages of development. This guide may be helpful in assisting families to move successfully through life stages, thereby reducing the risk for illness or crisis.

Stage	Possible nursing role
Couple	Counselor on sexual and role adjustment
	Teacher and counselor in family planning
	Teacher of parenting skills
	Coordinator for genetic counseling
	Facilitator in interpersonal relationships
Childbearing family	Monitor of prenatal care and referral for problems during pregnancy
	Counselor on prenatal nutrition
	Counselor on prenatal maternal habits
	Supporter of amniocentesis
	Counselor on breastfeeding
	Coordinator with pediatric services
	Supervisor of immunizations
	Referrer to social services
	Assistant in adjustment to parental role
Family with preschool and school-age children	Monitor of early childhood development; referrer when indicated
	Teacher in first-aid and emergency measures
	Coordinator with pediatric services
	Counselor on nutrition and exercise
	Teacher in problem-solving issues regarding health habits
	Participant in community organizations for environmental control
	Teacher of dental care hygiene
	Counselor on environmental safety in home
	Facilitator in interpersonal relationships
Family with adolescents	Teacher of risk factors to health
	Teacher in problem-solving issues regarding alcohol, smoking, diet, and exercise
	Facilitator of interpersonal skills with teenagers and parents
	Direct supporter, counselor, or referrer to mental health resources
	Counselor on family planning
	Referrer for sexually transmittable diseases

From Edelman CL, Mandle CL: *Health promotion throughout the lifespan,* ed 4, St Louis, 1998, Mosby.

Stage	Possible nursing role
Family with young or middle-age adults	Participant in community organizations on disease control habits
	Teacher in problem-solving issues regarding lifestyle and habits
	Participant in community organizations for environmental control
	Case finder in the home and community
	Screener for hypertension, Pap smear, breast examination, cancer signs, mental health, and dental care
	Counselor on menopausal transition
Family with older adults	Facilitator in interpersonal relationships among family members
	Referrer for work and social activity, nutritional programs, homemakers' services, and nursing home
	Monitor of exercise, nutrition, preventive services, and medications
	Supervisor of immunization
	Counselor on safety in the home
	Counselor on bereavement

Family Health Assessment Interview

General guidelines for family interview

Schedule the interview with the family at a time that is most convenient for all parties; include as many family members as possible; clearly state the purpose of the interview.

Begin the interview by asking each person's name and their relationship to each other.

Restate the purpose of the interview and the objective.

Keep the initial conversation general to put members at ease and to learn the "big picture" of the family.

Identify major concerns and reflect these back to the family to be certain that all parties perceive the same message.

Terminate the interview with a summary of what was discussed and a plan for additional sessions if needed.

From Wong D, et al: *Whaley and Wong's nursing care of infants and children,* ed 6, St Louis, 1999, Mosby.

Structural assessment areas

Family composition

Immediate members of the household (names, ages, and relationships)

Significant extended family members

Previous marriages, separations, death of spouses, or divorces

Home and community environment

Type of dwelling/number of rooms/occupants

Sleeping arrangements

Number of floors, accessibility of stairs, elevators

Adequacy of utilities

Safety features (fire escape, smoke detector, guardrails on windows, use of car restraint) and firearms

Environmental hazards (e.g., chipped paint, poor sanitation, pollution, heavy street traffic)

Availability and location of health facilities, schools, play areas

Relationship with neighbors

Recent crises or changes in home

Child's reaction/adjustment to recent stresses

Occupation and education of family members

Types of employment

Work schedules

Work satisfaction

Exposure to environmental/industrial hazards

Sources of income and adequacy

Effect of illness on financial status

Highest degree or grade level attained

Cultural and religious traditions

Religious beliefs and practices

Cultural/ethnic beliefs and practices

Language spoken in home

Assessment questions include:

Does the family identify with a particular religious/ethnic group? Are both parents from that group?

How is religious/ethnic background part of family life?

What special religious/cultural traditions are practiced in the home (e.g., food choices and preparation)?

Where were family members born and how long have they lived in this country?

What language does the family speak most frequently?

Do they speak/understand English?

What do they believe causes health or illness?

What religious/ethnic beliefs influence the family's perception of illness and its treatment?

What methods are used to prevent/treat illness?

How does the family know when a health problem needs medical attention?

Who is the person the family contacts when a member is ill?

Does the family rely on cultural/religious healers or remedies? If so, ask them to describe the type of healer or remedy.

Who does the family go to for support (clergy, medical healer, relatives)?

Does the family experience discrimination because of their race, beliefs, or practices? Ask them to describe.

Functional assessment areas

Family interactions and roles

Interactions refer to ways family members relate to each other

Chief concern is amount of intimacy and closeness among the members, especially spouses

Roles refer to behaviors of people as they assume a different status or position

Observations include:

Family members' responses to each other (cordial, hostile, cool, loving, patient, short-tempered)

Obvious roles of leadership vs submission

Support and attention shown to various members

Assessment questions include:

What activities do the family perform together?

Whom do family members talk to when something is bothering them?

What are members' household chores?

Who usually oversees what is happening with the children, such as at school or concerning their health?

How easy or difficult is it for the family to change or accept new responsibilities for household tasks?

Power, decision making, and problem solving

Power refers to individual member's control over others in family; manifested through family decision making and problem solving

Chief concern is clarity of boundaries of power between parents and children

One method of assessment involves offering a hypothetical conflict or problem, such as a child failing school, and asking family how they would handle this situation

Assessment questions include:

Who usually makes the decisions in the family?

If one parent makes a decision, can the child appeal to the other parent to change it?

What input do children have in making decisions or discussing rules?

Who makes and enforces the rules?

What happens when a rule is broken?

Communication

Concerned with clarity and directness of communication patterns

Observations include:

Who speaks to whom

If one person speaks for another or interrupts

If members appear disinterested when certain individuals speak

If there is agreement between verbal and nonverbal messages

Further assessment includes periodically asking family members if they understood what was just said and to repeat the message

Assessment questions include:

How often do family members wait until others are through talking before "having their say"?

Do parents or older siblings tend to lecture and preach?

Do parents tend to talk "down" to the children?

Expression of feelings and individuality

Concerned with personal space and freedom to grow with limits and structure needed for guidance

Observing patterns of communication offers clues to how freely feelings are expressed

Assessment questions include:

Is it OK for family members to get angry or sad?

Who gets angry most of the time? What do they do?

If someone is upset, how do other family members try to comfort this person?

Who comforts specific family members?

When someone wants to do something, such as try out for a new sport or get a job, what is the family's response (offer assistance, discouragement, or no advice)?

Eleven Functional Health-Pattern Assessment Guidelines for Families

Family assessment

The 11 functional health-pattern areas are applicable to the assessment of families. Families are the primary client in community health nursing. In some cases, a family assessment may be indicated (1) in the care of an infant or child whose development is influenced by family health patterns or (2) when an adult has certain health problems that can be influenced by family patterns. The following guidelines provide information on family functioning:

1. Health perception–health management pattern
   History:
   a. How has family's general health been (in last few years)?
   b. Colds in past year? Absence from work/school?
   c. Most important things you do to keep healthy? Think these make a difference to health? (Include family folk remedies, if appropriate.)
   d. Members' use of cigarettes, alcohol, drugs?
   e. Immunizations? Healthcare provider? Frequency of checkups? Accidents (home, work, school, driving)? (If appropriate: Storage of medicines, cleaning products, scatter rugs, etc.)
   f. In past, has it been easy to find ways to follow suggestions of doctors, nurses, social workers (if appropriate)?
   g. Things important in family's health that I could help with?
   Examination:
   a. General appearance of family members and home.
   b. If appropriate: Storage of medicines, cribs, playpens, stove, scatter rugs, hazards, etc.

2. Nutritional–metabolic pattern
   History:
   a. Typical family meal pattern/food intake? (Describe) Supplements (vitamins, types of snacks, etc.)?
   b. Typical family fluid intake? (Describe) Supplements: type available (fruit juices, soft drinks, coffee, etc.)?
   c. Appetites?
   d. Dental problems? Dental care (frequency)?
   e. Skin problems? Healing problems?
   Examination:
   a. If opportunity available: Refrigerator contents, meal preparation, contents of meal, etc.

3. Elimination pattern

From Gordon M: *Manual of nursing diagnosis: 1995-1996,* St Louis, 1995, Mosby.

History:
a. Family use of laxatives, other aids?
b. Problems in waste/garbage disposal?
c. Pet animals' waste disposal (indoor/outdoor)?
d. If indicated: Problems with flies, roaches, rodents?

Examination:
a. If opportunity available: Examine toilet facilities, garbage disposal, pet waste disposal; indicators of risk for flies, roaches, rodents.

4. Activity–exercise pattern

History:
a. In general, does family get a lot of/little exercise? Type? Regularity?
b. Family leisure activities? Active/passive?
c. Problems in shopping (transportation), cooking, keeping up the house, budgeting for food, clothes, housekeeping, house costs?

Examination:
a. Pattern of general home maintenance, personal maintenance.

5. Sleep–rest pattern

History:
a. Generally, family members seem to be well rested and ready for school/work?
b. Sufficient sleeping space and quiet?
c. Family finds time to relax?

Examination:
a. If opportunity available: Observe sleeping space and arrangements.

6. Cognitive–perceptual pattern

History:
a. Visual or hearing problems? How managed?
b. Any big decisions family has had to make? How made?

Examination:
a. If indicated: Language spoken at home.
b. Grasp of ideas and questions (abstract/concrete).
c. Vocabulatory level.

7. Self-perception–self-concept pattern

History:
a. Most of time family feels good (not so good) about themselves as a family?
b. General mood of family? Happy? Anxious? Depressed? What helps family mood?

Examination:

a. General mood state: nervous (5) or relaxed (1); rate from 1 to 5.

b. Members generally assertive (5) or passive (1); rate from 1 to 5.

8. Roles–relationship pattern

   History:

   a. Family (or household) members? Member age and family structure (diagram).

   b. Any family problems that are difficult to handle (nuclear/extended)? Child rearing? If appropriate: Spouse/parents (should be included if children are interviewed) ever get rough with you? The children?

   Family Assessment:

   c. Relationships good (not so good) among family members? Siblings? Support each other?

   d. If appropriate: Income sufficient for needs?

   e. Feel part of (or isolated from) community? Neighbors?

   Examination:

   a. Interaction among family members (if present).

   b. Observed family leadership roles.

9. Sexuality–reproductive pattern

   History:

   a. If appropriate (sexual partner within household or situation): Sexual relations satisfying? Changes? Problems?

   b. Use of family planning? Contraceptives? Problems?

   c. If appropriate (to age of children): Feel comfortable in explaining/discussing sexual subjects?

   Examination: None

10. Coping–stress-tolerance pattern

    History:

    a. Any big changes within family in last few years?

    b. Family tense or relaxed most of time? When tense what helps? Use of medicines, drugs, alcohol to decrease tension?

    c. When (if) family problems, how handled?

    d. Most of the time is this way(s) successful?

    Examination: None

11. Values–beliefs pattern

    History:

    a. Generally, family gets what it wants out of life?

    b. Important goals for the future?

    c. Any "rules" in the family that everyone believes are important?

    d. Religion important in family? Does this help when difficulties arise?

    Examination: None

Family Health and Functioning Assessment

I. Interview the family and obtain the following data:
   A. Demographic and family composition on a genogram
      1. Complete a three-generation genogram with legend and cultural heritage of all family members
      2. Identify the health status of each family member on the genogram
      3. Social networks of first generation members, including neighbor environment
   B. Family interactions
      Identify, discuss, and give examples for each of the following:
      1. Family structure
         a. Subsystems–identify all 5 subsystems
         b. Boundaries–include internal and external
         c. Roles of each family member
         d. Rules of the family–procedural and relational
         e. Triangles–identify all triangles [specify parentification and/or scapegoating]
      2. Family process
         a. Separateness/connectedness–describe this, including sexuality
         b. Enmeshment/disengagement–classify the family by one of these
         c. Communication–who communicates with whom and how
         d. Power–identify who has the power in the family
         e. Secrets/myths–how do they affect family process?
      3. Family spirituality
         a. Method by which family members express their spiritual domain
   C. Family development stage
      1. Identify Duvall's developmental stage[s] and family concerns within the stage[s]
   D. Family knowledge of health and illness
      1. Identify the family's knowledge in the following areas:
         a. Health maintenance and health promotion
         b. Physical and mental illnesses of members
         c. Management of illnesses of members, including medications and side effects
         d. Family coping methods

From Keltner N, Schwecke L, Bostrom C: *Psychiatric nursing,* ed 3, St Louis, 1999, Mosby.

      e. Resources such as family support, legal, financial, and community agencies

      f. Treatment options availability

II. Summary

  A. Discuss developmental and health problems in relationship to family (1) structure, (2) process, and (3) spirituality

  B. Discuss family strengths related to structure, process, spirituality, and social networks

  C. Discuss family problems related to structure, process, spirituality, and social networks

  D. Discuss the family's knowledge of health and illness

III. Goals for the family

As members of the treatment team, ask the family to identify the following:

  A. Changes to be made for a more effective functioning family

  B. Present needs of the family to better care for family members

  C. Family's and/or significant others' role in discharge planning

IV. Interventions

Indicate interventions and/or referrals related to specific assessment data and family goals

Family health assessment summary

Family's sociodemographic profile

Family's environment—strengths and problems regarding home, neighborhood, and community

Family structure, processes, functions—strengths and limitations, existing or potential problems

Family's coping profile

  Conflict management—strengths and limitations

  Life changes—strengths and limitations regarding coping with changes

  Support systems—strengths and limitations

  Life satisfaction profile

Family's health behavior profile

  Health history—existing or potential problems

  Health status—existing or potential problems

  Activities of daily living—strengths and limitations or problems

  Risk profile—for family unit and family members

  Health beliefs profile of values, attitudes, and beliefs regarding health and illness

Self-care—strengths and limitations

Healthcare resources—adequacy of availability, accessibility, attractiveness, and use; general practices

Community health nursing services—attitudes and expectations

Suggested Areas for Assessment of Family Health-Related Lifestyle

Nutrition
1. Meals prepared in the home are generally consistent with the food guide pyramid.
2. Healthy snacks are consumed in the home.
3. Knowledge about healthy eating habits is shared among family members.
4. Mutual assistance occurs among family members for maintenance of recommended weights and avoidance of overweight and underweight.
5. Family members praise each other for healthy eating.
6. Family members encourage each other to drink 6-8 glasses of water per day.
7. Family members base purchase decisions on nutritional labels on food.

Physical activity
1. Many family outings consist of vigorous or moderate physical activity.
2. Exercise equipment is available within the home.
3. Use of home exercise equipment is part of "family time."
4. Family members expect each other to be physically active.
5. A family membership is held in recreational facilities or programs.
6. Time together is seldom spent watching television or playing video games.
7. Family prefers to spend as much time out-of-doors as possible.

Stress control and management
1. Family manages time well to minimize stressful demands on members
2. Family often relaxes, shares stories, and laughs together.
3. Emotional expression is encouraged within the family.
4. Family members share stressful experiences with each other.
5. Family members offer each other assistance with difficult tasks.
6. Family members seldom "get on each other" about their faults.
7. Periods of relaxation and sleep are considered important by the family.

Health responsibility
1. A schedule for preventive care visits is maintained by the family.
2. Family often discusses news and articles about health topics.
3. Family members are encouraged to seek healthcare early if a problem develops.
4. Personal responsibility for health is encouraged by the family.
5. Family feels a sense of responsibility for the health of the family and each member.

From Pender MJ: *Health promotion in nursing practice,* ed 3, 1996, Appleton & Lange.

6. Health professionals are consulted about health promotion as well as care in illness.
7. Appropriate protective behaviors are openly discussed and encouraged (abstinence, use of condoms, hearing protection, eye protection, sunscreen).

Family resilience and resources
1. Worship or spiritual experiences are a regular part of family activities.
2. Family members share a sense of "togetherness" despite difficult life events.
3. Family has a common sense of purpose in life.
4. Family members encourage each other to "keep going" when life is difficult.
5. Growth in positive directions is mutually encouraged within the family.
6. Health is nurtured as a positive family resource.
7. Personal strengths and capabilities are nurtured.

Family support
1. Family has a number of friends or relatives that they see frequently.
2. Family is involved in community activities and groups.
3. Family members frequently praise each other.
4. In times of distress, the family can call on a number of other families or individuals for help.
5. Disagreements are settled through discussion rather than verbal abuse or physical violence.
6. Family members model healthy habits for each other.
7. Professional support services are sought when needed.

STAGES OF FAMILY LIFE CYCLES
Suggested use
The life cycle of the family consists of a series of periods characterized by states of movement or change and quiescence or stability. The times of change represent an instability in the structures and may lead to crisis or illness. The following is a guide to assist in assessing periods of family change which may affect health.

Family Career: Stages, Tasks, and Transitions

Period	Family stage	Family tasks	Family transitions
Early Adulthood	Families without children Families with infants Families with preschoolers	Provide economic resources that secure shelter, food, and clothing	Transitions or times of change are expected in families
Middle Adulthood	Families with school-age children Families with adolescents	Develop emotionally healthy individuals who manage crises and experience achievement	Families reorganize predictably when children grow
Late Adulthood	Launching children Middle-aged families Aging families	Ensure each member's socialization as a member of society in school, work, spiritual, and community life Give birth, adopt a child, or contribute to next generation Promote health and care for members experiencing injury, disease, and illness	Families reorganize when unpredictable changes occur in personal relationships, role and status, environment, physical and mental capabilities, and when there is loss of possessions Family routines change at transition points Family rituals acknowledge and celebrate family transition points

From Hanson S, Boyd S: *Family health care nursing: theory, practice, and research*, Philadelphia, 1996, FA Davis.

Family Stage-Specific Risk Factors and Related Health Problems

Stage	Risk factors	Health problem
Beginning childbearing family	Lack of knowledge about family planning	Premature baby
	Teenage marriage	Unsuccessful marriage
	Lack of knowledge concerning sexual and marital roles and adjustments	Low birth-weight infant
	Underweight or overweight	Birth defects
	Lack of prenatal care	Birth injuries
	Inadequate nutrition	Accidents
	Poor food habits	Sudden infant death syndrome (SIDS)
	Smoking, alcohol, drug abuse	Respiratory distress syndrome (RDS)
	Unmarried status	Sterility
	First pregnancy before age 16 or after age 35	Pelvic inflammatory disease (PID)
	History of hypertension and infections during pregnancy	Fetal alcohol syndrome (FAS)
	Rubella, syphilis, gonorrhea, and acquired immunodeficiency syndrome (AIDS)	Mental retardation
	Genetic factors present	Child abuse
	Low socioeconomic and educational levels	Injuries
	Lack of safety in the home	Birth defects
	Home unsafe	

Modified from US Department of Health and Human Services: *Healthy people 2000: national health promotion and disease prevention objectives,* Public Health Service 91-50212, Washington, DC, 1990, US Government Printing Office.

Continued

Family Stage-Specific Risk Factors and Related Health Problems—cont'd

Stage	Risk factors	Health problem
Family with school-age children	Home unstimulating Working parents with inappropriate use of resources for child care Poverty environment Abuse and/or neglect of children Generational pattern of using social agencies as a way of life Multiple, closely spaced children Low family self-esteem Children used as scapegoat for parental frustration Repeated infections, accidents, or hospitalizations Parents immature, dependent, and unable to handle responsibility Unrecognized or unattended health problems Strong beliefs about physical punishment Toxic substances unprotected in the home Poor nutrition (overeating and undereating)	Behavior disturbances Speech and vision problems Communicable diseases Dental caries School problems Learning disabilities Cancer Injuries Chronic diseases Homicide Violence
Family with adolescents	Racial and ethnic family origin Lifestyle and behavior patterns leading to chronic disease Lack of problem-solving skills Family values of aggressiveness and competition Socioeconomic factors contributing to peer relationships Family values rigid and inflexible Daredevil, risk-taking attitudes Denial behavior	Violent deaths and injuries Alcohol and drug abuse Unwanted pregnancy Sexually transmitted diseases Suicide Depression

Family with middle-age adults	Conflicts between parents and children	
	Pressure to live up to family expectations	
	Genetic predisposition	Cardiovascular disease, principally coronary artery disease and cerebrovascular accident (stroke)
	Hypertension	
	Smoking	
	High cholesterol level	
	Diabetes	
	Overweight	
	Physical inactivity	
	Personality patterns related to stress	
	Use of oral contraceptives	Cancer
	Sex, race, and other hereditary factors	Accidents
	Geographic area, age, occupational deficiencies	Homicide
	Habits (diet with low fiber, pickling, charcoal use, broiling)	Suicide
	Alcohol abuse	Abnormal fetus
	Exposure to certain substances (sunlight, radiation, water or air pollution)	Mental illness
	Socioeconomic class	
	Residence	
	Depression	
	Gingivitis	Periodontal disease and loss of teeth

Continued

Family Stage-Specific Risk Factors and Related Health Problems—cont'd

Stage	Risk factors	Health problem
Family with older adults	Age	Mental confusion
	Drug interactions	Reduced vision
	Depression	Hearing impairment
	Metabolic disorders	Hypertension
	Pituitary malfunctions	Acute illness
	Cushing's disease	Infectious disease
	Hypercalcemia	Influenza
	Chronic illness	Pneumonia
	Retirement	Injuries such as burns and falls
	Loss of spouse	Depression
	Reduced income	Chronic disease
	Poor nutrition	Elder abuse
	Lack of exercise	Death without dignity
	Past enviroments and lifestyle	
	Lack of preparation for death	

The Eight-Stage Family Life Cycle

Stage I	Beginning families (also referred to as married couples or the stage of marriage)
Stage II	Childbearing families (the oldest child is an infant through 30 months)
Stage III	Families with preschool children (oldest child is 2½ to 6 years of age)
Stage IV	Families with school children (oldest child is 6 to 13 years of age)
Stage V	Families with teenagers (oldest child is 13 to 20 years of age)
Stage VI	Families launching young adults (covering the first child who has left through the last child leaving home)
Stage VII	Middle-aged parents (empty nest through retirement)
Stage VIII	Family in retirement and old age (also referred to as aging family members or retirement to death of both spouses)

Hanson S, Boyd S: *Family health care nursing: theory, practice, and research,* Philadelphia, 1996, FA Davis.

Comparison of Family Life Cycle Stages of Duvall and Miller with Carter and McGoldrick

Family therapy perspective (Carter and McGoldrick)	Sociological perspective (Duvall and Miller)
1. Between families: the unattached young adult	No stage identified here, although Duvall considers young adult to be in process of "being launched." Because there is often a considerable time period between adolescence and marriage, addition of this "between stage" is indicated.
2. The joining of families through marriage: the newly married couple	1. Beginning families or the stage of marriage

Adapted from Carter B, McGoldrick M, editors: *The changing family life cycle,* ed 2, New York, 1988, Gardner Press; Duvall E, Miller B: *Marriage and family development,* ed 6, New York, 1985, Harper & Row.   *Continued*

Comparison of Family Life Cycle Stages of Duvall and Miller with Carter and McGoldrick—cont'd

Family therapy perspective (Carter and McGoldrick)	Sociological perspective (Duvall and Miller)
3. Families with young children (infancy through school age)	2. Childbearing families (oldest child up to 30 months of age)
	3. Families with preschool children (oldest child is 2½ to 5 years of age)
	4. Families with school-aged children (oldest child is 6 to 12 years of age)
4. Families with adolescents	5. Families with teenagers (oldest child is 13 to 20 years of age)
5. Launching children and moving on	6. Families launching young adults (all children leaving home)
	7. Middle-aged parents (empty nest up to retirement)
6. Families in later life	8. Families in retirement and old age (retirement to death of both spouses)

Dislocations of the Family Life Cycle by Divorce, Requiring Additional Steps to Restabilize and Proceed Developmentally

Phase	Emotional process of transition—prerequisite attitude	Developmental issues
Divorce		
1. The decision to divorce	Acceptance of inability to resolve marital tensions sufficiently to continue relationship	Acceptance of one's own part in the failure of the marriage
2. Planning the breakup of the system	Supporting viable arrangements for all parts of the system	Working cooperatively on problems of custody, visitation, and finances Dealing with extended family about the divorce
3. Separation	Willingness to continue cooperative co-parental relationship and joint financial support of children Work on resolution of attachment to spouse	Mourning loss of intact family Restructuring marital and parent-child relationships and finances, adaptation to living apart Realignment of relationships with extended family, staying connected with spouse's extended family

From Carter B, McGoldrick M, editors: *The changing family life cycle*, ed 2, New York, 1988, Gardner Press.

Continued

Dislocations of the Family Life Cycle by Divorce, Requiring Additional Steps to Restabilize and Proceed Developmentally—cont'd

Phase	Emotional process of transition— prerequisite attitude	Developmental issues
4. The divorce	More work on emotional divorce: overcoming hurt, anger, guilt, etc.	Mourning loss of intact family: giving up fantasies of reunion Retrieval of hopes, dreams, expectations from the marriage Staying connected with extended families
Postdivorce family		
1. Single-parent (custodial household or primary residence)	Willingness to maintain financial responsibilities, continue parental contact with ex-spouse, and support contact of children with ex-spouse and his or her family	Making flexible visitation arrangements with ex-spouse and his or her family Rebuilding own financial resources Rebuilding own social network
2. Single-parent (noncustodial)	Willingness to maintain parental contact with ex-spouse and support custodial parent's relationships with children	Finding ways to continue effective parenting relationship with children Maintaining financial responsibilities to ex-spouse and children Rebuilding own social network

Remarried Family Formation: A Developmental Outline

Steps	Prerequisite attitude	Developmental issues
1. Entering the new relationship	Recovery from loss of first marriage (adequate "emotional divorce")	Recommitment to marriage and to forming a family with readiness to deal with the complexity and ambiguity
2. Conceptualizing and planning new marriage and family	Accepting one's own fears and those of new spouse and children about remarriage and forming a stepfamily	Work on openness in the new relationships to avoid pseudomutuality
		Plan for maintenance of cooperative financial and coparental relationships with ex-spouse(s)
	Accepting need for time and patience for adjustment to complexity and ambiguity of: 1. Multiple new roles 2. Boundaries: space, time, membership, and authority 3. Affective issues: guilt, loyalty conflicts, desire for mutuality, unresolvable past hurts	Plan to help children deal with fears, loyalty conflicts, and membership in two systems
		Realignment of relationships with extended family to include new spouse and children
		Plan maintenance of connections for children with extended family of ex-spouse(s)
3. Remarriage and reconstitution of family	Final resolution of attachment to previous spouse and ideal of "intact" family; acceptance of a different model of family with permeable boundaries	Restructuring family boundaries to allow for inclusion of new spouse or step-parent
		Realignment of relationships and financial arrangements throughout subsystems to permit interweaving of several systems
		Making room for relationships of all children with biological (noncustodial) parents, grandparents, and other extended family
		Sharing memories and histories to enhance stepfamily integration

From Carter B, McGoldrick M, editors: *The changing family life cycle,* ed 2, New York, 1988, Gardner Press.

OTHER FAMILY ASSESSMENT TOOLS

Cultural Heritage Assessment Tool

This set of questions is to be used to describe a given client's—or your own—ethnic, cultural, and religious background. In performing a *heritage assessment* it is helpful to determine how deeply a given person identifies with his or her traditional heritage. This tool is most useful in setting the stage for assessing and understanding a person's traditional health and illness beliefs and practices and in helping to determine the community resources that will be appropriate to target for support when necessary. The greater the number of positive responses, the greater the degree to which the person may identify with his or her traditional heritage. The one exception to positive answers is the question about whether or not a person's name was changed.

1. Where was your mother born? _____
2. Where was your father born? _____
3. Where were your grandparents born? _____
   a. Your mother's mother? _____
   b. Your mother's father? _____
   c. Your father's mother? _____
   d. Your father's father? _____
4. How many brothers ____ and sisters ____ do you have?
5. What setting did you grow up in? Urban ____ Rural ____
6. What country did your parents grow up in?
   Father _____
   Mother _____
7. How old were you when you came to the United States? ____
8. How old were your parents when they came to the United States?
   Mother? ____ Father? ____
9. When you were growing up, who lived with you?
   _____
10. Have you maintained contact with
    a. Aunts, uncles, cousins?   (1) Yes ____ (2) No ____
    b. Brothers and sisters?   (1) Yes ____ (2) No ____
    c. Parents?   (1) Yes ____ (2) No ____
    d. Your own children?   (1) Yes ____ (2) No ____
11. Did most of your aunts, uncles, cousins live near your home?
    (1) Yes ____ (2) No ____
12. Approximately how often did you visit family members who lived outside of your home?
    (1) Daily ____ (2) Weekly ____ (3) Monthly ____
    (4) Once a year or less ____ (5) Never ____

From Spector R: *Cultural diversity in health and illness,* ed 5, Upper Saddle River, NJ, 2000, Prentice Hall Health.

13. Was your original family name changed?
    (1) Yes _____ (2) No _____
14. What is your religious preference?
    (1) Catholic _____ (2) Jewish _____
    (3) Protestant _____ Denomination _____
    (4) Other _____ (5) None _____
15. Is your spouse the same religion as you?
    (1) Yes _____ (2) No _____
16. Is your spouse the same ethnic background as you?
    (1) Yes _____ (2) No _____
17. What kind of school did you go to?
    (1) Public _____ (2) Private _____ (3) Parochial _____
18. Do you live in a neighborhood where the neighbors are the same religion and ethnic background as yourself?
    (1) Yes _____ (2) No _____
19. Do you belong to a religious institution?
    (1) Yes _____ (2) No _____
20. Would you describe yourself as an active member?
    (1) Yes _____ (2) No _____
21. How often do you attend your religious institution?
    (1) More than once a week _____ (2) Weekly _____
    (3) Monthly _____ (4) Special holidays only _____
    (5) Never _____
22. Do you practice your religion in your home?
    (1) Yes _____ (2) No _____ If yes, please specify:
    (3) Praying _____ (4) Bible reading _____ (5) Diet _____
    (6) Celebrating religious holidays _____
23. Do you prepare foods special to your ethnic background?
    (1) Yes _____ (2) No _____
24. Do you participate in ethnic activities?
    (1) Yes _____ (2) No _____ If yes, please specify:
    (3) Singing _____ (4) Holiday celebrations _____
    (5) Dancing _____ (6) Festivals _____
    (7) Costumes _____ (8) Other _____
25. Are your friends from the same religious background as you?
    (1) Yes _____ (2) No _____
26. Are your friends from the same ethnic background as you?
    (1) Yes _____ (2) No _____
27. What is your native language? _____
28. Do you speak this language?
    (1) Prefer _____ (2) Occasionally _____ (3) Rarely _____
29. Do you read your native language?
    (1) Yes _____ (2) No _____

Religious Beliefs That Affect Nursing Care

Beliefs about birth and death	Beliefs about diet and food practices	Beliefs regarding medical care	Comments
Adventist (Seventh-Day Adventist; Church of God; Christian church)			
Birth: Opposed to infant baptism Baptism in adulthood **Death:** Believe the dead are asleep until the return of Jesus Christ, at which time final rewards and punishments will be given **Organ donation/transplantation:** Individual and family have the right to receive or donate those organs that will restore any of the senses or will prolong life	Meat is prohibited in some groups No alcohol, coffee, or tea	Some believe in divine healing and practice anointing with oil and use of prayer May desire Communion or baptism when ill Believe in man's choice and God's sovereignty Some oppose hypnosis as therapy	Saturday is the biblical day of worship
Baptist (27 groups)			
Birth: Opposed to infant baptism Believers are baptized by immersion as adults **Death:** Clergy seeks to minister by counsel and prayer with patient and family	Some groups discourage coffee, tea, and alcohol	"Laying on of hands" (some) May encounter some resistance to some therapies, such as abortion Believe God functions through physician	Fundamentalist and conservative groups accept Bible as inspired word of God

Organ donation/transplantation: Both organ donation and transplantation are generally approved of when they do not seriously endanger donor and when they offer medical hope for recipient; a transplant must offer possibility of physical improvement and extension of human life		Some believe in predestination; may respond passively to care	
Black Muslim			General adherence to Moslem tenets is overlaid, in many instances, by antagonism to whites, especially Christians and Jews. Do not indulge in activities (such as sleeping) more than is necessary to health
Birth: No baptism	Prohibit alcohol, pork, and foods traditional among American blacks (e.g., corn bread, collard greens)	Faith healing is unacceptable. Always maintain personal habits of cleanliness	
Death: Have a carefully prescribed procedure for washing and shrouding the dead and performing funeral rites			
Organ donation/transplantation: To Muslims, life is precious; will accept a transplant if required to live			
Buddhist Churches of America			Optimistic outlook; teach ways to overcome fears, anxieties, apprehension
Birth: No infant baptism. Infant presentation	No requirements or restrictions. Some sects are strictly vegetarian	Illness is believed to be a trial to aid development of soul; illness due to Karmic causes	

Continued

Sources: Carpenito, 1992; Conley, 1990; Kozier and Erb, 1995; McQuay, 1995; Spector, 1985. In Wong D, et al: *Whaley and Wong's nursing care of infants and children*, ed 6, St Louis, 1999, Mosby.

Religious Beliefs That Affect Nursing Care—cont'd

Beliefs about birth and death	Beliefs about diet and food practices	Beliefs regarding medical care	Comments
Buddhist Churches of America—cont'd			
Death: "Last rite" chanting is often practiced at bedside soon after death; the deceased's Buddhist priest should be contacted, or family should contact him	Discourage use of alcohol and drugs	May be reluctant to have surgery or certain treatments on holy days Cleanliness is believed to be of great importance Family may request Buddhist priest for counseling	
Organ donation/transplantation: Believe that organ donation is a matter of individual conscience; there is no written resolution on the issue			
Church of Christ Scientist (Christian Science)			
Birth: No baptism	No requirements or restrictions	Deny the existence of health crisis; see sickness and sin as errors of the mind that can be altered by prayer Oppose human intervention with drugs or other therapies; however, accept legally required immunizations	Many desire services of practitioner or reader; will sometimes refuse even emergency treatment until they have consulted a reader
Death: No "last rites"; autopsy is not permitted except in cases of sudden death; it is an individual's decision to choose burial or cremation			Unlikely to donate organs for transplant
Organ donation/transplantation: Church takes no specific position on transplantation or donation as distinct from			

other medical or surgical procedures; members normally rely on spiritual rather than medical means for healing, but they are free to choose whatever form of medical treatment they desire, including organ transplantation

Many adhere to belief that disease is human mental concept that can be dispelled by "spiritual truth" to extent that they refuse all medical treatment

Church of Jesus Christ of Latter Day Saints (Mormon)

Birth:

No baptism at birth

Infant is "blessed" by church official at first opportunity after birth (in church)

Baptism by immersion at 8 years

Death: Believe that it is proper to bury the dead in the ground and cremation is discouraged; baptism of the dead is held as essential, although a living person may serve as proxy; preaching of the gospel to the dead is also practiced

Organ donation/transplantation: Question of whether one should will his or her organs to be used as transplants or for research after death must be answered from deep within conscience of the individual involved

Prohibit tea, coffee, alcohol

Some individuals avoid chocolate and other products that contain caffeine

Encourage sparing use of meats

Fasting for 24 hours on first Sunday of each month (from after evening meal Saturday until evening meal Sunday)

Devout adherents believe in divine healing through anointment with oil and "laying on of hands" by church officials (appointed church members)

Medical therapy is not prohibited

May request *Sacrament* on Sunday while in hospital

Financial support for sick is available through well-funded welfare system

Discourage cremation

Discourage use of tobacco

Married adults wear special undergarments

Continued

Religious Beliefs That Affect Nursing Care—cont'd

Beliefs about birth and death	Beliefs about diet and food practices	Beliefs regarding medical care	Comments
Eastern Orthodox (Turkey, Egypt, Syria, Rumania, Bulgaria, Cyprus, Albania, etc.)			
Birth: Most believe in infant baptism by immersion 8 to 40 days after birth **Death:** "Last rites" are obligatory if death is impending; cremation is discouraged **Organ donation/transplantation:** No religious conflict; both are permitted	Restrictions depend on specific sect	Anointment of the sick No conflict with medical science	Discourage cremation
Episcopal (Anglican)			
Birth: Infant baptism is mandatory; urgent if poor prognosis **Death:** "Last rites" (Rite for Anointing of the Sick) are not mandatory for all members; when death is imminent, family and pastor are gathered, and it is usually highly desirable to have Litany at the Time of Death read; infant baptism is mandatory and especially urgent if prognosis is poor, although aborted fetuses and stillborns are not baptized	Abstain from meat on fast days May fast on Wednesday, Friday, during Lent, and before Christmas Some fast for 6 hours before receiving Holy Communion	Some believe in spiritual healing Rite for anointing of the sick is available but not mandatory	Religious icons are very important Communion four times yearly: Christmas, Easter, June 30, and August 15; may be mandatory for some

Organ donation/transplantation: Find nothing offensive in organ donation/transplantation as long as moral integrity of donor is not violated

Friends (Quakers)

Birth:
No baptism
Infant's name is recorded in official book

Death: Do not believe in life after this life; God is in every person and can be approached directly

Organ donation/transplantation: Are in agreement with philosophy and concepts of organ donation/transplantation; both are permitted

No requirements or restrictions
Most practice moderation
Avoid alcohol and illicit drugs

No special rites or restrictions

Believe in plain speech and dress
Pacifists

Greek Orthodox

Birth:
Baptism is considered important; performed 40 days after birth
If not possible to baptize by sprinkling or immersion, church allows child baptism "in the air" by moving child in the form of a cross as appropriate words are said

Church-prescribed fast periods—usually occur on Wednesday, Friday, and during Lent; consist of avoiding meat and (in some cases) dairy products
If health is compromised, priest may be contacted to

Each health crisis is handled by ordained priest; deacon may also serve in some cases
Holy Communion is administered in hospital
Some may desire Sacrament of the Holy Unction per-

Oppose euthanasia
Believe every reasonable effort should be made to preserve life until termination by God
Discourage autopsies that may cause dismemberment

Continued

Religious Beliefs That Affect Nursing Care—cont'd

Beliefs about birth and death	Beliefs about diet and food practices	Beliefs regarding medical care	Comments
Greek Orthodox—cont'd			
Death: "Last rites" are Sacrament of Holy Communion; death rituals play a crucial role in life of family; death must be properly mourned, or else dead person may not be fully incorporated in world of the dead and may return to world of the living and inflict harm on close relatives	convince family to forego fasting	formed by priest	Prefer burial to cremation
Organ donation/transplantation: Organ transplantation such as skin grafting and blood transfusions from one human to another have always been acceptable; this is extended to include kidney transplants, heart transplants, etc.; life of donor, however, is of equal importance			

Hindu

Birth: No ritual

Death: Certain prescribed rites are followed after death; priest may tie thread around neck or wrist to signify blessing, and this should not be removed; immediately after death, priest will pour water into the mouth of the corpse, and family will wash the body; are particular about who touches their dead; bodies are to be cremated

Organ donation/transplantation: According to Hindu Temple of North America, they are not prohibited by religious laws from donating their organs; this is an individual decision

Many dietary restrictions
Beef and veal are not eaten
Some are strict vegetarians

Illness or injury is believed to represent sins committed in previous life
Accept most modern medical practices

Cremation is preferred

Continued

Religious Beliefs That Affect Nursing Care—cont'd

Beliefs about birth and death	Beliefs about diet and food practices	Beliefs regarding medical care	Comments
Islam (Muslim/Moslem)			
Birth: No baptism	Prohibit all pork products and any meat that is not ritually slaughtered	Faith healing is not acceptable unless psychologic condition of patient is deteriorating; performed for morale	Older Muslims often have a fatalistic view that may interfere with compliance to therapy
Death: Must confess sins and beg forgiveness before death, and family should be present; family washes and prepares the body and then turns it to face Mecca; only relatives and friends may touch the body and, unless required by law, there should be no autopsy; no body part should be removed unless for donation	Daylight fasting is practiced during ninth month of Muhammadan year (Ramadan) Strict Muslims do not use alcohol or mind-altering drugs	Ritual washing after prayer; prayer takes place five times daily (on rising, midday, afternoon, early evening, and before bed); during prayer, face Mecca and kneel on prayer rug	May oppose autopsy
Organ donation/transplantation: Moslem Religious Council initially rejected organ donation by followers of Islam, but it has since reversed its position, provided that donors consent in advance in writing; organs of Moslem donors must be transplanted immediately and not stored in organ banks			

Continued

Jehovah's Witness

Birth: No baptism

Death: No official "last rites" practiced when death occurs

Organ donation/transplantation: No definite statement related to this issue; do not encourage organ donation but believe it is a matter for individual conscience, according to Watch Tower Society (legal corporation for the religion); all organs and tissues, however, must be completely drained of blood before transplantation

Eat nothing to which blood has been added; can eat animal flesh that has been drained

Adherents are generally absolutely opposed to transfusions of whole blood, packed red blood cells, platelets, and fresh or frozen plasma, including banking of own blood; individuals can sometimes be persuaded in emergencies

May be opposed to use of albumin, globulin, factor replacement (hemophilia), vaccines

Not opposed to nonblood plasma expanders

Often possible to obtain a court order appointing a hospital official as temporary guardian to consent to a child's transfusion when parents refuse consent

Autopsy is approved only as required by law

No restrictions on giving blood sample

Judaism (Orthodox and Conservative)

Birth:

No baptism

Ritual circumcision of male infants on eighth day; performed by Mohel (ritual circumciser familiar with Jewish law and aseptic technique)

Reform Jews favor ritual circumcision, but not as a religious imperative

Numerous dietary kosher laws exist that may be influenced by local practices and family and cultural tradition

Are allowed only meat from animals that are vegetable eaters, are cloven hoofed,

May resist surgical procedures during Sabbath, which extends from sundown Friday until sundown Saturday

Seriously ill and pregnant women are exempt from fasting

Illness is grounds for violating

Oppose all forms of mutilation, including autopsy; amputated limbs, organs, or surgically removed tissues should be made available to family for burial

Donation or transplanta-

Religious Beliefs That Affect Nursing Care—cont'd

Beliefs about birth and death	Beliefs about diet and food practices	Beliefs regarding medical care	Comments
Judaism (Orthodox and Conservative)—cont'd			
Death: According to tradition, during last moments of life, relatives and close friends remain with the deceased; it is considered a matter of great respect to watch over a person as he or she passes from this world to the next	chew their cud, and are ritually slaughtered; fish that have scales and fins Prohibit any combination of meat and milk; milk products served first can be followed by meat in a few minutes, but milk may not be consumed for several hours after eating meat Fasting for 24 hours is part of Yom Kippur observance Matzo replaces leavened bread during Passover week	dietary laws (e.g., patient with congestive heart failure does not have to use kosher meats, which are high in sodium)	tion of organs requires rabbinical consent May oppose prolongation of life after irreversible brain damage
Organ donation/transplantation: Donation or transplantation of organs requires rabbinical consultation; sanctity of the human body covers each of its members and organs, so where any part of the body is separated from the corpus it, too, requires burial; where an organ is to be transplanted to save the life of a patient or improve his or her health, however, it is permitted; saving a human life takes precedence over maintaining sanctity of the human body			

Lutheran

Birth: Baptize only living infants shortly after birth

Death: "Last rites" are optional

Organ donation/transplantation: Ability to transplant organs from a deceased person to a living person is considered a genuine medical advancement; both are acceptable and encouraged

No requirements or restrictions

Church or pastor is notified of hospitalization

Communion may be given before or after surgery or similar crisis

Accept scientific developments

Mennonite (similar to Amish)

Birth:

No baptism in infancy

Baptism during early or middle teens

Death: No formal prescribed action; personal assistance and prayer as appropriate while patient is still conscious is necessary

Organ donation/transplantation: No religious conflict, so both organ donation and transplantation are acceptable

No requirements or restrictions

No illness rituals

Deep concern for dignity and self-determination of individual that would conflict with shock treatment or medical treatment affecting personality or will

Continued

Religious Beliefs That Affect Nursing Care—cont'd

Beliefs about birth and death	Beliefs about diet and food practices	Beliefs regarding medical care	Comments
Methodist **Birth:** No baptism at birth; performed on children or adults **Death:** Believe in divine punishment after death; good will be rewarded and evil punished **Organ donation/transplantation:** Church encourages "people of ethical concern in various relevant fields to get together to engage in study and direction of these developments," recognizing that they offer great potentialities for enhancing health while at the same time raising serious issues for traditional views of human nature and value	No requirements or restrictions	Communion may be requested before surgery or similar crisis	Encourage donations of body or body parts to medical science

Nazarene

Birth: Baptism optional
Death: No last rites

No requirements or restrictions
Alcohol is prohibited

Church official administers Communion and laying on of hands
Adherents believe in divine healing but not exclusive of medical treatment

Cremation is permitted

Pentecostal (Assembly of God, Four-Square)

Birth:
No baptism at birth
Baptism by complete immersion after age of accountability
Death: No official "last rites" practiced when death occurs
Organ donation/transplantation: No official position on organ donation/transplantation

Abstain from alcohol, eating blood, strangled animals, or anything to which blood has been added
Some individuals may resist pork

No restrictions regarding medical care
Deliverance from sickness is provided for in atonement; may pray for divine intervention in health matters and seek God in prayer for themselves and others when ill

Some insist illness is divine punishment; most consider it an intrusion of Satan
Practice glossolalia (speaking in tongues)

Orthodox Presbyterian

Birth: Infant baptism by sprinkling
Death: "Last rites" are not a sacramental procedure and are not performed; instead, they read scripture and pray

No requirements or restrictions

Communion is administered when appropriate and convenient
Blood transfusion is accepted

Full forgiveness is granted for any illness connected with a sin

Continued

Religious Beliefs That Affect Nursing Care—cont'd

Beliefs about birth and death	Beliefs about diet and food practices	Beliefs regarding medical care	Comments
Orthodox Presbyterian—cont'd			
Organ donation/transplantation: Encourage and endorse organ donation; respect individual conscience and a person's right to make decisions regarding his or her own body		when advisable Pastor or elder should be called for ill person Believe science should be used for relief of suffering	
Roman Catholic			
Birth: Infant baptism is mandatory; especially urgent if poor prognosis, when it may be performed by anyone	Fasting (eating only one full meal and no eating between meals) and abstaining from meat are mandatory on Ash Wednesday and Good Friday; fasting is optional during Lent; no meat on Fridays during Lent as a general rule Children and most hospital patients are exempt from fasting	Encourage anointing of the sick, although this may be interpreted by older members of church as equivalent to old terminology "extreme unction" or "last rites"; they may require careful explanation if reluctance is associated with fear of imminent death Traditional church teaching does not approve of contra-	Family may request that major amputated limb be buried in consecrated ground Transplantation is accepted as long as loss of organ does not deprive donor of life or functional integrity of body Autopsy is acceptable Religious articles are important
Death: Rite for Anointing of the Sick is a sacrament for the living; if prognosis is poor while patient is alive, patient or his or her family may request it			
Organ donation/transplantation: Transplantation of organs is viewed by Catholics as ethically and morally acceptable to Vatican; organ donation is an act of charity, fraternal love, and			

self-sacrifice; transplantation of organs from living donors is permissible when anticipated benefit to recipient is proportionate to harm done to donor (provided that loss of such organ[s] does not deprive donor of life itself or of functional integrity of his or her own body)	Some older Catholics may adhere to older rule of no meat on Friday	ceptives or abortion	
Russian Orthodox **Birth:** Baptism by priest only **Death:** Traditionally after death, arms are crossed, fingers set in a cross	No meat or dairy products on Wednesday, Friday, and during Lent	Cross necklace is important and should be removed only when necessary and replaced as soon as possible Adherents believe in divine healing, but not exclusive of medical treatment	Opposed to autopsy, embalming, or cremation
Unitarian Universalist **Birth:** Some practice infant baptism; most consider it unnecessary **Death:** No ritual	No requirements or restrictions	Most believe in general goodness of their fellow humans and appreciate expression of that goodness by visits from clergy and fellow parishioners during times of illness	Cremation is preferred to burial Believe in fully living this life as they know and understand it

Cultural Characteristics Related to Healthcare of Children and Families

Cultural group	Health beliefs	Health practices	Family relationships	Communication	Comments
Asians					
Chinese	A healthy body viewed as gift from parents and ancestors and must be cared for Health is one of the results of balance between the forces of *yin* (cold) and *yang* (hot)—energy forces that rule the world Illness caused by imbalance Believe blood is source of life and is not regenerated *Chi* is innate energy Lack of *chi* and blood results in deficiency that produces fatigue, poor constitution, and long illness	Goal of therapy is to restore balance of *yin* and *yang* Acupuncturist applies needles to appropriate meridians identified in terms of *yin* and *yang* Acupressure and *tai chi* replacing acupuncture in some areas *Moxibustion* is application of heat to skin over specific meridians Wide use of medicinal herbs procured and applied in prescribed ways	Extended family pattern common Strong concept of loyalty of young to old Respect for elders taught at early age—acceptance without questioning or talking back Children's behavior a reflection on family Family and individual honor and "face" important Self-reliance and self-restraint highly valued; self-expression repressed Males valued more highly than females; women submissive to men in family	Open expression of emotions unacceptable Often smile when do not comprehend	Do not react well to painful diagnostic workup; are especially upset by drawing of blood Deep respect for their bodies and believe it best to die with bodies intact; therefore may refuse surgery Believe in reincarnation Older members fear hospitals; often believe hospital is a place to go to die Children sometimes breast-fed for up to 4 or 5 years*

Japanese	Three major belief systems: *Shinto* religious influence Humans inherently good Evil caused by outside spirits Illness caused by contact with polluting agents (e.g., blood, corpses, skin diseases)	Believe evil removed by purification Energy restored by means of acupuncture, acupressure, massage, and moxibustion along affected meridians *Kampō* medicine—use of natural herbs Believe in removal of diseased parts Trend is to use both Western and Oriental	Folk healers are herbalist, spiritual healer, temple healer, fortune healer Meals may/may not be planned to balance hot/cold Milk intolerance relatively common Use of condiments (e.g., MSG and soy sauce) may create difficulty with some diet regimens (e.g., low-salt diets)	Close intergenerational relationships Family provides anchor Family tends to keep problems to self Value self-control and self-sufficiency Concept of *haji* (shame) imposes strong control; unacceptable behavior of children reflects on family Many adopt practices of	Issei—born in Japan; usually speak Japanese only Nisei, Sansei, and Yonsei have few language difficulties New immigrants able to read and write English better than able to speak or understand it Make significant use of nonverbal communication with subtle	Generational categories: *Issei*—1st generation to live in US *Nisei*—2nd generation *Sansei*—3rd generation *Yonsei*—4th generation Issei and Nisei—tolerant and permissive child-rearing until age 5 or 6, then emphasis on emotional reserve and control Cleanliness highly valued

*Most Asian cultures consider the child 1 year old at the time of birth. Traditional Chinese custom adds 1 year on January 1 regardless of the birthday—a child born in December is 2 years old the following January.

Sources: Anderson and Fenichel, 1989; Clark, 1981; DeSantis, 1988; Geissler, 1994; Giger and Davidhizar, 1995; Holland and Sweeney, 1985; Hollingsworth, Brown, and Brooten, 1980; Orgue, Bloch, and Monrroy, 1983; Randall-David, 1989; Sodetaini-Shibata, 1981. In Wong D, et al: *Whaley and Wong's nursing care of infants and children,* ed 6, St Louis, 1999, Mosby.

Continued

Cultural Characteristics Related to Healthcare of Children and Families—cont'd

Cultural group	Health beliefs	Health practices	Family relationships	Communication	Comments
Asians—cont'd					
Japanese—cont'd	Chinese and Korean influence Health achieved through harmony and balance between self and society Disease caused by disharmony with society and not caring for body Portuguese influence Upholds germ theory of disease	healing methods Care for disabled viewed as family's responsibility Take pride in child's good health Seek preventive care, medical care for illness May avoid some food combinations (e.g., milk and cherries, watermelon and crab) and believe pickled plums to have special properties	contemporary middle class Concern for child's missing school may result in sending to school before fully recovered from illness	gestures and facial expression Tend to suppress emotions Will often wait silently	Time considered valuable and used wisely Tendency to practice emotional control may make assessment of pain more difficult

Viet-namese	Good health considered to be balance between *yin* and *yang*	Family uses all means possible before using outside agencies for healthcare	Family is revered institution	Many immigrants are not proficient in speaking and understanding English	Consider status more important than money
	Believe person's life has been predisposed toward certain phenomena by cosmic forces	Fortune-tellers determine event that caused disturbance	Multigenerational families	May hesitate to ask questions	Children taught emotional control
	Health believed to be result of harmony with existing universal order; harmony attained by pleasing good spirits and avoiding evil ones	May visit temple to procure divine instruction	Family is chief social network	Questioning authority is sign of disrespect; asking questions considered impolite	Time concept more relaxed—consider punctuality less significant than other values (i.e., propriety)
	Belief in *am duc*, the amount of good deeds accumulated by ancestors	Use astrologer to calculate cyclic changes and forces	Children highly valued	Use indirectness rather than forthrightness in expressing disagreement	Place high value on social harmony
	Many use rituals to prevent illness	Regard health as family responsibility; outside aid sought when resources run out	Individual needs and interests are subordinate to those of a family group	May avoid eye contact with health professionals as a sign of respect	
	Practice some restrictions to prevent incurring wrath of evil spirits	Certain illnesses considered only temporary (such as pustules, open wounds) and ignored	Father is main decision maker		
		Seek generalist health healers	Women taught submission to men		
		May use special diets to prevent illness and promote health	Parents expect respect and obedience from children		
		Lactose intolerance prevalent			

Continued

Cultural Characteristics Related to Healthcare of Children and Families—cont'd

Cultural group	Health beliefs	Health practices	Family relationships	Communication	Comments
Filipinos	Believe God's will and supernatural forces govern universe Illness, accidents, and other misfortunes are God's punishment for violations of His will Widely accept "hot" and "cold" balance and imbalance as cause of health and illness	Some use amulets as a shield from witchcraft or as good luck pieces Catholics substitute religious medals and other items	Family is highly valued, with strong family ties Multigenerational family structure common, often with collateral members as well Personal interests are subordinated to family interests and needs Members avoid any behavior that would bring shame on the family	Immigrants and older persons may not be able to speak or understand English	Tend to have a fatalistic outlook on life Believe time and providence will solve all
African-American	Illness classified as: Natural—affected by forces of nature without adequate protection (e.g., cold air, pollution, food and water)	Self-care and folk medicine very prevalent Folk therapies usually religious in origin Attempt home remedies first; poorer people do	Strong kinship bonds in extended family; members come to aid of others in crisis group Less likely to view illness as a burden Augmented families com-	Alert to any evidence of discrimination Place importance on nonverbal behavior May use nonstandard English or "Black English"	High level of caution/distrust of majority group Social anxiety related to tradition of humiliation, oppression, and loss of dignity

Continued

Unnatural—evil influences (e.g., witchcraft, voodoo, hoodoo, hex, fix, root work); symptoms often associated with eating

Believe serious illness sent by God as punishment (e.g., parents punished by illness or death of child)

Believe serious illness can be avoided

May resist healthcare because illness is "will of God"

not seek help until illness serious

Usually seek help from: "old lady"—woman in community with a common knowledge of herbs; consulted regarding pediatric care

Spiritualist—has received gift from God for healing incurable diseases or solving personal problems; strongly based in Christianity

Priest (voodoo priest/priestess)—most powerful healer

Root doctor—meets need for herbs, oils, candles, and ointments

Prayer is common means for prevention and treatment

mon (unrelated persons living in same household)

Place strong emphasis on work and ambition

Sex-role sharing among parents

Elderly members respected

Use "testing" behaviors to assess personnel in healthcare situations before seeking active care

Best to use simple, direct, but caring approach

Will elect to retain dignity rather than seek care if values are compromised

Strong sense of peoplehood

High incidence of poverty

Black minister a strong influence in black community

Visits by family minister are sought, expected, and valued in helping to cope with illness and suffering

Cultural Characteristics Related to Healthcare of Children and Families—cont'd

Cultural group	Health beliefs	Health practices	Family relationships	Communication	Comments
African-American—cont'd					
Haitians*	Illnesses have a supernatural or natural origin	Health is a personal responsibility	Maintenance of family reputation is paramount	Recent immigrants and older persons may speak only Haitian creole	Will use biomedical and ethnomedical (folk) systems simultaneously
	Supernatural illnesses are caused by angry voodoo spirits, enemies, or the dead, especially deceased ancestors	Foods have properties of "hot"/"cold" and "light"/"heavy" and must be in harmony with one's life cycle and bodily states	Lineal authority supreme; children in a subordinate position in family hierarchy	May prefer family/friends to act as translators and confidants	Resistant to dietary and work restrictions
	Natural illnesses are based on conceptions of natural causation:	Natural illnesses are treated by home remedies first	Children valued for parental social security in old age and expected to contribute to family welfare at an early age	Often smile and nod in agreement when do not understand	Adherence to prescribed treatments directly related to perceived severity of illness
	Irregularities of blood volume, flow, purity, viscosity, color, and/ or temperature (hot/ cold)	Supernatural illness treated by healers: voodoo priest (houngan) or priestess (mambo), midwife (fam saj), and herbalist or leaf doctor (dokte fey)	Children viewed as "gifts from God" and treated with indulgence and affection	Quiet and gentle communication style and lack of assertiveness lead healthcare providers to falsely believe patients comprehend health teaching and are compliant	
	Gas (gaz)	Amulets and prayer used to protect against illness due to curses or willed by evil people		Will not ask questions if healthcare provider is busy or rushed	
	Movement and consistency of mother's milk				
	"Hot/cold" imbalance in the body				
	Bone displacement				
	Movement of diseases				

	Health is maintained by good dietary and hygienic habits				
Hispanics Mexicans (Latinos, Chicanos, Raza-Latinos)	Health beliefs have strong religious association Believe in body imbalance as a cause of illness, especially imbalance between *caliente* ("hot") and *frio* ("cold") or "wet" and "dry" Some maintain good health is a result of "good luck"—a reward for good behavior Illness prevented by performing properly, eating proper foods, and working proper amount of time; accomplished through prayer, wearing religious medals or amulets, and sleeping with relics at home	Seek help from *curandero* or *curandera*, especially in rural areas Curandero(a) receives his/her position by birth, apprenticeship, or a "calling" via dream or vision Treatments involve use of herbs, rituals, and religious artifacts Practice for severe illness—make promises, visit shrines, offer medals and candles, offer prayers Adhere to "hot" and "cold" food prescriptions and prohibitions for prevention and treatment of illness	Traditionally men considered breadwinners and key decision makers in matters outside the home; women considered homemakers Males considered big and strong (*macho*) Strong kinship; extended families include *compadres* (godparents) established by ritual kinship Children valued highly and desired, taken everywhere with family Many homes contain shrines with statues and pictures of saints Elderly treated with respect	May use nonstandard English Some bilingual; many speak only Spanish May have a strong preference for native language and revert to it in times of stress May shake hands or engage in introductory embrace Interpret prolonged eye contact as disrespectful	High degree of modesty—often a deterrent to seeking medical care and open discussions of sex Youngsters often reluctant to share communal showers in schools Relaxed concept of time—may be late for appointments More concerned with present than with future and therefore may focus on immediate solutions rather than long-term goals Magicoreligious practices common May view hospital as place to go to die

Continued

*This section was written by Lydia DeSantis, RN, PhD.

Cultural Characteristics Related to Healthcare of Children and Families—cont'd

Cultural group	Health beliefs	Health practices	Family relationships	Communication	Comments
Hispanics—cont'd					
Mexicans, etc.—cont'd	Illness is a punishment from God for wrongdoing, forces of nature, and the supernatural				
Puerto Ricans	Subscribe to the "hot–cold" theory of causation of illness Believe some illness caused by evil spirits and forces	Infrequent use of healthcare systems Seek folk healers—use of herbs, rituals Consult spiritualist medium for mental disorders *Santeria* is system, and practitioners are called *santeros* Treatments classified as "hot" or "cold"	Family usually large and home centered—the core of existence Father has complete authority in family—family provider and decision maker Wife and children subordinate to father Children valued—seen as a gift from God Children taught to obey and respect parents; corporal punishment to ensure obedience	May use nonstandard English Spanish speaking or bilingual Strong sense of family privacy—may view questions regarding family as impudent	Relaxed sense of time Pay little attention to *exact* time of day Suspicious and fearful of hospitals

| Cubans[†] | Prevention and good nutrition are related to good health | Diligent users of the medical model

Eclectic health-seeking practices, including preventive measures and, in some instances, folk medicine of both religious and nonreligious origins; home remedies; in many instances seek assistance of santeros and spiritualists to complement medical treatment

Nutrition is important; parents show overconcern with eating habits of their children and spend a considerable part of the budget on food; traditional Cuban diet is rich in meat and starch; consumption of fresh vegetables added in US | Strong family ties with mother and father kinships

Children supported and assisted by parents long after becoming adults

Elderly cared for at home | Most are bilingual (English/Spanish) except for segments of the senior population | In less than 30 years, Cubans have been able to obtain a higher standard of living than other Hispanic groups in US

Have been able to retain many of their former social institutions: bilingual and private schools, clinics, social clubs, the family as an extended network of support, etc.

Many do not feel discriminated against or harbor feelings of inferiority with respect to Anglo-Americans or "mainstream" population |

Continued

† This section was written by Mercedes Sandaval, PhD.

Cultural Characteristics Related to Healthcare of Children and Families—cont'd

Cultural group	Health beliefs	Health practices	Family relationships	Communication	Comments
Native Americans (numerous tribes)	Believe health is state of harmony with nature and universe Respect of bodies through proper management All disorders believed to have aspects of supernatural Violation of a restriction or prohibition thought to cause illness Fear of witchcraft May carry objects believed to guard against witchcraft	Medicine persons: Altruistic persons who must use powers in purely positive ways Persons capable of both good and evil—perform negative acts against enemies Diviner-diagnosticians—diagnose but do not have powers or skill to implement medical treatment Specialists—use herbs and curative but nonsacred	Extended family structure—usually includes relatives from both sides of family Elder members assume leadership roles	Most continue to speak their Indian lanuage, as well as English Nonverbal communication	Time orientation—present Respect for age Going to hospital associated with illness or disease; therefore may not seek prenatal care, since pregnancy viewed as natural process Tend to take time to form an opinion of professionals Sexual matters not openly discussed with members of opposite sex

Theology and medicine strongly interwoven

medical procedures

Medicine persons—use herbs and ritual

Singers—cure by the power of their song obtained from super-natural beings; affect cures by laying on of hands

Genogram Form

Family Name_____ Completed By_____

Date_____ Family Address_____

Generation 1

Generation 2

Generation 3

Key Hypotheses and Life Events   Significant Others

From McGoldrick M, Gerson R: Genograms in family assessment, *New York, 1985, WW Norton, p 156. Reprinted with permission.*

OUTLINE FOR A BRIEF GENOGRAM INTERVIEW
Index person, children, and spouses

Name? Date of birth? Occupation? Are they married? If so, give names of spouses, and the name and sex of children with each spouse. Include all miscarriages, stillbirths, adopted and foster children. Include dates of marriages, separations, and divorces. Also include birth and death dates, cause of death, occupations, and education of the above family members. Who lives in the household now?

Family of origin

Mother's name? Father's name? They were which of how many children? Give name and sex of each sibling. Include all miscarriages, stillbirths, adopted and foster siblings. Include dates of the parents' marriages, separations, and divorces. Also, include birth and death dates, cause of death, occupations, and education of the above family members. Who lived in the household when they were growing up?

From McGoldrick M, Gerson R: *Genograms in family assessment,* New York, 1985, WW Norton, pp. 157-158: Reprinted with permission.

Mother's family

The names of the mother's parents? The mother was which of how many children? Give name and sex of each of her siblings. Include all miscarriages, stillbirths, adopted and foster siblings. Include dates of grandparents' marriages, separations, and divorces. Also include birth and death dates, cause of death, occupations, and education of the above family members.

Father's family

The names of the father's parents? The father was which of how many children? Give name and sex of each of his siblings. Include all miscarriages, stillbirths, adopted and foster siblings. Include dates of grandparents' marriages, separations, and divorces. Also include birth and death dates, cause of death, occupations, and education of the above family members.

Ethnicity

Give the ethnic and religious background of family members and the languages they speak, if not English.

Major moves

Tell about major family moves and migrations.

Significant others

Add others who lived with or were important to the family.

For all those listed, note any of the following:

Serious medical, behavioral, or emotional problems
Job problems
Drug or alcohol problems
Serious problems with the law

For all those listed, indicate any who were:

Especially close
Distant or conflictual
Cut off from each other
Overly dependent on each other

Genogram Symbols

Symbols to describe basic family membership and structure. Include on genogram significant others who lived with or cared for family members and place them on the right side of the genogram with a notation about who they are.

Birthdate → 43-75 ← Death date

Death=X

Male: ☐   Female: ○

Index Person (IP): ☐ ◎

Marriage (give date) (Husband on left, wife on right):

Living together relationship or liaison:

Marital separation (give date):

Divorce (give date):

Children: List in birth order, beginning with oldest on left:

Adopted or foster children:

Fraternal twins: Identical twins: Pregnancy:

Spontaneous abortion: Induced abortion: Stillbirth:

Members of current IP household (circle them):
Please note where changes in custody have occurred:

Family interaction patterns. The following symbols are optional. The clinician may prefer to note them on a separate sheet. They are among the least precise information on the genogram, but may be key indicators of relationship patterns the clinician wants to remember:

Very close relationship: Conflictual relationship:

Distant relationship: Estrangement or cut off (give dates if possible):

Fused and conflictual:

From McGoldrick M, Gerson R: Genograms in family assessment, *New York, 1985, WW Norton, pp 154-155. Reprinted with permission.*

Ecomap Form

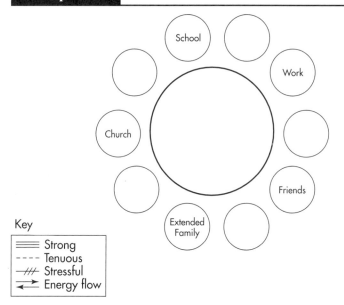

Key
≡≡≡	Strong
- - - -	Tenuous
—∦∦—	Stressful
⇄	Energy flow

Adapted from Friedman MM: Family nursing: theory and practice, *Norwalk, Conn, 1998, Appleton & Lange.*

INDIVIDUAL ASSESSMENT

The most common intervention by a nurse is at the individual level. Planning appropriate care to persons living in the community will enhance quality of life through prevention and health-promotion initiatives.

MENTAL HEALTH

Global Assessment of Functioning (GAF) Scale

Consider psychological, social, and occupational functioning on a hypothetical continuum of mental health–illness. Do not include impairment in functioning caused by physical (or environmental) limitations.

From American Psychiatric Association: *Diagnostic and statistical manual of mental disorders, (DSM IV),* ed 4, Washington, DC, 1994, The Association.

Code (**Note:** Use intermediate codes when appropriate, e.g., 45, 68, 72.)

100 **Superior functioning in a wide range of activities, life's problems never seem to get out of hand, is sought out by others because of his or her many positive qualities.**

91 **No symptoms.**

90 **Absent or minimal symptoms** (e.g., mild anxiety before an exam), **good functioning in all areas, interested and involved in a wide range of activities, socially effective, generally satisfied with life, no more than everyday problems or concerns** (e.g., an occasional argument

81 with family members).

80 **If symptoms are present, they are transient and expectable reactions to psychosocial stressors** (e.g., difficulty concentrating after family argument); **no more than slight impairment in social, occupational, or school functioning** (e.g., temporarily falling behind in

71 schoolwork).

70 **Some mild symptoms** (e.g., depressed mood and mild insomnia) **OR some difficulty in social, occupational, or school functioning** (e.g., occasional truancy, or theft within the household), **but generally functioning pretty**

61 **well, has some meaningful interpersonal relationships.**

60 **Moderate symptoms** (e.g., flat affect and circumstantial speech, occasional panic attacks) **OR moderate difficulty in social, occupational, or school functioning**

51 (e.g., few friends, conflicts with peers or coworkers).

50 **Serious symptoms** (e.g., suicidal ideation, severe obsessional rituals, frequent shoplifting) **OR any serious impairment in social, occupational, or school functioning**

41 (e.g., no friends, unable to keep a job).

40 **Some impairment in reality testing or communication** (e.g., speech is at times illogical, obscure, or irrelevant) **OR major impairment in several areas, such as work or school, family relations, judgment, thinking, or mood** (e.g., depressed man avoids friends, neglects family, and is unable to work; child frequently beats up younger children,

31 is defiant at home, and is failing at school).

30 **Behavior is considerably influenced by delusions or hallucinations OR serious impairment in communication or judgment** (e.g., sometimes incoherent, acts grossly inappropriately, suicidal preoccupation) **OR inability to function in almost all areas** (e.g., stays in bed all day; no
21 job, home, or friends).

20 **Some danger of hurting self or others** (e.g., suicide attempts without clear expectation of death; frequently violent; manic excitement) **OR occasionally fails to maintain minimal personal hygiene** (e.g., smears feces) **OR gross impairment in communication** (e.g., largely
11 incoherent or mute).

10 **Persistent danger of severely hurting self or others** (e.g., recurrent violence) **OR persistent inability to maintain minimal personal hygiene OR serious suicidal act**
 1 **with clear expectation of death.**
 0 Inadequate information.

Initial Patient Assessment

Demographic data: full name, sex, age, date of birth, address, marital status, family members' names and ages.

Admission data: date and time of admission, type of admission (voluntary or committed).

Reason for admission: current problems as perceived by the patient. These include stressors, difficulty with coping, developmental issues, "emergency behaviors" (suicidal or homicidal ideas/attempts, aggression, destructive behaviors, risk of escape), and family history.

Previous psychiatric history: dates, inpatient/outpatient, reasons for and types of treatment and their effectiveness, current medications, compliance, current medical problems and medications.

Drug and alcohol use/abuse: amount, frequency, duration of past and present use of legal/illegal substances, date and time of last use.

From Keltner N, Schwecke L, Bostrom C: *Psychiatric nursing,* ed 3, St Louis, 1999, Mosby.

Disturbances in patterns of daily living: sleep, intake, elimination, sexual activity, work, leisure, self-care, and hygiene.

Culture/spirituality: ethnicity, beliefs, practices, religious preference.

Support systems: amount of contact, nature/quality of relationships, and availability of support.

Mental status examination

General appearance: type and condition of clothing, cleanliness, physical condition, and posture.

Behaviors during the interview:

Expression of anger: covert, overt, verbal, or physical.

Degree of cooperation, resistance, or evasiveness.

Social skills: positive/unpleasant habits, shyness, withdrawal.

Amount/type of motor activity: psychomotor retardation, agitation, restlessness, tics, tremors, hypervigilance, lack of activity.

Speech patterns: amount, rate, volume, pressure, mutism, slurring, or stuttering.

Degree of concentration and attention span.

Orientation: to time, place, and person; and level of consciousness.

Memory: recent/remote, amnesia, blackouts, confabulation.

Thought clarity: coherence, confusion, vagueness.

Thought processes reflected in speech: blocking, circumstantiality, loose associations, flight of ideas, perseveration, tangential ideas, ambivalence, neologisms, or "word salad."

Thought content: helplessness, hopelessness, worthlessness, guilt, suicidal ideas/plans, homicidal ideas/plans, suspiciousness, phobias, obsessions, compulsions, preoccupations, antisocial attitudes, blaming of others, poverty of content, or denial.

Hallucinations: visual, auditory, or other.

Delusions: of reference, influence, persecution, grandeur, religious, or somatic.

Intellectual functioning: use of language and knowledge, abstract vs. concrete thinking (proverbs), or calculations (serial sevens), educational level.

Affect/mood: anxiety level; elevated or depressed mood; labile, blunted or flat affect; or inappropriate affect; specific feelings expressed.

Insight: degree of awareness of problems and their causes.

Judgment: soundness of problem solving and decisions.

Motivation: degree of motivation for treatment.

Family Health and Functioning Assessment

I. Interview the family and obtain the following data:
   A. Demographic and family composition on a genogram
      1. Complete a three-generation genogram with legend and cultural heritage of all family members
      2. Identify the health status of each family member on the genogram
      3. Social networks of first generation members, including neighbor environment
   B. Family interactions
      Identify, discuss, and give examples for each of the following:
      1. Family structure
         a. Subsystems—identify all 5 subsystems
         b. Boundaries—include internal and external
         c. Roles of each family member
         d. Rules of the family—procedural and relational
         e. Triangles—identify all triangles (specify parentification and/or scapegoating)
      2. Family process
         a. Separateness/connectedness—describe this, including sexuality
         b. Enmeshment/disengagement—classify the family by one of these
         c. Communication—who communicates with whom and how
         d. Power—identify who has the power in the family
         e. Secrets/myths—how do they affect family process?
      3. Family spirituality
         a. Method by which family members express their spiritual domain
   C. Family development stage
      1. Identify Duvall's developmental stage[s] and family concerns within the stage[s]
   D. Family knowledge of health and illness
      1. Identify the family's knowledge in the following areas:
         a. Health maintenance and health promotion
         b. Physical and mental illnesses of members
         c. Management of illnesses of members, including medications and side effects
         d. Family coping methods
         e. Resources, such as family support, legal, financial, and community agencies
         f. Treatment options availability
II. Summary
   A. Discuss developmental and health problems in relationship to family (1) structure, (2) process, and (3) spirituality

From Keltner N, Schwecke L, Bostrom C: *Psychiatric nursing,* ed 3, St Louis, 1999, Mosby.

   B. Discuss family strengths related to structure, process, spirituality, and social networks
   C. Discuss family problems related to structure, process, spirituality, and social networks
   D. Discuss the family's knowledge of health and illness
III. Goals for the family
   As members of the treatment team, ask the family to identify the following:
   A. Changes to be made for a more effectively functioning family
   B. Present needs of the family to better care for family members
   C. Family's and/or significant others' role in discharge planning
IV. Interventions
   Indicate interventions and/or referrals related to specific assessment data and family goals

Short Portable Mental Status Questionnaire (SPMSQ)

Mental assessment

The nurse can evaluate cognitive function with a simple bedside examination such as the Folstein mini-mental state examination. This brief examination covers orientation, registration, attention, calculation, recall, and language. The test is scored with a maximum of 30 points. A score below 24 is considered abnormal. Consideration for the client's education and life experience may influence the overall score. Early in a dementing illness, mild signs and symptoms of dementia may be difficult to identify. Thus, diagnosing dementia with certainty can be difficult. Detailed neuropsychologic testing may be helpful in evaluating higher cortical functions and providing a baseline for following the client over time.

Pertinent questions	Scoring
1. What is the date today (month/day/year)?	0-2 errors = intact
2. What day of the week is it?	3-4 errors = mild intellectual impairment
3. What is the name of this place?	5-7 errors = moderate intellectual impairment
4. What is your telephone number? (If no telephone, what is your street address?)	8-10 errors = severe intellectual impairment
5. How old are you?	
6. When were you born (month/day/year)?	Allow one more error if subject had no grade-school education

From Barker E: *Neuroscience nursing,* St Louis, 1994, Mosby.

From Kane R, Ouslander J, Abrass I: *Essentials of clinical geriatrics,* New York, 1994, McGraw-Hill.

Pertinent questions	Scoring
7. Who is the current president of the United States?	Allow one fewer error if subject has had education beyond high school
8. Who was the president just before him?	
9. What was your mother's maiden name?	
10. Subtract 3 from 20 and keep subtracting 3 from each new number all the way down.	

Mini-Mental LLC

NAME OF SUBJECT _____ Age _____
NAME OF EXAMINER _____ Years of School Completed _____
Date of Examination _____

Approach the patient with respect and encouragement.
Ask: Do you have any trouble with your memory?   ☐ Yes ☐ No
May I ask you some questions about your memory?   ☐ Yes ☐ No

Score   Item

5 ( )   Time Orientation

Ask:
What is the year _____ (1), season _____ (1),
month of the year _____ (1), date _____ (1),
day of the week _____ (1)?

5 ( )   **Place Orientation**

Ask:
Where are we now? What is the state _____ (1), city
_____ (1), part of the city _____ (1), building
_____ (1), floor of the building _____ (1)?

3 ( )   **Registration of three words**

Say: Listen carefully. I am going to say three words. You say them back after I stop. Ready? Here they are... PONY (wait one second), QUARTER (wait one second), ORANGE (wait one second). What were those words?
_____ (1) _____ (1) _____ (1)
Give one point for each correct answer, then repeat them until the patient learns all three.

5 ( )   **Serial 7s as a test of attention and calculation**

Ask: Subtract 7 from 100 and continue to subtract 7 from each subsequent remainder until I tell you to stop. What is 100 take away 7? _____ (1)
Say:
Keep Going _____ (1), _____ (1),
_____ (1), _____ (1).

Score	Item

3 ( ) Recall of three words

Ask:

What were those three words I asked you to remember?

Give one point for each correct answer _____ (1),

_____ (1), _____ (1).

2 ( ) Naming

Ask:

What is this? (show pencil) _____ (1). What is this? (show watch) _____ (1).

1 ( ) Repetition

Say:

Now I am going to ask you to repeat what I say. Ready? No ifs, ands, or buts. Now you say that. _____ (1)

3 ( ) Comprehension

Say:

Listen carefully because I am going to ask you to do something:

Take this piece of paper in your left hand (1), fold it in half (1), and put it on the floor. (1)

1 ( ) Reading

Say:

Please read the following and do what it says, but do not say it aloud. (1)

Close your eyes

1 ( ) Writing

Say:

Please write a sentence. If patient does not respond, say: Write about the weather. (1)

---

1 ( ) Drawing

Say: Please copy this design.

Total score _____

Assess level of consciousness along a continuum

Alert	Drowsy	Stupor	Coma

	Yes	No
Cooperate:	☐	☐
Depressed:	☐	☐
Anxious:	☐	☐
Poor Vision:	☐	☐
Poor Hearing:	☐	☐
Native Language:	_____	

	Yes	No
Deteriorate from previous level of functioning:	☐	☐
Family History of Dementia:	☐	☐
Head Trauma:	☐	☐
Stroke:	☐	☐
Alcohol Abuse:	☐	☐
Thyroid Disease:	☐	☐

Function by Proxy
Please record date when patient was last able to perform the following tasks.
Ask caregiver if patient independently handles:

	Yes	No	Date
Money/Bills:	☐	☐	_____
Medication:	☐	☐	_____
Transportation:	☐	☐	_____
Telephone:	☐	☐	_____

Mental Status Test (Mini-Mental State) and Directions

I. Orientation (maximum score 10)

Points

Ask "What is today's date?" Then ask specifically for parts omitted; e.g., "Can you also tell me what season it is?"

Date (e.g., Jan. 21) . ___
Year . . . . ___
Month . . . . ___
Day (e.g., Monday) . ___
Season . . . . ___

Ask "Can you tell me the name of this hospital or where we are?"
"What floor are we on?" (if applicable)
"What town (or city) are we in?"
"What county are we in?"
"What state are we in?"

Hospital (home). . . . ___
Floor . . . . ___
Town/City . . . . ___
County . . . . ___
State . . . . ___

II. Registration (maximum score 3)

Ask the subject if you may test his or her memory, then say "ball," "flag," "tree" clearly and slowly, about 1 second for each. After you have said all three words, ask subject to repeat them. This first repetition determines the score (0 to 3) but keep saying them (up to 6 trials) until the subject can repeat all three words. If subject does not eventually learn all three, recall cannot be meaningfully tested.

"ball" . . . . ___
"flag" . . . . ___
"tree" . . . . ___

From Kane R, Ouslander J, Abrass I: *Essentials of clinical geriatrics.* New York, 1994, McGraw-Hill.

III. Attention and calculation (maximum score 5)

Ask the subject to begin at 100 and count backward by 7. Stop after five subtractions (93, 86,
79, 72, 65). Score 1 point for each correct
number.

"93" . . . . ___
"86" . . . . ___
"79" . . . . ___
"72" . . . . ___
"65" . . . . ___

or

If the subject cannot or will not perform this task,
ask him or her to spell the word "world"
backwards (D,L,R,O,W). The score is 1 point
for each correctly placed letter, e.g.,
DLROW = 5, DLORW = 3. Record how the
subject spelled "world" backwards: _____

No. of correctly
placed letters . . . . . . ___

D L R O W

IV. Recall (maximum score 3)

Ask the subject to recall the three words you
previously asked him or her to remember
(learned in Registration)

"ball" . . . . ___
"flag" . . . . ___
"tree" . . . . ___

V. Language (maximum score 9)

Naming: Show the subject a wristwatch and ask
"What is this?" Repeat for pencil. Score 1 point
for each item named correctly.

Watch. . . . . ___
Pencil. . . . . ___

Repetition: Ask the subject to repeat, "No ifs,
ands, or buts." Score 1 point for correct
repetition.

Repetition . . . . ___

Three-Stage Command: Give the subject a piece
of blank paper and say, "Take the paper in your
right hand, fold it in half, and put it on the
floor." Score 1 point for each action performed
correctly.

Takes in rt. hand . . . ___
Folds in half . . . . . . ___
Puts on floor . . . . . . ___

Reading: On a blank piece of paper, print the
sentence "Close your eyes" in letters large
enough for the subject to see clearly. Ask subject to read it and do what it says. Score correct
only if subject actually closes his or her eyes.

Closes eyes . . . . ___

Writing: Give the subject a blank piece of paper
and ask him or her to write a sentence. It is to
be written spontaneously. It must contain a
subject and verb and make sense. Correct
grammar and punctuation are not necessary.

Writes sentence . . . . ___

Copying: On a clean piece of paper, draw inter-
secting pentagons, each side about 1 inch, and
ask subject to copy it exactly as it is. All 10
angles must be present and two must intersect
to score 1 point. Tremor and rotation are
ignored. For example,

Draws pentagons . . . ___

TOTAL SCORE ___

DEVELOPMENT

Flow Chart Showing Growth and Development Changes Throughout the Life Cycle*

Overview of developmental changes	Prenatal →	Infancy →	Childhood →	Puberty and adolescence →	Adulthood →	Middle age →	Old age
Heart and circulatory system							
Action of heart and circulatory system is under control of autonomic nervous system. Throughout life, cardiac rate is responsive to organ needs and emotional states (fear, anxiety, tension, depression)	Heart formed and begins to beat about third week	Heart grows a little more slowly than rest of body (weight doubled by 1 year, body weight tripled) Grows steadily during childhood With birth, considerable change in paths and relative volumes of blood flow, reflected in loss of certain fetal structures and changes in heart and major vessels		At puberty, heart takes part in rapid growth, reaching mature size with rest of body	Heart weight remains relatively constant after age 25 (only organ other than prostate that does not decrease in weight with age) Cardiac output decreases 30% to 40% between age 25 and 65 Cardiac power is less with age, whereas expenditure of energy is more than in youth. Capacity to increase rate and strength of beat during physical work is diminished		

*This chart indicates only general trends and directions of growth and development; it is not all-inclusive. No distinct ages, absolute values, or ranges of normal variations are intended in this flow chart.

Adapted from Sutterly D, Donneley G: *Perspectives in human development: nursing throughout the life cycle*, Philadelphia, 1973, Lippincott. In Edelman CL, Mandle CL: *Health promotion throughout the lifespan*, ed 3, St Louis, 1994, Mosby.

Continued

Flow Chart Showing Growth and Development Changes Throughout the Life Cycle*—cont'd

Overview of developmental changes	Prenatal →	Infancy →	Childhood →	Puberty and adolescence →	Adulthood →	Middle age →	Old age
Heart and circulatory system—cont'd							
	Heart rate high, approximately 150 beats/min	Heart rate falls steadily throughout childhood 130 beats/min	70-80 beats/min Heart rate more variable during childhood—regular	60 beats/min in adolescence; rates differ between sexes		After maturity, women have slightly higher pulse rate than men, 65 beats/min; men maintain same pulse rate in maturity (slightly lower body temperature than women)	
			Not until mid-childhood does peripheral blood picture become same as adult (girls' temperature remains stationary, higher than boys')				
Urinary system							
As a whole, parallels growth of body as a whole. Proportion of body water and solids follows pattern related to growth—tendency for human organism	Young fetus is about 90% water Urinary system begins in first month	Newborn is about 70% water Urinary system does not complete full development until end of first year All renal units	Composition of urine in healthy child (after age 2) changes little as child matures; thus renal function and urinalysis can be used as monitor of well-being		Adult is about 58% water Glomerular filtration rate decreases about 57% from age 20 to 90	Renal mass decreases with age; renal flow decreases 53% (some researchers believe this is an adaptive change, compensating for declining cardiac output)	

to dry out as life progresses	immature at birth; thus fluid and electrolyte imbalance occurs readily Kidney function adequate at birth if not subject to undue stress		
Function of kidneys, with other organ systems, is to help in regulation of internal environment of the body			
Digestive system			
As a whole grows as total body grows, although evidence suggests that various parts of gastrointestinal (GI) system undergo separate periods of growth, maturity, and senescence	Before birth, nutrients are supplied through placental circulation; digestion and absorption do not occur in the GI tract	Stomach size increases rapidly first months, then grows steadily through childhood Spurt of growth of puberty Digestive apparatus immature at birth (food passes through rapidly, reverse peristalsis common)	All actions of the GI tract (food intake, digestion, absorption, elimination) not only respond to physiologic needs but from birth to old age are sensitive to tensions and anxiety Available data suggest generalized atrophy of entire GI tract with advancing age Nutritional needs vary according to individual variation—decreasing metabolism →decreasing enzyme production →HCl →stomach volume—tone of large intestine may become impaired

Continued

Flow Chart Showing Growth and Development Changes Throughout the Life Cycle—cont'd

Overview of developmental changes	Prenatal →	Infancy →	Childhood →	Puberty and adolescence →	Adulthood →	Middle age →	Old age
Digestive system—cont'd		Activity of gastric juices varies over life span; low during infancy, rises in childhood; plateau about age 10, rise in puberty					Until decrease with senescence (also diminished taste)
		Free gastric acid (HCl) more pronounced in boys					
		Salivary glands small at birth					
		Increase rapidly during first 3 mo; reach relative adult proportions by age 2					
Special senses Most are well developed at birth, although their association with higher	Begin early in embryonic development— 3-6 wk	Sense of touch is developed first, then hearing and vision					
		Vision: infant can perceive simple differences in shape but not complex patterns (greater proportion of total growth before birth); various dimensions of vision develop at various ages, eye muscles function at mature level first year, fusion begins 9 mo until 6 yr; refractive power changes over life cycle—hyperopia increases until eyeball reaches adult size (approximately 8 yr), then reverses trend toward emmetropia—postpubertal years—toward total myopia until 30—myopia decreases—hyperopia increases					

centers comes about gradually during early life and diminishes with advancing age

Adipose tissue

Although adipose tissue varies greatly from individual to individual, overall lifetime pattern exists. Fat accumulation varies greatly with body build and constitution	Accumulates rapidly before birth; peak at seventh prenatal month	Increases rapidly during first 6 mo	Decreases from first to seventh year in both sexes	Begins to increase slowly to puberty	Typically both sexes tend to gain weight in fifties and sixties but do not maintain same body contours of earlier years at same weight (increase deposit on abdomen and hips)	Usually fat stores are lost after seventh decade in both sexes Sharpness in contours, increasingly

Continued

Flow Chart Showing Growth and Development Changes Throughout the Life Cycle—cont'd

Overview of developmental changes	Prenatal →	Infancy →	Childhood →	Puberty and adolescence →	Adulthood →	Middle age →	Old age
Adipose tissue—cont'd							
Relationship between caloric intake, amount of exercise, and utilization and accumulation of fat is not yet fully understood but is basis of much interrelated research	Premature infant may look wrinkled and scrawny because of lack of adipose tissue	(Gender differences are not noted in the body shape of prepubescent children)		Fat begins to accumulate slowly and continues uninterrupted in girls, producing feminine curves; accounts for much of weight gain	Some girls slim down after full maturation; many maintain about same amount of adipose tissue as at puberty		prominent bony land marks
				Deposition of fat differs in body—amount decreases sharply at time of maximum growth	After full maturation, fat accumulation begins →		

(Continues →)

Lymphoid tissue

Lymphoid tissue is scattered widely throughout body and includes lymph nodes, tonsils, adenoids, thymus, spleen, and lymphocytes of the blood; follows unique pattern of growth, rapid in infancy and puberty

Begins in last month of uterine life—immunoglobulins cross placenta at levels equal to mother's and continue for several months after delivery

Grows most rapidly during infancy and childhood, reaching maximum size a few years before puberty; parallels development of immunity

Increased incidence of disease with increasing age of child

spurt (increased weight caused by increase in muscle mass and bones)

Atrophies and is smaller in volume at full maturity than during childhood

Thymus so small that it is difficult to locate in older people

Respiratory system

Growth parallels that of total body growth. Respira-

Before birth, air sacs do not contain

When umbilical cord is cut, infant must use own breathing apparatus—breathing irregular at first both in rate and depth—fast in infancy—gradually slowing through

No sex difference in respiratory rate at any time of life

Basal metabolism rate declines

Continued

Flow Chart Showing Growth and Development Changes Throughout the Life Cycle—cont'd

Overview of developmental changes	Prenatal →	Infancy →	Childhood →	Puberty and adolescence →	Adulthood →	Middle age →	Old age
Respiratory system—cont'd							
tory apparatus is a highly organized system of organs under nervous and hormonal regulation which functions in coordination with rest of body. Sex difference in gaseous exchange becomes apparent during puberty	air; oxygen supplied through maternal circulation	childhood until full maturity is reached				(rate higher in men than women)	

Respiratory exchange gradually becomes more efficient as life advances. Actual volume of air inhaled with each breath increases as lung size expands with general body growth. Vital capacity and maximum breathing capacity rise gradually in both sexes, increasing more in boys during puberty; men have more efficient respiratory exchange, are capable of greater feats of muscular exertion without exhaustion than women

Skeletal system

Bone growth passes through successive stages of development from connective tissue to cartilage to osseous tissue; completion of calcification indicates end of growing period and is thus a useful measure of growth rate and physiologic maturity. Most growth ceases in adolescence	Follows cephalocaudal law of development	Reserved during growth spurt	Maximum height in early twenties to thirties	Gradual decline until onset of senescence. Thinning of vertebral disk beginning in middle years, most rapid in last decade
	70% of head growth before birth; bones of hands and wrist laid down in cartilage	After first year, legs fastest growing, 66% of total increase in height; longer puberty is delayed, greater the leg length		
		Trunk fastest growing, 60% of total increase		
		Length of trunk and depth of chest reach peak growth speeds last		
	At birth, shafts of metacarpals are ossified (and visible by radiograph);	Growth of both sexes nearly even until onset of puberty in girls first (approximately 10½ yr). Boys begin approximately 2½ yr later, but noticeably greater. Peak in height comes before peak in weight		Spinal column shortens (osteoporosis) with thinning vertebrae—shortening of trunk with long extremities—reversal of growth proportions in infancy

Continued

Flow Chart Showing Growth and Development Changes Throughout the Life Cycle—cont'd

Overview of developmental changes	Prenatal →	Infancy →	Childhood →	Puberty and adolescence →	Adulthood →	Middle age →	Old age
Skeletal system—cont'd		carpal bones begin to ossify					
Muscular system							
Number of striated muscle fibers is roughly same in all human beings. Tremendous difference in size, not only from fetus to adult but among adults, is caused by ability of individual muscle fibers to increase in size. Growth potential, however, is influ-	Muscle formation begins early, assuming final shape by end of second month	Increases rapidly during infancy but slowly during childhood. Growth in both sexes is same in childhood		With onset of puberty, muscle strength is greater in boys (when muscle growth is stimulated by testosterone) Greatest increase begins in puberty; muscle size precedes muscle strength in boys	Muscle mass continues to increase gradually—maximum strength in early adulthood—then declines slight—according to use and genetic constitution Will increase in bulk and strength as used		Until onset of senescence—

enced by genes, nutrition, exercise, and possibly other unknown factors		Increase in muscle size means increasing strength in children; increase in skill is more intimately related to maturation of nervous system		atrophy and loss of muscle tone
Nervous system Growth and maturation of central nervous system (CNS) (brain, cord, peripheral nerves, many sense organs) follow pattern reflected by changing size of the head	Growth rapid during intrauterine development; head increases at greater rate than rest of body	Has all the brain cells of first year, which will continue to increase in size; number and complexity of axons and dendrites will continue to increase	Function continues with use	Possible decrease in size and number of brain cells in senescence (subject of study)

Continued

Flow Chart Showing Growth and Development Changes Throughout the Life Cycle*—cont'd

Overview of developmental changes	Prenatal →	Infancy →	Childhood →	Puberty and adolescence →	Adulthood →	Middle age →	Old age
Nervous system—cont'd							Decrease in myelin sheath, impulses decrease; slow down speed of action and reaction
		All neural tissues grow rapidly during infancy and early childhood		(No neural growth spurt at puberty)			
		Brain grows rapidly after birth, reaching 90% of total size by age 2	By midchildhood, almost reaches adult size	Slow increase to full maturity	Brain weight decreases with age		
		Segmented spinal nerves are mature, fully myelinated, and functioning at term (e.g., knee jerk), but acquisition of myelin in cortex, brain stem, and cord is closely correlated with observed behavior (myelinization of this tract follows cephalocaudal, proximodistal law)					
		Equipment for sense of taste and smell present at birth and perhaps most acute at that time				Taste less acute, less discrimatory with advancing age Structural changes in CNS result in impaired perception	

Reproductive system

Organs of reproductive system show little increase during early life but rapid development just before and coincident with puberty. Maturation and fulfillment of reproductive functions of maturity (in female) are followed by involution in later years	Genital organs form during uterine life; uterus undergoes growth spurt before birth (hormone stimulation from mother)	Female sex organs well formed but not functioning at birth (but have full quota of sensory nerves)	Quiescent during childhood →	Maturation at puberty (menstruation) →		Involution after menopause
		Uterus undergoes involution to half its birth weight	Regained size by age 10-11 →	Adult size at puberty →	Maximum increase with pregnancy →	
		In male—testes, as with ovary, remain dormant and small, not even growing in pro-	Until puberty, interstitial cells of Leydig reappear and secrete testosterone; so testes and penis continue increase in size (pubic hair appears)			Begins to atrophy with advancing age

Continued

Flow Chart Showing Growth and Development Changes Throughout the Life Cycle—cont'd

Overview of developmental changes	Prenatal →	Infancy →	Childhood →	Puberty and adolescence →	Adulthood →	Middle age →	Old age
Reproductive system—cont'd							
		portion to rest of body (with sensory nerves)					
	Mammary glands develop in both sexes during fetal life	Enlargement of breasts at birth (both sexes) →	Nonsecretory during childhood until puberty →	Development rapid →	Enlarge during pregnancy, developing alveoli →		Atrophy with advanced age
	Sex hormones; until puberty girls and boys produce male hormones (androgens) and female hormones (chiefly estrogens) in small and roughly equal amounts						
Integumentary system							
Includes skin and its appendages and adnexa (nails, hair, sebaceous glands, eccrine and apocrine sweat glands). Al-	Hair, skin, and sebaceous glands fully formed in utero	Skin contains all its adult structures at birth but immature in function	Matures slowly until puberty (children prone to rashes)	Rapid spurt in maturation of skin and all its structures		Changes in skin most obvious sign of aging (exposure and environmental conditions)	

though all skin is similar, this organ shows considerable variability in different parts of body (and between individuals) and varies greatly during the life span

Lanugo begins to decrease before birth and continues regression few weeks postnatally →

Activity of sebaceous decreases after birth →

Replaced by body hair, less extensive distribution; large difference in type and distribution of hair at puberty → Increases rapidly at puberty (more prone to acne)

Decrease in regenerative and growth power decreases and skin loses elasticity

Endocrine system

Consists of a number of glandular structures scattered throughout the body. Although small in size, their

Immaturity of entire endocrine system puts infant at disadvantage if required to adjust to wide fluctuations in concentration of water, electrolytes, glucose, amino acids. All are interrelated, but each organ develops at own rate:

Thyroid—increases from midfetal life to maturity: little larger in boys than girls; growth spurt at adolescence

Adrenals—after birth decreases in size and continues throughout first year, increases again during childhood (but smaller than at birth); spurts at puberty, reaching maturity with rest of body: greater increase in male gonads and testes and female ovaries—are endocrine glands as well as reproductive organs; follow genital type of growth pattern

Hypophysis or pituitary gland—produces or stimulates hormones that influence growth

Parathyroids—produce hormones that maintain homeostasis of calcium and phosphorus

Islets of Langerhans—dispersed through pancreas; produce insulin and glucagon

Continued

Flow Chart Showing Growth and Development Changes Throughout the Life Cycle—cont'd

Overview of developmental changes	Prenatal →	Infancy →	Childhood →	Puberty and adolescence →	Adulthood →	Middle age →	Old age
Endocrine system—cont'd hormones influence all growth and development of whole organism						With age, decline occurs in all endocrine gland functions	

Erikson's Eight Stages of Human Development

Stage (approximate)	Psychosocial stages	Lasting outcomes
1. Infancy	Basic trust versus basic mistrust	Drive and hope
2. Toddlerhood	Autonomy versus shame and doubt	Self-control and willpower
3. Preschool	Initiative versus guilt	Direction and purpose
4. Middle childhood (school age)	Industry versus inferiority	Method and competence
5. Adolescence	Identity versus role confusion	Devotion and fidelity
6. Young adulthood	Intimacy versus isolation	Affiliation and love
7. Middle adulthood	Generativity versus stagnation	Production and care
8. Older adulthood	Ego integrity versus despair	Renunciation and wisdom

Adapted from Erikson EH: *Childhood and society,* New York, 1993, Norton, with permission of WW Norton. In Edelman CL: Mandle CL: *Health promotion throughout the lifespan,* ed 4, St Louis, 1998, Mosby.

Piaget's Levels of Cognitive Development

Stage	Age	Characteristics
Sensorimotor	0-2 yr	Thought dominated by physical manipulation of objects and events
Substage 1	0-1 mo	Pure reflex adaptations
Substage 2	1-4 mo	Primary circular reactions
Substage 3	4-8 mo	Secondary circular reactions
Substage 4	8-12 mo	Coordination of secondary schemata
Substage 5	12-18 mo	Tertiary circular reactions
Substage 6	18-24 mo	Invention of new solutions through mental combinations
Preoperational	2-7 yr	Functions symbolically using language as major tool
Preconceptual	2-4 yr	Uses representational thought to recall past, represent present, and anticipate future
Intuitive	4-7 yr	Increased symbolic functioning
Concrete operations	7-11 yr	Mental reasoning processes assume logical approaches to solving concrete problems
Formal operations	11-15 yr	True logical thought and manipulation of abstract concepts emerge

Adapted from Schuster C, Ashburn S: *The process of human development: a holistic lifespan approach,* Boston, 1992, Lippincott. In Edelman CL, Mandle CL: *Health promotion throughout the lifespan,* ed 4, St Louis, 1998, Mosby.

Kohlberg's Stages of Moral Development

The responses to moral dilemmas indicate that there are distinct sequential stages of moral thinking. These stages depend greatly on cognitive development and always follow the same sequence. There are three levels of moral judgment, and each consists of two stages. These levels and stages are outlined in the table following.

In our society, progression through the successive stages of moral development generally takes place during the school-age, adolescent, and young adult years. Not everyone progresses through all stages. In fact, only a minority of adults operate in stage 6 or even stage 5. Beyond the very young adult years, a stabilization or increased consistency of thought and perhaps an increased correlation between moral judgment and moral action can occur.

Level and stage	What is right	Reasons for doing right
Level A: preconventional Stage 1: punishment and obedience	Avoiding breaking rules, to obey for obedience's sake, and to avoid doing physical damage to people and property	Avoiding punishment and the superior power of authorities
Stage 2: individual instrumental purpose and exchange	Following rules when it is in someone's immediate interest Using fairness, equal exchange, agreement	Serving one's own needs or interests in a world where one must recognize that other people have interests as well
Level B: conventional Stage 3: mutual interpersonal expectations, relationships, and conformity	Living up to what is expected by relatives and friends or what is generally expected in one's role as son, sister, friend, and so on; "being good" is important	Needing to be good in one's own eyes and those of others Following the "golden rule"
Stage 4: social system and conscience maintenance	Fulfilling actual duties to which one has agreed Laws are to be upheld unless they conflict with other fixed social duties and rights Contributing to society, the group, or institution	Keeping institution going as a whole Using self-respect or conscience to meet one's defined obligations
Level B/C: transition		Basing reasons on emotions; conscience is arbitrary and relative

Continued

Compiled from Kohlberg L: *The philosophy of moral development,* San Francisco, 1981, Harper & Row. From Edelman CL, Mandle CL: *Health promotion throughout the lifespan,* ed. 4, St Louis, 1998, Mosby.

Level and stage	What is right	Reasons for doing right
Level C: postconventional and principled Stage 5: prior rights and social contract or utility	Being aware that people hold a variety of values and opinions, most of which are relative to one's group Realizing that some nonrelative values and rights, such as life and liberty, must be upheld in any society	Feeling obligated to obey the law because one has made a social contract to make and abide by laws for good of all; the greatest good for the greatest number
Stage 6: universal ethical principles	Acting in accordance with the principle when laws violate universal ethical principles Understanding the equality of human rights and respecting dignity of human beings as individuals	As a rational person, seeing validity of principles and becoming committed to them

Life Strengths Interview Guide

Introduction
What is it about your life:
  . . . that is most worth living for?
  . . . that makes you feel most alive?
  . . . that makes you feel most like yourself?

[Probe: These can be things that may seem quite small, like brewing Earl Grey tea in your familiar china teapot, or working at your computer, or cooking the dishes you've been making for decades. Or they may be things that seem larger, like making sure your grandchildren learn good values, or writing letters for Amnesty International, or voting, or working for causes you believe in.]

Hope and faith (trust and mistrust)
What is it in your life that gives you hope?
  How do moral beliefs and values fit into your life?
  How have they fit in earlier times?
  What is your religious affiliation?
  What about religion is most important to you?
  How do you like to express your religious beliefs?
  Is religion something you practice in private? Is some group religious activity important to you?
  What is it in your life that gives you a sense of security?
  What do you tell yourself or think about when you're afraid and you need to believe that things will be all right?

Willfulness, independence, and control (autonomy and shame/doubt)
(We all like to be in control of ourselves and our lives. And when you think about it, we spend most of our lives trying to strike a tolerable balance between being independent and having things the way we want them, on one hand, and accepting help and going along with other people's wishes, on the other hand.)
  How is your health these days?
  Do you:
  . . . have any physical limitations?
  . . . have any diseases or conditions for which you're being treated?
  . . . take medications?

From Kivnick H: Everyday mental health: guide to assessing life strengths, *Generations* Winter/Spring, 1993.

. . . rely on aids such as glasses, hearing aid, cane/walker/wheelchair, etc.?

. . . rely on assistance with homemaking, personal care, etc.?

What parts of your life is it most important that *you* stay in charge of?

What kinds of control are easier to give up, as long as you remain in charge of what's really important?

[Probe: To prioritize autonomy-related issues in daily life. Levels of probe vary, depending on whether elder currently lives independently or in some kind of protected environment.

For example: What you eat; where you eat; when you eat; making your own food; feeding yourself; what you wear; dressing yourself; walking, toileting, and bathing yourself; who assists you with ADLs?]

Daily routine:

Listen to radio and TV as you wish
Use the telephone when you wish
Go out and come back when you wish
Have access to preferred reading materials
Get-up time; mealtime; nap time; bedtime

Living in your own home:

Decorate as you wish
Save belongings as you wish
Lock your door to keep out whomever you want to keep out
Leave your house to whomever you choose

Medical treatment:

Following doctor's orders as you wish
Hospitalization vs. outpatient treatment
Surgery vs. noninvasive treatment
Respirators; artificial nutrition; artificial hydration

Spending money:

Spend money on your own enjoyment
Spend money on your own care
Save money for a rainy day (What is a rainy day?)
Save money to leave it to your heirs

What kinds of independence would you find especially painful to give up?

What do you think might make it easier to accept help, when you wish you didn't need help in the first place?

What is it that has always given you confidence in yourself?

What kinds of decisions are absolutely most important that you make for yourself?

What kinds of decisions are you willing to have someone else make for you? Who?

Purposefulness, pleasure, and imagination (initiative and guilt)

What kinds of things do you enjoy doing? What kinds of activities give you pleasure?

What kinds of activities have always given you pleasure?

[Probe: Eating; movies; walking; cooking; concerts; museums; library; parks; shopping; visiting with friends; travel; reading; writing; helping; babysitting; radio; music; work with hands; caring for plants; charity; volunteer work; church work; arts; sports; house-cleaning; making things for people]

What do you do for fun these days?

What would you do for fun if you could do anything in the world?

What have you done, in your life, that makes you proudest?

What is there that you've always been curious about?

What do you want to do, most of all, with the rest of your life?

Competence and hard work (industry and inferiority)

1. What have you worked hard at?

   What would you like to be working at now, if you were able?

2. What kinds of things have you always been good at?

   What kinds of things are you good at now? What skills do you have? Or areas of expertise?

   [Probe: These may be professionally related skills like accounting or photography, or they may be personal skills like reading poetry, or cooking certain special dishes, or making phone calls.]

3. What is there that you've always wanted to learn, but never quite gotten around to?

   What do you wish you could do better?

   Would you find it easier to accept assistance if you could trade some skill or activity in return?

Values and sense of self (identity and confusion)

What is it about life that makes you feel most like yourself? Why do you think this activity or belief or relationship makes you feel this way?

What do you believe in?

Do you have a philosophy of life that has guided the way you live your life? That guides your life today?

What kind of person would you say:

. . . you are?

. . . you have always been?

What is the image that you carry around inside about who you are in the world?

When people describe you, what do they say? What would you like them to say?

Love and friendship (intimacy and isolation)

Who is important to you in your life today? Where do they live?

Whom do you count on these days? Who counts on you?

Whom do you have contact with these days?

Who, among these, are people you contact by choice?

Tell me about someone you've loved at some point in your life.

Can you tell me about:

. . . your marriage?

. . . your best friend?

What do the people who know you best like most about you? What do they respect most in you?

Who, in which relationships, has brought out the best in you?

How do you feel about being alone these days?

Care and productivity (generativity and self-absorption)

Whom or what do you especially care about?

[Probe: What people, pets, ideas, activities, organizations and issues concern you? What plants and objects, people and issues are you sure to take care of?]

How do you show your caring?

Who is there that you lean on, these days? Who leans on you?

Who is there that it's important to you to be good for? Or to be nice to? Or to set a good example for?

What is there about yourself and your life that you want to make sure people remember?

Who and what have you cared about over the years? Whom have you cared for? Taken care of? Tell me about them.

What's the most important thing for you to do with your life these days?

Who is the person who makes you think, "This is the one who will carry on for me when I'm gone"?

Wisdom and perspective (integrity and despair)

What is there about your life that you wish had been different?

What is there that you're struggling to make sense of about the world?

What has been most meaningful about your life so far?

How do you deal with disappointment? How do you experience joy?

What strategies have you used for coping with fear?

Let's talk a bit about death:

What are your thoughts about:

. . . your own death?

. . . how you'd like to die?

. . . where you'd like to die?

. . . who should be there with you?

. . . anything you'd want to be sure and get done first?

. . . anything you'd want to be sure to say to anyone first?

. . . who should take what kinds of measures to prolong your life?

Have these thoughts changed over the years?

Are you afraid of dying?

Do you know what you're afraid of?

Do you have any ideas about what might help you be less afraid?

Putting it all together again

What is it about your life today that:

. . . makes you feel most alive?

. . . is most worth living for?

. . . makes you feel most like yourself?

I'd like you to think back over your whole life. Over everything you've seen and everything that's happened to you. And I'd like you to tell me a story about something in your life. Anything. But a story from your life that is somehow meaningful for you.

SOCIAL NETWORK

Social network assessments are recommended as a regular part of a client health assessment, because of the recognized link between social networks and morbidity and mortality. If the client is at risk, the nurse should be aware of the impact on health and progress in care. The nurse may want to consider a referral to an appropriate community agency.

Lubben Social Network Scale

Family networks

Q1. How many relatives do you see or hear from at least once a month? (NOTE: Include in-laws with relatives.)   Q1 ____

    0 = zero   3 = three or four
    1 = one   4 = five to eight
    2 = two   5 = nine or more

Q2. Tell me about the relative with whom you have the most contact. How often do you see or hear from that person?   Q2 ____

    0 = <monthly   3 = weekly
    1 = monthly   4 = a few times per week
    2 = a few times 5 = daily
         per month

Q3. How many relatives do you feel close to? That is, how many of them do you feel at ease with, can talk to about private matters, or can call on for help?   Q3 ____

    0 = zero   3 = three or four
    1 = one   4 = five to eight
    2 = two   5 = nine or more

Friends networks

Q4. Do you have any close friends? That is, do you have any friends with whom you feel at ease, can talk to about private matters, or can call on for help? If so, how many?   Q4 ____

    0 = zero   3 = three or four
    1 = one   4 = five to eight
    2 = two   5 = nine or more

Q5. How many of these friends do you see or hear from at least once a month?   Q5 ____

    0 = zero   3 = three or four
    1 = one   4 = five to eight
    2 = two   5 = nine or more

From Lubben I: Assessing social networks among elderly populations, *Fam Comm Health* 11(3): 1988.

Q6. Tell me about the friend with whom you have the most contact. How often do you see or hear from that person?   Q6 ____

      0 = <monthly   3 = weekly
      1 = monthly   4 = a few times per week
      2 = a few times   5 = daily
         per month

Confidant relationships

Q7. When you have an important decision to make, do you have someone you can talk to about it?   Q7 ____

Always	Very often	Often	Sometimes	Seldom	Never
5	4	3	2	1	0

Q8. When other people you know have an important decision to make, do they talk to you about it?   Q8 ____

Always	Very often	Often	Sometimes	Seldom	Never
5	4	3	2	1	0

Helping others

Q9a. Does anybody rely on you to do something for them each day? For example: shopping, cooking dinner, doing repairs, cleaning house, providing child care, etc.

      NO—if no, go on to Q9b.
      YES—if yes, Q9 is scored "5" and skip to Q10

Q9b. Do you help anybody with things like shopping, filling out forms, doing repairs, providing child care, and so on?   Q9 ____

Always	Very often	Often	Sometimes	Seldom	Never
5	4	3	2	1	0

Living arrangements

Q10. Do you live alone or with other people? (NOTE: Include in-laws with relatives.)   Q10 ____

5 · Live with spouse
4   Live with other relatives or friends
1   Live with other unrelated individuals (e.g., paid help)
0   Live alone

TOTAL LSNS SCORE: ____

Scoring:

The total LSNS score is obtained by adding up scores from each of the 10 individual items. Thus, total LSNS scores can range from 0 to 50. Scores on each item were anchored between 0 and 5 to permit equal weighting of the 10 items. It is suggested that a score below 20 indicates an extreme risk for limited social networks.

Social Assessment of the Elderly

Social assessment is an important indicator of the level of independent functioning of the elderly. It is recommended that this be a part of the comprehensive client assessment.

1. Has any of the following happened in the last year? (Describe if yes):

Death of spouse   ____
Death of other close family member   ____
Change in health of family member   ____
Change in living situation   ____
Divorce or separation   ____
Marriage or "pairing up"   ____
Change in financial state   ____

2. Living situation

   a. House   ____
        Apartment   ____
        Other   ____

   b. Alone   ____
        With another person or others   ____
        If so, who lives with client?

Name	Relationship
1.	
2.	
3.	

From Kane R, Ouslander J, Abrass I: *Essentials of clinical geriatrics,* New York, 1994, McGraw-Hill.

c. Telephone

None   ____

Yes [phone number (____) ____ - _____]   ____

d. Stairs

No ____

Yes ____

If yes, how many? ____

Is elevator available? No ____ Yes ____

3. a. Does client require help in any of the following? If so, who provides it?

	Help needed	Provided by
Meal preparation	_____	_____
Shopping	_____	_____
Light housecleaning	_____	_____
Laundry	_____	_____
Getting out of bed	_____	_____
Getting into bed	_____	_____
Dressing	_____	_____
Bathing	_____	_____

b. Describe what the client ate yesterday:

Breakfast	Lunch	Dinner
_____	_____	_____
_____	_____	_____

4. How often in past week did client leave the house (other than this visit)?

At least daily ____ Several times ____ Once ____ Never ____

5. How often do visitors come to client's house?

Daily ____ Weekly ____ Less often ____ Never ____

6. Whom would client call in an emergency (nonprofessional)?

_____

7. Does client have a legal guardian or durable power of attorney for healthcare?

No ____ Yes ____ (If yes, list name/address/telephone number.)

_____

_____

8. Is client's care covered by

Medicaid   ____

Supplemental private insurance (beyond Medicare)   ____

9. Does the client receive

Social Security   ____

Supplemental Security Income (SSI)   ____

Private pension   ____

Other income   ____

10. Does income permit purchase of needed

Food   ____
Clothing   ____
Housing   ____
Heating   ____
Transportation ____
Drugs   ____

Is money a problem for the client? No ____ Yes ____

11. Does client receive services from any social agency?

Yes ____ No ____

Name and phone number of agency _____

Primary Changes of Aging

Skin	Wrinkling, sagging of subcutaneous support, hair loss, ↓ in sebaceous secretions, epidermal thinning, degeneration of the elastic fibers providing dermal support, ↓ in vascularity
Skeletal	↓ in bone density, shrinkage of vertebral disks, deterioration of cartilage
Muscular	↓ in muscle mass strength, and endurance, ↓ in myofibrils; impaired coordination and reflexes
Cardiovascular	↑ in blood pressure, ↓ in cardiac contractile function, ↓ in cardiac output under stress, progressive stiffening of arteries, development of atherosclerotic plaques
Urinary	↓ in peak bladder capacity, ↑ in residual urine, ↓ in renal blood flow, ↓ in glomerular filtration rate, ↑ in urinary frequency including nocturia, benign prostatic hypertrophy, ↓ in pelvic muscle tone
Gastrointestinal	Dental changes, ↓ in number of taste buds, ↓ in peristalsis, ↓ in gastric acid secretion, ↓ in absorption
Endocrine	↓ in utilization of insulin, ↓ in estrogen and testosterone
Special senses	Impaired night vision and color discrimination, ↓ in peripheral vision, ↑ in sensitivity to glare, lens opacity, ↓ in high-frequency hearing ability, difficulty in speech discrimination of such high-pitched sounds as *s, z, sb,* and *ch*
Sexual	↓ in penile sensitivity, slower and weaker erection, ↓ in ejaculatory volume, ↑ in refractory period in men, ↓ in vascularity and fat content of vaginal walls, ↓ in size of vagina, atrophic vaginitis

Adapted from Sloane PD: Normal aging. In Ham RJ, Sloane PD, editors: *Primary care geriatrics,* ed 3, St Louis, 1997, Mosby. Also adapted from Lincoln R: Promotion of health in the elderly. In Long BC, Phipps WJ, Cassemeyer VL, editors: *Medical-surgical nursing: a nursing process approach,* ed 3, St Louis, 1993, Mosby.

NUTRITIONAL ASSESSMENT

Nutrition is one of the most essential aspects in life for all. Diet, whether therapeutic or regular, has a major impact on a person's health, maintenance, and recovery from an illness. Nutritional behavior is a lifestyle that is influenced by culture; it must be considered as the nurse provides advice and guidance to individuals and families.

Anthropometric Measurements

Muscle mass measurements are obtained by measuring the arm circumference of the nondominant upper arm. The arm hangs freely at the side, and a measuring tape is placed around the midpoint of the upper arm, between the acromion of the scapula and the olecranon of the ulna. The centimeter circumference is recorded and compared with standard values in the table below.

The combined midarm circumference and triceps skinfold calculations provide an estimate of midarm muscle areas that can be a useful indicator for determining protein-energy malnutrition. These measurements can also be used to monitor interventions and changes in the nutritional status of elders regardless of race.

Percentage of standard	Male	Female
Mid-upper arm circumference (in cm)		
90	26.33	25.7
80	23.4	22.8
70	20.5	20.0
60	17.6	17.1
STANDARD	29.3	28.5
Tricep skinfold (in mm)		
90	11.3	11.9
80	10.0	13.2
70	8.8	11.6
60	7.5	9.9
STANDARD	12.5	16.5

Modified from Keithley JK, Proper nutritional assessment can prevent hospital malnutrition, *Nurs '79* 92:70, 1979. In Ebersole P: Hess P: *Toward healthy aging: human needs and nursing response,* ed 5, St Louis, 1998, Mosby.

Body fat is assessed by measuring specific skinfolds with Lange or Harpenden calipers. Two areas are accessible for measurement. One area is the midpoint of the upper arm, the triceps area, which is also used to obtain arm circumference. The nondominant arm is again used. The nurse lifts the skin with the thumb and forefinger so that it parallels the humerus. The calipers are placed around the skinfold, 1 cm below where the fingers are grasping the skin. Two readings are averaged to the nearest half centimeter. Results should be compared with standard values. If there is a neuropathologic condition or hemiplegia after a stroke, the unaffected arm should be used for obtaining measurements.

The second and more accurate site is immediately below the tip of the scapula. This area provides uniformity of the fat layer. The skin immediately below the tip of the scapula is grasped with the thumb and forefinger, the calipers applied, and two consecutive readings obtained and averaged in the same manner as the triceps measurement.

Nutritional Status Percentiles

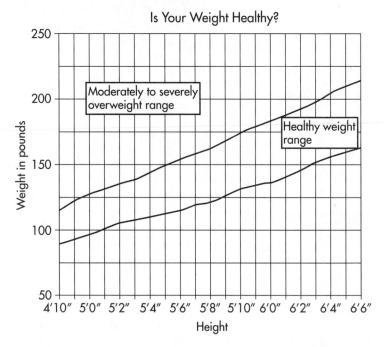

From Williams S: Nutrition and diet therapy, *ed 8, St Louis, 1997, Mosby.*

Mid–upper-arm circumference percentiles (cm)

Age (yr)	Female percentiles					Male percentiles				
	5th	25th	50th	75th	95th	5th	25th	50th	75th	95th
1	13.8	14.8	15.6	16.4	17.7	14.2	15.0	15.9	17.0	18.3
2	14.2	15.2	16.0	16.7	18.4	14.1	15.3	16.2	17.0	18.5
3	14.3	15.8	16.7	17.5	18.9	15.0	16.0	16.7	17.5	19.0
4	14.9	16.0	16.9	17.7	19.1	14.9	16.2	17.1	18.0	19.2
5	15.3	16.5	17.5	18.5	21.1	15.3	16.7	17.5	18.5	20.4
6	15.6	17.0	17.6	18.7	21.1	15.5	16.7	17.9	18.8	22.8
7	16.4	17.4	18.3	19.9	23.1	16.2	17.7	18.7	20.1	23.0
8	16.8	18.3	19.5	21.4	26.1	16.2	17.7	19.0	20.2	24.5
9	17.8	19.4	21.1	22.4	26.0	17.5	18.7	20.0	21.7	25.7
10	17.4	19.3	21.0	22.8	26.5	18.1	19.6	21.0	23.1	27.4
11	18.5	20.8	22.4	24.8	30.3	18.6	20.2	22.3	24.4	28.0
12	19.4	21.6	23.7	25.6	29.4	19.3	21.4	23.2	25.4	30.3
13	20.2	22.3	24.3	27.1	33.8	19.4	22.8	24.7	26.3	30.1
14	21.4	23.7	25.2	27.2	32.2	22.0	23.7	25.3	28.3	32.3
15	20.8	23.9	25.4	27.9	32.2	22.2	24.4	26.4	28.4	32.0
16	21.8	24.1	25.8	28.3	32.4	24.4	26.2	27.8	30.3	34.3
17	22.0	24.1	26.4	29.5	35.0	24.6	26.7	28.5	30.8	34.7
18	22.2	24.1	25.8	28.1	32.5	24.5	27.6	29.7	32.1	37.9
19-25	21.1	24.7	26.5	29.0	34.5	26.2	28.8	30.8	33.1	37.2
25-35	23.3	25.6	27.7	30.4	36.8	27.1	30.0	31.9	34.2	37.5
35-45	24.1	26.7	29.0	31.7	37.8	27.8	30.5	32.6	34.5	37.4
45-55	24.2	27.4	29.9	32.8	38.4	26.7	30.1	32.2	34.2	37.6
55-65	24.3	28.0	30.3	33.5	38.5	25.8	29.6	31.7	33.6	36.9
65-75	24.0	27.4	29.9	32.6	37.3	24.8	28.5	30.7	32.5	35.5

Data derived from the Health and Nutrition Examination Survey data of 1971-1974, using same population samples as those of the National Center for Health Statistics (NCHS) growth percentiles for children. Adapted from Frisancho AR: New norms of upper limb fat and muscle areas for assessment of nutritional status, *Am J Clin Nutr* 34:2540, 1981. In Williams S: *Nutrition and diet therapy,* ed 8, St Louis, 1997, Mosby.

Triceps skinfold percentiles (mm)

Age (yr)	Female percentiles					Male percentiles				
	5th	25th	50th	75th	95th	5th	25th	50th	75th	95th
1	6	8	10	12	16	6	8	10	12	16
2	6	9	10	12	16	6	8	10	12	15
3	7	9	11	12	15	6	8	10	11	15
4	7	8	10	12	16	6	8	9	11	14
5	6	8	10	12	18	6	8	9	11	15
6	6	8	10	12	16	5	7	8	10	16
7	6	9	11	13	18	5	7	9	12	17
8	6	9	12	15	24	5	7	8	10	16
9	8	10	13	16	22	6	7	10	13	18
10	7	10	12	17	27	6	8	10	14	21
11	7	10	13	18	28	6	8	11	16	24
12	8	11	14	18	27	6	8	11	14	28
13	8	12	15	21	30	5	7	10	14	26
14	9	13	16	21	28	4	7	9	14	24
15	8	12	17	21	32	4	6	8	11	24
16	10	15	18	22	31	4	6	8	12	22
17	10	13	19	24	37	5	6	8	12	19
18	10	15	18	22	30	4	6	9	13	24
19-25	10	14	18	24	34	4	7	10	15	22
25-35	10	16	21	27	37	5	8	12	16	24
35-45	12	18	23	29	38	5	8	12	16	23
45-55	12	20	25	30	40	6	8	12	15	25
55-65	12	20	25	31	38	5	8	11	14	22
65-75	12	18	24	29	36	4	8	11	15	22

From Williams S: *Nutrition and diet therapy,* ed 8, St Louis, 1997, Mosby.

Mid–upper-arm muscle circumference percentiles (cm)

Age (yr)	Female percentiles					Male percentiles				
	5th	25th	50th	75th	95th	5th	25th	50th	75th	95th
1	10.5	11.7	12.4	13.9	14.3	11.0	11.9	12.7	13.5	14.7
2	11.1	11.9	12.6	13.3	14.7	11.1	12.2	13.0	14.0	15.0
3	11.3	12.4	13.2	14.0	15.2	11.7	13.1	13.7	14.3	15.3
4	11.5	12.8	13.8	14.4	15.7	12.3	13.3	14.1	14.8	15.9
5	12.5	13.4	14.2	15.1	16.5	12.8	14.0	14.7	15.4	16.9
6	13.0	13.8	14.5	15.4	17.1	13.1	14.2	15.1	16.1	17.7
7	12.9	14.2	15.1	16.0	17.6	13.7	15.1	16.0	16.8	19.0
8	13.8	15.1	16.0	17.1	19.4	14.0	15.4	16.2	17.0	18.7
9	14.7	15.8	16.7	18.0	19.8	15.1	16.1	17.0	18.3	20.2
10	14.8	15.9	17.0	18.0	19.7	15.6	16.6	18.0	19.1	22.1
11	15.0	17.1	18.1	19.6	22.3	15.9	17.3	18.3	19.5	23.0
12	16.2	18.0	19.1	20.1	22.0	16.7	18.2	19.5	21.0	24.1
13	16.9	18.3	19.8	21.1	24.0	17.2	19.6	21.1	22.6	24.5
14	17.4	19.0	20.1	21.6	24.7	18.9	21.2	22.3	24.0	26.4
15	17.5	18.9	20.2	21.5	24.4	19.9	21.8	23.7	25.4	27.2
16	17.0	19.0	20.2	21.6	24.9	21.3	23.4	24.9	26.9	29.6
17	17.5	19.4	20.5	22.1	25.7	22.4	24.5	25.8	27.3	31.2
18	17.4	19.1	20.2	21.5	24.5	22.6	25.2	26.4	28.3	32.4
19-25	17.9	19.5	20.7	22.1	24.9	23.8	25.7	27.3	28.9	32.1
25-35	18.3	19.9	21.2	22.8	26.4	24.3	26.4	27.9	29.8	32.6
35-45	18.6	20.5	21.8	23.6	27.2	24.7	26.9	28.6	30.2	32.7
45-55	18.7	20.6	22.0	23.8	27.4	23.9	26.5	28.1	30.0	32.6
55-65	18.7	20.9	22.5	24.4	28.0	23.6	26.0	27.8	29.5	32.0
65-75	18.5	20.8	22.5	24.4	27.9	22.3	25.1	26.8	28.4	30.6

Values derived by formula calculation. Data derived from the Health and Nutrition Examination Survey data of 1971-1974, using same population samples as those of the National Center for Health Statistics (NCHS) growth percentiles for children. Adapted from Frisancho AR: New norms of upper limb fat and muscle areas for assessment of nutritional status, *Am J Clin Nutr* 34:2540, 1981. In Williams S: *Nutrition and diet therapy,* ed 8, St Louis, 1997, Mosby.

Nutritional Self-Assessment

As the risk of malnutrition among the elderly became recognized, the American Dietetic Association, the American Academy of Family Physicians, and the National Council on Aging developed the Nutrition Screening Initiative (NSI) project to identify individuals over age 65 who are at nutritional risk. A simple-to-use screening tool is based on key risk factors that may represent determinants of undernutrition or malnutrition. The tool can be used by the individual or caregiver who can then consult a health professional for further guidance.

Determine your nutritional health

The warning signs of poor nutritional health are often overlooked. Use this checklist to find out if you or someone you know is at nutritional risk.

Read the statements below. Circle the number in the *yes* column for those that apply to you or someone you know. For each *yes* answer, score the number in the box. Total your nutritional score.

	YES
I have an illness or condition that made me change the kind and/or amount of food I eat.	2
I eat fewer than 2 meals per day.	3
I eat few fruits or vegetables, or milk products.	2
I have 3 or more drinks of beer, liquor, or wine almost every day.	2
I have tooth or mouth problems that make it hard for me to eat.	2
I don't always have enough money to buy the food I need.	4
I eat alone most of the time.	1
I take 3 or more different prescribed or over-the-counter drugs per day.	1
Without wanting to, I have lost or gained 10 pounds in the last 6 months.	2
I am not always physically able to shop, cook and/or feed myself.	2
	Total

Total Your Nutritional Score. If it's

0-2	*Good!* Recheck your nutritional score in 6 months.
3-5	*You are at moderate nutritional risk.* See what can be done to improve your eating habits and lifestyle. Your office on aging, senior nutrition program, senior citizens center or health department can help. Recheck your nutritional score in 3 months.
6 or more	*You are at high nutritional risk.* Bring this checklist the next time you see your doctor, dietitian, or other qualified health or social service professional. Talk with them about any problems you may have. Ask for help to improve your nutritional health.

From the Nutrition Screening Initiative, a project of American Academy of Family Physicians, American Dietetic Association, and National Council on the Aging and funded in part by a grant from Ross Laboratories, Division of Abbott Laboratories. For additional information see Grodner M, Anderson S, DeYoung S: *Foundations and clinical applications of nutrition: a nursing approach,* ed 2, St Louis, 2000, Mosby.

Family Nutritional Assessment Tool

To be completed by the nurse

Family members	Age	Educational level	Developmental level
1.			
2.			
3.			
4.			
5.			
6.			

Family's perception of health status (describe)

Nutritional practices

Who decides on the menu?

Who does the grocery shopping?

Who prepares the meals?

Number of meals consumed per day?

Describe mealtime (Who is present, when, where, and atmosphere)

Does mealtime serve a particular function? (For example, are the day's activities planned? Are problems discussed?)

Snacks consumed and frequency

Knows food sources from the food pyramid

24-hour food recall

Dietary fat

Use of red meat, fish, and poultry (once a week, three times, etc.)

How often do you eat cheese? What kinds do you purchase?

How often do you use cold cuts?

How often do you use fish/chicken? (Describe preparation)

How often do you use processed foods such as bakery products, frozen dinners?

How much milk or other dairy products do you consume? What types?

Cholesterol and saturated fat

How many eggs does the family eat per week?

What kind of fat do you use in cooking?

What kind of vegetable oil do you use?

From Bomar P: *Nurses and family health promotion: concepts, assessment and interventions,* ed 2, Philadelphia, 1996, WB Saunders.

Complex carbohydrates and fiber

How often do you eat fruit? How do you eat it (juices, fresh, canned)?

What kind of vegetables do you eat (canned, frozen, fresh)?

What kind of bread do you eat (whole grain, white)?

Sugar consumption

Do you use sugar in cooking? Do you buy candy, pastries, sweetened cereals?

Sodium

How often do you use processed foods (canned or packaged, such as macaroni and cheese)?

Do you add salt to food?

Alcohol consumption

How often do you use alcohol?

Caffeine

How much coffee and tea do you drink per day?

Supplements

Do you take vitamins or mineral supplements? What and how much? Reason.

Cultural influences

"Special" foods

Eating habits unique to culture

Family food preferences or restrictions

Economics

Do you receive any supplementary income to purchase food items?

Eating problems

Do you have problems with indigestion, vomiting, nausea, sore mouth?

Do you have any difficulty swallowing liquids or solids or chewing and feeding yourselves?

Medications

Are you on any medications? Do they affect your appetite or weight?

Weight

Has weight changed in the last 6 months? How much? Describe events associated with the change.

Elimination pattern
Describe bowel and urinary patterns

Activity and exercise patterns
Usual daily/weekly activities of family members

Source of nutrition information
Magazines, family member, schools, health food store

Family work patterns
Do family members work outside of the home? Type of work and hours

Physical assessment
Describe appearance of the family
Height
Weight
Blood pressure
Pulse/respirations
Percent body fat (or body mass index)

$$\text{Relative weight} = \frac{\text{actual weight} \times 100}{\text{ideal weight}}$$

Example: 160 (actual weight) × 100 = 16,000
(16,000 divided by ideal weight of 140 = 114%)
The closer relative weight is to 100%, the better.
120-139% mild obesity
140-159% moderate obesity
160+ severe obesity
Family strengths/weaknesses
(Identify nutritional concerns of the family)
Barriers to change? Are there reasons why the family cannot change the problem area?

Assessment summary
Check problem area or potential problems

1. Dietary fat
2. Cholesterol and saturated fat
3. Complex carbohydrates and fiber
4. Sugar
5. Sodium
6. Alcohol
7. Caffeine

8. Supplements
9. Cultural influences
10. Economics
11. Eating problems
12. Medications
13. Weight changes
14. Elimination pattern
15. Activity and exercise
16. Nutrition resources
17. Work patterns
18. Notes of concern

Nursing diagnosis:

Plan and intervention

Evaluation

Supplementary assessment for obesity problems

Physical assessment (height, weight, body fat composition, blood pressure, pulse, respirations)
Highest and lowest weight
Why do you want to lose?
What are the contributing factors to weight gain?
Family weight history
   Maternal
   Paternal
Eating patterns
Diets and attempts
Medical problems associated with obesity
Activity level
Developmental stage, stresses, significant life events
Nursing diagnosis
Goal
Plan
Evaluation

Nutritional Screening Assessment Guide

Level I screen

	Value	Measurement abnormal	
		Yes	No
Height (in.)	_____	_____	_____
Weight (lb)	_____	_____	_____
Percent desirable body weight	_____	_____	_____
Weight loss or gain in 6 mo	_____	_____	_____
Dietary data			
Does not have enough food each day	_____	_____	_____
Number of days per month without any food	_____	_____	_____
Poor appetite	_____	_____	_____
Usually eats alone	_____	_____	_____
Difficulty chewing or swallowing	_____	_____	_____
Problems with mouth, teeth, or gums	_____	_____	_____
Housebound	_____	_____	_____
Eats milk or milk products daily	_____	_____	_____
Eats fruits and vegetables daily	_____	_____	_____
On a special diet	_____	_____	_____
Usual daily food intake (optional)			
Less than 2 servings of milk or dairy products	_____	_____	_____
Less than 2 servings of meat/poultry/fish/eggs	_____	_____	_____
Less than 2 servings of fruit/juice	_____	_____	_____
Less than 3 servings of vegetables	_____	_____	_____
Less than 6 servings of bread/cereals/grains	_____	_____	_____
More than 2 ounces of alcohol for men	_____	_____	_____
More than 1 ounce of alcohol for women	_____	_____	_____
Living environment			
Income less than $6000/year/person	_____	_____	_____
Lives alone	_____	_____	_____
Concerned about home security	_____	_____	_____
Inadequate heating or cooling	_____	_____	_____

From Ebersole P, Hess P: *Toward healthy aging: human needs and nursing response,* ed 5, St Louis, 1998, Mosby.

| | | Measurement abnormal | |
	Value	Yes	No
No stove or refrigerator	_____	_____	_____
Unable or prefers not to spend money on food	_____	_____	_____

Functional status—needs assistance with:

Bathing	_____	_____	_____
Dressing	_____	_____	_____
Continence	_____	_____	_____
Toileting	_____	_____	_____
Eating	_____	_____	_____
Ambulation	_____	_____	_____
Transportation	_____	_____	_____
Food preparation	_____	_____	_____

Identified problems should be referred to the appropriate healthcare professional such as physician, nurse, social worker, dietitian, dentist, or case manager.

Refer to a physician if there is:

An involuntary increase or decrease in weight of greater than 10 lb in the past 6 mo
A body weight that is 20% above or below desirable body weight

Refer to a dietitian for food-related problems.
Repeat this screen yearly or if a major change in status occurs.

Level II screen. In-depth assessment (performed in medical settings). Additional information to be obtained after referral to a physician or other qualified healthcare professional

| | | Measurement abnormal | |
	Value	Yes	No
Height (in.)	_____	_____	_____
Weight (lb)	_____	_____	_____
Percent desirable body weight	_____	_____	_____
Body mass index	_____	_____	_____
Weight loss or gain in 6 mo	_____	_____	_____

Level II screen—cont'd

	Value	Measurement abnormal	
		Yes	**No**
Dietary data			
Does not have enough food each day	_____	_____	_____
Number of days per month without any food	_____	_____	_____
Poor appetite	_____	_____	_____
Usually eats alone	_____	_____	_____
Special dietary needs	_____	_____	_____
Self-defined	_____	_____	_____
Prescribed	_____	_____	_____
Problems with compliance/ meeting special needs	_____	_____	_____
Multiple diet prescriptions	_____	_____	_____
Other unusual dietary practices	_____	_____	_____
Usual daily food intake (optional)			
Less than 2 servings of milk or dairy products	_____	_____	_____
Less than 2 servings of meat/ poultry/fish/eggs	_____	_____	_____
Less than 2 servings of fruit/juice	_____	_____	_____
Less than 3 servings of vegetables	_____	_____	_____
Less than 6 servings of bread/ cereals/grains	_____	_____	_____
More than 2 ounces of alcohol for men	_____	_____	_____
More than 1 ounce of alcohol for women	_____	_____	_____
Laboratory and anthropometric data			
Serum albumin less than 3.5 g/dL	_____	_____	_____
Serum cholesterol less than 160 mg/dL	_____	_____	_____
Serum cholesterol greater than 240 mg/dL	_____	_____	_____
Triceps skinfold thickness below 10% of desirable	_____	_____	_____
Midarm muscle circumference below 10% of desirable	_____	_____	_____
Clinical features			
Difficulty chewing or swallowing	_____	_____	_____
Problems with mouth, teeth, or gums	_____	_____	_____

	Value	Measurement abnormal	
		Yes	No
Skin changes that suggest malnu-trition	___	___	___
Angular stomatitis	___	___	___
Glossitis	___	___	___
History of bone pain	___	___	___
Bone fractures	___	___	___

Living environment

	Value	Yes	No
Income less than $6,000/year/person	___	___	___
Lives alone	___	___	___
Concerned about home security	___	___	___
Inadequate heating or cooling	___	___	___
No stove or refrigerator	___	___	___
Unable or prefers not to spend money on food	___	___	___

Functional status—needs assis-tance with

	Value	Yes	No
Bathing	___	___	___
Dressing	___	___	___
Continence	___	___	___
Toileting	___	___	___
Eating	___	___	___
Ambulation	___	___	___
Transportation	___	___	___
Food preparation	___	___	___
Shopping	___	___	___

Mental/cognitive status

	Value	Yes	No
Mini-mental examination indicates impairment (score <26)	___	___	___
Depression scale suggests depress-sion (Beck <15, GDS >5)	___	___	___

Drug use

	Value	Yes	No
More than 3 prescription drugs	___	___	___
More than 3 nonprescription drugs	___	___	___
Vitamin and mineral supplements	___	___	___

Criteria for the recognition of common problems from comple-tion of the screen

Is there weight loss or is the client underweight?

Weight loss greater than 10% in last 6 months
Body weight less than 80% of desirable weight
Triceps skinfold thickness below the 10th percentile
Midarm muscle circumference below 10th percentile

Level II screen—cont'd

Is there evidence of protein energy (hypoalbuminemic) malnutrition?
Serum albumin less than 3.5 g/dL

Is there evidence suggesting osteoporosis or mineral deficiency?
History of bone pain or bone fractures
Patient housebound

Is there evidence of hypovitaminosis or mineral deficiency?
Angular stomatitis, glossitis, or bleeding gums
Inadequate intakes of fruit and vegetables
Pressure ulcers

Is there evidence of obesity or hypercholesterolemia?
Weight greater than 120% of desirable weight
Serum cholesterol greater than 240 mg/dL

Should the client be referred to a dietitian or community nutrition program?
Food intake inappropriate, inadequate, or excessive
Problems complying with specialized diet
Need for nutrition-specific counseling or education, related to
   specific diseases
Functionally dependent for eating or food-related activities of daily
   living
Identified problems should be referred to the appropriate healthcare professional such as a physician, nurse, social worker, dietitian, dentist, or case manager.

Nutritional Screening Over the Life Span

	Medical and socioeconomic	Dietary	Anthropometric measurements	Clinical evaluation	Laboratory evaluation
Infants	Birth weight Length of gestation	Bottle- or breast-fed Supplemental feedings (fluids, solids, method of preparation, weaning, self-feeding) Source of iron Vitamin supplements	Weight Length Overall rate of growth Head circumference	Skin color, turgor Malformations	Hematocrit Hemoglobin
Children	Birth weight Chronic/recent illness Physical activity	Food intake* Appetite Feeding jags, pica Snacking habits Vitamin/mineral supplements Arrangements for eating away from home	Weight Height Arm circumference Overall rate of growth	Skin color, turgor Muscle tone Subcutaneous fat Dental caries	Hematocrit Hemoglobin BUN
Adolescents	Medical history/allergies Socioeconomic data Physical activity Family history Medications	Food intake* (assess for excessive salt or sugar) Where and when foods are eaten Snacking habits Fad diets (especially girls) Vitamin/mineral supplements Alcohol intake	Weight Height Recent weight changes	General appearance of hair, skin, eyes Muscle tone Subcutaneous fat Dental caries	Hemoglobin Urine protein Blood glucose

Adults	Medical history Age Number in family Socioeconomic data Physical activity Family history Medications	Food intake* (assess for saturated fat, cholesterol, sugar, salt; iron and calcium in women) Snacking habits Vitamin/mineral supplements Alcohol intake	Weight Height Recent weight changes	General appearance and maintenance of hair, skin, eyes, muscles Dental caries Blood pressure	Hemoglobin Albumin Transferrin Blood glucose Urinary pH Cholesterol
Elderly persons	Chronic illness or disability Use of tobacco, alcohol, drugs Source of income; amount for food Any physical changes (bleeding, bowel/urinary patterns, fainting, headaches)	Food intake* and patterns Supplements (protein, vitamins, minerals) Who purchases and prepares food Changes in food habits Taste changes Dietary restrictions	Weight Height Recent weight changes	Skin color, pallor Blood pressure Dentition	Hemoglobin Blood glucose Urinalysis Feces

*Question about the frequency of use of foods in the Food Guide Pyramid.

From Davis J, Sherer K: *Applied nutrition and diet therapy for nurses*, ed 2, Philadelphia, 1994, WB Saunders.

Nutritional Self-Care Activities Throughout the Life Span

Developmental stage	Nutritional considerations	Self-care activities
Infancy	Feeding experiences promote bonding with significant others.	Hold baby close during feeding. Feed promptly when hunger noticed.
	Iron stores are depleted by 4-5 mo.	Add iron supplement 4-5 mo.
	Primary teeth begin erupting at about 6 mo	Introduce solid foods 4-6 mo. Begin with strained, mushy foods. Progress to bite-size food by 10-12 mo.
		Introduce new foods one at a time at weekly intervals to screen for allergy.
		Offer foods from six exchanges by end of first year.
	Overweight infants have increased incidence of lower respiratory infection and an increased number of fat cells.	Allow child to determine quantity of foods.
	Underweight infants have slow bone growth, delayed calcification, slow fat deposition, retarded growth of lean body mass, smaller reserve, and higher susceptibility to illness.	Allow, encourage child to self-feed when able. Encourage physical activity.
	Infants who drink cows' milk are subject to dehydration during hot weather or during illness with vomiting, fever, or diarrhea.	Give fluid supplements: water or electrolyte solution.
	Skim milk lacks calories and linoleic acid and results in an increased renal solute load for infants.	Limit use of skim milk before 1 yr of age.

Stage	Characteristics	Self-Care Activities
Toddler	Toddlers eat less than infants because of change in rate of growth.	Use serving size rule: one teaspoon or bite of each food for each year of age.
	Coordination can be poor and eating messy.	Offer finger foods.
		Offer praise for self-feeding.
	Molars may not have erupted.	Avoid inappropriate foods: tough, stringy foods, nuts, popcorn, peanut butter, raw carrots, hot dogs.
	Iron is often deficient in diet.	Offer iron supplements, foods high in iron.
	Toddler begins to identify and model food habits.	Provide good modeling of nutritional self-care.
Preschool	Activity level strongly influences amount of foods consumed. May "play too hard to eat."	Make nutritious snacks.
	Likes to make choices and help prepare foods.	Offer foods cut in finger-sized pieces.
		Have child help prepare meal, set table.
	Suspicious of new foods.	Begin nutrition education.
		Arouse interest in foods. Talk about it when buying, storing, preparing.
		Model good nutritional self-care.
	May dislike "strong-tasting" foods.	Introduce small amounts of spicy foods, broccoli, cabbage, and so forth.
School-age	Appetite may be low or fluctuate.	*Child*
	Sedentary children become overweight.	Gain new skills in balancing own energy input and output.
	Beginning to eat away from nuclear family.	Learn to avoid foods with caffeine and stimulants.
	Stable mealtimes may be difficult to maintain as activities increase.	Choose healthy snacks.

Adapted from Ebersole P, Hess P: *Toward healthy aging,* ed 5, St Louis, 1998, Mosby; Grodner M, Anderson S, DeYoung S: *Foundations and clinical applications of nutrition: a nursing approach,* ed 2, St Louis, 2000, Mosby; Williams S: *Essentials of nutrition and diet therapy,* ed 7, St Louis, 1999, Mosby; Davis J, Sherer K: *Applied nutrition and diet therapy for nurses,* ed 2, Philadelphia, 1994, WB Saunders; Murray R, Zentner J: *Health assessment and promotion strategies through the life span,* ed 6, Stanford, CT, 1997, Appleton & Lange; Wong D, et al.: *Whaley and Wong's nursing care of infants and children,* ed 6, St Louis, 1999, Mosby.

Continued

Nutritional Self-Care Activities Throughout the Life Span—cont'd

Developmental stage	Nutritional considerations	Self-care activities
	Nutrition may affect school performance. Some nutritious snacks, such as peanut butter or dried fruit, may also promote tooth decay.	*Parent* Provide for dental self-care. Provide nutritious snacks. Model nutrition self-care. Praise wise choices. Encourage physical activity.
Adolescence	Most common nutritional problems are tooth decay, anemia, and obesity. Key period in acquiring adult habits. American obsession with thinness may precipitate fad diets, bulimia, or anorexia nervosa. Strenuous physical activity requires additional calories, fluids. Growth spurts and periods of heavy appetite vary widely. Many adolescents have sound nutritional knowledge.	*Adolescent* Provide for own iron intake. Balance own energy input/output. Model nutrition self-care for peers/family. Provide for adequate fluid/caloric intake. *Parent* Provide for dental self-care. Support self-care activities. Continue nutrition education. Praise wise choices. Allow to budget, plan, shop, and prepare family foods.
Young adulthood	Leaving home for college, job, marriage. New responsibility for budgeting, planning, preparing foods. Metabolic rate leveling off. Caloric intake tied to activity level.	Model nutrition self-care for peers/family. Plan eating out carefully. Increase skills in budgeting and shopping. Alter intake in response to changes in exercise and stress levels.

Pregnancy/lactation	Mother's nutritional status affects the health of fetus, infant.	Increase water intake to 6-8 glasses per day, more in hot weather.
	Adequate calories, fluid, nutrient intake to meet demands of developing fetus and nursing infant.	Eat regularly 5-6 times per day to develop regular supply of nutrients, fluids, calories.
		Balance energy input and output.
		Avoid alcohol, caffeine, over-the-counter drugs.
		Use LaLeche League for additional information, support.
Middle age	Nutrition-related conditions may surface during this time: cardiovascular disease, diabetes mellitus, gallbladder disease, liver disease.	Maintain exercise program to offset decreasing metabolic rate.
	Changing lifestyle: decreased child-care responsibilities, career involvement, slower physical pace.	Keep alcohol, caffeine intake at a minimum.
		Provide for regular mealtimes and break times.
	Metabolic rate decreasing.	Balance energy input and output.
	Body image changing.	Maintain calcium intake to prevent osteoporosis.
Later adulthood	Aging process affects nutritional planning: decrease in taste sensitivity, decrease in gastric secretion, decrease in metabolic rate, declining body mass.	Balance energy input and output.
		Limit fatty, spicy foods as needed.
	Food selection may be attached to memories: e.g., may like dill pickles because of the memory of growing and canning cucumbers.	Limit sugar intake.
		Eat small, more frequent meals.

Continued

Nutritional Self-Care Activities Throughout the Life Span—cont'd

Developmental stage	Nutritional considerations	Self-care activities
	Food purchases are influenced by changing financial status, ability to get to and from marketplace, physical stamina to prepare foods, interest in food preparation (particularly if living alone), ability to chew and digest foods, and beliefs of nutritional models. Aging adults generally need more protein, iron, calcium, vitamins A and C, folic acid, and fiber. They usually need less fat, sugar, sodium, and fewer calories.	Use available services such as Meals-on-Wheels, senior centers, food stamp programs to provide supplementary assistance. Consider strengths and limitations when planning diet. Use selected convenience foods when necessary. Encourage eating with another, sharing of food preparation.

Nutritional Assessment of the Elderly

Dietary history	Medical and socioeconomic history	Clinical evaluation	Laboratory evaluation
1. Number of daily meals; regularity	1. Chronic disease or disability; occupational hazard exposure; use of tobacco, alcohol, or drugs	1. Height and weight; obesity or physical wasting	1. Hemoglobin level or hematocrit ratio
2. Usual daily diet	2. Symptoms such as bleeding, fainting, loss of memory, shortness of breath, headache, pain, changed bowel habits; altered sight or hearing and condition of teeth or dentures	2. Blood pressure, pulse rate, and rhythm	2. Blood or urine glucose analysis
3. Supplemental vitamins or minerals; protein concentrate	3. Self-administered or prescribed therapy such as vitamins, alcohol, drugs, food fads, prescription items, eyeglasses, or hearing aids	3. Skin color and texture	3. Urinalysis (color, odor, bile, and sediment by gross inspection), pH, glucose, albumin, blood, and acetone by stick test
4. General nutritional knowledge; sources of information	4. Names, addresses, and phone numbers of persons providing medical or healthcare	4. Anthropometric measurement of mid-upper-arm circumference and tricep or subscapular skin-fold	4. Feces (color, texture, gross blood; occult blood by guaiac test)
	5. Living situation: lives alone or with spouse or companion; house, apartment or senior citizen housing	5. Condition of teeth or dentures and oral hygiene	
	6. Sources of income	6. Mental state during interview and examination	
		7. Vision and hearing assessments	
		8. Any gross evidence of neglect	

From Nutritional assessment in health programs, *Am J Public Health* 63(suppl):74, Nov, 1973; Miller CA: *Nursing care of older adults*, Glenview, Ill, 1990, Scott Foresman/Little Brown Higher Education; Cape ROT. In *The Merck manual of geriatrics*, Rahway, NJ, 1990, Merck Sharpe & Dohme Research Laboratories.

Age-Related Gastrointestinal Changes, Outcomes, and Illness Prevention, Health Promotion, and Maintenance Approaches

Age-related changes	Outcomes	Illness prevention, health promotion, and maintenance
Decreased acuity of taste	Dry mouth	Take in adequate fiber in diet
Decreased salivary production with increased alkalinity	Diminished taste	Adequate exercise
Brittle teeth/retracted gingiva	Pale gums	Bowel training
Less effective chewing	Vermilion border of mouth missing	No or little use of laxative
Decreased esophageal and intestinal motility	Atrophy of gums with loss of teeth or decay	Good oral care
Decrease in gastric secretions	Difficulty chewing	Suck on ice chips or hard candy
Loss of elasticity in intestinal wall	Decreased appetite	Hold cold water in mouth before swallowing
Decreased blood flow to intestines	Thirst	Use sodium-free flavorings
Reduced blood flow to liver	Coughing or choking	Consult dentist once or twice a year
Loss or diminished anal sphincter control	Dysphagia	Use soft-bristled toothbrush and dental floss
	Nausea/vomiting	For dentures, brush to clean between teeth

Weaker neural impulses to lower bowel	Heartburn/indigestion	Cut food into small pieces, chew thoroughly
	Diarrhea	Have abdominal pain evaluated
	Constipation	Increase dietary fiber, fluids, and exercise
	Fecal impaction	Have a regular meal pattern
	Malnutrition	Respond promptly to the urge to defecate
	Drug toxicity	Report any change in bowel routine
		Manage diet within budget
		Use Meals on Wheels if needed
		Use dietary supplements
		Recognize signs of drug toxicity for drugs taken
Fewer taste buds	Food tastes bland	Encourage social dining
	Overseasoning of food	Nutritional supplementation
		Use herbs for seasoning, lemons, spices (nonsalty)

From Ebersole P, Hess P: *Toward healthy aging: human needs and nursing response*, ed 5, St Louis, 1998, Mosby.

Foodborne Disease

Foodborne disease	Causative organisms (genus and species)	Food source	Symptoms and course
Bacterial food infections			
Salmonellosis	Salmonella S. typhi S. paratyphi	Milk, custards, egg dishes, salad dressings, sandwich fillings, polluted shellfish	Mild to severe diarrhea, cramps, vomiting; appears 12-24 hours or more after eating; lasts 1-7 days
Shigellosis	Shigella S. dysenteriae	Milk and milk products, seafood, salads	Mild diarrhea to fatal dysentery (especially in young children); appears 7-36 hours after eating; lasts 3-14 days
Listeriosis	Listeria L. monocytogenes	Soft cheese, poultry, seafood, raw milk, meat products (paté)	Severe diarrhea, fever, headache, pneumonia, meningitis, endocarditis; symptoms begin after 3-21 days
Bacterial food poisoning (Enterotoxins)			
Staphylococcal	Staphylococcus S. aureus	Custards, cream fillings, processed meats, ham, cheese, ice cream, potato salad, sauces, casseroles	Severe abdominal pain, cramps, vomiting, diarrhea, perspiration, headache, fever, prostration; appears suddenly 1-6 hours after eating; symptoms subside generally within 24 hours

Clostridial Perfringens enteritis	Clostridium C. perfringens	Cooked meats, meat dishes held at warm or room temperature	Mild diarrhea, vomiting; appears 8-24 hours after eating; lasts a day or less
Botulism	C. botulinum	Improperly home-canned foods; smoked and salted fish, ham, sausage, shellfish	Symptoms range from mild discomfort to death within 24 hours; initial nausea, vomiting, weakness, dizziness, progressing to motor and sometimes fatal breathing paralysis

From Williams S: *Essentials of nutrition and diet therapy*, ed 7, St Louis, 1999, Mosby.

Recommended Dietary Allowances (National Research Council, 1989 Version)

Age (years)	Weight* kg	Weight* lb	Height cm	Height in	Protein (g)	Vitamin A (RE)†	Vitamin D (µg)‡	Vitamin E (mg)α §	Vitamin K (µg)	Vitamin C (mg)	Thiamin (mg)	Riboflavin (mg)	Niacin (mg NE)||	Vitamin B-6 (mg)	Folate (µg)	Vitamin B-12 (µg)	Calcium (mg)	Phosphorus (mg)	Magnesium (mg)	Iron (mg)	Zinc (mg)	Iodine (µg)
Infants																						
0.0-0.5	6	13	60	24	13	375	7.5	3	5	30	0.3	0.4	5	0.3	25	0.3	400	300	40	6	5	40
0.5-1.0	9	20	71	28	14	375	10	4	10	35	0.4	0.5	6	0.6	35	0.5	600	500	60	10	5	50
Children																						
1-3	13	29	90	35	16	400	10	6	15	40	0.7	0.8	9	1.0	50	0.7	800	800	80	10	10	70
4-6	20	44	112	44	24	500	10	7	20	45	0.9	1.1	12	1.1	75	1.0	800	800	120	10	10	90
7-10	28	62	132	52	28	700	10	7	30	45	1.0	1.2	13	1.4	100	1.4	800	800	170	10	10	120
Men																						
11-14	45	99	157	62	45	1000	10	10	45	50	1.3	1.5	17	1.7	150	2.0	1200	1200	270	12	15	150
15-18	66	145	176	69	59	1000	10	10	65	60	1.5	1.8	20	2.0	200	2.0	1200	1200	400	12	15	150
19-24	72	160	177	70	58	1000	10	10	70	60	1.5	1.7	19	2.0	200	2.0	1200	1200	350	10	15	150
25-50	79	174	176	70	63	1000	5	10	80	60	1.5	1.7	19	2.0	200	2.0	800	800	350	10	15	150
51+	77	170	173	68	63	1000	5	10	80	60	1.2	1.4	15	2.0	200	2.0	800	800	350	10	15	150

	(kg)	(lb)	(cm)	(in)																	
Women																						
11-14	46	101	157	62	46	800	10	8	45	50	1.1	1.3	15	1.4	150	2.0	1200	1200	280	15	12	150
15-18	55	120	163	64	44	800	10	8	55	60	1.1	1.3	15	1.5	180	2.0	1200	1200	300	15	12	150
19-24	58	128	164	65	46	800	10	8	60	60	1.1	1.3	15	1.6	180	2.0	1200	1200	280	15	12	150
25-50	63	138	163	64	50	800	5	8	65	60	1.1	1.3	15	1.6	180	2.0	800	800	280	15	12	150
51+	65	143	160	63	50	800	5	8	65	60	1.0	1.2	13	1.6	180	2.0	800	800	280	10	12	150
Pregnant					60	800	10	10	65	70	1.5	1.6	17	2.2	400	2.2	1200	1200	320	30	15	175
Lactating																						
1st 6 months					65	1300	10	12	65	95	1.6	1.8	20	2.1	280	2.6	1200	1200	355	15	19	200
2nd 6 months					62	1200	10	11	65	90	1.6	1.7	20	2.1	260	2.6	1200	1200	340	15	16	200

*Weights and heights of Reference Adults are actual medians for the US population of the designated age, as reported by NHANES II. The use of these figures does not imply that the height-to-weight ratios are ideal.

†Retinol equivalents. 1 retinol equivalent = 1 μg retinol or 6 μg β-carotene.

‡As cholecalciferol. 10 μg cholecalciferol = 400 IU of vitamin D.

§α-Tocopherol equivalents. 1 mg d-α tocopherol = 1 α-TE.

‖1 NE (niacin equivalent) is equal to 1 mg of niacin or 60 mg of dietary tryptophan.

From Williams S: *Nutrition and diet therapy*, ed 8, St Louis, 1997, Mosby.

Recommended Nutrient Intakes for Canadians

Summary examples of recommended nutrient intake based on age and body weight expressed as daily rates

Age	Sex	Energy (kcal)	Thiamin (mg)	Riboflavin (mg)
0-4 mo	Both	600	0.3	0.3
5-12 mo	Both	900	0.4	0.5
1 yr	Both	1100	0.5	0.6
2-3 yr	Both	1300	0.6	0.7
4-6 yr	Both	1800	0.7	0.9
7-9 yr	M	2200	0.9	1.1
	F	1900	0.8	1.0
10-12 yr	M	2500	1.0	1.3
	F	2200	0.9	1.1
13-15 yr	M	2800	1.1	1.4
	F	2200	0.9	1.1
16-18 yr	M	3200	1.3	1.6
	F	2100	0.8	1.1
19-24 yr	M	3000	1.2	1.5
	F	2100	0.8	1.1
25-49 yr	M	2700	1.1	1.4
	F	1900	0.8	1.0
50-74 yr	M	2300	0.9	1.2
	F	1800	0.8†	1.0†
75+ yr	M	2000	0.8	1.0
	F‡	1700	0.8†	1.0†
Pregnancy (additional)				
First trimester		100	0.1	0.1
Second trimester		300	0.1	0.3
Third trimester		300	0.1	0.3
Lactation (additional)		450	0.2	0.4

NE, Niacin equivalents; *PUFA*, polyunsaturated fatty acids; *RE*, retinol equivalents.
*Protein is assumed to be from breast milk and must be adjusted for infant formula.
†Level below which intake should not fall.
‡Assumes moderate physical activity.
§Infant formula with high phosphorus should contain 375 mg of calcium.

From Scientific Review Committee: Nutrition recommendations, *Health & Welfare*, Ottawa, 1990.

Niacin NE	n-3 PUFA (g)	n-6 PUFA (g)	Weight (kg)	Protein (g)	Vit. A RE
4	0.5	3	6.0	12*	400
7	0.5	3	9.0	12	400
8	0.6	4	11	13	400
9	0.7	4	14	16	400
13	1.0	6	18	19	500
16	1.2	7	25	26	700
14	1.0	6	25	26	700
18	1.4	8	34	34	800
16	1.2	7	36	36	800
20	1.5	9	50	49	900
16	1.2	7	48	46	800
23	1.8	11	62	58	1000
15	1.2	7	53	47	800
22	1.6	10	71	61	1000
15	1.2	7	58	50	800
19	1.5	9	74	64	1000
14	1.1	7	59	51	800
16	1.3	8	73	63	1000
14†	1.1†	7§	63	54	800
14	1.1	7	69	59	1000
14†	1.1†	7§	64	55	800
0.11	0.05	0.3		5	0
0.22	0.16	0.9		20	0
0.22	0.16	0.9		24	0
0.33	0.25	1.5		20	400

Continued

Summary examples of recommended nutrient intake based on age and body weight expressed as daily rates—cont'd

Age	Sex	Vit. D (μg)	Vit. E (mg)	Vit. C (mg)	Folate (μg)	Vit. B$_{12}$ (μg)
0-4 mo	Both	10	3	20	25	0.3
5-12 mo	Both	10	3	20	40	0.4
1 yr	Both	10	3	20	40	0.5
2-3 yr	Both	5	4	20	50	0.6
4-6 yr	Both	5	5	25	70	0.8
7-9 yr	M	2.5	7	25	90	1.0
	F	2.5	6	25	90	1.0
10-12 yr	M	2.5	8	25	120	1.0
	F	2.5	7	25	130	1.0
13-15 yr	M	2.5	9	30	175	1.0
	F	2.5	7	30	170	1.0
16-18 yr	M	2.5	10	40¶	220	1.0
	F	2.5	7	30¶	190	1.0
19-24 yr	M	2.5	10	40¶	220	1.0
	F	2.5	7	30¶	180	1.0
25-49 yr	M	2.5	9	40¶	230	1.0
	F	2.5	6	30¶	185	1.0
50-74 yr	M	5	7	40¶	230	1.0
	F	5	6	30¶	195	1.0
75+ yr	M	5	6	40¶	215	1.0
	F	5	5	30¶	200	1.0
Pregnancy (additional)						
First trimester		2.5	2	0	200	1.2
Second trimester		2.5	2	10	200	1.2
Third trimester		2.5	2	10	200	1.2
Lactation (additional)		2.5	3	25	100	0.2

§Infant formula with high phosphorus should contain 375 mg of calcium.

‖Breast milk is assumed to be the source of the mineral.

¶Smokers should increase vitamin C by 50%.

Calcium (mg)	Phosphorus (mg)	Magnesium (mg)	Iron (mg)	Iodine (μg)	Zinc (mg)
250§	150	20	0.3‖	30	2‡
400	200	32	7	40	3
500	300	40	6	55	4
550	350	50	6	65	4
600	400	65	8	85	5
700	500	100	8	110	7
700	500	100	8	95	7
900	700	130	8	125	9
1100	800	135	8	110	9
1100	900	185	10	160	12
1000	850	180	13	160	9
900	1000	230	10	160	12
700	850	200	12	160	9
800	1000	240	9	160	12
700	850	200	13	160	9
800	1000	250	9	160	12
700	850	200	13	160	9
800	1000	250	9	160	12
800	850	210	8	160	9
800	1000	230	9	160	12
800	850	210	8	160	9
500	200	15	0	25	6
500	200	45	5	25	6
500	200	45	10	25	6
500	200	65	0	50	6

Summary of Nutrients for Health

Function	Signs and symptoms of deficiencies/individuals at increased risk for deficiencies (if applicable)	Food sources
Water		
Solvent for many chemical reactions in metabolism, participant in some chemical reactions (e.g., sugar digestion), temperature regulation, removal of wastes, lubrication and cushioning, transport of nutrients throughout the body	Dehydration, or fluid volume deficit: thirst, flushed skin, sense of apprehension, nausea, heat exhaustion, increased pulse rate and temperature, mental confusion, cyanosis, poor skin turgor, loss of body weight *At risk:* Infants and young children with diarrhea or vomiting, elderly	Water and other beverages; water contained in foods (esp. fruits, vegetables); metabolic water, released from the oxidation of nutrients in the body
Carbohydrates		
Glucose and carbohydrates that yield glucose: Energy (4 kcal/g carbohydrate from food, 3.4 kcal/g IV glucose), protein sparing*	Ketosis (excessive production of ketones from incomplete metabolism of fat): increased urination and thirst, dehydration (see above), flushed dry skin, rapid shallow respirations, fruity odor of breath *At risk:* Individuals with diabetes	Grain products, vegetables, fruits, milk, yogurt, ice cream, sugar, honey, syrup, jelly, jam, candy, other sweets

Fiber, insoluble†: Improve elimination by increasing fecal mass	Constipation, diverticula (herniations that protrude through the musculature of the large intestine and can become inflamed; hemorrhoids; possibly increased risk of colon cancer	Legumes, whole grain breads and cereals, vegetables, fruits
Fiber, soluble: Delay gastric emptying, slow glucose absorption, inhibit cholesterol absorption	Hyperglycemia; hypercholesterolemia	Citrus fruits, oat bran, legumes
Amino acids/nitrogen‡ Constituents of structural proteins (muscles, bones), enzymes, antibodies, hormones, chromosomes; transport oxygen, nutrients, and wastes in the blood; acid-base balance; energy (provide 4 kcal/g)	Hypoalbuminemia, edema, lymphopenia, hair easily pluckable, skin lesions, poor wound healing *At risk:* Serious acute or chronic disease, elderly	Meats, poultry, fish, eggs, milk, yogurt, cheese, legumes, grain products

*IV, Intravenous. Protein sparing refers to the fact that protein can be used for glucose formation via gluconeogenesis (formation of glucose from noncarbohydrates). Adequate carbohydrate intake spares protein to be used for vital functions, rather than energy production.

†Insoluble fiber does not dissolve in water; soluble fiber forms a gel or swells when combined with water.

‡We usually speak of a requirement for protein, but the requirement is actually for nitrogen in the form of amino acids, which are essential (needed in the diet because the body does not produce a sufficient amount) or nonessential (not necessary in the diet because the body synthesizes it). Essential amino acids are histidine, isoleucine, leucine, lysine, methionine, phenylalanine, threonine, tryptophan, valine, and possibly glutamine. In addition, infants require dietary arginine, cysteine (cystine), and taurine.

From Moore MC: *Pocket guide to nutritional care,* ed 3, St Louis, 1997, Mosby.

Continued

Summary of Nutrients for Health—cont'd

Function	Signs and symptoms of deficiencies/individuals at increased risk for deficiencies (if applicable)	Food sources
Lipids (fats and oils)		
Energy (9 kcal/g): insulation and protection of body organs; essential fatty acids (EFA): precursors of eicosanoids (hormonelike compounds)—prostaglandins, thromboxanes, prostacyclins, and leukotrienes; linoleic acid is the primary EFA; omega-3 fatty acids are also involved in eicosanoid formation and are being intensively studied at present	Essential fatty acid deficiency: dry scaly skin, poor wound healing, delayed growth in children *At risk:* Premature infants, individuals receiving total parenteral nutrition (TPN)	Nuts, seeds, and their oils; meat, poultry, fish, eggs, whole milk, cream, and their products—butter, yogurt, ice cream, cheese Essential fatty acids: safflower, sunflower, corn, cottonseed, and soybean oils Omega-3 fatty acids: canola and soybean oils, fatty fish such as salmon, tuna, sardines
Fat-soluble vitamins *Vitamin A*		
Formation and maintenance of epithelial tissue, formation of visual rods and cones, antioxidant (a substance that prevents damage to cells from "free radicals"—oxygen-containing compounds that can disrupt proteins and lipids in cells, possibly contributing to aging and development of cancers)	Night blindness, growth retardation, Bitot's spots, corneal drying and damage (xerophthalmia), follicular hyperkeratosis *At risk:* Individuals with fat malabsorption, poor vegetable intake	Liver; fortified milk; β-carotene (vitamin A precursor): deep yellow vegetables and fruits (e.g., carrot, sweet potato, butternut squash, apricot, cantaloupe); deep green leafy vegetables (e.g., spinach, broccoli, greens)

Vitamin D Forms the hormone calcitriol, which increases calcium and phosphorus absorption in the intestine, decreases urinary loss of calcium, and regulates bone calcium	Rickets (children): bowed legs, enlarged joints, knobby deformities on rib cage Osteomalacia (adults): weakening of bones, bony pain *At risk:* People with little sun exposure (institutionalized elderly or children, cultural clothing practices that cover most skin), dark-skinned individuals	Nondiet source: sun exposure Fortified milk, fatty fish (tuna, salmon, sardines), fortified cereals
Vitamin E Antioxidant, protects cell membranes from free-radical damage	Anemia due to red blood cell hemolysis, neuropathy, and myopathy *At risk:* Premature infants, individuals with fat malabsorption	Plant oils and margarine made from them, whole grains, wheat germ, nuts, peanuts, sweet potato, avocado
Vitamin K Activation of clotting factors II (prothrombin), VII, IX, and X	Increased prothrombin time, ecchymoses, bleeding *At risk:* Individuals receiving prolonged courses of antibiotics (rare)	Egg yolk, liver, green leafy vegetables, synthesized by gut bacteria

Continued

Summary of Nutrients for Health—cont'd

Function	Signs and symptoms of deficiencies/individuals at increased risk for deficiencies (if applicable)	Food sources
Water-soluble vitamins (vitamin C and B complex)		
Vitamin C (ascorbic acid)		
Formation of collagen, thyroxine, epinephrine, norepinephrine, steroid hormones; antioxidant	Scurvy: petechiae, easy bruising, bleeding gums, painful joints, poor wound healing. *At risk:* Smokers, individuals with poor fruit and vegetable intake, oral contraceptive users, alcoholism, increased stress of illness, surgery, trauma	Citrus fruits, strawberries, kiwifruit, broccoli, peppers (red, green, or chili), cantaloupe, Brussels sprouts, cauliflower, papaya, tomatoes, potatoes
Thiamin (B₁)		
Component of coenzyme (thiamin pyrophosphate or TPP) in carbohydrate metabolism	Beriberi: weakness, irritability, peripheral neuropathy, deep muscle pain; wet beriberi: enlarged heart, tachycardia, congestive heart failure; Wernicke-Korsakoff syndrome: confusion, ataxia, eye muscle paralysis. *At risk:* Alcoholics	Pork, whole grain and enriched breads and cereals, legumes, liver, nuts
Riboflavin (B₂)		
Component of coenzymes (flavin mononucleotide [FMN] and flavin adenine dinucleotide [FAD]) in carbohydrate, protein, and fat metabolism	Cheilosis (cracking at mouth corners), glossitis (inflamed tongue), seborrheic dermatitis (scaly, greasy skin). *At risk:* Alcoholics	Milk, yogurt, enriched breads and cereals, liver

Niacin (B₃) Components of coenzymes (nicotinamide adenine dinucleotide [NAD] and nicotinamide adenine dinucleotide phosphate [NADP]) in energy production from carbohydrates, fats, and protein and fat synthesis	Pellagra: anorexia, skin lesions in areas exposed to sunlight, confusion; classic symptoms, "4 Ds," are dermatitis, diarrhea, dementia, death *At risk:* Alcoholics, poverty causing corn and rice to be major protein sources in the diet	Meats, peanuts, enriched breads and cereals, potato with skin
Pantothenic acid Component of coenzyme A, involved in fatty acid and cholesterol synthesis and lipid, protein, and carbohydrate synthesis	Rarely seen; occurs only experimentally or with other B vitamin deficiencies: burning sensation in feet, fatigue *At risk:* Alcoholics	Widespread, especially in organ meats, meat, poultry, fish, mushrooms, avocado, milk
Pyridoxine (B₆) Component of coenzyme (pyridoxal phosphate [PLP]) involved in transamination reactions, synthesis of hemoglobin	Neuropathy, microcytic anemia *At risk:* Alcoholics, oral contraceptive users, pregnant women, people receiving isoniazid (for tuberculosis)	Whole grains, meat, poultry, fish, bananas, potatoes

Continued

Summary of Nutrients for Health—cont'd

Function	Signs and symptoms of deficiencies/individuals at increased risk for deficiencies (if applicable)	Food sources
Biotin Cofactor for enzymes in synthesis of fat and purines (DNA, RNA), glucose metabolism	Rarely seen; dermatitis, atrophy of papillae on tongue, hypercholesterolemia *At risk:* Unusually high regular intake of raw egg white, alcoholics, prolonged use of antibiotics	Liver, egg yolk, cauliflower, cheese, whole grains, synthesized by gut bacteria
Folic acid (Folacin, Folate) One-carbon transfer reactions (e.g., DNA and RNA synthesis), amino acid synthesis	Megaloblastic (macrocytic) anemia, glossitis, diarrhea *At risk:* Alcoholics, pregnant women	Green leafy vegetables, liver, orange juice, legumes
Cobalamin (B_{12}) Methylation reactions (e.g., synthesis of DNA and RNA), folic acid metabolism	Megaloblastic (macrocytic) anemia, especially pernicious anemia caused by lack of intrinsic factor produced in the stomach, neuropathy, glossitis *At risk:* Elderly, postgastrectomy patients, strict vegetarians, individuals taking >10 times the RDA of vitamin C	Animal products only: liver, meat, fish, poultry, milk, egg, cheese

Continued

Component of bones, teeth, cell membranes; involved in all energy producing reactions as ATP	Muscle weakness, cardiorespiratory failure, red blood cell hemolysis *At risk:* Individuals with rapid tissue synthesis after starvation (refeeding syndrome)	Milk, cheese, yogurt, meats, whole grains, legumes, nuts, food additives, carbonated beverages
Magnesium (Mg) Component of bones, cofactor in many enzyme systems (glucose, fat, nucleic acid metabolism), involved in nerve transmission and muscle contraction	Paresthesias, tremor, muscle spasms, tetany, seizures, coma *At risk:* Alcoholics, those using diuretic therapy	Nuts, legumes, whole grains, dried fruits
Sodium (Na) Major cation in extracellular fluid, water balance, nerve transmission	Muscle cramps, nausea, vomiting, dizziness, shock, coma *At risk:* People with excessive perspiration or other fluid loss replaced with plain water	Table salt, processed foods, salted snack foods, condiments, meats, milk, cheese, breads
Potassium (K) Major cation in intracellular fluid, water balance, nerve transmission, protein synthesis	Weakness, diminished reflexes, confusion, ileus, cardiac dysrhythmia (heart block) *At risk:* Severe diarrhea or vomiting; thiazide diuretics, diabetic ketoacidosis treated with insulin and glucose	Fruits, vegetables, legumes, nuts, whole grains, meats, milk

Summary of Nutrients for Health—cont'd

Function	Signs and symptoms of deficiencies/individuals at increased risk for deficiencies (if applicable)	Food sources
Chloride (Cl) Major anion in extracellular fluid, water balance, hydrochloric acid in stomach	Hypochloremic alkalosis *At risk:* Prolonged vomiting, nasogastric suction	Table salt, salt added in food processing
Trace Minerals or Elements (<100 mg/day)		
Chromium (Cr) Cofactor for insulin in glucose metabolism	Glucose intolerance, neuropathy, weight loss, hypercholesterolemia and hypertriglyceridemia *At risk:* Heavy users of highly processed foods	Whole grains, brewer's yeast, meats
Copper (Cu) Hemoglobin synthesis, cofactor for many enzymes (e.g., in protein synthesis)	Microcytic anemia, low neutrophil count *At risk:* Excessive supplementation with Zn	Liver, meat, shellfish, legumes, nuts, cocoa, copper cookware or water pipes
Fluoride (F) Makes tooth enamel resistant to decay	Dental caries *At risk:* People not receiving fluoridated water or dental treatments	Fluoridated water, toothpaste, dental treatments, tea

Continued

Iodine (I)

Component of thyroid hormones

Goiter: enlarged thyroid, hypothyroidism
Cretinism: infant with short stature and mental retardation born to woman iodine-deficient during pregnancy
At risk: None in US

Iodized salt, seafood, food colorings, bread (from dough conditioner), milk (from cleaning agent in dairies)

Iron (Fe)

Oxygen transport in hemoglobin and myoglobin, cytochrome enzyme system

Microcytic anemia
At risk: Infants, children, adolescents, pregnant women, some endurance athletes, individuals with blood loss, postgastrectomy, vegetarians

Liver, meats, eggs, whole and en-riched grains, legumes, dark-green leafy vegetables, iron cookware

Manganese (Mn)

Cofactor in protein, carbohydrate, and fat metabolism

Rare and symptoms uncertain: weight loss, hypocholesterolemia, dermatitis
At risk: Long-term TPN without supple-mentation

Whole grains, legumes, nuts, dark-green leafy vegetables

Molybdenum (Mo)

Cofactor in oxidase enzymes

Very rare: tachycardia, stupor, central scotomas (loss of vision), coma
At risk: Long-term TPN without supple-mentation

Legumes, whole grains

Summary of Nutrients for Health—cont'd

Function	Signs and symptoms of deficiencies/individuals at increased risk for deficiencies (if applicable)	Food sources
Selenium (Se) Component of glutathione peroxidase (an antioxidant)	Cardiomyopathy, sudden death *At risk:* People eating food grown in selenium-deficient soil (Keshan province of China, New Zealand), long-term TPN without supplementation	Seafoods, whole grains, meats, legumes, milk (meat, milk, and plant Se content depend on soil content)
Zinc (Zn) Cofactor in more than 70 enzyme systems involved in growth, sexual maturation, reproduction, taste acuity, immune function	Impaired sense of taste and smell, anorexia, dermatitis, growth retardation, delayed sexual maturity, poor wound healing, impaired immune function *At risk:* Excessive Fe supplementation or Cu intake, vegetarian diet, severe diarrhea, intestinal drainage	Shellfish, meats, liver, milk, cheese, eggs, whole grains, legumes

Dietary Guidelines for All Americans

What should Americans eat to stay healthy? These guidelines, published by the US departments of Agriculture and Health and Human Services, reflect recommendations of nutrition authorities who agree that enough is known about the effect of diet on health to encourage certain dietary practices. The guidelines are as follows:

Eat a variety of foods.
Maintain a healthy weight.
Choose a diet low in fat, saturated fat, and cholesterol.
Choose a diet with plenty of vegetables, fruits, and grain products.
Use sugars only in moderation.
Use salt and sodium only in moderation.
Children and adolescents should not drink alcoholic beverages.

The *Dietary Guidelines* suggest at least the following number of servings from each of these food groups:

Vegetables	3-5 servings
Fruits	2-4 servings
Breads, cereals, rice, and pasta	6-11 servings
Milk, yogurt, and cheese	2-3 servings*
Meats, poultry, fish, dried beans and peas, eggs, and nuts	2-3 servings

---

*People aged 12 through 24 years should have three or more servings daily of foods rich in calcium.

From Center for Food Safety and Applied Nutrition: *Dietary guidelines for all Americans*, ed 4, 1995, US Food and Drug Administration.

Signs That Suggest Nutritional Imbalance

Area of concern	Possible deficiency	Possible excess
Hair		
Dull, dry, brittle	Pro	
Easily plucked (with no pain)	Pro	
Hair loss	Pro, Zn, biotin	Vit A
Flag sign (loss of hair pigment in strips around the head)	Pro, Cu	
Head and neck		
Bulging fontanel (infants)		Vit A
Headache		Vit A, D
Epistaxis (nosebleed)	Vit K	
Thyroid enlargement	Iodine	
Eyes		
Conjunctival and corneal xerosis (dryness)	Vit A	
Pale conjunctiva	Fe	
Blue sclerae	Fe	
Corneal vascularization	Vit B_2	
Mouth		
Cheilosis or angular stomatitis (lesions at corners of mouth)	Vit B_2	
Glossitis (red, sore tongue)	Niacin, folate, vit B_{12}, other B vit	
Gingivitis (inflamed gums)	Vit C	
Hypogeusia, dysgeusia (poor sense of taste, bad taste)	Zn	
Dental caries	Fluoride	
Mottling of teeth		Fluoride
Atrophy of papillae on tongue	Fe, B vit	
Skin		
Dry, scaly	Vit A, Zn, EFA	Vit A
Follicular hyperkeratosis (resembles goose-flesh)	Vit A, EFA, B vit	
Eczematous lesions	Zn	
Petechiae, ecchymoses	Vit C, K	
Nasolabial seborrhea (greasy, scaly areas between nose and upper lip)	Niacin, vit B_2, B_6	
Darkening and peeling of skin in areas exposed to sun	Niacin	
Poor wound healing	Pro, Zn, vit C	

Pro, Protein; *Vit,* vitamin(s); *EFA,* essential fatty acids; *Ca,* calcium; *Cu,* copper; *Fe,* iron; *K,* potassium; *Mg,* magnesium; *Na,* sodium; *P,* phosphorus; *Se,* selenium; *Zn,* zinc.

From Moore MC: *Pocket guide to nutritional care,* ed 3, St Louis, 1997, Mosby.

Signs That Suggest Nutritional Imbalance—cont'd

Area of concern	Possible deficiency	Possible excess
Nails		
Koilonychia (spoon-shaped nails)	Fe	
Brittle, fragile	Pro	
Heart		
Enlargement, tachycardia, failure	Vit B_1	
Small size	kcal	
Sudden failure, death	Se	
Arrhythmia	Mg, K, Se	
Hypertension	Ca, K	Na
Abdomen		
Hepatomegaly	Pro	Vit A
Ascites	Pro	
Musculoskeletal, extremities		
Muscle wasting (especially temporal area)	kcal	
Edema	Pro, vit B_1	
Calf tenderness	Vit B_1 or C, biotin, Se	
Beading of ribs, or "rachitic rosary" (child)	Vit C, D	
Bone and joint tenderness	Vit C or D, Ca, P	Vit A
Knock knees, bowed legs, fragile bones	Vit D, Ca, P, Cu	
Neurologic		
Paresthesias (pain and tingling or altered sensation in the extremities)	Vit B_1, B_6, B_{12}, biotin	
Weakness	Vit C, B_1, B_6, B_{12}, kcal	
Ataxia, decreased position and vibratory senses	Vit B_1, B_{12}	
Tremor	Mg	
Decreased tendon reflexes	Vit B_1	
Confabulation, disorientation	Vit B_1	
Drowsiness, lethargy	Vit B_1	Vit A, D
Depression	Vit B_1, biotin	

THE FOOD GUIDE PYRAMID

What Is the Food Guide Pyramid?

The Pyramid is an outline of what to eat each day. It is not a rigid prescription but a general guide that lets you choose a healthful diet that is right for you.

The Pyramid calls for eating a variety of foods to get the nutrients you need and at the same time the right amount of calories to maintain a healthy weight.

The Pyramid also focuses on fat because most American diets are too high in fat, especially saturated fat.

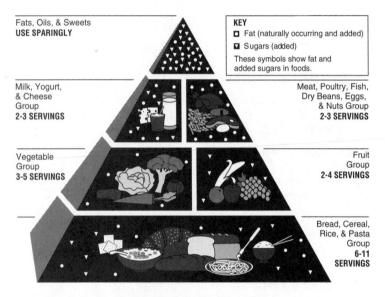

Fats, Oils, & Sweets
USE SPARINGLY

KEY
□ Fat (naturally occurring and added)
◪ Sugars (added)
These symbols show fat and added sugars in foods.

Milk, Yogurt, & Cheese Group
2-3 SERVINGS

Meat, Poultry, Fish, Dry Beans, Eggs, & Nuts Group
2-3 SERVINGS

Vegetable Group
3-5 SERVINGS

Fruit Group
2-4 SERVINGS

Bread, Cereal, Rice, & Pasta Group
6-11 SERVINGS

The Food Guide Pyramid

From the Center for Food Safety & Applied Nutrition, 1995, US FDA.

How To Make the Pyramid Work for You

How many servings are right for me?

The Pyramid shows a range of servings for each major food group. The number of servings that are right for you depends on how many calories you need, which in turn depends on your age, sex, size, and

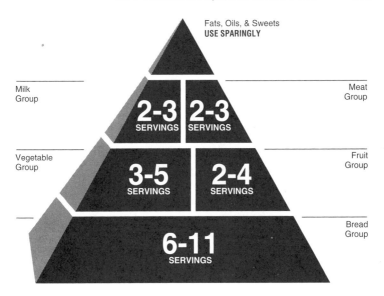

Fats, Oils, & Sweets
USE SPARINGLY

Milk Group

Meat Group

2-3 SERVINGS

2-3 SERVINGS

Vegetable Group

Fruit Group

3-5 SERVINGS

2-4 SERVINGS

Bread Group

6-11 SERVINGS

activity level. Almost everyone should have at least the lowest number of servings in the ranges.

The following calorie level suggestions are based on recommendations of the National Academy of Sciences and on calorie intakes reported by people in national food consumption surveys.

For adults and teens

1600 calories is about right for many sedentary women and some older adults.

2200 calories is about right for most children, teenage girls, active women, and many sedentary men. Women who are pregnant or breast-feeding may need somewhat more.

2800 calories is about right for teenage boys, many active men, and some very active women.

For young children

It is hard to know how much food children need to grow normally. If you're unsure, check with your doctor. Preschool children need the same variety of foods as older family members do but may need less than 1,600 calories. For fewer calories they can eat smaller servings.

From the Center for Food Safety & Applied Nutrition: *How to make the pyramid work for you,* ed 4, 1995, US FDA.

However, it is important that they have the equivalent of 2 cups of milk per day.

For you

Now, take a look at the following table. It tells you how many servings you need for your calorie level. For example, if you are an active woman who needs about 2,200 calories per day, 9 servings of breads, cereals, rice, or pasta would be right for you. You would also want to eat about 6 ounces of meat or alternates per day. Keep total fat (fat in the foods you choose as well as fat used in cooking or added at the table) to about 73 grams per day.

If you are between calorie categories, estimate servings. For example, some less active women may need only 2,000 calories to maintain a healthy weight. At that calorie level, 8 servings of breads would be about right.

Sample Diets for a Day at Three Calorie Levels

	Lower (about 1600)	Moderate (about 2200)	Higher (about 2800)
Bread group servings	6	9	11
Vegetable group servings	3	4	5
Fruit group servings	2	3	4
Milk group servings	2-3*	2-3*	2-3*
Meat group (ounces)	5†	6†	7†
Total fat (grams)	53	73	93
Total added sugars (teaspoons)	6	12	18

*Women who are pregnant or breast-feeding, teenagers, and young adults to age 24 need 3 servings.

†Meat group amounts are in total ounces.

From US Dept of Agriculture, No 252, Rockville, Md, 1992.

What Counts As a Serving?

Food groups

Bread, cereal, rice, and pasta

1 slice of bread	1 ounce of ready-to-eat cereal	½ cup of cooked cereal, rice, or pasta

Vegetable

1 cup of raw leafy vegetables	½ cup of other vegetables, cooked or chopped raw	¾ cup of vegetable juice

Fruit

1 medium apple, banana, orange	½ cup of chopped, cooked, or canned fruit	¾ cup of fruit juice

Milk, yogurt, and cheese

1 cup of milk or yogurt	1½ ounces of natural cheese	2 ounces of processed cheese

Meat, poultry, fish, dry beans, eggs, and nuts

2-3 ounces of cooked lean meat, poultry, or fish	½ cup of cooked dry beans, 1 egg, or 2 tablespoons of peanut butter count as 1 ounce of lean meat

From US Dept of Agriculture, No 252, Rockville, Md, 1992.

PART THREE

INDICATORS OF RISK

Indicators of risk are valuable as predictors of potential health problems. The nurse is always aware of changes in behavior, state of usual (normal) lifestyle, and resulting health status of clients. Risk indicators can cue the nurse toward appropriate anticipatory guidance and interactions.

ABUSE

SUBSTANCE ABUSE

Characteristics of Substances of Abuse

Substance	Route (most common first)	Common street names	Dependence: physical/psychological	Use signs and symptoms	Overdose signs and symptoms	Withdrawal signs and symptoms	Special considerations/consequences of use
Depressants							
Alcohol	Ingestion	Booze, brew, juice, spirits	Yes/Yes	Depression of major brain functions such as mood, cognition, attention, concentration, insight, judgment, memory, affect, and emotional rapport in interpersonal relationships. Extent of depression is dose dependent and ranges from lethargy through anesthesia and death.	Unconsciousness, coma, respiratory depression, death	*General depressant withdrawal syndrome:* Tremors, agitation, anxiety, diaphoresis, increased pulse and blood pressure, sleep disturbance, hallucinosis, seizures, delusions, DTs. *Postacute withdrawal:* Mood swings, difficulty sleeping, impaired cognitive functioning, increased emotionality, overreaction to stress.	Chronic alcohol use leads to serious disruptions in most organ systems: malnutrition and dehydration; vitamin deficiency leading to Wernicke's encephalopathy and alcoholic amnestic syndrome; impaired liver function, including hepatitis and cirrhosis; esophagitis, gastritis, pancreatitis; osteoporosis; anemia; peripheral neuropathy; impaired pulmonary function; cardiomyopathy;
Barbiturates	Ingestion, injection	Barbs, beans, black beauties, blue angels, candy, downers, goof balls, G.B., nebbies, reds, sleepers, yellow jackets, yellows	Yes/Yes	Psychomotor impairment, increased reaction time, interruption of hand-eye coordination, motor ataxia, nystagmus. Decreased REM sleep leading to more dreams and sometimes nightmares.			
Benzodiazepines	Ingestion, injection	Downers	Yes/Yes			*Low-dose benzodiazepine withdrawal:* Therapeutic	

Drug	Route	Dependence Physical/Psychological	Signs of use	Effects of overdose	Withdrawal syndrome	Comments
					doses for no more than 6 months; subtle symptoms, peak in about 12 days; wax and wane for 6-12 months; several symptom-free days, followed by acute anxiety, dilated pupils, and elevated pulse and blood pressure. *High-dose benzodiazepine withdrawal:* Peaks in 2 to 3 days for short-acting drugs and 5 to 8 days for longer-acting; symptoms usually gone in 2 weeks.	myopathy; disrupted immune system; and brain damage. High susceptibility to other dependencies. Dependence on barbiturates and benzodiazepines may develop insidiously; users may underreport the actual amount taken because of guilt about multiple prescriptions and abuse.
Stimulants						
Amphetamines	Ingestion, injection	Yes/Yes	A, AMT, bam, bennies, crystal, diet pills, dolls, eye-openers, lid poppers, pep pills, purple hearts, speed, uppers, wake-ups	Sudden rush of euphoria, abrupt awakening, increased energy, talkativeness, elation. Agitation, hyperactivity, irritability, grandiosity, pressured speech. Diaphoresis, anorexia, weight loss, insomnia. Increased temperature, blood pressure, and pulse. Tachycardia, ectopic heartbeats, chest pain. Urinary retention, constipation, dry mouth.	Seizures. Cardiac arrhythmias, coronary artery spasms, myocardial infarctions, marked increase in blood pressure and temperature that can lead to cardio-	*Crash:* Depression, agitation, anxiety, and intense drug craving followed by fatigue, depression, loss of drug desire, insomnia, desire for sleep followed by prolonged sleep then extreme hunger, renewed drug cravings, anergia, and anhedonia, which may increase for 1 to 4 days.	Certain amphetamines prescribed for attention deficit hyperactivity disorder in children because of a paradoxical depressant action. Sometimes these medications are stolen and abused. May be used alternately with depressants.

Continued

From Stuart G, Laraia M: *Stuart & Sundeen's principles and practice of psychiatric nursing,* ed 6, St Louis, 1998, Mosby.

Characteristics of Substances of Abuse—cont'd

Substance	Route (most common first)	Common street names	Dependence: physical/ psychological	Use signs and symptoms	Overdose signs and symptoms	Withdrawal signs and symptoms	Special considerations/ consequences of use
Stimulants —cont'd							
Cocaine	Inhalation, smoking, injection, topical	Bernice, bernies, big C, blow, C, charlie, coke, dust, girl, heaven, jay, lady, nose candy, nose powder, snow, sugar, white lady Crack = conan, freebase, rock, toke, white cloud, white tomado	Yes/Yes	*High dose:* Slurred, rapid, incoherent speech. Stereotypic movements, ataxic gait, teeth grinding, illogical thought processes, headache, nausea, vomiting. *Toxic psychosis:* Paranoid delusions in clear sensorium; auditory, visual, or tactile hallucinations. Very labile mood. Unprovoked violence.	vascular shock and death	Pattern varies widely among patients; anxiety, depression, irritability, fatigue may last several weeks; craving may return; relapse is a risk. Sometimes a user stops stimulants purposely to decrease tolerance, decreasing the amount needed to get high.	Cocaine use may lead to multiple physical problems: destruction of the nasal septum related to snorting, coronary artery vasoconstriction, seizures, cerebrovascular accidents; transient ischemic episodes, sudden death related to respiratory arrest, and myocardial infarction. Intravenous use of stimulants may lead to the serious physical consequences described under Opiates

Opiates

Heroin	Injection, ingestion, inhalation	H, horse, harry, boy, scag, shit, smack, stuff, white junk, white stuff	Yes/Yes	Euphoria, relaxation, relief from pain, "nodding out" (apathy, detachment from reality, impaired judgment, and drowsiness); constricted pupils, nausea, constipation, slurred speech, respiratory depression.	Unconsciousness, coma, respiratory depression, circulatory depression, respiratory arrest, cardiac arrest, death. Anoxia can lead to brain abscess	*Initially:* Drug craving, lacrimation, rhinorrhea, yawning, diaphoresis. *In 12-72 hr:* Sleep disturbance, mydriasis, anorexia, piloerection, irritability, tremor, weakness, nausea, vomiting, diarrhea, chills, fever, muscle spasms, flushing, spontaneous ejaculation, abdominal pain, hypertension, increased rate and depth of respirations. *Protracted withdrawal:* Changes in respirations and temperature, decreased self-esteem, anxiety, depression, drug hunger, and abnormal responses to stressful situations. Lasts up to 6 months.	Intravenous use leads to risk for infection with bloodborne pathogens, such as HIV or hepatitis B. Other infections (skin abscesses, phlebitis, cellulitis, and septic emboli causing pneumonia, pulmonary abscess, or subacute bacterial endocarditis) may occur as a result of lack of asepsis or contaminated substances. Chronic use leads to lack of concern about physical well-being, resulting in malnutrition and dehydration. Criminal behavior may occur to acquire money for drugs.
Morphine	Injection						
Meperidine	Injection, ingestion						
Codeine	Ingestion, injection						
Opium	Smoking, ingestion						
Methadone	Ingestion						

Continued

Characteristics of Substances of Abuse—cont'd

Substance	Route (most common first)	Common street names	Dependence: physical/ psychological	Use signs and symptoms	Overdose signs and symptoms	Withdrawal signs and symptoms	Special considerations/ consequences of use
Marijuana	Smoking, ingestion	Acapulco gold, aunt mary, broccoli, dope, grass, grunt, hay, hemp, herb, J, joint, joy stick, killer weed, maryjane, pot, ragweed, reefer, smoke, weed	No/Yes	Altered state of awareness, relaxation, mild euphoria, reduced inhibition, red eyes, dry mouth, increased appetite, increased pulse, decreased reflexes, panic reaction.	Toxic psychosis	None	Pulmonary problems. Interference with reproductive hormones. May cause fetal abnormalities.
Hallucinogens	Ingestion, smoking	Acid, big D, blotter, blue heaven, cap, D, deeda, flash, L, mellow yellows, microdots, paper acid, sugar, ticket, yello	No/No	Distorted perceptions and hallucinations in the presence of a clear sensorium. Distortions of time and space, illusions, depersonalization, mystical experiences, heightened sense of awareness. Extreme mood lability. Tremor, dizziness, piloerection, paresthesias, synesthesia, nausea, and vomiting. Increased temperature, pulse, blood	Rare with LSD: convulsions, hyperthermia, death	None	Flashbacks may last for several months. Permanent psychosis may occur.

Drug	Route	Street Names	Physical/Psychological Dependence	Effects	Overdose	Withdrawal	Flashbacks
Phencyclidine (PCP)	Smoking, ingestion	Angel dust, DOA, dust, elephant, hog, peace pill, supergrass, tic tac	No/No	pressure, and salivation. Panic reaction, "bad trip." Intensely psychotic experience characterized by bizarre perceptions, confusion, disorientation, euphoria, hallucinations, paranoia, grandiosity, agitation. Anesthesia. Apparent enhancement of strength and endurance. Rage reactions. May be agitated and hyperactive with tendency toward violence or catatonic and withdrawn or vacillate between the two conditions. Red, dry skin; dilated pupils, nystagmus, ataxia, hypertension, rigidity, and seizures.	Seizures, coma, and death	None	If flashbacks occur, they are mild and usually not disturbing.
Inhalants	Inhalation	Spray, rush, bolt, huffing, bagging, sniffing	Yes/Yes	*Psychological:* Belligerence, assaultiveness, apathy, impaired judgment. *Physical:* Dizziness, nystagmus, incoordination, slurred speech, unsteady gait, depressed reflexes, tremor, blurred vision, euphoria, anorexia.	Lethargy, stupor/coma, respiratory arrest, cardiac arrhythmia	Headaches, chills, abdominal cramps, delirium, tremors (not common)	Death from inhalants can occur in different ways: Sudden death is caused by cardiac arrhythmia—sometimes this happens the first time an inhalant is used.

Continued

Characteristics of Substances of Abuse—cont'd

Substance	Route (most common first)	Common street names	Dependence: physical/ psychological	Use signs and symptoms	Overdose signs and symptoms	Withdrawal signs and symptoms	Special considerations/ consequences of use
Inhalants— cont'd							Suicide may be a result of impaired judgment. Injury: Under the influence of inhalants, the user feels invulnerable. Burns and frostbite can also be caused by these chemicals. Permanent cognitive impairment may require an individual to reside in a structured setting.

The Five Stages of Substance Abuse

Stage	Drugs	Sources	Frequency	Feelings	Behavior	Treatment
1. Curiosity	None	Available—but not used	—	Curiosity	Risk taking, desire for acceptance	Optimal time; anticipatory guidance to develop good coping skills and strong self-esteem; clear family guidelines on drug and alcohol use; drug education
2. Experimentation	Tobacco, alcohol, marijuana	House supply, friends, siblings	Weekend use for recreational purposes	Excitement, pleasure, few consequences; learning how easy it is to feel good	Lying, little change	Drug education; attention to societal messages; reduction of supply; strict, loving rules at home; establishment of drug-free alternative activities
3. Regular use	As above, plus hashish or oil, tranquilizers, sedatives, amphetamines	Buying	Progresses to midweek use; purpose is to get high	Excitement followed by guilt	Mood swings, faltering school performance, truancy, changing peer groups, changing style of dress	Drug-free self-help groups (Alcoholics or Narcotics Anonymous); family involvement; psychiatric counseling unhelpful unless family therapy and aftercare provided

Adapted from MacDonald DI: *Pediatric Rev* 10:89, 1988. In Stuart G, Laraia M: *Stuart & Sundeen's principles and practice of psychiatric nursing*, ed 6, St Louis, 1998, Mosby.

Continued

The Five Stages of Substance Abuse—cont'd

Stage	Drugs	Sources	Frequency	Feelings	Behavior	Treatment
4. Psychologic or chemical dependency	As above, plus stimulants, hallucinogens	Selling to support habit; possibly stealing or prostitution in exchange for drugs	Daily	Euphoric highs followed by depression, shame, guilt, and perhaps suicidal thoughts	Pathologic lying; school failure; family fights; involvement with the law over curfew, truancy, vandalism, shoplifting, driving under the influence, breaking and entering, violence	Inpatient or foster care programs that require family involvement and provide aftercare
5. Using drugs to feel "normal"	As above; any available drug, including opiates	Any way possible	All day	Euphoria rare and harder to achieve; chronic depression	Drifting, with repeated failures and psychologic symptoms of paranoia and aggression; frequent overdosing, blackouts, amnesia, chronic cough, fatigue, malnutrition	Inpatient or foster care programs that require family involvement and provide aftercare

Brief Drug Abuse Screening Test (B-DAST)

Instructions: The following questions concern information about your involvement with and abuse of drugs. Drug abuse refers to (1) the use of prescribed or over-the-counter drugs in excess of the directions and (2) any nonmedical use of drugs. Carefully read each statement and decide whether your answer is YES or NO. Then circle the appropriate response. Give one point for all YES answers and zero points for NO answers. Items 4 and 5 get one point for NO response. Scores of 6 or above suggest significant drug abuse problems. Patients who score above established cut-off scores are considered to be addicted. Since tools can be incorrect, all people screened positive for addiction should be further assessed according to diagnostic criteria.

YES	NO	1. Have you used drugs other than those required for medical reasons?
YES	NO	2. Have you abused prescription drugs?
YES	NO	3. Do you abuse more than one drug at a time?
YES	NO	4. Can you get through the week without using drugs (other than those required for medical reasons)?
YES	NO	5. Are you always able to stop using drugs when you want to?
YES	NO	6. Have you had "blackouts" or "flashbacks" as a result of drug use?
YES	NO	7. Do you ever feel bad about your drug abuse?
YES	NO	8. Does your spouse (or parents) ever complain about your involvement with drugs?
YES	NO	9. Has drug abuse ever created problems between you and your spouse?
YES	NO	10. Have you ever lost friends because of your use of drugs?
YES	NO	11. Have you ever neglected your family or missed work because of your use of drugs?
YES	NO	12. Have you ever been in trouble at work because of drug abuse?
YES	NO	13. Have you ever lost a job because of drug abuse?
YES	NO	14. Have you gotten into fights when under the influence of drugs?
YES	NO	15. Have you engaged in illegal activities in order to obtain drugs?

From Skinner HA: *Addict Behav* 7:363, 1982.

YES	NO	16. Have you ever been arrested for possession of illegal drugs?
YES	NO	17. Have you ever experienced withdrawal symptoms as a result of heavy drug intake?
YES	NO	18. Have you had medical problems as a result of your drug use (e.g., memory loss, hepatitis, convulsions, bleeding)?
YES	NO	19. Have you ever gone to anyone for help for a drug problem?
YES	NO	20. Have you ever been involved in a treatment program specifically related to drug use?

The CAGE Questionnaire

- Have you ever felt you ought to **C**ut down on your drinking?
- Have people **A**nnoyed you by criticizing your drinking?
- Have you ever felt bad or **G**uilty about your drinking?
- Have you ever had a drink first thing in the morning to steady your nerves or get rid of a hangover (**E**ye-opener)?

Scoring: One "yes" answer calls for further inquiry. Two "yes" answers suggest an alcohol abuse problem.

From Ewing JA: *JAMA* 252(14):1905-1907, 1984. Copyright 1984 by the American Medical Association. Reprinted by permission.

Selected Drugs Commonly Abused and Symptoms of Abuse

Drug category	Street names	Methods of use	Symptoms of use	Hazards of use
Marijuana/hashish	Pot, grass, reefer, weed, Columbian, hash, hash oil, sinsemilla, joint	Most often smoked; can also be swallowed in solid form	Sweet, burnt odor Neglect of appearance Loss of interest, motivation Possible weight loss	Impaired memory, perception Interference with psychologic maturation Possible damage to lungs, heart, and reproduction and immune systems Psychologic dependence
Alcohol	Booze, hooch, juice, brew	Swallowed in liquid form	Impaired muscle coordination, judgment	Heart and liver damage Death from overdose Death from car accidents Addiction
Amphetamines* Amphetamine Dextroamphetamine Methamphetamine	Speed, uppers, pep pills Bennies Dexies Meth, crystal Black beauties	Swallowed in pill or capsule form, or injected into veins	Excess activity Irritability; nervousness Mood swings Needle marks	Loss of appetite Hallucinations; paranoia Convulsions; coma Brain damage Death from overdose

*Includes look-alike drugs resembling amphetamines that contain caffeine, phenylpropanolamine (PPA), and ephedrine.

Continued

Selected Drugs Commonly Abused and Symptoms of Abuse—cont'd

Drug category	Street names	Methods of use	Symptoms of use	Hazards of use
Cocaine	Coke, snow, toot, white lady, crack	Most often inhaled (snorted); also injected or swallowed in powder form, smoked	Restlessness, anxiety Intense, short-term high followed by dysphoria	Intensive psychologic dependence Sleeplessness; anxiety Nasal passage damage Lung damage Death from overdose
Nicotine	Coffin nail Butt, smoke	Smoked in cigarettes, cigars, and pipes, snuff, chewing tobacco	Smell of tobacco High carbon monoxide blood levels Stained teeth	Cancers of the lung, throat, mouth, eso-phagus Heart disease; emphysema
Barbiturates Pentobarbital Secobarbital Amobarbital	Barbs, downers Yellow jackets Red devils Blue devils	Swallowed in pill form or injected into veins	Drowsiness Confusion Impaired judgment Slurred speech Needle marks Constricted pupils	Infection Addiction with severe, life-threatening with-drawal symptoms Loss of appetite Death from overdose Nausea
Narcotics Dilaudid, Percodan Demerol, Methadone		Swallowed in pill or liq-uid form, injected	Drowsiness Lethargy	Addiction with severe withdrawal symptoms Loss of appetite Death from overdose

Drug	Street Names	How Used	Symptoms
Morphine Heroin Codeine	Dreamer, junk, smack, horse School boy	Injected into veins, smoked Swallowed in pill or liquid form	Needle marks
Hallucinogens PCP (Phencyclidine)	Angel dust, killer weed, supergrass, hog, peace pill	Most often smoked; can also be inhaled (snorted), injected, or swallowed in tablets	Slurred speech; blurred vision, uncoordination Confusion, agitation Aggression Anxiety; depression Impaired memory, perception Death from accidents Death from overdose
LSD	Acid, cubes, purple haze	Injected or swallowed in tablets	
Mescaline	Mesc, cactus	Usually ingested in their natural form	Dilated pupils Delusions; hallucinations Mood swings Breaks from reality Emotional breakdown Flashback
Psilocybin	Magic mushrooms		
Inhalants Gasoline Airplane glue Paint thinner		Inhaled or sniffed, often with use of paper or plastic bag or rag	Poor motor coordination Impaired vision, memory, and thought processes Abusive, violent behavior Slowed thought Headache High risk of sudden death Drastic weight loss Brain, liver, and bone marrow damage Anemia, death by anoxia
Nitrites Amyl Butyl	Poppers, locker room, rush, snappers		

Leading Drugs Abused in the United States*

Males	Females
1. alcohol in combination	1. alcohol in combination
2. cocaine	2. cocaine
3. heroin/morphine	3. acetaminophen (Tylenol)
4. marijuana/hashish	4. heroin/morphine
5. acetaminophen (Tylenol)	5. aspirin
6. methamphetamine/speed	6. alprazolam (Xanax)
7. aspirin	7. ibuprofen (Motrin)
8. ibuprofen (Motrin)	8. marijuana/hashish
9. diazepam (Valium)	9. diazepam (Valium)
10. PCP/PCP combinations	10. lorazepam (Ativan)
11. benzodiazepine (unspecified)	11. clonazepam (Klonopin)
12. alprazolam (Xanax)	12. amitriptyline (Elavil)
13. clonazepam (Klonopin)	13. D-propoxyphene (Darvon products)
14. amitriptyline (Elavil)	14. acetaminophen with codeine
15. amphetamine	15. diphenhydramine (Benadryl)

*Trade names are in parentheses; many of these products are also available under other trade or generic names. Statistics are based on drug episodes caused by an illegal drug or nonmedical use of a legal drug resulting in emergency department visits.

CHILD ABUSE

Types of Child Abuse

Physical neglect
Suggestive physical findings

Failure to thrive

Signs of malnutrition, such as thin extremities, abdominal distention, lack of subcutaneous fat

Poor personal hygiene, especially of teeth

Unclean and/or inappropriate dress

Evidence of poor healthcare, such as nonimmunized status, untreated infections, frequent colds

Frequent injuries from lack of supervision

From Wong D, et al: *Whaley and Wong's nursing care of infants and children,* ed 6, St Louis, 1999, Mosby.

Suggestive behaviors

Dull and inactive; excessively passive or sleepy

Self-stimulatory behaviors, such as finger-sucking or rocking

Begging or stealing food ⎫

Absenteeism from school ⎬ in older child

Drug or alcohol addiction ⎪

Vandalism or shoplifting ⎭

Emotional abuse and neglect

Suggestive physical findings

Failure to thrive

Feeding disorders, such as rumination

Enuresis

Sleep disorders

Suggestive behaviors

Self-stimulatory behaviors such as biting, rocking, sucking

During infancy, lack of social smile and stranger anxiety

Withdrawal

Unusual fearfulness

Antisocial behavior, such as destructiveness, stealing, cruelty

Extremes of behavior, such as overcompliant and passive or aggressive and demanding

Lags in emotional and intellectual development, especially language

Suicide attempts

Physical abuse

Suggestive physical findings

Bruises and welts

On face, lips, mouth, back, buttocks, thighs, or areas of torso

Regular patterns descriptive of object used, such as belt buckle, hand, wire hanger, chain, wooden spoon, squeeze or pinch marks

May be present in various stages of healing

Burns

On soles of feet, palms of hands, back, or buttocks

Patterns descriptive of object used, such as round cigar or cigarette burns, "glovelike" sharply demarcated areas from immersion in scalding water, rope burns on wrists or ankles from being bound, burns in the shape of an iron, radiator, or electric stove burner

Absence of "splash" marks and presence of symmetric burns

Stun gun injury—lesions circular, fairly uniform (up to

0.5 cm), and paired approximately 5 cm apart (Frechette and Rimsza, 1992)

Fractures and dislocations
    Skull, nose, or facial structures
    Injury may denote type of abuse, such as spiral fracture or dislocation from twisting of an extremity or whiplash from shaking the child
    Multiple new or old fractures in various stages of healing

Lacerations and abrasions
    On backs of arms, legs, torso, face, or external genitalia
    Unusual symptoms, such as abdominal swelling, pain, and vomiting from punching
    Descriptive marks such as from human bites or pulling out of hair

Chemical
    Unexplained repeated poisoning, especially drug overdose
    Unexplained sudden illness, such as hypoglycemia from insulin administration

Suggestive behaviors

Wariness of physical contact with adults
Apparent fear of parents or of going home
Lying very still while surveying environment
Inappropriate reaction to injury, such as failure to cry from pain
Lack of reaction to frightening events
Apprehensiveness when hearing other children cry
Indiscriminate friendliness and displays of affection
Superficial relationships
Acting-out behavior, such as aggression, to seek attention
Withdrawal behavior

Sexual abuse

Suggestive physical findings

Bruises, bleeding, lacerations or irritation of external genitals, anus, mouth, or throat
Torn, stained, or bloody underclothing
Pain on urination or pain, swelling, and itching of genital area
Penile discharge
Sexually transmitted disease, nonspecific vaginitis, or venereal warts
Difficulty in walking or sitting
Unusual odor in the genital area
Recurrent urinary tract infections
Presence of sperm
Pregnancy in young adolescent

Suggestive behaviors

Sudden emergence of sexually related problems, including excessive or public masturbation, age-inappropriate sexual play, promiscuity, or overtly seductive behavior

Withdrawn behavior, excessive daydreaming

Preoccupation with fantasies, especially in play

Poor relationships with peers

Sudden changes, such as anxiety, loss or gain of weight, clinging behavior

In incestuous relationships, excessive anger at mother for not protecting daughter

Regressive behavior, such as bed-wetting or thumb-sucking

Sudden onset of phobias or fears, particularly fears of the dark, men, strangers, or particular settings or situations (e.g., undue fear of leaving the house or staying at the daycare center or the babysitter's house)

Running away from home

Substance abuse, particularly of alcohol or mood-elevating drugs

Profound and rapid personality changes, especially extreme depression, hostility, and aggression (often accompanied by social withdrawal)

Rapidly declining school performance

Suicidal attempts or ideation

Components of Report of Child Maltreatment

History of injury

1. Date, time, and place of occurrence
2. Sequence of events with recorded times
3. Presence of witnesses, especially person caring for child at time of incident
4. Time lapse between occurrence of injury and initiation of treatment
5. Interview with child when appropriate, including verbal quotations and information from drawing or other play activities
6. Interview with parent, witnesses, or other significant persons, including verbal quotations
7. Description of parent-child interactions (verbal interactions, eye contact, touching, parental concern)
8. Name, age, and condition of other children in home (if possible)

From Wong D, et al: *Whaley and Wong's nursing care of infants and children,* ed 6, St Louis, 1999, Mosby.

Physical examination

1. Location, size, shape, and color of bruises; approximate location, size, and shape on drawing of body outline
2. Distinguishing characteristics, such as a bruise in the shape of a hand; round burn (possibly caused by cigarette)
3. Symmetry or asymmetry of injury; presence of other injuries
4. Degree of pain; any bone tenderness
5. Evidence of past injuries; general state of health and hygiene
6. Developmental level of child; perform screening test

Parental Risk Factors for Child Maltreatment

Physical indicators	Behavioral indicators in child	Parental behaviors/characteristics
Indicators of physical abuse		
Bruises and welts	Believes deserves punishment	Offers illogical, contradicting, or changing explanation of injury
On face, lips, mouth	May be wary of adult contacts	Seems unconcerned about child
On torso, back, buttocks, thighs	Becomes apprehensive when other children cry	Blames injury on child or someone else (e.g., sibling)
In various stages of healing	Exhibits behavioral extremes	Does not respond to child's crying or needs
Red/purple 2-4 hours	Withdrawal	Uses harsh discipline inappropriate to child's age, condition, or behavior
Green 5-7 days	Aggressiveness	Is unable to supply history of child's development, milestones, etc.
Yellow 8-14 days	Inappropriate maturity	Delays bringing child in for treatment
Brown/fading 2-4 weeks	Much manipulative behavior	Refuses to consent to diagnostic studies
Clustered, forming regular patterns	Exhibits fear of parents or of going home	"Hospital shops"
Reflecting shape of article used to inflict injury (e.g., electrical cord, belt buckle, hand)	May report injury by parent	Is emotionally immature
On several surfaces	Does not cry when approached by examiner or during painful procedures	Has low self-esteem
Burns	Forms only superficial relationships	Is isolated—no support system
Circular burns (i.e., cigarette) especially on soles, palms, back, or buttocks	Engages in indiscriminate displays of affection	Has unrealistic expectations of children
Immersion burns (socklike, glovelike, perineal) symmetrical, absence of "splash" marks	Responds to questions in monosyllables	Expects children to meet emotional needs (role reversal)
Patterned object used (iron, radiator, stove burner)	Demonstrates poor self-concept	Sees the child as "bad" or "different"

Continued

From Scipien G, et al: *Pediatric nursing care,* St Louis, 1990, Mosby.

Parental Risk Factors for Child Maltreatment—cont'd

Physical indicators	Behavioral indicators in child	Parental behaviors/characteristics
Rope burns on arms, legs, neck, or torso		
Infected burns indicating a delay in seeking treatment		
Fractures/dislocations		
To skull, nose, facial structures, ribs, clavicle		
Femural fractures in the nonambulatory child		
Multiple, in various stages of healing		
Spiral fractures indicative of twisting of extremity		
Lacerations and abrasions		
To face, torso, back of arms or legs, external genitals		
Bite mark appearance		
Abdominal injuries		
External bruises		
Internal		
Renal		
Pancreatic		
Ruptured liver, spleen, intestinal perforation		

Head injuries
  Subdural hematomas
  Skull fractures
  Scalp swelling
  Bald patches on scalp
  Retinal hemorrhages
  Black eyes
Chemical
  Unexplained repeat poisoning, drug overdose, or other unusual substance

Indicators of physical neglect

Underweight, poor growth patterns, failure-to-thrive	Begs, steals food	Has chaotic home life
Hunger, poor hygiene, inappropriate clothing	Arrives early and stays late at school or is frequently absent from school	Has inadequate, unsafe living conditions
Abdominal distention	Fatigued and listless, falls asleep in class	Lacks knowledge of child's needs
Wasting of subcutaneous tissue	Inappropriately seeks affection	Has low self-esteem
Unattended physical problems or medical needs	States he has no caretaker	Is passive, has little motivation to effect change in lives
Abandonment	Assumes adult responsibilities and concerns	Lives isolated from friends, neighbors, and relatives
	Delinquent	
	Abuses alcohol and drugs	

Indicators of emotional abuse and neglect

Failure-to-thrive	Infant—lack of social smile and stranger anxiety	Blames and belittles the child
Feeding disorders	Withdrawal	Withhold love
Speech disorders	Self-stimulating behaviors such as sucking, biting, rocking	Is cold and rejecting
Sleep disorders		Has unrealistic expectations
Enuresis		

Continued

Parental Risk Factors for Child Maltreatment—cont'd

Physical indicators	Behavioral indicators in the child	Parental behaviors/characteristics
Lags in physical development	Antisocial behaviors—destructiveness, cruelty, stealing Lags in emotional and intellectual development Behavior extremes: passive and compliant to aggressive and demanding Unusual fearfulness Psychoneurotic reactions—phobias, obsession, compulsions Suicide attempts	Is verbally abusive (name-calling, constant criticism) Treats children in home unequally Minimizes child's problems Has personality disorders
Indicators of sexual abuse		
Difficulty in walking or sitting Torn, stained, or bloody underclothing Pain on urination Bruises or lacerations of external genital, vaginal, or anal areas Pain, swelling, or itching in genital area Mouth and throat injuries Sexually transmitted disease in child under 12 years of age	Infant/toddler Irritability Sleep disturbances Altered level of activity Preschool child Nightmares Regression in development Explicit knowledge of sexual acts Clinging/whining to nonabusive parent Fear of places, persons, or situations of which not previously afraid	Has low self-esteem Has unmet emotional needs Lacks social and emotional contacts outside the family—isolated May have marital problems with spouse and seek affection from child May have experienced loss of spouse through death or divorce

School-age child
  Behavioral problems
  Frightening dreams, sleep disturbances
  Withdrawal, regression, fantasy
  Unwilling to change for or participate
    in physical education
  Poor peer relationships
  Decreased school performance
  Truancy, running away
  Bizarre sexual knowledge and behavior
Adolescent
  Fright, confusion
  Anger, acting out
  Truancy, running away, promiscuity,
    prostitution
  Depression
  Drug and alcohol abuse
  Poor peer relationships
  Suicide

Paraphilias

Disorder	Definition	Distinguishing characteristics
Transvestic fetishism	Recurrent or persistent cross-dressing in the clothes of the opposite sex for release of tension or for sexual pleasure	Some transvestites are transsexuals, whereas some are homosexuals, cross-dressing to attract other homosexuals. Intense frustration is experienced when there is interference with cross-dressing. Cross-dressing is generally used for the purpose of sexual excitement.
Zoophilia (Bestiality)	The act of deriving sexual pleasure from animals	Sexual activity with animals is the exclusive method of achieving sexual pleasure.
Pedophilia (Child molesting)	The act of obtaining sexual pleasure by molesting a child in the prepubertal stage of development	Pedophiles are often male and in their late thirties or early forties. The offender is often familiar to the child and may be a relative, friend, or acquaintance. The child is generally at least 10 years younger than the offender, who may be oriented toward children of the same or opposite sex.
Exhibitionism	The act of deriving erotic pleasure from briefly exposing the genitals to a surprised victim	The act generally occurs in a public place. Pleasure stems from seeing the shocked reaction of the viewer. Masturbation sometimes accompanies the act of exposure. Victims are generally female children or adults.
Voyeurism	The act of deriving sexual pleasure through viewing sex organs or sex acts of an unsuspecting victim	The voyeur's primary sex activity is viewing the sexual behavior of others. Generally occurs in early adulthood and is a chronic condition.
Sexual masochism	The act of deriving sexual pleasure and gratification by experiencing physical or mental pain and humiliation	The masochist desires to be dominated in the sexual relationship and is excited by the idea of being the recipient of pain. It involves being humiliated, bound, beaten, or otherwise made to suffer.

From Haber J, et al: *Comprehensive psychiatric nursing,* ed 5, St Louis, 1997, Mosby.

Disorder	Definition	Distinguishing characteristics
Sexual sadism	The act of receiving sexual pleasure and erotic gratification through infliction of physical or psychological pain on another	The sadist achieves orgasm from sadistic acts even when other sexual outlets are available. The desire to dominate is a primary dynamic. Generally, it involves a nonconsenting partner but may sometimes involve a consenting partner. Rape may be committed by persons with this disorder.

Methods Used to Pressure Children into Sexual Activity

The child is offered gifts or privileges.

The adult misrepresents moral standards by telling the child that it is "okay to do."

Isolated and emotionally and socially impoverished children are enticed by adults who meet their needs for warmth and human contact.

The successful sex offender pressures the victim into secrecy regarding the activity by describing it as a "secret between us" that other people may take away if they find out.

The offender plays on the child's fears, including fear of punishment by the offender, fear of repercussions if the child tells, and fear of abandonment or rejection by the family.

From Wong DL, et al: *Whaley and Wong's nursing care of infants and children,* ed 6, St Louis, 1999, Mosby.

Talking with Children Who Reveal Abuse

Provide a private time and place to talk.

Do not promise not to tell; tell them that you are required by law to report the abuse.

Do not express shock or criticize their family.

Use their vocabulary to discuss body parts.

Avoid using any leading statements that can distort their report.

Reassure them that they have done the right thing by telling.

Tell them that the abuse is not their fault, that they are not bad or to blame.

Determine their immediate need for safety.

Let the child know what will happen when you report.

Warning Signs of Child Abuse

Physical evidence of abuse or neglect, including previous injuries

Conflicting stories about the "accident" or injury from the parents or others

Cause of injury blamed on sibling or other party

An injury inconsistent with the history, such as a concussion and broken arm from falling off a bed

History inconsistent with child's developmental level, such as a 6-month-old turning on the hot water

A complaint other than the one associated with signs of abuse (e.g., a chief complaint of a cold when there is evidence of first- and second-degree burns)

Inappropriate response of caregiver, such as an exaggerated or absent emotional response; refusal to sign for additional tests or agree to necessary treatment; excessive delay in seeking treatment; absence of the parents for questioning

Inappropriate response of child, such as little or no response to pain; fear of being touched; excessive or lack of separation anxiety; indiscriminate friendliness to strangers

Child's report of physical or sexual abuse

Previous reports of abuse in the family

Repeated visits to emergency facilities with injuries

From Wong DL, et al: *Whaley and Wong's nursing care of infants and children,* ed 6, St Louis, 1999, Mosby.

Child History—Indicators of Potential or Actual Child Abuse and Neglect

Area of assessment	At-risk responses
Primary concern/ reason for visit	Historical data that do not fit with physical findings
	Vague complaints about child
	Inappropriate delay in bringing child to healthcare facility
	Reluctance on the part of the parent to give information
	Inappropriate parental reaction to nurse's concern (overreacts or underreacts)
	Hyperactivity
Family health history	
Parents	Grew up in a violent home (abused as child, observed mother or siblings abused)
	Low self-esteem
	Violence between adults
	Little knowledge of child development and care
	Substance abuse
	Adolescent birth of child
Siblings	History of abuse or neglect of siblings
	Large family
	History of sudden infant death
	Several young, dependent children in family
Other family members	Other history of violence or violent death
Household	Violence and aggression used to resolve conflicts and solve problems
	Poverty
	Single parent
	Very young parent (early teens)
	No friends, neighbors, or other support systems available
	Problems between parents, especially over children
	Other stressors
	Unemployment
	Illness in the family
	History of child foster home or other institutional placement for abuse/neglect
Child health history	
Prenatal	Unwanted pregnancy
	Difficult or complicated pregnancy
	Early adolescent parent
	Wanted a baby so that "I would have someone to love"
	Little or no prenatal care

From Campbell J, Humphreys J: *Nursing care of survivors of family violence,* St Louis, 1993, Mosby.   *Continued*

Child History—Indicators of Potential or Actual Child Abuse and Neglect—cont'd

Area of assessment	At-risk responses
Birth	Cesarean section
	Prematurity
	Low birth weight
	Birth defect
	Immediate separation of parents and child
	Child not of preferred sex or appearance
Neonatal	Separation of parents and child
	Complications or identification of health problem
Nutrition (if necessary include 24-hour dietary recall)	History of feeding problems (frequent change of formula, colic, difficult to feed)
	Inappropriate food, drink, or drugs
	Dietary intake that does not fit with physical findings
	Inadequate or excessive food or fluid intake
	Obesity, anorexia, or bulimia
Personal/social	Negative description of child (different, troublesome, difficult)
	Parent has unrealistic expectations of child
	Multiple school absences
	Difficulty in school
	Depression
	History of phobias, running away from home, or delinquent acts
	Poor peer relationships or no peer relations
	Sexual problems in child (excessive or public masturbation, age-inappropriate sexual play, promiscuity)
	History of pregnancy
	Substance abuse
Discipline	Use of physical punishment, especially in an infant or adolescent
	Use of an object to administer physical punishment
	Excessive, inappropriate, inconsistent physical punishment
	History of parent "losing control" or "hitting too hard"
Sleep	"Doesn't sleep," "Awake all night"
	Consistent history of inadequate sleep for age
Elimination	Inappropriate, excessive home treatment of constipation
	Enuresis
	Violent or excessively severe toilet training

Area of assessment	At-risk responses
Growth and development	History of excessive autostimulation
	"Hyperactivity"
	Learning disability
	Developmental delays
	Excessive aggression or passivity
Illness	Disability requiring special treatment from parents
	History of multiple, unexplained illnesses
	History of menstrual disorders
Operations/ hospitalization	Surgery or illness that required extended hospitalization
	Surgery for rupture of internal organs (spleen, liver)
	Parent refusal to have child hospitalized
	Significant delay in seeking hospitalization
	History of suicide attempt
	History of overdose, even in young children
	History of multiple, unexplained operations or hospitalizations
Diagnostic tests	Evaluation for failure-to-thrive or other problem that would explain injuries or lack of weight gain
	History of multiple evaluations or diagnostic tests for unexplained illnesses
	Severe anemia
	Elevated lead level
	Parent refusal for further diagnostic studies
	Parent insistence on further, unwarranted diagnostic studies
Accidents	Repeated
	History of preceding events does not support actual injuries
Area of assessment	At-risk responses
Safety	No age-appropriate safety precautions
	History of poisoning
Immunizations	None or only a few
Healthcare utilization	Parent "shops" for hospital care
	No consistent provider
	Significant delay in seeking healthcare for serious problems
Review of body systems	Changes in previously reported data
	Pertinent data not previously reported

Parenting Profile Assessment

	Yes	No	Unsure

Assessment made of client (via mother)
Moderate to severe discipline as a child (5)
Past or present spousal abuse (3)
Perception of stress (4, 5)
Moderate to severe life change unit score (4, 5)**
High school education or less (3)
Rare involvement out of home (1.25)
Little or no prenatal care (2.5)
Does not feel good about herself (3.5)
Feels like running away (3)
Age at first birth under 20 (2)

Assessment made of family (via mother)
Unlisted or no phone (1)
Difficulty communicating with family members (3.5)
History of unemployment over a two-month period
   (of usual provider) (2)
Currently under or unemployed (usual provider) (2)
Family involvements with police (2)
Less than $20,000 per year income (2.5)

Assessment made of discipline methods
  (via mother)***
Curses at child(ren) when disciplining (3.5)
Child(ren) shows evidence of punishment
   postdisciplining (3) (cuts, bruises, missed school)
Perceives discipline of children as harsh (3)
Calls child(ren) names when disciplining (3.5)

Scoring of risk assessment:

Scores for each variable are located in parenthesis beside the variable. The scores match the scoring value on the original data collection instrument.

For each yes answer add in the appropriate score. Unsure statements are not scored. Over 3 unsures question the validity of the risk assessment score.

After totaling the score for each individual variable, review the assessment for the presence of all the following five variables:

    Income under $20,000 per year
    High school education or less
    Family involvements with police
    Perceives discipline of child(ren) as harsh
    Moderate or severe life change unit score**

From Anderson CL: *Appl Nurs Res* 6(1):31-38, 1993.

Alert for abuse:

*Possible parenting problems and risk for child abuse: over 21 points or the presence of all the above five variables (these families require a follow-up home visit).

Minimal parenting problems and low risk for child abuse: under 21 points and a lack of one to five of the above variables. (Follow-up for families is optional).

Uncertain risk: no additional children at home for immediate assessment of discipline methods by mother or three or more unsures checked. (Follow-up required for additional information.)

*Timing of a repeat home assessment is indicated by the at-risk status of the mother. A reassessment of variables may be required to determine additional areas of risk and necessary interventions.

**Tool to assess life change unit score must accompany this tool.

***If assessment made in hospital between mother and first newborn, observations of this area will need to be deferred until home follow-up.

Check appropriate box:
☐ Possible parenting problems
☐ Risk for child abuse
☐ Minimal parenting problems
☐ Low risk for child abuse
☐ Uncertain risk
☐ Follow-up schedule for child abuse

Administering the parenting profile assessment

The majority of questions can be answered yes/no by the mother (or father) through a simple interview (either in the hospital or in the home). Observations of disciplining techniques with children at home or in other settings may be necessary along with observations of children for documentable signs of abuse, such as bruises. To determine moderate to severe Life Change Unit (LCU) scores, the Social Readjustment Rating Scale (SRRS) is used.

The SRRS, developed by Holmes and Rahe (1967), is useful in determining stressful life events. The 43 life events listed indicate or require some change and consequent coping behavior in the life of the individual. Each event has been assigned an LCU value depending on the amount of social readjustment one needs in the face of the event. Events listed include such items as death of a spouse (100 LCU), marriage (50 LCU), trouble with in-laws (29 LCU), or change in social activities (18 LCU). Holmes and Rahe found that LCU scores of 150 to 199 indicate mild stress; LCU scores of 200 to 299 indicate moderate stress; and LCU scores of 300+ indicate high stress and major life crises.

As a frequently used tool to assess stress levels, the SRRS was selected as a companion tool with the parenting profile assessment (PPA) to assess potential parenting problems. When assessing families, both tools can be presented with content in a yes/no format providing easily administered tools in a short period of time.

LCU scores for each individual are totaled and determined as mild, moderate, or severe. A check in the appropriate place of the PPA under the "yes" column indicates moderate or severe stress. A check in the "no" column indicates mild stress (or a score of under 200). After all items of the PPA are assessed, a risk assessment is made. Unsure answers are not scored, and three or more unsure answers will question the validity of the tool and the accuracy of the information. All items on the PPA have scores. Total the scores for the items according to the "yes" answers checked. Follow-up for families is indicated if a score of over 21 or if a "yes" answer applies to the following five items: (a) income under $20,000/year, (b) high school education or less, (c) family involvements with police, (d) disciplining of children perceived as harsh, and (e) moderate or severe LCU score.

First-time parents will need assessments made when the child is older. Clinicians must be cautioned that the PPA is a guideline for potential services and not a diagnostic tool. It is possible that parents who are not or never will be abusive will have high scores, and parents who abuse their children may score low. Tools may be obtained from the author.

ELDER ABUSE

Definitions of Elder Abuse

Source	Definition
O'Malley, Segal, and Perez (1979), adapted from Connecticut Department of Aging	Abuse: the willful infliction of physical pain, injury, or debilitating mental anguish; unreasonable confinement; or deprivation by a caretaker of services that are necessary to maintain mental and physical health.
Block and Sinnott (1979)	1. Physical abuse: malnutrition; injuries (e.g., bruises, welts, sprains, dislocations, abrasions, or lacerations). 2. Psychologic abuse: verbal assault, threat, fear, isolation. 3. Material abuse: theft, misuse of money or property. 4. Medical abuse: withholding of medications or aids required.
Douglass, Hickey, and Noele (1980)	1. Passive neglect: being ignored, left alone, isolated, forgotten. 2. Active neglect: withholding of companionship, medicine, food, exercise, assistance to bathroom. 3. Verbal or emotional abuse: name calling, insults, treating as a child, frightening, humiliation, intimidation, threats. 4. Physical abuse: being hit, slapped, bruised, sexually molested, cut, burned, physically restrained.
Lau and Kosberg (1979)	1. Physical abuse: direct beatings; withholding personal care, food, medical care; lack of supervision. 2. Psychologic abuse: verbal assaults, threats, provoking fear, isolation. 3. Material abuse: monetary or material theft or misuse. 4. Violation of rights: being forced out of one's dwelling or forced into another setting.
Wolf and Pillemer (1984)	1. Physical abuse: infliction of physical pain or injury, physical coercion (confinement against one's will), e.g., slapped, bruised, sexually molested, cut, burned, physically restrained.

From Fulmer T, O'Malley FA: *Inadequate care of the elderly: a health care perspective on abuse and neglect,* New York, 1987, Springer.   *Continued*

Definitions of Elder Abuse—cont'd

Source	Definition
	2. Psychologic abuse: the infliction of mental anguish (e.g., called names, treated as child, frightened, humiliated, intimidated, threatened, isolated).
	3. Material abuse: the illegal or improper exploitation or use of funds or other resources.
	4. Active neglect: refusal or failure to fulfill a caretaking obligation, including a conscious and intentional attempt to inflict physical or emotional stress on the elder (e.g., deliberate abandonment or deliberate denial of food or health-related services).
	5. Passive neglect: refusal or failure to fulfill a caretaking obligation, excluding a conscious and intentional attempt to inflict physical or emotional distress on the elder (e.g., abandonment, nonprovision of services).

Signs of Elder Mistreatment

Contusions

Lacerations

Abrasions

Fractures

Sprains

Dislocations

Burns

Oversedation

Anxiety

Overmedication or undermedication

Decubiti

Untreated but previously treated conditions

Dehydration

Misuse of medications

Malnutrition

Freezing

Poor hygiene

Depression

Adapted from O'Malley TA, et al: *Ann Intern Med* 98:998, 1983; Fulmer T, O'Malley TA: *Inadequate care of the elderly: a health care perspective on abuse and neglect,* New York, 1987, Springer.

History of Elder—Possible Indicators of Potential or Actual Elder Abuse

Area of assessment	At-risk responses or indicators of possible abuse/neglect
Primary concern/reason for visit	Historical data that conflict with physical findings
	Acute or chronic psychologic or physical disability
	Inability to participate independently in activities of daily living
	Inappropriate delay in bringing elder to healthcare facility
	Reluctance on the part of caregiver to give information on elder's condition
	Inappropriate caregiver reaction to nurse's concern (overreacts, underreacts)
Family health	
Elder	Substance abuse
	Grew up in a violent home (abused as child, spouse; abused children)
	Excessive dependence of elder on child(ren)
Child(ren) of elder	Were abused by parents as children
	Antagonistic relationship with elder
	Excessive dependence on elder
	Substance abuse
	History of violent relationship with other siblings or spouse
Siblings	Antagonistic relationship between siblings
	Excessive dependence of one or more siblings on another or each other
	Other history of abuse or neglect or violent death
Other family members and family relations	Violence and aggression used to resolve conflicts and solve problems
	History of abuse or neglect among family members
Household	Poverty
	Few or no friends or neighbors or other support systems available

From Campbell J, Humphreys J: *Nursing care of survivors of family violence*, St Louis, 1993, Mosby.

Continued

History of Elder—Possible Indicators of Potential or Actual Elder Abuse—cont'd

Area of assessment	At-risk responses or indicators of possible abuse/neglect
	Excessive number of stressful situations encountered during a short period of time (unemployment, death of a relative or significant other, etc.)
Health history of elder	
Child	History of chronic physical or psychologic disability
Midlife	History of chronic physical or psychologic disability
Nutrition	History of feeding problems (gastrointestinal disease, food preference idiosyncracies)
	Inappropriate food or drink
	Dietary intake that does not fit with findings
	Inadequate food or fluid intake
Drugs/medications	Drugs/medications not indicated by physical condition
	Overdose of drugs or medications (prescribed or over-the-counter)
	Medications not taken as prescribed
Personal/social	Caregiver has unrealistic expectations of elder
	Social isolation (little or no contact with friends, neighbors, or relatives; lack of outside activity)
	Substance abuse
	History of spouse abuse (as victim or abuser)
	History of antagonistic relationships among family members (between family members in general, including elder)
	Large age difference between elder and spouse
	Large number of family problems
	Excessive dependence on spouse, children, or significant others
Discipline	
Physical	Belief that the use of physical punishment is appropriate
	Threats with an instrument as a means to punish
	Use of an instrument to administer physical punishment

Emotional/violation of rights	Excessive, inappropriate inconsistent physical punishment
	History of caregiver or others "losing control" or "hitting too hard"
	Fear-provoking threats
	Infantilization
	Berating
	Screaming
	Forced move out of home
	Forced institutionalization
	Prohibiting marriage
	Prevention of free use of money
	Isolation
Sleep	—
Elimination	—
Illness	Chronic illness or handicap
	Disability requiring special treatment from caregiver and others
Operations/hospitalization	Operations or illness that require extended or repeated hospitalizations
	Caregiver's refusal to have elder hospitalized
	Caregiver overanxious to have elder hospitalized
Diagnostic tests	Caregiver's refusal for further diagnostic tests
	Caregiver's overreaction or underreaction to diagnostic findings
Accidents	Repeated
	History of preceding events that do not support actual injuries
Safety	Appropriate safety precautions not taken, especially in elder known to be confused, disoriented, or with physical disabilities restricting mobility
Healthcare utilization	Infrequent
	Caregiver overanxious to have elder hospitalized
	Healthcare "shopping"
Review of body systems	—

PARTNER ABUSE

Abuse Assessment Screen

1. Have you ever been emotionally or physically abused by your partner or someone important to you? Yes No

2. Within the last year, have you been hit, slapped, kicked, or otherwise physically hurt by someone? Yes No
   If *yes,* by whom _____
   Number of times _____

3. Since you have been pregnant, have you been hit, slapped, kicked or otherwise physically hurt by someone? Yes No
   If *yes,* by whom _____
   Number of times _____
   Mark the area of injury on body map.

4. Within the last year, has anyone forced you to have sexual activities? Yes No
   If *yes,* by whom _____
   Number of times _____

5. Are you afraid of your partner or anyone you listed above? Yes No

From Creasia JL, Parker B: *Conceptual foundations of professional nursing practice,* ed 2, St Louis, 1996, Mosby.

Danger Assessment

Several risk factors have been associated with homicides (murder) of both batterers and battered women in research that has been conducted after the killings have taken place. We cannot predict what will happen in your case, but we would like for you to be aware of the danger of homicide in situations of severe battering and for you to see how many of the risk factors apply to your situation. (The "he" in the questions refers to your husband, partner, ex-husband, ex-partner, or whoever is currently physically hurting you).

___ **1.** Has the physical violence increased in frequency over the past year?

___ **2.** Has the physical violence increased in severity over the past year or has a weapon or threat with weapon been used?

___ **3.** Does he ever try to choke you?

___ **4.** Is there a gun in the house?

___ **5.** Has he ever forced you into sex when you did not wish to do so?

___ **6.** Does he use drugs? By drugs I mean "uppers" or amphetamines, speed, angel dust, cocaine, "crack," street drugs, heroin, or mixtures.

___ **7.** Does he threaten to kill you or do you believe he is capable of killing you?

___ **8.** Is he drunk every day or almost every day? (In terms of quantity of alcohol.)

___ **9.** Does he control most or all of your daily activities? For instance, does he tell you who you can be friends with, how much money you can take with you shopping, or when you can take the car? (If he tries, but you do not let him, check here ___)

___ **10.** Have you ever been beaten by him while you were pregnant? (If never pregnant by him, check here ___)

___ **11.** Is he violently and constantly jealous of you? (For instance, does he say, "If I can't have you, no one can.")

___ **12.** Have you ever threatened or tried to commit suicide?

___ **13.** Has he ever threatened or tried to commit suicide?

___ **14.** Is he violent toward the children?

___ **15.** Is he violent outside of the home?

___ **Total *yes* answers**

Thank you. Please talk to your nurse, advocate, or counselor about what the danger assessment means in terms of your situation.

From Campbell J, Humphreys J: *Nursing care of survivors of family violence,* St Louis, 1993, Mosby.

Indicators of Potential or Actual Wife Abuse From History

Area of assessment	At-risk responses*
Primary concern/reason for visit	Unwarranted delay between time of injury and seeking treatment
	Inappropriate spouse reactions (lack of concern, overconcern, threatening demeanor, reluctance to leave wife, etc.)
	Vague information about cause of injury or problem; discrepancy between physical findings and verbal description of cause; obviously incongruous cause of injury given
	Minimizing serious injury
	Seeking emergency department treatment for vague stress-related symptoms and minor injuries
	Suicide attempt; history of previous attempts
Family health history	
Family of origin	Traditional values about women's role taught
	Spouse abuse or child abuse (may not be significant for wife but should be noted)
Children	Children abused
	Physical punishment used routinely and severely with children
	Children are hostile toward or fearful of father
	Father perceives children as an additional burden
	Father demands unquestioning obedience from children
Partner	Alcohol or drug abuse
	Holds machismo values
	Experience with violence outside of home, including violence against women in previous relationships
	Low self-esteem; lack of power in workplace or other arenas outside of home
	Uses force or coercion in sexual activities
	Unemployment or underemployment
	Extreme jealousy of female friendships, work, and children, as well as other men; jealousy frequently unfounded
	Stressors such as death in family, moving, change of jobs, trouble at work
	Abused as a child or witnessed father abusing mother

Household	Poverty
	Conflicts solved by aggression or violence
	Isolated from neighbors, relatives; few friends; lack of support systems
Woman's health history	Fractures and trauma injuries
	Depression, anxiety symptoms, substance abuse
	Injuries while pregnant
	Spontaneous abortions
	Psychophysiological complaints
	Previous suicide attempts
Nutrition	Evidence of overeating or anorexia as reactions to stress
	Sudden changes in weight
Personal/social	Low self-esteem; evaluates self poorly in relation to others and ideal self, has trouble listing strengths, makes negative comments about self frequently, doubts own abilities
	Expresses feelings of being trapped, powerlessness, that the situation is hopeless, that it is futile to make future plans
	Chronic fatigue, apathy
	Feels responsible for spouse's behavior
	Holds traditional values about home, wife's prescribed role, husband's prerogatives, strong commitment to marriage
	External locus of control orientation, feels no control over situation, believes fate or other forces determine events
	Major decisions in household made by spouse, indicates far less power than he has in relationship, activities controlled by spouse, money controlled by spouse
	Few support systems, few supportive friends, little outside home activity, outside relationships have been discouraged by spouse or curtailed by self to deal with violent situation
	Physical aggression in courtship
Sleep	Sleep disturbances, insomnia, sleeping more than 10 to 12 hours per day
Elimination	Chronic constipation, diarrhea, or elimination disturbances related to stress
Illness	Frequent psychophysiologic illnesses
	Treatment for mental illness
	Use of tranquilizers, mood elevators, or antidepressants

Continued

*At-risk responses are derived from clinical experiences and review of the literature.
From Campbell J, Humphreys J: *Nursing care of survivors of family violence,* St Louis, 1993, Mosby.

Indicators of Potential or Actual Wife Abuse From History—cont'd

Area of assessment	At-risk responses*
Operations/hospitalization	Hospitalizations for trauma injuries
	Suicide attempts
	Hospitalization for depression
	Refusals of hospitalization when suggested by physician
Personal safety	Handgun(s) in home
	History of frequent accidents
	Does not take safety precautions
Healthcare utilization	No regular provider
	Indicates mistrust of healthcare system
Review of systems	Headache, undiagnosed gastrointestinal symptoms, palpitations, other possible psychophysiologic complaints
	Sexual difficulties, feels husband is "rough" in sexual activities, lack of sexual desire, pain with intercourse
	Joint pain or other areas of tenderness, especially at the extremities
	Chronic pain
	Pelvic inflammatory disease

Indicators of Potential or Actual Violence in a Family From Nursing History

Area of assessment	At-risk responses
Information from genogram	Severe physical punishment or husband-wife violence in parental families of origin
	Violent death or serious injury from violence in genogram
	Family members in parental families of origin using violence outside the home
	Wife abuse in husband's previous marital relationship
Family structure	Single-parent home
	Dependent grandparent in home
	Blended family (involving stepparents or stepchildren)
Family resources	Unemployment; poverty
	Inadequate housing
	Elderly member with controlled resources
	Financial problems
	Total control of monetary resources by male head of household
	Perception of inadequate "fit" of family resources to family demands
Family role	Rigid traditional sex roles
	Individual or family dissatisfaction with roles family expects individuals to fulfill
	Roles incompatible
	Roles rigid, unchangeable
Family boundaries	Boundaries rigid; mistrust of all outsiders
Family communication patterns	Family communications nonnurturing; destructive to some members
	Communications ambiguous
	Lack of communication among family members

From Campbell J, Humphreys J: *Nursing care of survivors of family violence*, St Louis, 1993, Mosby.

Continued

Indicators of Potential or Actual Violence in a Family From Nursing History—cont'd

Area of assessment	At-risk responses
Family conflict resolution patterns	Extensive use of verbal aggression; many threats of violence
	Evidence of physical aggression used in husband-wife, parent-child, sibling-sibling, or parent-grandparent conflict resolution
Family power distribution	Autocratic decision making by father
	Children have no power
	Grandparent in home who is powerless
	Frequent power struggles
Family values	Violence considered acceptable or valued
	Great incongruence of values among family members or between family and society
	Differing values among family members considered intolerable
Emotional climate	High tension in home
	Lack of visible affection
	Scapegoating
	High anxiety in family member(s)
	Lack of support between family members
	Frequent disparagement between family members
Division of labor	Rigid division of labor according to sex
	Members highly dissatisfied with division of labor
Support systems	Family isolation
	Family inhibitions to helpseeking
	Children not forming close, supportive peer relationships (especially same-sex peer relationships)
	Lack of support systems considered useful for direct aid, emotional support, or affirmation

Developmental stages	Relatives are highly critical; tension among extended family
	Sudden withdrawal by adolescent from social activity and peers
	Violence in extended family
	More than one family member facing difficult developmental crisis
	Lack of knowledge in parents of what to expect at various developmental stages in children, selves, and grandparents
Stressors	At-risk scores on stress scale
	Lack of successful coping mechanisms to deal with stress in the past
	Situational crises
	Stress-related physical symptoms in family members
Socialization of children	Physical punishment used
	Only one parent disciplines children
	Lack of nurturance of children
	Children displaying aggressive behavior, at home or outside of home
	Juvenile delinquency or sexual promiscuity in children
Health history	Frequent trauma injuries to family members
	Adolescent suicide attempts
	Serious illness in a family member
	History of treatment for mental illness or vaginal trauma
	History of sexually transmitted disease or genital trauma in children
	Drug or alcohol abuse
	Substance abuse in adolescents

Indicators of Potential or Actual Violence in a Family From Nursing Observation

Area of assessment	
General considerations	Observations differ significantly from information gathered on history
Family resources	Family members inadequately clothed and groomed
	One family member inadequately clothed or groomed, but the rest are not
	Household totally disorganized and family members indicate displeasure with the lack of organization
Family roles	One parent looks to the other to hold major interaction with children
	One parent answers all questions
	One parent looks to other for approval before answering questions
Family communication patterns	Members continually interrupt each other
	Members answer questions for each other; one member never talks for himself or herself
	Negative nonverbal behavior in other members when one family member is speaking
	Members frequently misunderstand each other
	Members do not listen to each other
Family conflict resolution	Verbal aggression used in front of nurse
Family power distribution	Members act afraid of another member
	One person makes all decisions
	Power struggles
	At-risk responses
Emotional climate	Nonverbals unhappy, anxious, fearful
	Excessive physical distance maintained between members
	Members never touch each other
	Tense atmosphere
	Secretive atmosphere
	Voice tones sharp, nonaffectionate, disparaging

From Campbell J, Humphreys J: *Nursing care of survivors of family violence*, St Louis, 1993, Mosby.

Criteria for Possible Aggression

	Passive	Assertive	Aggressive
Content of speech	Negative Self-derogatory "Can I?" "Will you?"	Positive Self-enhancing "I can," "I will"	Exaggerated Other-derogatory "You always," "You never"
Tone of voice	Quiet, weak, whining	Modulated	Loud, demanding
Posture	Drooping, bowed head	Erect, relaxed	Tense, leaning forward
Personal space	Allows invasion of space by others	Maintains a comfortable distance; claims right to own space	Invades space of others
Gestures	Minimal, weak gesturing, fidgeting	Demonstrative gestures	Threatening, expansive gestures
Eye contact	Little or none	Intermittent, appropriate to relationship	Constant stare

From Stuart G, Laraia M: *Stuart & Sundeen's principles and practice of psychiatric nursing*, ed 6, St Louis, 1998, Mosby.

MENTAL HEALTH

Behaviors Associated With Low Self-Esteem

Criticism of self or others
Decreased productivity
Destructiveness toward others
Disruptions in relatedness
Exaggerated sense of self-importance
Feelings of inadequacy
Guilt
Irritability or excessive anger
Negative feelings about one's body
Perceived role strain
Pessimistic view of life
Physical complaints
Polarizing view of life
Rejection of personal capabilities
Self-derision
Self-destructiveness
Self-diminution
Social withdrawal
Substance abuse
Withdrawal from reality
Worrying

From Stuart GW, Laraia MT: *Principles and practice of psychiatric nursing,* ed 6, St Louis, 1998, Mosby.

Behavioral Characteristics of Borderline Personality Disorder

Types	Mood	Self-image	Behavior	Relatedness	Cognitive mode	Defense mechanism
Borderline	**LABILE:** Mood has either marked shifts from normality to depression to excitement or has extended periods of dejection and apathy, interspersed with brief spells of anger, anxiety, or euphoria	**UNCERTAIN:** Experiences the confusions of an immature, nebulous, or wavering sense of identity; seeks to redeem actions with expression of contrition and self-punitive behaviors	**PRECIPITATE:** Displays a desultory energy level with sudden, unexpected, and impulsive outbursts; abrupt, endogenous shifts in drive state and in inhibitory control places activation equilibrium in constant jeopardy	**PARADOXICAL:** Although needing attention and affection, is unpredictably contrary, manipulative, and volatile, frequently eliciting rejection rather than support; reacts to fears of separation and isolation in angry, mercurial, and often self-damaging ways	**CAPRICIOUS:** Experiences rapidly changing, fluctuating, and antithetical perceptions of thoughts concerning passing events; contradictory reactions are evoked in others, creating, in turn, conflicting and confusing social feedback	**REGRESSION:** Retreats under stress to developmentally earlier levels of anxiety tolerance, impulse control, and social adaptation; among adolescents, is unable to cope with adult demands and conflicts, as evident in immature, if not increasingly infantile, behaviors

From Haber J, et al: *Comprehensive psychiatric nursing*, ed 5, St Louis, 1997, Mosby.

NANDA Nursing Diagnosis: Altered Family Processes (Specify)*

Definition

Inability of family system (household members) to meet needs of members, carry out family functions, or maintain communications for mutual growth and maturation.

Defining characteristics

- Inability of family members to relate to each other for mutual growth and maturation
- Failure to send and receive clear messages
- Poorly communicated family rules, rituals, symbols; unexamined myths
- Unhealthy family decision-making processes
- Inability of family members to express and accept wide range of feelings
- Inability to accept and receive help
- Does not demonstrate respect for individuality and autonomy of members
- Rigidity in functions and roles
- Fails to accomplish current (or past) family developmental tasks
- Inappropriate (nonproductive) boundary maintenance
- Inability to adapt to change
- Inability to deal with traumatic or crisis experience constructively
- Parents do not demonstrate respect for each other's views on child-rearing practices
- Inappropriate (nonproductive) level and direction of energy
- Inability to meet needs of members (physical, security, emotional, spiritual)
- Family uninvolved in community activities

Etiology or related factors

Situational crisis or transition (e.g., alcoholism of a member)
Developmental crisis or transition

---

*This is a broad taxonomic category. Specify the processes that are altered.

From Gordon M: *Manual of nursing diagnosis, 1997-1998,* St Louis, 1997, Mosby, p 377.

Families With Disturbances in Internal Dynamics

Developmental stages and tasks: The family has difficulty achieving tasks at the stage-appropriate time. Situational and maturational crises occur simultaneously. Tasks for the next stage are delayed or not accomplished.

Roles: Patterns of expected behavior are not appropriate to age and ability, are rigidly assigned, and are unable to support family functioning.

Boundaries: Boundaries are closed and impermeable or completely diffuse. They fail to allow appropriate exchange with the environment or fail to define the family unit. Boundaries between subsystems have no clear generational lines and do not support a strong parental coalition. Subsystem boundaries may be unclear, rigid, or diffuse.

Subsystems: As in most families, each member of the family belongs to several subsystems simultaneously: spouse, parent-child, sibling, grandparent. However, subsystems may include inappropriate members.

Patterns of interaction: Repetitive and fixed. Focused on one member who is blamed, left out, or put down in the interaction. Family cohesion is extremely enmeshed or disengaged. Communication patterns of placater, blamer, superresponsible one, and distractor are often used. Distance, conflict, projection, and overresponsibility/underresponsibility are common.

Power: No clarity of role definition and appropriate rules. Power is not shared, appropriate to age, or within the parental subsystem until the children are independent.

External stressors: Are very intense, numerous, and occur simultaneously. The family has little chance to adapt. Chronic illness adds to family stress.

Open/closed system: As the system closes, all variables and patterns become fixed and less able to adapt. Energy is used in dysfunctional ways.

Communication: Is unclear, not honest, and indirect; contains incongruency of feelings and words; and is nonspecific. The family is not able to use it as a mechanism to resolve conflict.

Values: Do not provide guidelines for behavior acceptable to society and culture. Unable to be modified to adapt to changing times.

From Smith CM, Maurer FA: *Community health nursing: theory and practice,* ed 2, Philadelphia, 2000, WB Saunders, p 294.

Encouragement of autonomy/acceptance of difference: A balance does not exist between autonomy of members and the need to be a cohesive group. There are strong pressures to conform and to sacrifice individual needs for the purpose of the group.

Level of anxiety: Is extremely high. People in the family have difficulty thinking and problem-solving. Long-term anxiety tends to wear down the ability of the family to function well.

Resources/social support: Family has few internal and external sources of support. Those that are available are not used to their capacity or are overused. All families have some strengths, but the strengths may be different from those expected by society.

Meaning, perception, and paradigm: The family agrees to allow myths and secrets to structure the meaning of many situations. Life problems are viewed as unsolvable problems rather than challenges. The family views itself as powerless.

Adaptability: Resilience is necessary for a family to be able to cope with changing demands. These families are not able to be flexible or are so chaotic that cohesiveness and predictability are missing.

Early Warning Signs of Mental Health Problems in Children and Adolescents

Enhancing a child's self-esteem

Targeted area	Strategy
Caregiver expectations	Describe expectations for the child
	Assess anticipated developmental milestones
	Review family patterns and influences
Personal value	Communicate confidence in the child
	Structure situations to promote success of the child
	Implement effective ways of praising the child
	Be a role model of valuing self
Communication	Listen attentively
	Encourage openness to feelings
	Avoid using judgmental statements
	Elicit different points of view
Discipline	Use effective methods of limit setting
	Discuss and implement appropriate consequences
	Review problem-solving techniques
	Discourage use of physical punishment

Modified from Sieving R, Ziebel-Donisch S: *J Ped Health Care* 2(4): 290, 1990. In Haber J, et al: *Comprehensive psychiatric nursing,* ed 5, St Louis, 1997, Mosby.

Targeted area	Strategy
Guidance	Encourage open exchange with the child
	Know the child's activities away from home
	Express interest in school events
	Become familiar with the child's friends
Autonomy	Demonstrate respect for the child
	Promote the child's responsible decision making
	Expect reciprocal respect

Risks for adolescent mental disorders
- Poverty
- Crowded inner-city neighborhoods
- Racial inequality
- Large family size
- Unstable families
- Marital discord
- Inconsistent caretakers
- Prolonged parent-child separation
- Foster care
- Maternal mental illness
- Paternal criminality
- Depressed parents
- Parents with substance abuse disorders
- Rejection by parents
- Physical, sexual, emotional abuse
- Homelessness
- Catastrophic events
- Bereavement
- Aberrant peer groups
- Models for deviant behavior

Vulnerabilities for adolescent mental disorders
- Low birth weight
- Prematurity
- Early difficult temperament
- Developmental disabilities
- Mental retardation
- Brain damage
- Epilepsy
- Chronic illnesses
- Physical disabilities
- Low perceived life chances

Continued

Early Warning Signs of Mental Health Problems in Children and Adolescents—cont'd

- Low self-esteem
- Risk-taking propensity
- Poor school performance

Resilience to adolescent mental disorders
- Easy temperament
- Good problem-solving abilities
- High intelligence
- Supportive family
- Caring adults outside the home
- Compensatory experiences outside the home
- Models for conventional behavior
- Neighborhood resources
- Supports for coping and values
- Intolerance of deviance
- Values on achievement
- Values on health
- Good schools
- Good school performance
- Involvement in church and school clubs

DEPRESSION

Major Depressive Disorder Subgroups

Subgroup	Essential features	Diagnostic implications	Treatment implications	Prognostic implications
Psychotic	Hallucinations Delusions	More likely to become bipolar than nonpsychotic types May be misdiagnosed as schizophrenia	Antidepressant medication plus a neuroleptic is more effective than are antidepressants alone ECT is very effective	Usually a recurrent illness Subsequent episodes are usually psychotic Psychotic subtypes run in families Mood-incongruent features have a poorer prognosis
Melancholic	Anhedonia Unreactive mood Severe vegetative symptoms	May be misdiagnosed as dementia More likely in older patients	Antidepressant medication is essential ECT is 90% effective	If recurrent, consider maintenance medications

ECT, Electroconvulsive therapy; *MAOIs*, monoamine oxidase inhibitors; *SSRIs*, selective serotonin reuptake inhibitors; *TCAs*, tricyclic antidepressants.

From Depression Guideline Panel: *Depression in primary care*, vol 1, *Detection and diagnosis, clinical practice guideline*, No 5, Publication No 93-0550, Rockville, Md, 1993, US Department of Health and Human Services, Public Health Service Agency for Health Care Policy and Research.

Continued

Major Depressive Disorder Subgroups—cont'd

Subgroup	Essential features	Diagnostic implications	Treatment implications	Prognostic implications
Atypical	Reactive mood Overeating/weight gain Oversleeping Rejection sensitivity Heavy limb sensation Fewer episodes	Common in younger patients May be misdiagnosed as personality disorder	TCAs may be less effective; MAOIs are preferred ?SSRIs preferred	Unclear
Seasonal	Onset, fall Offset, spring Recurrent	More frequent in non-equatorial latitudes Pattern occurs in major depressive and bipolar disorders	Medications have questionable efficacy Psychotherapy has questionable efficacy Phototherapy is an option	Recurs
Postpartum psychosis/depression	Acute onset (<30 days) in postpartum period Severe labile mood symptoms 1/1000 is psychotic form	Often heralds a bipolar disorder	Hospitalize Treat medically	50% chance of recurring in next postpartum period

Behaviors Associated With Depression

Affective	Physiologic	Cognitive	Behavioral
Anger	Abdominal pain	Ambivalence	Aggressiveness
Anxiety	Anorexia	Confusion	Agitation
Apathy	Backache	Inability to concentrate	Alcoholism
Bitterness	Chest pain	Indecisiveness	Altered activity level
Dejection	Constipation	Loss of interest and motivation	Drug addiction
Denial of feelings	Dizziness	Self-blame	Intolerance
Despondency	Fatigue	Self-depreciation	Irritability
Guilt	Headache	Self-destructive thoughts	Lack of spontaneity
Helplessness	Impotence	Pessimism	Overdependency
Hopelessness	Indigestion	Uncertainty	Poor personal hygiene
Loneliness	Insomnia		Psychomotor retardation
Low self-esteem	Lassitude		Social isolation
Sadness	Menstrual changes		Tearfulness
Sense of personal worthlessness	Nausea		Underachievement
	Overeating		Withdrawal
	Sexual nonresponsiveness		
	Sleep disturbances		
	Vomiting		
	Weight change		

From Stuart GW, Laraia, MT: *Stuart & Sundeen's principles and practice of psychiatric nursing*, ed 6, St Louis, 1998, Mosby.

Illnesses Associated With Depression

Central nervous system disorders
Alzheimer's disease (senile and presenile)
Amyotrophic lateral sclerosis
Brain tumor (especially nondominant lobe)
Cerebrovascular accident (stroke)
Chronic subdural hematoma
Multiple sclerosis
Normal-pressure hydrocephalus
Parkinson's disease
Subarachnoid hemorrhage

Infections
Acquired immunodeficiency syndrome
Encephalitis
Hepatitis
Infectious mononucleosis
Influenza
Syphilis
Tuberculosis
Viral pneumonia

Collagen vascular disease
Polymyalgia rheumatica
Rheumatoid arthritis
Systemic lupus erythematosus
Temporal arteritis

Neoplastic disorders
Carcinoma of head of pancreas
Chronic myelogenous leukemia
Lymphoma
Other malignant diseases
Small-cell carcinoma of lung

Adapted from Ford CV, Folks DG: Psychiatric disorders in geriatric medical/surgical patients, II. Review of clinical experience in consultation, *South Med J* 78(4):397, 1985. In Keltner N, Schwecke L, Bostrom C: *Psychiatric nursing,* ed 3, St Louis, 1999, Mosby.

Illnesses Associated With Depression

Toxic–metabolic disturbances and endocrinopathies

Addison's disease
Apathetic hyperthyroidism
Cushing's disease
Diabetes mellitus
Electrolyte disorders
Hypoglycemia
Hypothyroidism
Metal intoxication
Parathyroid disorders
Uremia

Other

Chronic fatigue syndrome
Chronic obstructive pulmonary disease

Differences Between Anxiety and Depression

Anxiety	Depression
Predominantly fearful or apprehensive with feelings of dread	Predominantly sad or hopeless with feelings of despair
Difficulty falling asleep (initial insomnia)	Early-morning awakening (late insomnia) or hypersomnia
Phobic avoidance behavior	Diurnal variation (feels worse in the morning)
Rapid pulse and psychomotor and autonomic hyperactivity	Slowed speech and thought processes
Breathing disturbances	Delayed response time
Tremors and palpitations	Psychomotor retardation (agitation may also occur)
Sweating and hot or cold spells	Loss of interest in usual activities
Faintness, light-headedness, dizziness	Inability to experience pleasure
Depersonalization (feelings of detachment from one's body)	Thoughts of death or suicide
Derealization (feeling that one's environment is strange, unreal, or unfamiliar)	Negative appraisals are pervasive, global, and exclusive
Negative appraisals are selective and specific and do not include all areas of life	Sees the future as blank and has given up all hope
Sees some prospects for the future	Regards mistakes as beyond redemption
Does not regard defects or mistakes as irrevocable	Absolute in negative evaluations
Uncertain in negative evaluations	Global view that nothing will turn out right
Predicts that only certain events may go badly	

From Stuart GW, Laraia MT: *Stuart & Sundeen's principles and practice of psychiatric nursing,* ed 6, St Louis, 1998, Mosby.

Dealing With Depression: The Nursing Process and Maslow's Hierarchy of Need

Needs	Assessment	Identifying problems	Establishing goals	Intervention	Evaluation
Physiologic needs Food/fluid Shelter/warmth Air Rest/sleep Avoidance of pain Sex	Usual and present nutritional, elimination, sleep, and sexuality patterns Physical activity—exercise pattern Emotional pain and discomfort Suicide potential Physical health Medications	Nutritional deficit Dehydration Constipation Sleep pattern disturbance Sexual dysfunction Self-destructive behavior Medications or physical illnesses that may cause depression	Establishing and maintaining adequate biologic functioning in areas of sleep, nutrition, and elimination Relief from emotional pain and discomfort Elimination of drug- or disease-induced depression	Assist with ADLs Support of self-care abilities Encouragement to start a physical activity regimen Teach side effects of anti-depressants Treat medical problems under poor control Change medications that may cause depression	Feelings of physical satiation Homeostasis Optimal physical health
Safety and security needs Feel free from danger Need for a predictable, lawful, orderly world	Home environment assessment Mental status examination Assessment of visual acuity and hearing Knowledge of disease process	Perceived inability to control feelings or behavior Perceived powerlessness Translocation syndrome Cognitive impairment	Establish predictability and structure in environment Maintenance of a safe environment Realistic understanding of disease course and expected outcome	ECT, hospitalization, antidepressive medications for the severely depressed Avoid relocations when possible Correct environmental hazards	Feeling in control of one's disease and optimistic about the future Confidence in the future Feelings of safety, peace, security,

Continued

ADLs, activities of daily living; *ECT*, electroconvulsive therapy.
From Ronsman K: *J Gerontol Nurs* 13(12):21, 1987.

Dealing With Depression: The Nursing Process and Maslow's Hierarchy of Need—cont'd

Needs	Assessment	Identifying problems	Establishing goals	Intervention	Evaluation
Need to feel in control	Physical mobility	Alteration in sensory perceptions Impaired physical mobility	Reversal of treatable confusion	Encourage a structured daily routine Instruct about disease course and prognosis	protection, lack of danger and threat
Need for love, belonging, and affection Need for contact and intimacy Need for friends Need for a feeling of having a place, "belonging" Need for interactions with others	Family relationships and members Friends that are supportive Recent losses Present and past social interaction	Disruption in significant relationships Social isolation Lack of contact with or absence of significant others Alterations in socialization with reduced social interactions	Maintenance of significant relationships with family and friends Establish community support system Resumption of previous level of social activity	Encourage social interactions that have been enjoyed in the past Encourage interactions with family members, friends, and healthcare providers Provide reassuring, supportive atmosphere	Feelings of loving and being loved, of being one of a group, of acceptance

Need	Assessment	Nursing Diagnosis	Outcomes	Intervention	Characteristics
Need for esteem and self-respect Need for achievement, mastery, and competence Need for reputation or prestige, appreciation, and dignity Need for love of self	Amount of pleasurable pursuits Emotional or mood assessment Role patterns Coping—stress tolerance pattern Attitude about self, the world, the future	Negative feelings or conception of self Loss of significant roles Unrealistic self-expectations Anxiety Lifestyle change Dependency on others	Acceptance of realistic limitations Establish appropriate roles Achieve self-acceptance Accept ownership of consequences of one's own behavior	Teach problem-solving skills Cognitive therapy Promote self-care Counseling Behavior therapy Relaxation techniques	Feelings of self-confidence, worth, strength, capability, and adequacy, of being useful and necessary in the world
Need for self-actualization Need for beauty Need for self-expression Need for new situations and stimulation	Occupation, job history Value-belief patterns	Distress of human spirit Loss of zest for life	Expression of self through meaningful recreational activities Exploring new interests	Encourage a nonrestrictive environment Provide beauty in environment Read to the sick or hard of hearing Music	Autonomy Freshness of appreciation Creativeness Spontaneity Feelings of self-fulfillment

Changes Symptomatic of Depression

Physiological	Cognitive	Affective	Behavioral
Amenorrhea	Ambivalence	Anger	Aggressiveness
Changes in appetite and weight	Confusion	Anxiety	Agitation
(anorexia and weight loss,	Inability to concentrate	Apathy	Alcoholism
overeating and weight gain)	Indecisiveness	Bitterness	Changes in activity level
Dizziness	Loss of interest and motivation	Dejection	Drug addiction
Gastrointestinal upset:	Obsessional thoughts	Despair	Flat affect
• Constipation	Pessimism	Despondency	Intolerance
• Indigestion	Self-blame	Fatigue	Irritability
• Nausea	Self-destructive thoughts	Gloom	Lack of spontaneity:
• Vomiting	Self-doubt	Guilt	• Robotlike movements
Lethargy	Slow cognition	Helplessness	• Unchanging facial
Pain:	Suicidal thoughts	Hopelessness	expression
• Backache	Uncertainty	Ineffectiveness	Poor personal hygiene
• Chest pain			Poverty of speech:
• Headache			• Marked decrease in amount
Sexual changes:		Isolation	of speech
• Decreased sexual desire		Joylessness	• Long pauses
• Decreased responsiveness		Loneliness	• Low monotone vocal pitch
• Impotence			

Sleep disturbances:
- Difficulty falling asleep (initial insomnia)
- Waking up during the night (middle insomnia)
- Early-morning awakening (late insomnia)
- Hypersomnia (excessive sleeping)

Weakness

Low self-esteem

Overwhelmed

Powerless

Sadness

Worthlessness

Psychomotor retardation:
- Slowing of movement and speech

Social withdrawal and/or isolation

Suicidal gestures and attempts:
- Repeated car accidents
- Self-inflicted lacerations or abrasions
- Food bingeing, purging, or starvation

From Haber J, et al: *Comprehensive psychiatric nursing*, ed 5, St Louis, 1997, Mosby.

SUICIDE

Risk Factors Related to Suicide

Family history of suicide
Family history of substance abuse
Previous suicide attempts
History of mood disorder
Depression
Psychosis (hallucinations, delusions)
Substance abuse (use of or withdrawal from)
General medical illnesses
Organic brain disorders (delerium, dementia)
Personality disorders
Impulse control disorders
Anxiety
Stress (acute or chronic)
Isolation
Loss of a significant other
Loss of self-esteem
Loss of social and economic resources
Guilt
Ambivalence
Sex and age (white males over age 60)

From Haber J, et al: *Comprehensive psychiatric nursing,* ed 5, St Louis, 1997, Mosby.

Assessing Risk for Suicide

Assessment factor	Low risk (1 point)	Moderate risk (2 points)	High risk (3 points)
Suicidal ideation	No current suicidal thoughts	Intermittent or fleeting suicidal thoughts	Constant suicidal thoughts
Previous suicide attempts	No previous attempts	Past attempts of low lethality	Past attempts of high lethality
Suicide plan	No plan	Has plan without access to planned method	Has carefully thought out plan with actual or potential access to method
Lethality of plan	Low lethality of plan (e.g., superficial scratching)	Moderate lethality (e.g., swallowing 20 aspirin; reckless driving)	High lethality of plan (e.g., hanging, gun, jumping, carbon monoxide)
Current morbid thoughts (e.g., preoccupation with death, reunion fantasies)	Rarely	Intermittent	Constantly
No Harm Contract	Reliably signs No Harm Contract	Signs No Harm Contract, but is ambivalent	Unwilling or unable to sign No Harm Contract
Current alcohol and/or drug use	Infrequently to excess	Frequently to excess	Continual abuse

Adapted from Hatten, CI, Valente, SM: (1984). *Suicide assessment and intervention*, ed 2, Norwalk, CT, Appleton-Century Crofts. In Haber, J, et al: *Comprehensive psychiatric nursing*, ed 5, St Louis, 1997, Mosby.

Continued

Assessing Risk for Suicide—cont'd

Assessment factor	Low risk (1 point)	Moderate risk (2 points)	High risk (3 points)
Behavioral symptoms: • Anxiety • Anger/rage • Guilt/shame • Helplessness • Hopelessness • Impulsivity • Isolation	None to two symptoms present	Three to four symptoms present	Five to seven symptoms present
Support systems	Several friends, coworkers, and relatives available	Few or only one friend, coworker, or relative available	None available
Coping mechanisms	Generally constructive	Some are constructive	Predominantly destructive

Total score _____
RN signature _____
Date and time _____

Scoring directions

1. Assess each assessment factor.
2. Circle one descriptor for each assessment factor that *best* describes the client.
3. Assign appropriate points (1, 2, or 3) to each factor.
4. Add the points for each assessment factor to arrive at a total score.

Scoring key

10–13 = No precautions
14–19 = Moderate risk precautions (15-min. checks)
20 or above = High risk precautions (1 : 1 constant observation) above

Clues of Suicidal Risk in Adolescents

Depressive equivalents are symptoms associated with depression: delinquency, aggressiveness, sexual promiscuity, running away, drug or alcohol use, headaches, abdominal pain, accident proneness, fatigue, slow speech, anorexia, sloppiness, and preoccupation with death.

Verbal clues are statements that indicate the adolescent is thinking of suicide: "This world would be better off without me"; "I won't be around anymore."

Behavioral clues are actions that indicate the adolescent might be contemplating suicide: resigning from organizations, giving away cherished belongings, writing suicide notes, or exhibiting sudden changes in usual patterns of behavior (e.g., the good student who begins to fail, the quiet student who becomes aggressive).

From Edelman CL, Mandle CL: *Health promotion throughout the lifespan,* ed 4, St Louis, 1998, Mosby.

Suicide/Self-Harm Assessment

Directions:

1. Assess each key factor and current admission precipitated by attempt.
2. Circle one (of three) descriptor for each key factor that BEST describes the client.
3. Add the points for each circled item plus current admission precipitated by suicide attempt to obtain the total score.
4. Add RN's subjective appraisal of risk score to total score.

Key factors	High risk (1:1)	Moderate risk (q15min observation)	No precautions
Contract for safety	Unwilling to contract OR Unable to contract because of impaired reality testing (e.g., hallucinations, delusions, dementia, delirium, dissociation) 2	Contracts but is ambivalent or guarded 1	Reliably contracts for safety 0
Suicide plan	Has plan with actual OR potential access to planned method 2	Has plan without access to planned method 1	No plan 0
Plan lethality	Highly lethal plan (e.g., gun, hanging, jumping, carbon monoxide) 2	Low lethality of plan 1	Low lethality of plan (e.g., superficial scratching, head banging, pillow over face, biting, holding breath) 0
Elopement risk	High elopement risk 2	Low elopement risk 1	No elopement risk 0
Suicidal ideation	Constant suicidal thoughts 2	Intermittent or fleeting suicidal thoughts 1	No current suicidal thoughts 0

Attempt history	Past attempts of high lethality	Past attempts of low lethality	No previous attempts
	2	1	0
Symptoms (circle those that apply) Hopelessness Helplessness Anhedonia Guilt/shame Anger/rage Impulsivity	5-6 symptoms present 2	3-4 symptoms present 1	0-2 symptoms present 0
Current morbid thoughts (e.g., reunion fantasies, preoccupation with death)	Constantly 2	Frequently 1	Rarely 0

Current admission precipitated by suicide attempt   Yes 2
                                                       No 1

RN's subjective appraisal of risk:
Client replies not trustworthy, several nonverbal cues   4
Client replies questionably, trustworthy, at least 1 nonverbal cue   3
Client replies trustworthy   0

Scoring key: high risk precautions   = 10 or more
               moderate risk precautions = 4-9
               no precautions   = 0-3

Total score _____

Assessed by (RN): _____

Date: _____

Time: _____

From Division of Psychiatric Nursing, Medical University of South Carolina.

STRESS

Dealing With Stress

Stress and stressors

Quick! Can you identify which of the following are causes of stress: the fender bender during rush hour or getting a new car? Too much chocolate or a ringing telephone? Facing retirement or having a baby? Getting laid off or getting that incredible job you dreamed of? The correct answer: all of the above. In fact, the word "Quick!" at the beginning of this paragraph can cause stress in the tense, worried, or even enthusiastic reader. Stress is neither good nor bad. Stress is a general term used to describe change, and a stressor is anything that can cause a response in you, whether physically, mentally, or emotionally. Stressors, like stress, are neither good nor bad. They take on meaning only as you react to them. Stressors fall into three categories: environmental (that ringing telephone), physical (too much chocolate!), or psychologic (having a baby or a fender bender; both of these stressors tend to provoke an emotional response).

The stress response

So what happens when you're hit by a stressor? Physiologically, your body enters a state of arousal. For example, blood is diverted from the digestive functions to muscles to prepare the body for action. Nerve impulses signal the heart to beat harder and faster; blood pressure and pulse rate both rise. Changes occur in the movements of the stomach and intestines, and hormones secreted into the body mobilize glucose and blood, making more energy available to the brain and muscles. All of this is your body's effort to defend itself. Psychologically, you respond by trying to evaluate the emotional impact of the situation. This can calm you down or make you even more upset. This often depends, too, on the kind of stress you're experiencing: short-term or long-term. Short-term stress is a healthy kind of stress, because it represents a challenge or a threat, which causes an alarm reaction and elicits a response, which resolves the situation and eliminates the stress. Short-term stress is the kind of stress we were designed to deal with. Long-term stress is what causes the most trouble. All of us have a certain amount of long-term stress—experiences or situations that may never be resolved in our lifetime, such as coping with a chronic illness of a family member, financial problems, or conflict in the work

From *Mosby's patient teaching guides,* St Louis, 1996, Mosby.

site. But if this level of emotional arousal continues over a prolonged period, the body pays a price for the strain.

In a crisis, your doctor may prescribe therapy or medication. But for ongoing, daily stress situations, a variety of relaxation techniques or exercises can provide the individual in stress with nonmedical relief. These can range from passive or concentration responses (e.g., meditation, progressive relaxation, imagery, yoga, positive health promotion, vacations, and biofeedback) to active coping techniques (e.g., humor, reading, socializing with friends, exercising, and engaging in sports, music, art, or a craft). A few specific stress management techniques are outlined below. You can get more details on any of these from your physician or a stress management clinic or workshop.

Stress charting.   A good first step is to "chart" or track down the stressors in your life, so that you are aware of where they come from. Sometimes the individual under stress discovers stressors that simply don't need to *be* stressors—causes that had simply not been noticed. The first step is to list all the stressors present and the area of life in which each stressor occurs (e.g., family members, friends, work, health, finances, social concerns, recreation, or church). Then each stressor is rated as to effect, using a scale of 1 to 5. Awareness gained from this exercise may motivate you to making decisions about lifestyle changes or in choosing relaxation techniques.

Progressive relaxation.   A simple relaxation technique that can be done anywhere and at any time is progressive relaxation. Find a quiet, soothing, private place and, with eyes closed, concentrate on relaxing each part of the body, beginning with the toes and concentrating on each muscle and joint, moving up the body and ending with the head. Some people like to imagine all the stress or pain leaving each muscle as it relaxes, finally visualizing the stress leaving the body through the top of the head. Others like to incorporate deep-breathing exercises into this practice. However you choose to do it, try to allow yourself time after this exercise to sit quietly for a few minutes before resuming your daily activities.

Acupuncture, acupressure, shiatsu, and reflexology.   *Acupuncture* is based on the Chinese philosophy that all life is a microcosm of a vast, constantly changing, flowing circle of energy. The body can reach a balanced state only if both the "rising" energy (yang) and "descending" energy (yin) are flowing smoothly. *Acupressure,* the predecessor of acupuncture, is the term applied to a number of techniques of applying pressure to stimulate acupuncture points on the body. Both techniques release tension and relieve pain and are used to balance energy by applying needles or pressure to specific points. *Shiatsu* is an ancient form of manipulation administered by the thumbs, fingers, and palms, without any instruments, to correct internal malfunctioning, maintain health, and treat disease. *Reflexology* is a technique based on the premise that body organs have corresponding reflex points on other parts of the body.

Biofeedback.   Biofeedback is a means of receiving feedback or a message from the body about internal physiologic processes using specific techniques or equipment to read tension, and to learn ways of releasing that tension when cues of stress response are identified.

Massage.   Massage is a systematic manipulation of the body tissue that benefits the nervous and muscular systems, local and general circulation, skin, viscera, and metabolism. During massage the hands stimulate the sensory receptors of the skin and subcutaneous tissues, causing a series of reflex effects, including capillary vasodilation or constriction, relaxation or stimulation of voluntary muscle contraction, and possible sedation or stimulation of pain in an area far from the area touched.

Yoga.   This Indian philosophic system emphasizes the practice of special techniques to attain the highest degree of physical, emotional, and spiritual integration. Its practice can reduce blood pressure, lower pulse rate, reduce serum cholesterol, regulate menstrual flow and thyroid function, increase range of motion, reduce joint pain, and increase the feeling of well-being.

Self-hypnosis.   Self-hypnosis allows the individual to induce the feeling of warmth and heaviness associated with a trance state. The exercises can be used to increase resistance to stressors, reduce or eliminate sleep disorders, and modify pain reactions. The system has been found to be effective in treating disorders of the respiratory, gastrointestinal, circulatory, and endocrine systems, and also in alleviating anxiety and fatigue.

Thought stopping.   This behavioral modification technique is useful when nagging, repetitive thoughts interfere with behavior and wellness. Such unwanted thoughts are interrupted with the command "Stop," and a positive thought is substituted.

Refuting irrational ideas.   Everyone engages in almost continuous self-talk during waking hours. When this internal dialogue is accurate and realistic, wellness is enhanced; when it is irrational and untrue, stress occurs. Refuting these irrational ideas requires a series of steps: identifying what brought on the stress-inducing thought; writing down and identifying the negative thought and the emotion it brought on; writing down all evidence that the idea is false; predicting both the worst and best possible outcomes if the negative, irrational idea *were* true; and substituting alternative self-talk with positive, rational statements.

Centering. Centering refers to separating from outside influences to gain an inner reference or thought of stability, calm, and self-awareness; a sense of self-relatedness, a quiet place within the self where the individual can feel integrated, unified, and focused. Centering reduces fatigue, stress, depression, or anger when working with others and increases self-control. It involves sitting quietly, relaxing tense spots in the body as you inhale and exhale, and concentrating on breathing until you feel calm.

Assertive communication/behavior. Assertiveness means expressing personal thoughts, feelings, and desires, defining and making known personal rights that are reasonable while respecting the other person. Workshops frequently help people learn this way of behaving. Assertive techniques are particularly helpful in the face of criticism and other negative reactions. These include admitting mistakes, without defensiveness but without agreeing to a specific change that you may not want; asking what specifically is bothersome about a behavior for which you are criticized; shifting the conversation back to the subject and away from an intense expression of negative emotions; postponing a conversation when it reaches an impasse; not responding to an inappropriate or irrational attack; and using humor or deflection.

Guided imagery. This practice can be defined as focused attention on an inner, mental picture or a statement of belief of what the individual wants to accomplish by being open to and responding to the language of the unconscious or the deeper body levels. It is similar to self-hypnosis in that it involves sitting in a quiet place, relaxing, and envisioning a peaceful, soothing scene that can maintain relaxation and a positive attitude. Guided imagery promotes emotional health by building self-awareness and increasing coping resources.

Symptoms of Stress

Physiological/behavioral
Increased heart rate
Rise in blood pressure
Dryness of mouth and throat
Sweating
Tightness of chest
Headache
Nausea, vomiting
Indigestion
Diarrhea
Trembling, twitching
Grinding of teeth
Insomnia
Anorexia
Fatigue
Slumped posture
Pain, tightness in neck and back muscles
Urinary frequency
Missed menstrual cycle
Reduced interest in sex
Accident proneness
Startle reaction
Hyperventilation
Accidents
Altered food intake
Poor concentration
Disinterest in activities
Decreased involvement with others
Bickering
Smoking
Use of alcohol and drugs
Increased use of sarcasm
Tendency to cry easily
Nightmares
Complaining, criticizing

Affective
Irritability
Depression
Angry outbursts
Emotional instability
Withdrawal
Restlessness
Anxiety
Suspiciousness
Jealousy
Tendency to be easily startled

Cognitive
Forgetfulness
Poor judgment
Poor concentration
Reduced creativity
Less fantasizing
Errors in arithmetic and grammar
Preoccupation
Inattention to details
Blocking
Reduced productivity
Diminished problem solving

Spiritual
Expressed concerns about belief system
Expressed concerns about relationship with a clergy (representation of religion)
Separation from cultural and religious relationship

From Edelman CL, Mandle CL: *Health promotion throughout the lifespan*, ed 4, St Louis, 1998, Mosby.

Strategies for Managing Stress

- Evaluate sources of stress at work and attempt to change them.
- Learn to manage time effectively.
- Limit overtime.
- Discuss and try to solve problems with co-workers.
- Try not to personalize criticisms. Remember, it is often the situation that is the problem, although you may be the target of others' emotions.
- Rotate assignments of those who are difficult to care for.
- Recognize the symptoms of stress in yourself and seek the help of an objective party to assist you in discussing and managing your feelings.
- Learn techniques for controlling your response to stress (e.g., deep breathing, repeating a saying in your mind that helps you stay calm, counting to 25).
- Withdraw from the situation and seek help when you feel you may lose control.
- When you feel "burned out" or as though you cannot cope, talk to your supervisor about scheduling time off.
- Instead of coffee and cigarette breaks, enjoy breaks in which you do short relaxation exercises, recline in a quiet area, or listen to relaxation tapes.
- Eat a well-balanced diet; avoid junk foods.
- Exercise regularly.
- Do something for yourself to unwind between work and home.
- Take naps; allow ample time for sleep.
- Schedule leisure activities into your life; develop a hobby.
- Do not rely on cigarettes, alcohol, or drugs to assist in relaxation.
- Learn about meditation and relaxation exercises and attempt to build them into your life.

From Edelman CL, Mandle CL: *Health promotion throughout the lifespan,* ed 4, St Louis, 1998, Mosby.

Family Systems Stressor-Strength Inventory (FS³I)

INSTRUCTIONS FOR ADMINISTRATION

The Family Systems Stressor-Strength Inventory (FS³I) is an assessment/measurement instrument intended for use with families. It focuses on identifying stressful situations occurring in families and the strengths families use to maintain healthy family functioning. Each family member is asked to complete the instrument on an individual form prior to an interview with the clinician. Questions can be read to members unable to read.

Following completion of the instrument, the clinician evaluates the family on each of the stressful situations (general and specific) and the available strengths they possess. This evaluation is recorded on the family member form.

The clinician records the individual family member's score and the clinician perception score on the Quantitative Summary. A different color code is used for each family member. The clinician also completes the Qualitative Summary, synthesizing the information gleaned from all participants. Clinicians can use the Family Care Plan to prioritize diagnoses, set goals, develop prevention/intervention activities, and evaluate outcomes.

Family name _____ Date _____

Family member(s) completing assessment _____

Ethnic background(s) _____

Religious background(s) _____

Referral source _____

Interviewer _____

Family members	Relationship in family	Age	Marital status	Education (highest degree)	Occupation
1. ___	___	___	___	___	___
2. ___	___	___	___	___	___
3. ___	___	___	___	___	___
4. ___	___	___	___	___	___
5. ___	___	___	___	___	___
6. ___	___	___	___	___	___

Family's current reasons for seeking assistance?

_____

_____

_____

From Berkey KM, Hanson SMH: *Pocket guide to family assessment and intervention,* St Louis, 1991, Mosby.

Part I: Family Systems Stressors: General

DIRECTIONS: Each of the 25 situations/stressors listed here deals with some aspect of normal family life. Each stressor has the potential for creating stress within families or between families and the world in which they live. We are interested in your overall impression of how these situations affect your family life. Please circle a number (0 through 5) that best describes the amount of stress or tension they create for you.

Stressors:	Not apply	Little stress	Medium stress	High stress	Clinician perception Score
1. Family member(s) feel unappreciated	0	1	2	3	4	5	_____
2. Guilt for not accomplishing more	0	1	2	3	4	5	_____
3. Insufficient "me" time	0	1	2	3	4	5	_____
4. Self-image/self-esteem/ feelings of unattractiveness	0	1	2	3	4	5	_____
5. Perfectionism	0	1	2	3	4	5	_____
6. Dieting	0	1	2	3	4	5	_____
7. Health/illness	0	1	2	3	4	5	_____
8. Communication with children	0	1	2	3	4	5	_____
9. Housekeeping standards . .	0	1	2	3	4	5	_____
10. Insufficient couple time . .	0	1	2	3	4	5	_____
11. Insufficient family playtime	0	1	2	3	4	5	_____
12. Children's behavior/discipline/sibling fighting	0	1	2	3	4	5	_____
13. Television	0	1	2	3	4	5	_____
14. Over-scheduled family calendar	0	1	2	3	4	5	_____
15. Lack of shared responsibility in the family	0	1	2	3	4	5	_____
16. Moving	0	1	2	3	4	5	_____
17. Spousal relationship (communication, friendship, sex)	0	1	2	3	4	5	_____
18. Holidays	0	1	2	3	4	5	_____
19. In-laws	0	1	2	3	4	5	_____
20. Teen behaviors (communication, music, friends, school)	0	1	2	3	4	5	_____
21. New baby	0	1	2	3	4	5	_____
22. Economics/finances/ budgets	0	1	2	3	4	5	_____

Stressors:	Family perception score				Clinician perception
	Not apply	Little stress	Medium stress	High stress	Score
23. Unhappiness with work situation	0	1	2	3	4	5	_____
24. Overvolunteerism	0	1	2	3	4	5	_____
25. Neighbors	0	1	2	3	4	5	_____

Additional Stressors: _____

_____

Family Remarks: _____

_____

Clinician: Clarification of stressful situations/concerns with family members. Prioritize in order of importance to family members:

_____

Part II: Family Systems Stressors: Specific

DIRECTIONS: The following 12 questions are designed to provide information about your specific stress-producing situation/problem, or area of concern influencing your family's health. Please circle a number (1 through 5) that best describes the influence this situation has on your family's life and how well you perceive your family's overall functioning.

The specific stress-producing situation/problem or area of concern at this time is: _____

_____

Stressors:	Family perception score			Clinician perception
	Little	Medium	High	Score
1. To what extent is your family bothered by this problem or stressful situations? (e.g., effects on family interactions, communication among members, emotional and social relationships)	1 2	3 4	5	_____

Family Remarks: _____

_____

Stressors:	Family perception score			Clinician perception
	Little	Medium	High	Score
2. How much of an effect does this stressful situation have on your family's usual pattern of living? (e.g., effects on lifestyle patterns and family developmental task)	1	2 3 4	5	_____

Family Remarks: _____

_____

Clinician Remarks: _____

_____

| 3. How much has this situation affected your family's ability to work together as a family unit? (e.g., alteration in family roles, completion of family tasks, following through with responsibilities) | 1 | 2   3   4 | 5 | _____ |

Family Remarks: _____

_____

Clinician Remarks: _____

_____

Has your family ever experienced a similar concern in the past?
1. YES   If YES, complete question 4
2. NO   If NO, complete question 5

| 4. How successful was your family in dealing with this situation/ problem/concern in the past? (e.g., workable coping strategies developed, adaptive measures useful, situation improved) | 1 | 2   3   4 | 5 | _____ |

Family Remarks: _____

_____

Clinician Remarks: _____

_____

Stressors:	Family perception score			Clinician perception
	Little	Medium	High	Score

5. How strongly do you feel this current situation/problem/concern will affect your family's future?
(e.g., anticipated consequences)

   1   2   3   4   5   _____

   Family Remarks: _____

   _____

   Clinician Remarks: _____

   _____

6. To what extent are family members able to help themselves in this present situation/problem/concern?
(e.g., self-assistive efforts, family expectations, spiritual influence, and family resources)

   1   2   3   4   5   _____

   Family Remarks: _____

   _____

   Clinician Remarks: _____

   _____

7. To what extent do you expect others to help your family with this situation/problem/concern?
(e.g., what roles would helpers play; how available are extra-family resources)

   1   2   3   4   5   _____

   Family Remarks: _____

   _____

   Clinician Remarks: _____

   _____

8. How would you rate the way your family functions overall?
(e.g., how your family members relate to each other and to larger family and community)

   1   2   3   4   5   _____

Stressors:	Poor	Family perception score Satisfactory	Excellent	Clinician perception Score

Family Remarks: _____

_____

Clinician Remarks: _____

_____

9. How would you rate the overall physical health status of each family member by name? (Include yourself as a family member; record additional names on back.)

a. _____	1	2	3	4	5	_____
b. _____	1	2	3	4	5	_____
c. _____	1	2	3	4	5	_____
d. _____	1	2	3	4	5	_____
e. _____	1	2	3	4	5	_____

10. How would you rate the overall physical health status of your family as a whole?   1   2   3   4   5 _____

Family Remarks: _____

_____

Clinician Remarks: _____

_____

11. How would you rate the overall mental health status of each family member by name? (Include yourself as a family member; record additional names on back.)

a. _____	1	2	3	4	5	_____
b. _____	1	2	3	4	5	_____
c. _____	1	2	3	4	5	_____
d. _____	1	2	3	4	5	_____
e. _____	1	2	3	4	5	_____

12. How would you rate the
    overall mental health status
    of your family as a whole?　　1　　2　　3　　4　　5 _____

    Family Remarks: _____

    _____

    Clinician Remarks: _____

    _____

Part III: Family Systems Strengths

DIRECTIONS: Each of the 16 traits/attributes listed below deals with some aspect of family life and its overall functioning. Each one contributes to the health and well-being of family members as individuals and to the family as a whole. Please circle a number (0 through 5) that best describes the extent that the trait applies to your family.

My family:	Not apply	Seldom	Usually	Always	Score
		Family perception score			**Clinician perception**
1. Communicates and listens to one another ...	0	1 2	3	4	5 ____
2. Affirms and supports one another	0	1 2	3	4	5 ____
3. Teaches respect for others	0	1 2	3	4	5 ____

1. Communicates and
   listens to one another ...　0　　1　　2　　3　　4　　5 _____

   Family Remarks: _____

   _____

   Clinician Remarks: _____

   _____

2. Affirms and supports
   one another ....　0　　1　　2　　3　　4　　5 _____

   Family Remarks: _____

   _____

   Clinician Remarks: _____

   _____

3. Teaches respect for
   others ....　0　　1　　2　　3　　4　　5 _____

   Family Remarks: _____

   _____

My family:	Family perception score				Clinician perception
	Not apply	Seldom	Usually	Always	Score

Clinician Remarks: _____

_____

4. Develops a sense of
   trust in members 0   1   2   3   4   5 _____

   Family Remarks: _____

   _____

   Clinician Remarks: _____

   _____

5. Displays a sense of play
   and humor 0   1   2   3   4   5 _____

   Family Remarks: _____

   _____

   Clinician Remarks: _____

   _____

6. Exhibits a sense of shared
   responsibility 0   1   2   3   4   5 _____

   Family Remarks: _____

   _____

   Clinician Remarks: _____

   _____

7. Teaches a sense of right
   and wrong 0   1   2   3   4   5 _____

   Family Remarks: _____

   _____

   Clinician Remarks: _____

   _____

My family:	Not apply	Family perception score			Clinician perception
		Seldom	Usually	Always	Score

8. Has a strong sense of
    family in which rituals
    and traditions abound ... 0   1   2   3   4   5 _____

   Family Remarks: _____

   _____

   Clinician Remarks: _____

   _____

9. Has a balance of inter-
    action among members .. 0   1   2   3   4   5 _____

   Family Remarks: _____

   _____

   Clinician Remarks: _____

   _____

10. Has a shared religious
    core 0   1   2   3   4   5 _____

   Family Remarks: _____

   _____

   Clinician Remarks: _____

   _____

11. Respects the privacy of
    one another 0   1   2   3   4   5 _____

   Family Remarks: _____

   _____

   Clinician Remarks: _____

   _____

12. Values service to others .. 0   1   2   3   4   5 _____

   Family Remarks: _____

   _____

| My family: | Not apply | Family perception score | | | Clinician perception |
		Seldom	Usually	Always	Score
Clinician Remarks: _____					

13. Fosters family table time
and conversation 0   1   2   3   4   5 _____

Family Remarks: _____

Clinician Remarks: _____

14. Shares leisures time 0   1   2   3   4   5 _____

Family Remarks: _____

Clinician Remarks: _____

15. Admits to and seeks help
with problems 0   1   2   3   4   5 _____

Family Remarks: _____

Clinician Remarks: _____

16a. How would you rate the
overall strengths that
exist in your family? . . . 0   1   2   3   4   5 _____

Family Remarks: _____

Clinician Remarks: _____

16b. Additional family strengths: _____

_____

_____

16c. Clinician: Clarification of family strengths with individual members:

_____

_____

_____

SCORING SUMMARY
Section 1: Family Perception Scores
INSTRUCTIONS FOR ADMINISTRATION: The Family Systems Stressor-Strength Inventory (FS^3I) Scoring Summary is divided into two sections: Section 1, Family Perception Scores and Section 2, Clinician Perception Scores. These two sections are further divided into three parts: Part I, Family Systems Stressors: General; Part II, Family Systems Stressors: Specific; and, Part III, Family Systems Strengths. Each part contains a Quantitative Summary and a Qualitative Summary.

Quantifiable family and clinician perception scores are both graphed on the Quantitative Summary. Each family member has a designated color code. Family and clinician remarks are both recorded on the Qualitative Summary. Quantitative summary scores, when graphed, suggest a level for initiation of prevention/intervention modes: Primary, Secondary, and Tertiary. Qualitative summary information, when synthesized, contributes to the development and channeling of the Family Care Plan.

Part I: Family Systems Stressors: General.   Add scores from questions 1 to 25 and calculate an overall numerical score for Family System Stressors (General). Ratings are from 1 (most positive) to 5 (most negative). The Not Apply (0) responses are omitted from the calculations. Total scores range from 25 to 125.

Family Systems Stressor Score: General

$$\frac{(\quad)}{25} \times 1 = \underline{\quad}$$

Graph score on Quantitative Summary, Family Systems Stressors: General, Family Member Perception. Color code to differentiate family members.

Record additional stressors and family remarks in Part I, Qualitative Summary: Family and Clinician Remarks.

Part II: Family Systems Stressors: Specific.   Add scores from questions 1-8, 10 and 12 and calculate a numerical score for Family Systems through Stressors: Specific. Ratings are from 1 (most positive) to 5 (most negative). Questions 4, 6, 7, 8, 10, and 12 are reverse scored.* Total scores range from 10 to 50.

Family Systems Stressor Score: Specific

$$\frac{(\quad\quad)}{10} \times 1 = \underline{\quad\quad}$$

Graph score on Quantitative Summary: Family Systems Stressor: Specific (Family Member Perceptions). Color code to differentiate family members.

Summarize data from questions 9 and 11 (reverse scored) and record family remarks in Part II, Qualitative Summary: Family and Clinician Remarks

Part III: Family Systems Strengths.   Add scores from questions 1 to 16 and calculate a numerical score for Family Systems Strengths. Ratings are from 1 (seldom) to 5 (always). The Not Apply (0) responses are omitted from the calculations. Total scores range from 16 to 80.

$$\frac{(\quad\quad)}{16} \times 1 = \underline{\quad\quad}$$

Graph score on Quantitative Summary: Family Systems Strengths (Family Member Perception).

Record Additional Family Strengths and Family Remarks in Part III, Qualitative Summary: Family and Clinician Remarks.

Section 2: Clinician Perception Scores

Part I: Family Systems Stressors: General.   Add scores from questions 1 to 25 and calculate an overall numerical score for Family System Stressors: General. Ratings are from 1 (most positive) to 5 (most negative). The Not Apply (0) responses are omitted from the calculations. Total scores range from 25 to 125.

---

*Reverse Scoring:

   Question answered as (1) is scored 5 points

   Question answered as (2) is scored 4 points

   Question answered as (3) is scored 3 points

   Question answered as (4) is scored 2 points

   Question answered as (5) is scored 1 point

Family Systems Stressor Score: General

$$\frac{(\quad)}{25} \times 1 = \underline{\qquad}$$

Graph score on Quantitative Summary, Family Systems Stressors: General (Clinician Perception).

Record Clinicians' clarification of general stressors in Part I, Qualitative Summary: Family and Clinician Remarks.

Part II: Family Systems Stressors: Specific.   Add scores from questions 1-8, 10, and 12 and calculate a numerical score for Family Systems Stressors: Specific. Ratings are from 1 (most positive) to 5 (most negative). Questions 4, 6-8, 10, and 12 are reverse scored.* Total scores range from 10 to 50.

Family Systems Stressor Score: Specific

$$\frac{(\quad)}{10} \times 1 = \underline{\qquad}$$

Graph score on Quantitative Summary: Family Systems Stressor: Specific (Clinician Perceptions).

Summarize data from questions 9 and 11 (reverse order) and record Clinician Remarks in Part II, Qualitative Summary: Family and Clinician Remarks

Part III: Family Systems Strengths.   Add scores from questions 1 to 16 and calculate a numerical score for Family Systems Strengths. Ratings are from 1 (seldom) to 5 (always).

The Not Apply (0) responses are omitted from the calculations. Total scores range from 16 to 80.

$$\frac{(\quad)}{16} \times 1 = \underline{\qquad}$$

Graph score on Quantitative Summary: Family Systems Strengths (Clinician Perception).

---

*Reverse Scoring:
   Question answered as (1) is scored 5 points
   Question answered as (2) is scored 4 points
   Question answered as (3) is scored 3 points
   Question answered as (4) is scored 2 points
   Question answered as (5) is scored 1 point

Record Clinicians' clarification of family strengths in Part III, Qualitative Summary: Family and Clinician Remarks.

Quantitative Summary Family Systems Stressors: General and Specific Family and Clinician Perception Scores

DIRECTIONS: Graph the scores from each family member inventory by placing an "X" at the appropriate location. (Use first name initial for each different entry and different color code for each family member.) See pp. 400-401 following.

Scores for wellness and stability	Family Systems Stressors: General	
	Family member perception score	Clinician perception score
5.0		
4.8		
4.6		
4.4		
4.2		
4.0		
3.8		
3.6		
3.4		
3.2		
3.0		
2.8		
2.6		
2.4		
2.2		
2.0		
1.8		
1.6		
1.4		
1.2		
1.0		

*PRIMARY Prevention/Intervention Mode: Flexible Line 1.0-2.3
*SECONDARY Prevention/Intervention Mode: Normal Line 2.4-3.6
*TERTIARY Prevention/Intervention Mode: Resistance Lines 3.7-5.0
*Breakdowns of numerical scores for stressor penetration are suggested values

	Family Systems Stressors: Specific	
Scores for wellness and stability	**Family member perception score**	**Clinician perception score**
5.0 _____		
4.8 _____		
4.6 _____		
4.4 _____		
4.2 _____		
4.0 _____		
3.8 _____		
3.6 _____		
3.4 _____		
3.2 _____		
3.0 _____		
2.8 _____		
2.6 _____		
2.4 _____		
2.2 _____		
2.0 _____		
1.8 _____		
1.6 _____		
1.4 _____		
1.2 _____		
1.0 _____		

*PRIMARY Prevention/Intervention Mode: Flexible Line 1.0-2.3
*SECONDARY Prevention/Intervention Mode: Normal Line 2.4-3.6
*TERTIARY Prevention/Intervention Mode: Resistance Lines 3.7-5.0
*Breakdowns of numerical scores for stressor penetration are suggested values

Family Systems Strengths: Family and Clinician Perception Scores

DIRECTIONS: Graph the scores from the inventory by placing an "X" at the appropriate location and connect with a line. (Use first name initial for each different entry and different color code for each family member.)

	Family systems: strengths	
Scores for wellness and stability	Family member perception score	Clinician perception score
5.0		
4.8		
4.6		
4.4		
4.2		
4.0		
3.8		
3.6		
3.4		
3.2		
3.0		
2.8		
2.6		
2.4		
2.2		
2.0		
1.8		
1.6		
1.4		
1.2		
1.0		

*PRIMARY Prevention/Intervention Mode: Flexible Line 1.0-2.3
*SECONDARY Prevention/Intervention Mode: Normal Line 2.4-3.6
*TERTIARY Prevention/Intervention Mode: Resistance Lines 3.7-5.0
*Breakdowns of numerical scores for stressor penetration are suggested values

Qualitative Summary Family and Clinician Remarks

Part I: Family Systems Stressors: General

Summarize general stressors and remarks of family and clinician.
Prioritize stressors according to importance to family members.

_____
_____
_____
_____

Part II: Family Systems Stressors: Specific

A. Summarize specific stressor and remarks of family and clinician.

_____
_____
_____
_____

B. Summarize differences (if discrepancies exist) between how family members and clinician view effects of stressful situation on family.

_____
_____
_____
_____

C. Summarize overall family functioning.

_____
_____
_____
_____

D. Summarize overall significant physical health status for family members.

_____
_____
_____
_____

E. Summarize overall significant mental health status for family members.

_____
_____
_____
_____

Part III: Family Systems Strengths

Summarize family systems strengths and family and clinician remarks that facilitate family health and stability.

_____
_____
_____
_____

Family care plan*

Diagnosis general & specific family system stressors	Family systems strengths supporting family care plan	Goals family & physician	Prevention/intervention mode		Outcomes evaluation and replanning
			Primary, secondary, or tertiary	Prevention/ intervention activities	

*Prioritize the three most significant diagnoses.

The Worry Scale

Instructions: Below is a list of problems that often concern many Americans. Please read each one carefully. After you have done so, please fill in one of the spaces to the right with a check that describes how much that problem worries you. Make only one check mark for each item.

Things that worry me . . .

	Never	Rarely (1-2 times per month)	Sometimes (1-2 times per week)	Often (1-2 times a day)	Much of the time (more than 2 times a day)
Finances					
1. I'll lose my home					
2. I won't be able to pay for the necessities of life (such as food, clothing, or medicine)					
3. I won't be able to support myself independently					
4. I won't be able to enjoy the "good things" in life (such as travel, recreation, entertainment)					
5. I won't be able to help my children financially					
Health					
6. My eyesight or hearing will get worse					
7. I'll lose control of my bladder or kidneys					
8. I won't be able to remember important things					
9. I won't be able to get around by myself					
10. I won't be able to enjoy my food					

Continued

From Powers CB, Wisocki PA, Whitbourne SK: *Gerontologist* 32(1):82, 1992.

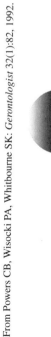

The Worry Scale—cont'd

	Never	Rarely (1-2 times per month)	Sometimes (1-2 times per week)	Often (1-2 times a day)	Much of the time (more than 2 times a day)
11. I'll have to be taken care of by my family					
12. I'll have to be taken care of by strangers					
13. I won't be able to take care of my spouse					
14. I'll have to go to a nursing home or hospital					
15. I won't be able to sleep at night					
16. I may have a serious illness or accident					
17. My spouse or a close family member may have a serious illness or accident					
18. I won't be able to enjoy sex					
19. My reflexes will slow down					
20. I won't be able to make decisions					
21. I won't be able to drive a car					
22. I'll have to use a mechanical aid (such as a hearing aid, bifocals, a cane)					
Social conditions					
23. I'll look "old"					
24. People will think of me as unattractive					
25. No will want to be around me					
26. No one will love me anymore					

27. I'll be a burden to my loved ones
28. I won't be able to visit my family and friends
29. I may be attacked by muggers or robbers on the streets
30. My home may be broken into and vandalized
31. No one will come to my aid if I need it
32. My friends and family won't visit me
33. My friends and family will die
34. I'll get depressed
35. I'll have serious psychological problems

Other worries

36.
37.
38.
39.
40.

CRISIS

Family Crisis-Oriented Personal Evaluation Scales (F-COPES)

The Family Crisis-Oriented Personal Evaluation Scales is designed to record effective problem-solving attitudes and behavior that families develop to respond to problems or difficulties.

Directions

First, read the list of "Response Choices" one at a time. Second, decide how well each statement describes your attitudes and behavior in response to problems or difficulties. If the statement describes your response *very well,* then circle the number 5 indicating that you STRONGLY AGREE; if the statement does not describe your response at all, then circle the number 1 indicating that you STRONGLY DISAGREE; if the statement describes your response to some degree, then select a number 2, 3, or 4 to indicate how much you agree or disagree with the statement about your response.

When we face problems or difficulties in our family, we respond by	Strongly disagree	Moderately disagree	Neither agree nor disagree	Moderately agree	Strongly agree
1. Sharing our difficulties with relatives	1	2	3	4	5
2. Seeking encouragement and support from friends	1	2	3	4	5
3. Knowing we have the power to solve major problems	1	2	3	4	5
4. Seeking information and advice from persons in other families who have faced the same or similar problems	1	2	3	4	5
5. Seeking advice from relatives (grandparents, etc.)	1	2	3	4	5
6. Seeking assistance from community agencies and programs designed to help families in our situation	1	2	3	4	5
7. Knowing that we have the strength within our own family to solve our problems	1	2	3	4	5
8. Receiving gifts and favors from neighbors (food, taking in mail, etc.)	1	2	3	4	5
9. Seeking information and advice from the family doctor	1	2	3	4	5
10. Asking neighbors for favors and assistance	1	2	3	4	5
11. Facing the problems "head-on" and trying to get solutions right away	1	2	3	4	5
12. Watching television	1	2	3	4	5
13. Showing that we are strong	1	2	3	4	5
14. Attending church services	1	2	3	4	5
15. Accepting stressful events as a factor of life	1	2	3	4	5
16. Sharing concerns with close friends	1	2	3	4	5

From McCubbin HI, Olson DH, Larsen A: F-COPES: Family Crisis-Oriented Personal Evaluation Scales. In McCubbin HI, Thompson AI, McCubbin MA: *Family assessment: resiliency, coping, and adaptation—inventories for research and practice,* Madison, 1996, University of Wisconsin.

Continued

When we face problems or difficulties in our family, we respond by	Strongly disagree	Moderately disagree	Neither agree nor disagree	Moderately agree	Strongly agree
17. Knowing luck plays a big part in how well we are able to solve family problems	1	2	3	4	5
18. Exercising with friends to stay fit and reduce tension	1	2	3	4	5
19. Accepting that difficulties occur unexpectedly	1	2	3	4	5
20. Doing things with relatives (get-togethers, dinners, etc.)	1	2	3	4	5
21. Seeking professional counseling and help for family difficulties	1	2	3	4	5
22. Believing we can handle our own problems	1	2	3	4	5
23. Participating in church activities	1	2	3	4	5
24. Defining the family problem in a more positive way so that we do not become too discouraged	1	2	3	4	5
25. Asking relatives how they feel about problems we face	1	2	3	4	5
26. Feeling that no matter what we do to prepare, we will have difficulty handling problems	1	2	3	4	5
27. Seeking advice from a clergyperson	1	2	3	4	5
28. Believing if we wait long enough, the problem will go away	1	2	3	4	5
29. Sharing problems with neighbors	1	2	3	4	5
30. Having faith in God	1	2	3	4	5

Scoring the instrument is done by summing the numbers circled for items in each subscale, except for items 17, 26, and 28, which are reversed. The subscales are acquiring social support (1, 2, 5, 8, 10, 16, 20, 25, 29); reframing (3, 7, 11, 13, 15, 19, 22, 24); seeking spiritual support (14, 23, 27, 30); mobilizing the family to acquire and accept help (4, 6, 9, 21); and passive appraisal (12, 17, 26, 28). A total coping score is the sum of the subscales and has a possible range from 29 to 145. The mean scores reported range from 91.24 to 95.64, and standard deviations are from 12.06 to 14.05.

Assessment Data for Crisis Intervention

The following instrument will assist the nurse and client in naming the problem that has resulted in a client crisis. It will help the nurse determine both the effect of the crisis on the client's normal level of functioning and potential dangers to the client's health. The data collected may indicate a need for referral.

Date _____

Name _____   Next of kin _____
Age _____   Address _____
Address _____   _____
_____   Telephone no. _____
Telephone no. _____   Information obtained from:
Reliable historian   Client _____
   Yes _____   Next of kin _____
   No _____   Other _____
      Name _____
      Address _____
      _____
      Telephone no. _____

1. Identification of problem or crisis event
    Reason for seeking help:

    Time event occurred:
      Sudden onset _____
      Gradual onset _____

From Detherage KS, Johnson SS. In Edelman CL, Mandle CL: *Health promotion throughout the lifespan,* ed 4, St Louis, 1998, Mosby.

Effects of crisis on client:

Effects of crisis on client's significant others:

Response to crisis event:

2. Perception of crisis event
Meaning of crisis to client:

Meaning of crisis to client's significant others:

Changes in client's life because of the crisis:

Effects of crisis on client's goals:

Is client perceiving crisis in realistic manner?

3. Identification of external support resources available to client
(Note supports that are most meaningful to client.)
Family:

Friends:

Clergy:

Community agencies:

Others:

4. Coping abilities
Usual methods of coping:

Coping behaviors that can be used to relieve present crisis:

5. Is client homicidal? _____ If yes, give details:

6. Is client suicidal? _____ If yes, give details:

7. Ego functioning
Memory:

Judgment:

Problem-solving ability:

Perceptions:

8. Mood (happy, sad, etc.)

9. Level of anxiety
Mild _____
Moderate _____
Severe _____

Problems Exhibited by the Crisis-Prone Person

Difficulty in learning from experience
History of frequent crises, ineffectively resolved because of poor coping ability
History of mental disorder or other serious emotional disturbances
Low self-esteem, which may be masked by provocative behavior
Tendency toward impulsive "acting out" behavior (doing without thinking)
Marginal income
Lack of regular, fulfilling work
Unsatisfying marriage and family relations
Heavy drinking or other substance abuse
History of numerous accidents
Frequent encounters with law-enforcement agencies
Frequent changes in address

From Detherage KS, Johnson SS. In Edelman CL, Mandle CL: *Health promotion throughout the lifespan,* ed 4, St Louis, 1998, Mosby.

EATING DISORDERS

Areas of Disordered Functioning in Anorexia Nervosa

1. Disturbed body image and delusional body concept. The young girl identifies with her emaciation, defending the skeleton-like ap-

Modified from Bruch H: *Nutr Today* 13(5):14-18, 1978. In Wong DL, et al: *Whaley and Wong's nursing care of infants and children,* ed 6, St Louis, 1999, Mosby.

pearance as normal, actively maintains it, and denies that it is abnormal. She indicates that it is rewarding to achieve and maintain this emaciated state. She is increasingly fearful of weight gain and interprets the concern of others as attempts to make her fat.

2. **Inaccurate and confused perception and interpretation of inner stimuli.** Inaccurate hunger awareness is pronounced. The adolescent does not recognize signs of nutritional need in herself and is unable to assess the amounts of food taken. She may feel "full" after only a few bites and derives pleasure from the refusal of food. A preoccupation and tremendous involvement with food and related activities are associated with this eating behavior; the girl frequently assumes all meal planning and preparation for others. Girls with anorexia nervosa often increase their activity to help counteract the possibility of weight gain. This hyperactivity may continue until emaciation is far advanced.

3. **Paralyzing sense of ineffectiveness that pervades all aspects of daily life.** Teenagers with anorexia nervosa are overwhelmed by a deep sense of ineffectiveness. They are convinced that they function only in response to demands and wishes of others, rather than doing as they want or choose. They have always been compliant children, but careful analysis reveals this to be mechanical obedience and overconformity that is not recognized as a reflection of a serious problem—a self-doubt regarding their ability to stand up for themselves or even the right for self-assertion.

Some Characteristics of Eating Disorders

Factors	Anorexia nervosa	Bulimia
Food	Turns away from food to cope	Turns to food to cope
Personality	Introverted	Extroverted
	Avoids intimacy	Seeks intimacy
	Negates feminine role	Aspires to feminine role
Behavior	"Model" child	Often "acts out"
	Compulsive/obsessive	Impulsive
School	High achiever	Variable school performance
Control	Maintains rigid control	Loses control
Body image	Body distortion	Less frequent body distortion
Health	Denies illness	Recognizes illness
		Fluctuates
Weight	Body weight less than 85% of expected norm	Within 5 to 15 lb of normal body weight
Sexuality	Usually not sexually active	Often sexually active

From Wong DL, et al: *Whaley and Wong's nursing care of infants and children,* ed 6, St Louis, 1999, Mosby.

Early Signs of Anorexia Nervosa

The adolescent

Consumes an inappropriate diet (excessively strict) or may refuse to eat altogether

Develops peculiar eating habits such as toying with food, food "rituals," preparing and forcing food on family members without eating any herself

Engages in excessive exercise, such as compulsive jogging, running up and down stairs, rigorous calisthenics to burn off calories—often to the point of exhaustion

Withdraws from social interaction—starts to spend all her time in her room studying, exercising, or otherwise occupied

Ceases to have menstrual periods after sudden or excessive weight loss—sometimes almost as soon as dieting begins

Takes laxatives, diuretics, or enemas to speed intestinal transit time to lose added weight and empty intestines to flatten abdomen

Vomits deliberately—may go to bathroom after a meal and turn on faucets to avoid being heard

Denies hunger even after eating practically nothing for days or even weeks

Develops a distorted body image—states she "feels fat" as she becomes increasingly thinner

Loses weight—growing girls fail to achieve the 25th percentile on normal growth curves

From Wong DL, et al: *Whaley and Wong's nursing care of infants and children,* ed 6, St Louis, 1999, Mosby.

Diagnostic Criteria for Anorexia Nervosa

1. Refusal to maintain body weight at or above a minimally normal weight for age and height (e.g., weight loss leading to maintenance of body weight less than 85% of that expected; or failure to make expected weight gain during period of growth, leading to body weight less than 85% of that expected)
2. Intense fear of gaining weight or becoming fat, even though underweight

From American Psychiatric Association: *Diagnostic and statistical manual of mental disorders (DSM-IV),* ed 4, Washington, DC, 1994, The Association.

3. Disturbance in the way in which one's body weight or shape is experienced, undue influence of body weight or shape on self-evaluation, or denial of the seriousness of the current low body weight

4. In postmenarcheal females, amenorrhea (i.e., the absence of at least three consecutive menstrual cycles) (a woman is considered to have amenorrhea if her periods occur only after hormone, e.g., estrogen, administration)

Specify type:

Restricting: During the current episode of anorexia nervosa, the person has not regularly engaged in binge-eating or purging behavior (i.e., self-induced vomiting or the misuse of laxatives, diuretics, or enemas).

Binge eating/purging: During the current episode of anorexia nervosa, the person has regularly engaged in binge eating or purging behavior (i.e., self-induced vomiting or the misuse of laxatives, diuretics, or enemas).

Diagnostic Criteria for Bulimia Nervosa

1. Recurrent episodes of binge eating. An episode of binge eating is characterized by both of the following:
   a. Eating, in a discrete period of time (e.g., within any 2-hour period), an amount of food that is definitely larger than most people would eat during a similar period of time and under similar circumstances
   b. A sense of lack of control over eating during the episode (e.g., a feeling that one cannot stop eating or control what or how much one is eating)
2. Recurrent inappropriate compensatory behavior to prevent weight gain, such as self-induced vomiting; misuse of laxatives, diuretics, enemas, or other medications; fasting; or excessive exercise.
3. The binge eating and inappropriate compensatory behaviors both occur, on average, at least twice a week for 3 months.
4. Self-evaluation is unduly influenced by body shape and weight.
5. The disturbance does not occur exclusively during episodes of anorexia nervosa.

From American Psychiatric Association: *Diagnostic and statistical manual of mental disorders (DSM-IV),* ed 4, Washington, DC, 1994, The Association.

Specify type:

Purging: During the current episode of bulimia nervosa, the person has regularly engaged in self-induced vomiting or the misuse of laxatives, diuretics, or enemas.

Nonpurging: During the current episode of bulimia nervosa, the person has used other inappropriate compensatory behaviors, such as fasting or excessive exercise, but has not regularly engaged in self-induced vomiting or the misuse of laxatives, diuretics, or enemas.

LIFESTYLE

Social Readjustment Rating Scale

Holmes and Rahe developed this scale to rate the amount of stress caused by many changes in life: major and minor, pleasant and unpleasant. To obtain your score, circle the ones that apply to you and then add up the total. Follow-up studies show that people who accumulate more than 200 points in a year are at high risk for physical or psychologic stress-related illnesses.

Life event	Mean value
1. Death of spouse	100
2. Divorce	73
3. Marital separation from mate	65
4. Detention in jail or other institution	63
5. Death of a close family member	63
6. Major personal injury or illness	53
7. Marriage	50
8. Being fired at work	47
9. Marital reconciliation with mate	45
10. Retirement from work	45
11. Major change in the health or behavior of a family member	44
12. Pregnancy	40
13. Sexual difficulties	39
14. Gaining a new family member (e.g., through birth, adoption, or elder moving in)	39
15. Major business readjustment (e.g., merger, reorganization, bankruptcy)	39

From Holmes TH, Rahe RH: *J Psychosom Res* 11(8), 213-217, 1967.

Continued

Life event	Mean value
16. Major change in financial state (e.g., a lot worse off or a lot better off than usual)	38
17. Death of a close friend	37
18. Changing to a different line of work	36
19. Major change in the number of arguments with spouse (e.g., either a lot more or a lot less than usual regarding child rearing, personal habits)	35
20. Taking out a mortgage or loan for a major purchase (e.g., for a home, business)	31
21. Foreclosure on a mortgage or loan	30
22. Major change in responsibilities at work (e.g., promotion, demotion, lateral transfer)	29
23. Son or daughter leaving home (e.g., marriage, attending college)	29
24. Trouble with in-laws	29
25. Outstanding personal achievement	28
26. Spouse beginning or ceasing work outside the home	26
27. Beginning or ceasing formal schooling	26
28. Major change in living conditions (e.g., building a new home, remodeling, deterioration of home or neighborhood)	25
29. Revision of personal habits (dress, manners, associations, etc.)	24
30. Trouble with the boss	23
31. Major change in working hours or conditions	20
32. Change in residence	20
33. Changing to a new school	20
34. Major change in usual type or amount of recreation	19
35. Major change in church activities (e.g., a lot more or a lot less than usual)	19
36. Major change in social activities (e.g., clubs, dancing, movies, visiting)	18
37. Taking out a mortgage or loan for a lesser purchase (e.g., for a car, TV, freezer)	17
38. Major change in sleeping habits (a lot more or a lot less sleep, or a change in part of day when asleep)	16
39. Major change in number of family get-togethers (e.g., a lot more or a lot less than usual)	15
40. Major change in eating habits (a lot more or a lot less food intake, or very different meal hours or surroundings)	15
41. Vacation	13
42. Christmas	12
43. Minor violations of the law (e.g., traffic lights, jaywalking, disturbing the peace)	11

Family Inventory of Life Events and Changes (FILE)

Scoring for FILE* is done by totaling the numbers assigned for each item the client checks *yes*.

High score	= over 750	Inform family of high stress and offer
Moderate score	= 501–749	assistance in coping
Low score	= under 500	

Purpose

Over their life cycle, all families experience many changes as a result of normal growth and development of members and due to external circumstances. The following list of family life changes can happen in a family at any time. Because family members are connected to each other in some way, a life change for any one member affects all the other persons in the family to some degree.

> "Family" means a group of two or more persons living together who are related by blood, marriage, or adoption. This includes persons who live with you and to whom you have a long term commitment.

Directions

"Did the change happen in your family?"

Please read each family life change and decide whether it happened to any member of your family—including you.

- During the last year

  First, decide if it happened any time during the last 12 months and check

  Yes or No.

During last 12 months
Yes ☐   No ☐

---

*Developed by HI McCubbin, JM Patterson, and LR Wilson.

From McCubbin HI, Thompson AI, McCubbin MA, *Family assessment: resiliency, coping, and adaptation—inventories for research and practice,* Madison, 1996, University of Wisconsin.

Family life changes		Did the change happen in your family?		Score
		During last 12 months		
		Yes	No	
I. Intrafamily strains				
1. Increase of husband/father's time away from family	46	☐	☐	
2. Increase of wife/mother's time away from family	51	☐	☐	
3. A member appears to have emotional problems	58	☐	☐	
4. A member appears to depend on alcohol or drugs	66	☐	☐	
5. Increase in conflict between husband and wife	53	☐	☐	
6. Increase in arguments between parent(s) and child(ren)	45	☐	☐	
7. Increase in conflict among children in the family	48	☐	☐	
8. Increased difficulty in managing teenage child(ren)	55	☐	☐	
9. Increased difficulty in managing school-age child(ren) (6-12 yr)	39	☐	☐	
10. Increased difficulty in managing preschool-age child(ren) (2½-6 yr)	36	☐	☐	
11. Increased difficulty in managing toddler(s) (1-2½ yr)	36	☐	☐	
12. Increased difficulty in managing infant(s) (0-1 yr)	35	☐	☐	
13. Increase in the amount of "outside activities" that the child(ren) are involved in	25	☐	☐	
14. Increased disagreement about a member's friends or activities	35	☐	☐	
15. Increase in the number of problems or issues that do not get resolved	45	☐	☐	
16. Increase in the number of tasks or chores that do not get done	35	☐	☐	
17. Increased conflict with in-laws or relatives	40	☐	☐	
II. Marital strains				
18. Spouse/parent was separated or divorced	79	☐	☐	
19. Spouse/parent has an "affair"	68	☐	☐	
20. Increased difficulty in resolving issues with a "former" or separated spouse	47	☐	☐	
21. Increased difficulty with sexual relationship between husband and wife	58	☐	☐	

Subtotal 1 _____

Family life changes		Did the change happen in your family? During last 12 months		Score
		Yes	No	
III. Pregnancy and childbearing strains				
22. Spouse had unwanted or difficult pregnancy	45	☐	☐	
23. An unmarried member became pregnant	65	☐	☐	
24. A member had an abortion	50	☐	☐	
25. A member gave birth to or adopted a child	50	☐	☐	
IV. Finance and business strains				
26. Took out a loan or refinanced a loan to cover increased expenses	29	☐	☐	
27. Went on welfare	55	☐	☐	
28. Change in conditions (economic, political, weather) that hurts the family business	41	☐	☐	
29. Change in agriculture market, stock market, or land values that hurts family investments or income	43	☐	☐	
30. A member started a new business	50	☐	☐	
31. Purchased or built a home	41	☐	☐	
32. A member purchased a car or other major item	19	☐	☐	
33. Increasing financial debts caused by overuse of credit cards	31	☐	☐	
34. Increased strain on family "money" for medical/ dental expenses	23	☐	☐	
35. Increased strain on family "money" for food, clothing, energy, home care	21	☐	☐	
36. Increased strain on family "money" for child(ren) education	22	☐	☐	
37. Delay in receiving child support or alimony payments	41	☐	☐	
V. Work-family transitions and strains				
38. A member changed to a new job/career	40	☐	☐	
39. A member lost or quit a job	55	☐	☐	
40. A member retired from work	48	☐	☐	
41. A member started or returned to work	41	☐	☐	
42. A member stopped working for extended period (e.g., laid off, leave of absence, strike)	51	☐	☐	
43. Decrease in satisfaction with job/career	45	☐	☐	

Family life changes		Did the change happen in your family? During last 12 months		Score
		Yes	No	
44. A member had increased difficulty with people at work	32	☐	☐	
45. A member was promoted at work or given more responsibilities	40	☐	☐	
46. Family moved to a new home/apartment	43	☐	☐	
47. A child/adolescent member changed to a new school	24	☐	☐	

Subtotal 2 _____

VI. Illness and family "care" strains

48. Parent/spouse became seriously ill or injured	44	☐	☐	
49. Child became seriously ill or injured	35	☐	☐	
50. Close relative or friend of the family became seriously ill	44	☐	☐	
51. A member became physically disabled or chronically ill	73	☐	☐	
52. Increased difficulty in managing a chronically ill or disabled member	58	☐	☐	
53. Member or close relative was committed to an institution or nursing home	44	☐	☐	
54. Increased responsibility to provide direct care or financial help to husband's or wife's parent(s)	47	☐	☐	
55. Experienced difficulty in arranging for satisfactory child care	40	☐	☐	

VII. Losses

56. A parent/spouse died	98	☐	☐	
57. A child member died	99	☐	☐	
58. Death of husband's or wife's parent or close relative	48	☐	☐	
59. Close friend of the family died	47	☐	☐	
60. Married son or daughter was separated or divorced	58	☐	☐	
61. A member "broke up" a relationship with a close friend	35	☐	☐	

VIII. Transitions "in and out"

62. A member was married	42	☐	☐	
63. Young adult member left home	43	☐	☐	

64. A young adult member began college (or post-high school training)	28	☐	☐
65. A member moved back home or a new person moved into the household	42	☐	☐
66. A parent/spouse started school (or training program) after being away from school for a long time	38	☐	☐
IX. Family legal violations			
67. A member went to jail or juvenile detention	68	☐	☐
68. A member was picked up by police or arrested	57	☐	☐
69. Physical or sexual abuse or violence in the home	75	☐	☐
70. A member ran away from home	61	☐	☐
71. A member dropped out of school or was suspended from school	38	☐	☐

Subtotal 3 _____

Grand Total _____

Personal Health Assessment

Section I: Personal Health Habits

What you put into your body—nutrition—how you take care of your body—rest, relaxation, and exercise—and your general level of awareness, love, and acceptance of your body are the major factors important in health. To investigate your health behavior, you might keep a weekly diary of food, exercise, sleep, relaxation, and stress. In this way you create an accurate record of your behavior, which is the first step in a program of modification and change. The following pages are *aids* for that process and ask important questions about your health behavior.

1. Lester Breslow of UCLA, after observing the health and behavior of thousands of adults, has demonstrated that a person's life expectancy and health are related to the following basic health habits:
   __ Three meals per day at regular times and no snacking
   __ Breakfast every day
   __ Moderate exercise two or three times per week
   __ Adequate sleep (7 to 8 hours, not more or less per night)
   __ No smoking
   __ Moderate weight
   __ No alcohol or only in moderation

From Edelman C, Mandle C: *Health promotion throughout the lifespan,* ed 4, St Louis, 1998, Mosby.

Check off how many you observe regularly, giving yourself two checks if you are nearly perfect in that category. Statistically, each habit adds a few years to your life.

Nutrition

2. How much awareness do you have of your particular diet and its effects on your body?

3. In a sentence or two, describe your relationship to food.

4. My favorite foods are:

5. I eat _____ meals per day.

6. My smoking habits are

_____

7. My drinking habits are

_____

8. Do you see a relationship among stress and tension, emotional upsets, and your diet or eating habits?
   Describe:

_____

Exercise and relaxation

A person needs to (1) exercise the body regularly to the point of sweating, (2) get adequate rest in the form of sleep, and (3) practice frequently a form of relaxation response, meditation, self-hypnosis, or related technique that elicits deep relaxation. The more stressful and demanding your life, the more you need both relaxation and exercise: the basic pair of methods of keeping the body healthy and in tune.

Exercise

9. I exercise vigorously approximately _____ hours per week.

10. The type of regular exercise in my life are:

   __ active walking

   __ jogging

   __ sport (which) _____

   __ heavy labor

   __ other (describe) _____

11. Describe your exercise habits and patterns:

12. My attitude toward exercise is:

   __ I love it

   __ I hate it

   __ I'll do it if I have to

   __ other _____

13. I would feel better about exercise, or exercise more, if

_____

_____

Sleep

14. I average _____ hours of sleep per night.

15. My sleep is usually

___ restful and refreshing

___ fitful

___ interrupted

___ other _____

16. I most often awaken feeling

___ refreshed

___ anxious

___ exhausted

___ unfinished

___ other _____

17. I fall asleep

___ easily

___ with difficulty

___ with difficulty when I am under stress

___ regularly using food _____, drink _____, or medication _____

18. Are there any problems, dissatisfactions, or difficulties connected with your sleep patterns? What aspects would you like to change?

Body awareness

19. I consider my normal energy level to be

___ high

___ moderate

___ adequate for most of what I do

___ barely adequate

___ low

___ other descriptive term that seems appropriate _____

_____

20. I consider myself to be

___ tuned into my body's functioning, rhythms, special needs

___ unaware of my body's functioning, rhythms, special needs

___ other _____

21. When I experience my body right now, what does it tell me?

22. How do I feel about my body? (Check all that apply)

___ I like it

___ I dislike it

___ I am proud of it

___ I am a little ashamed or self-conscious about it
___ I barely tolerate it
___ I have no special feelings or awareness
___ I am not sure I have one
___ other feelings and attitudes

23. In a sentence, describe your relationship to your body.

24. The part or parts of my body I like best are

Why, or what about them?

25. What do you want to change about your body awareness or relationship to your body?
26. Draw a picture of yourself as you see or feel yourself now.

Section II: Health History

How aware are you of your history of illness? How much do you know about what is or was going on physically in your body when you were ill with each of your illnesses? Are you aware of the parts of your body, organs, and organ systems that are weak and tend to be the first to feel the effects of the stress in your life? Each person has one or more target organs, the weak links in his or her physical chain, that are the first to break down.

Knowing your health history, knowing your illnesses and target organs, and looking for patterns can be useful in preparing your own health program. In question 27, fill in as well as you can your personal health history, including dates, severity, organ affected, treatment, and also others in your family who may have had that or a similar illness (include the age at which they had it).

27. **Personal Health History** (give most recent first):

MONTH, YEAR	DIAG-NOSIS	SYMP-TOMS	SEVERITY, DURATION	ORGAN AFFECTED	TREAT-MENTS	OTHER FAMILY MEMBERS WITH ILLNESS AND AGE AT ONSET

Section III: Family and Life History

28. Please write something about each member of your family of origin, mentioning perhaps such things as how important they were to you, how close or distant you were, where they are now, and the quality of your relationship.

    Father:

    Mother:

    Brothers and sisters:

    Other important family members:

29. Describe the general health and/or serious illness of each of your parents. If deceased, mention when and the cause of death.

30. Mention something about your childhood home life and family environment, including stressful or traumatic events, family crises, degree of conflict or tension, and any special memories.

31. How do you remember your family responded to illness? What do you remember about your health or illness as a child and how your family reacted to it?

32. List the most important events, crises, transitions, changes (negative or positive), or developments in your life. Take time to do this, because hopefully it should lead to a period of reflection on your life history and how it created you as you are today. List the events and briefly, in a sentence or two, describe what they were and their effect in you. Place an asterisk or two in front of those events that seem especially central to your life. Some of the important events will be childhood traumas, changes in the family through birth and death, important relationships or emotional changes, and so on.

33. Describe briefly your educational history.

34. Comment on its importance and meaningfulness to your life.

35. Starting with your present work or major life activity (not necessarily for profit), describe the work or jobs you have done.

36. In your life now, what is your most meaningful or central activity?

37. What are the other important jobs or activities that you do?

38. Right now, how do you feel about your work, career? What are your most common feelings about it?

39. How would you like your work or career to change?

Section IV: Leisure and Social Activities

40. Write five things that you do to play.

41. Describe something that you laughed about during the week.

42. What things do you do that make you feel good?

43. How many people, outside your immediate family, do you see in a typical week?

44. What sort of friendships do you have? Are they especially close? Do you have few or many? Are they primarily of the same or opposite sex? Please write about your friendships.

45. Describe your present living conditions—whom you live with, how long you have lived there.

46. Please list some of the main satisfactions and dissatisfactions with your living conditions.

Satisfactions:

Dissatisfactions:

47. List the most important people in your life right now and indicate their relationship to you, and in a few words, describe the nature of the relationship or how it feels to you or why its important in your life.

PERSON   **RELATIONSHIP/DESCRIPTION**

Sex

48. Is sex an important aspect of your life? _____ How important, and what role, would you say sex plays in your current life?

49. Are you currently in a sexual relationship? _____ Please write something about it. How satisfying is it for you?

50. Please write something about your sexual history, attitudes, and feelings about sex in your family, sexual awakening, and previous sexual relationships.

51. Did you feel particularly sexually attractive or unattractive at times in your life? _____ During what periods or times?

52. What would you most want to change about your current sexual relationships?

Group or community

53. Every person derives meaning and identity from the human community of which they are a part. A person may identify with many communities—a neighborhood, professional group, friendship network, extended family, religious or ethnic group, political group, and so on. List, in order of their centrality to your life, your communities and affiliations and their importance to you.

---

54. List some of the ways that you affect your environment or one of your communities. How powerful do you feel in making changes in your world?

Section V: Life Stress and Coping Patterns
Recurrent daily stresses

55. Often specific times, activities, or events are the most regular sources of stress in your life. Think about the past few weeks and which stressful situations occurred regularly, how you usually respond to them (what you did, how you felt), and how you might modify them to make them less stressful or destructive to you.

DESCRIPTION OF STRESSFUL EVENT	YOUR RESPONSE (INTERNAL AND EXTERNAL)	POTENTIAL WAYS TO MODIFY EVENT

---

56. What seems to be your usual response to stressful situations? For example, do you blow up, withdraw, take it out on others, get sick, get anxious, cry, become afraid, avoid situations, try to forget, or some combination of these?

57. What situations make you feel calm, relaxed, at peace, or comfortable?

58. What situations make you feel anxious, tense, depressed, fearful, or upset?

59. When you are in such situations, how do you make yourself feel better?

60. Underline any of the following symptoms or difficulties that apply to you:

Headaches	Dizziness	No appetite
Palpitations	Stomach trouble	Insomnia
Bowel disturbances	Fatigue	Alcoholism
Nightmares	Take sedatives	Tremors
Feel tense	Feels panicky	Take drugs
Depression	Suicidal ideas	Shy with people
Unable to relax	Sexual problems	Can't make decisions
Don't like weekends or vacations	Overambitious	Home conditions bad
	Inferiority feelings	Unable to have a good
Can't make friends	Memory problems	time
Can't keep a job	Fainting spells	Concentration
Financial problems		difficulties
Others:		

61. Which of these symptoms cause you the most concern? Which would you be willing to work on changing?

62. Life change index.

For past and anticipated future life events, add up the mean values assigned to each life event listed in Family Inventory of Life Events (FILE) on page 419 to get your life change units for both the past year and the coming year. If your total for the past year is over 150, research suggests that you are at risk for a health change or illness, and you need to take steps to counteract the buildup of stress.

Section VI: Personality and Personal Identity

Personality

63. Please write a few words that help to describe you and tell the kind of person you are.

64. What are the most important, or most regular, emotions in your life?

65. What emotions would you say control you?

66. Do you have trouble expressing

___ anger	___ joy	___ happiness
___ sadness	___ love	___ other (specify)
___ crying	___ sexuality	

67. What do you feel are your major strengths as a person, your most important personal qualities?

68. What are your weaknesses, your negative aspects?

Personal identity

69. Who am I?

A person has many identities, which embody activities, feelings, and powers within and in the environment and personal relationships. List as many as you can of the ways that you would answer the question, "Who am I?" letting yourself respond freely to any way that you might interpret or experience an answer to that question—in terms of role; in metaphoric or feeling terms; or in terms of job, accomplishment, or way you think of yourself. Afterward, go back and rank them, starting with 1, in order of their centrality or importance to you.

Section VII: Values and Inner Life

70. The external events in your life are intimately affected by your inner world, beliefs, and world view. In the first column, write one of the 10 things that you most value in life. Next, describe how you actualize these values or how or why you fail to actualize them. In doing this, you will begin to see how closely you are living your life according to your values.

VALUE	HOW ACTUALIZED	HOW NOT ACTUALIZED

71. In what way would you say you are a religious or spiritual person?

72. What is your religious background?

73. Has your religious or spiritual faith been of help to you during your life? _____ In what ways?

74. Do you meditate, pray, or perform a regular religious ritual? _____ What sort and how frequently?

75. Has your religious or spiritual practice been helpful during times of illness or difficulty? _____ In what ways?

Section VIII: Change Goals and the Future

76. How many more years do you expect to live, and how do you expect to die?

77. Please write your own epitaph, about how you would like to be remembered.

78. Please write several reasons—things to accomplish, desires, interests, areas of life to explore, relationships, obligations—that you have to overcome or get relief from your current difficulties. Please do this carefully, and be specific.

79. What emotional feeling do you have when you imagine your future?

80. Please write the specific goals and achievements you expect to accomplish in your future.

81. What are some of the specific changes, things you will have to learn or give up, that you will have to make to achieve these goals?

82. How completely do you expect to overcome your current major and minor health, emotional, and life difficulties? (If experiencing any.)

83. How long do you expect this process to take?

Section IX: Inquiry Into Illness

This section is to be answered if you are currently experiencing an illness or if you want to explore an illness that you had previously.

84. Thinking back to the time of the first onset of the illness or symptoms you wish to explore and your life situation at the time, write down several factors or reasons in your psychological and family life that may have made you susceptible to that illness.

85. Before the initial symptoms or your decision to seek help, did you have any premonitions, dreams, thoughts, expectations, or worries that you might be, or become, ill? _____ Describe them.

86. List a few of the factors in your life today that might tend to maintain you in a state of illness or make it difficult to become well. These may be things that you do, things that you feel, fears of the future, benefits of being ill, feelings about yourself, or things that you can't do. These are the major obstacles to your getting well.

87. Draw a picture that represents to you, either literally or symbolically, your symptom or illness. Then look at your picture regularly, and become familiar with your feelings about it.

88. Draw a representation of the potential healing forces or powers within you that might have an effect on or the power to heal your illness. You might draw the healing forces in action against your illness. Use this image as part of your healing meditation to depict your healing forces in action.

Mortality Risk Appraisal

In each row, place a check in the box that best describes your current life situation or behavior.

Risk for cardiovascular disease

→ Increasing risk →

Risk factor:		Female under 40	Female 40-50	Male 25-40	Female after menopause	Male 40-60	Male 61 or over
Sex and age		Female under 40	Female 40-50	Male 25-40	Female after menopause	Male 40-60	Male 61 or over
Family history (mother, father, brothers, sisters)	High blood pressure	No relatives with condition			One relative	Two relatives	Three relatives
	Heart attack	No relatives with condition		One relative with condition after age 60	Two relatives with condition after age 60	One relative with condition before age 60	Two relatives with condition before age 60
	Diabetes	No relatives with condition			One or more relatives with maturity onset diabetes	One or more relatives with preadolescent or adolescent onset	
Blood pressure*	Systolic	≤120	121-140	141-160	161-180	181-200	>200
	Diastolic	≤70	71-80	81-90	91-100	101-110	>110

Continued

From Pender NJ: *Health promotion in nursing practice*, ed 3, Norwalk, Conn., 1996, Appleton & Lange.

Mortality Risk Appraisal—cont'd

In each row, place a check in the box that best describes your current life situation or behavior.

Risk for cardiovascular disease

→ Increasing risk →

Risk factor:						
Diabetes*	No diagnosis	Maturity onset, controlled	Maturity onset, uncontrolled	Adolescent onset, controlled	Adolescent onset, uncontrolled	
Weight*	At or slightly below recommended weight	10% overweight	20% overweight	30% overweight	40% overweight	50% overweight
Cholesterol*† level (mg/100 mL)	Below 180		200-239		240+	
Serum triglycerides* fasting (mg/100 mL)	Below 150		200-400		400+	
Percent of fat in diet*	20%-30%	31%-40%		41%-50%	Above 50%	
Frequency of exercise* (Recreational)	Intensive recreational exertion 35-45 min at least 4 times/wk	Moderate recreational exertion		Minimal recreational exertion	No recreational exertion	

	Intensive occupational exertion		Moderate occupational exertion	Minimal occupational exertion		Sedentary occupation
Occupational						
Sleep patterns*	7 or 8 hr sleep/night		More than 8 hr sleep/night			4-6 hr sleep/night
Cigarette smoking* — No./day	Nonsmoker	1-10/day	11-20/day	21-30/day	31-40/day	Over 40/day
Cigarette smoking* — No. of yr smoked	Nonsmoker	Less than 10 yr	11-15/yr	16-20/yr	21-30/yr	31 yr or more
Stress* — Domestic	Minimal		Moderate	High		Very high
Stress* — Occupational	Minimal		Moderate	High		Very high
Behavior pattern* (particularly men)	**Type B** Relaxed, appropriately assertive, not time dependent, moderate to slow speech			**Type A** Excessively competitive, aggressive, striving, hyperalert, time dependent, loud, explosive speech		
Air pollution*	Low		Moderate		High	
Use of oral contraceptives* (women)	Do not use oral contraceptives		Under age 40 and use oral contraceptives		Over age 40 and use oral contraceptives	

*Indicates risk factors that can be fully or partially controlled.

†Serum lipid analysis is also recommended to determine low-density (beta) and high-density (alpha) lipoprotein levels. Evidence suggests that high-density lipoprotein (HDL) carries cholesterol from tissues for metabolism and excretion. An inverse correlation appears to exist between HDL and coronary artery disease. National Institutes of Health and the American Heart Association suggest complete lipid profiles before actual risk is assigned.

Continued

Mortality Risk Appraisal—cont'd

In each row, place a check in the box that best describes your current life situation or behavior.

Risk for cardiovascular disease

→ Increasing risk →

Risk factor:						
Breast cancer (Women)						
Age	20-29		30-39	40-49		50 or over
Race	Asian		Black		White	
Family history (grandmother, mother, sister)	None	Mother, sister, or grandmother		Mother and grandmother		Mother and sister
Onset of menstruation	>12 yr of age				<12 yr of age	
Onset of menopause	>55 yr of age		45-55 yr of age		<45 yr of age	
Pregnancy* — Time	First pregnancy before age 25		First pregnancy after age 25		No pregnancies	
Pregnancy* — No.	Three or more		One or two		None	
Weight*	0%-40% overweight			>40% overweight		
Personal history	No evidence of dysplasia or previous breast cancer		Breast dysplasia		Previous breast cancer	
Lung cancer — Cigarette smoking* — No./day	Nonsmoker	1-10/day	11-20/day	21-30/day	21-40/day	Over 40/day

Risk factor						
Occupational exposure to toxic chemicals*‡						
No. of yr smoked	Nonsmoker	Less than 10 yr	11-15 yr	16-20 yr	21-30 yr	31 or more yr
Length of exposure	Less than one yr	1-5 yr	6-10 yr		11-15 yr	Over 15 yr
Frequency and intensity of exposure	Low frequency and low intensity	Low frequency, moderate intensity	Moderate frequency, moderate intensity		Moderate frequency, high intensity (or vice versa)	High frequency, high intensity
Cervical cancer						
Onset of sexual activity*	After 28 yr of age		22-27 yr of age	16-21 yr of age		Before 16 yr of age
No. of sexual partners*	Two		Three			Four or more
Marital status*		Single			Married	
Sexual partner*		Circumcised		Uncircumcised		
Colorectal cancer						
Age		<45 yr of age			>45 yr of age	
Personal history	No history of ulcerative colitis		Ulcerative colitis under 10 yr			Ulcerative colitis more than 10 yr
Fiber content of diet*	High		Moderate			Low
Weight* (men)		<40% overweight			>40% overweight	

*Indicates risk factors that can be fully or partially controlled.

‡Chemicals such as asbestos, nickel, chromates, arsenic, chlormethyl ethers, radioactive dust, petroleum or coal products, and iron oxide.

Continued

Mortality Risk Appraisal—cont'd

In each row, place a check in the box that best describes your current life situation or behavior.

Risk for cardiovascular disease

→ Increasing risk →

Risk factor:			
Rectal bleeding or black bowel movement	Never	Occasionally	Frequently
Uterine and ovarian cancer Age	<45 yr of age		>45 yr of age
Weight*	Less than 40% overweight		More than 40% overweight
Vaginal bleeding other than during menstrual period	Never	Occasionally	Frequently
Skin cancer Complexion	Dark	Medium	Fair
Sun exposure (without protection)	Never or seldom	Occasionally	Frequently

Risk for auto accidents

Risk factor:				
Alcohol consumption*	Nondrinker	Occasionally small to moderate consumption	Frequently small to moderate consumption	Occasionally heavy consumption	Frequently heavy consumption

Mileage driven/yr*	<5000 miles/yr	5001-10,000 miles/yr	10,001-20,000 miles/yr	>20,000 miles/yr
Use of seat belt*	Always	Usually	Occasionally	Never
Use of shoulder harness*	Always	Usually	Occasionally	Never
Use of drugs or medication that decrease alertness*	No use	Occasional use	Moderate use	Frequent use

Risk for suicide

Family history	No history		One family member		Two or more family members
Personal history*	Seldom experience depression	Periodically experience mild depression	Frequently experience mild depression	Periodically experience deep depression	Frequently experience deep depression
Access to hypnotic medication*	No access		Access to small or limited dosages		Unlimited access to large dosages

Risk for diabetes

Weight*	Desired weight	15% overweight	30% overweight	45% overweight	>45% overweight
Family history (parent or sibling)	None		Either parent or sibling		Both parents and sibling

Continued

*Indicates risk factors that can be fully or partially controlled.

Mortality Risk Appraisal—cont'd

In each row, place a check in the box that best describes your current life situation or behavior.

| Risk factor: | **Risk for cardiovascular disease** | | |
| | | → Increasing risk | → |
Health problem	(1) Total no. of risk factors	(2) No. for which client is in highest risk level(s)§	(3) Percent for which client is in highest risk level(s) (col. 2 ÷ col. 1)
Cardiovascular disease	21‖		
Breast cancer	8		
Lung cancer	4		
Cervical cancer	4		
Colorectal cancer	5		
Uterine or ovarian cancer	3		
Skin cancer	2		
Auto accidents	5		
Suicide	3		
Diabetes	2		

§*High risk* is risk within highest level of two to three levels within risk factor, or risk within highest two levels of four or more levels within risk factor.
‖All subcategories under a given heading are counted individually. For example, Pregnancy—Time and Pregnancy—Number each count as a separate factor.

Healthier People Health Risk Appraisal

Health Risk Appraisal is an education tool. It shows you choices you can make to keep good health and avoid the most common causes of death for a person your age and sex. This Health Risk Appraisal is not a substitute for a checkup or physical exam that you get from a doctor or nurse. It only gives you some ideas for lowering your risk of getting sick or injured in the future. It is NOT designed for people who already have HEART DISEASE, CANCER, KIDNEY DISEASE, OR OTHER SERIOUS CONDITIONS. If you have any of these problems and you want a Health Risk Appraisal anyway, ask your doctor or nurse.

DIRECTIONS: To get the most accurate results answer as many questions as you can and as best you can. If you do not know the answer leave it blank. Questions with a * (star symbol) are important to your health but are not used to calculate your risks. However, your answers may be helpful in planning your health and fitness program.

1. SEX	❏ Male	❏ Female
2. AGE	[＿＿＿] Years	
3. HEIGHT (Without shoes)	[＿＿] Feet [＿＿] Inches	
4. WEIGHT (Without shoes)	[＿＿＿] lbs	
5. Body frame size	❏ Small ❏ Medium ❏ Large	
6. Have you ever been told that you have diabetes	❏ Yes ❏ No	
7. Are you now taking medicine for high blood pressure?	❏ Yes ❏ No	
8. What is your blood pressure now?	[＿＿＿] / [＿＿＿] Systolic (High number)/Diastolic (Low number)	
9. If you *do not* know the numbers, check the box that describes your blood pressure.	❏ High ❏ Normal or Low ❏ Don't Know	
10. What is your TOTAL cholesterol level (based on a blood test)?	[＿＿＿] mg/dL	
11. What is your HDL cholesterol (based on a blood test)?	[＿＿＿] mg/dL	

From The Carter Center of Emory University, Decatur, Georgia. *Continued*

Healthier People Health Risk Appraisal—cont'd

12. How many cigars do you usually smoke per day?　　[   ] cigars per day

13. How many pipes of tobacco do you usually smoke per day?　　[   ] pipes per day

14. How many times per day do you usually use smokeless tobacco? (Chewing tobacco, snuff, pouches, etc.)　　[   ] times per day

15. CIGARETTE SMOKING
How would you describe your cigarette smoking habits?
- ❏ Never smoked　Go to 18
- ❏ Used to smoke　Go to 17
- ❏ Still smoke　Go to 16

16. STILL SMOKE
How many cigarettes a day do you smoke?
[   ] cigarettes per day　Go to 18

　　　　GO TO QUESTION 18

17. USED TO SMOKE
   a. How many years has it been since you smoked cigarettes fairly regularly?　[   ] years
   b. What was the average number of cigarettes per day that you smoked in the 2 years before you quit?　[   ] cigarettes per day

18. In the next 12 months how many thousands of miles will you probably travel by each of the following:
(NOTE: US average = 10,000 miles)
   a. Car, truck, or van:　[   ] ,000 miles
   b. Motorcycle:　[   ] ,000 miles

19. On a typical day, how do you USUALLY travel?
(Check one only)
- ❏ Walk
- ❏ Bicycle
- ❏ Motorcycle
- ❏ Subcompact or compact car
- ❏ Midsize or full-size car
- ❏ Truck or van
- ❏ Bus, subway, or train
- ❏ Mostly stay home

20. What percent of the time do you usually buckle your safety belt when driving or riding?　[   ] %

Healthier People Health Risk Appraisal—cont'd

21. On the average, how close to the speed limit do you usually drive?
- ❏ Within 5 mph of limit
- ❏ 6-10 mph over limit
- ❏ 11-15 mph over limit
- ❏ More than 15 mph over limit

22. How many times in the last month did you drive or ride when the driver perhaps had too much alcohol to drink?

[____] times last month

23. How many drinks of alcoholic beverages do you have in a typical week?

(Write the number of each type of drink)
- [____] Bottles or cans of beer
- [____] Glasses of wine
- [____] Wine coolers
- [____] Mixed drinks or shots of liquor

(MEN GO TO QUESTION 33)

WOMEN

24. At what age did you have your first menstrual period?

[____] years old

25. How old were you when your first child was born?

[____] years old
(If no children write 0)

26. How long has it been since your last breast x-ray (mammogram)?
- ❏ Less than 1 year ago
- ❏ 1 year ago
- ❏ 2 years ago
- ❏ 3 or more years ago
- ❏ Never

27. How many women in your natural family (mother and sisters only) have had breast cancer?

[____] women

28. Have you had a hysterectomy?
- ❏ Yes
- ❏ No
- ❏ Not sure

29. How long has it been since you had a Pap smear?
- ❏ Less than 1 year ago
- ❏ 1 year ago
- ❏ 2 years ago
- ❏ 3 or more years ago
- ❏ Never

***30.** How often do you examine your breasts for lumps?
- ❏ Monthly
- ❏ Once every few months
- ❏ Rarely or never

Continued

Healthier People Health Risk Appraisal—cont'd

*31. About how long has it been since you had your breasts examined by a physician or nurse?

❑ Less than 1 year ago
❑ 1 year ago
❑ 2 years ago
❑ 3 or more years ago
❑ Never

*32. About how long has it been since you had a rectal exam?

(WOMEN GO TO QUESTION 34)

❑ Less than 1 year ago
❑ 1 year ago
❑ 2 years ago
❑ 3 or more years ago
❑ Never

MEN
*33. About how long has it been since you had a rectal or prostate exam?

❑ Less than 1 year ago
❑ 1 year ago
❑ 2 years ago
❑ 3 or more years ago
❑ Never

*34. How many times in the last year did you witness or become involved in a violent fight or attack where there was a good chance of a serious injury to someone?

❑ 4 or more times
❑ 2 or 3 times
❑ 1 time or never
❑ Not sure

*35. Considering your age, how would you describe your overall physical health?

❑ Excellent
❑ Good
❑ Fair
❑ Poor

*36. In an average week, how many times do you engage in physical activity (exercise or work which lasts at least 20 minutes without stopping and which is hard enough to make you breathe heavier and your heart beat faster)?

❑ Less than 1 time per week
❑ 1 or 2 times per week
❑ At least 3 times per week

*37. If you ride a motorcycle or all-terrain vehicle (ATV) what percent of the time do you wear a helmet?

❑ 75% to 100%
❑ 25% to 74%
❑ Less than 25%
❑ Does not apply to me

*38. Do you eat some food every day that is high in fiber, such as whole grain bread, cereal, fresh fruits or vegetables?

❑ Yes   ❑ No

*39. Do you eat foods every day that are high in cholesterol or fat, such as fatty meat, cheese, fried foods, or eggs?

❑ Yes   ❑ No

Healthier People Health Risk Appraisal—cont'd

*40. In general, how satisfied are you with your life?	❏ Most satisfied ❏ Partly satisfied ❏ Not satisfied
*41. Have you suffered a personal loss or misfortune in the past year that had a serious impact on your life? (For example, a job loss, disability, separation, jail term, or the death of someone close to you.)	❏ Yes, 1 serious loss or misfortune ❏ Yes, 2 or more ❏ No
*42a. Race	❏ Aleutian, Alaska native, Eskimo or American Indian ❏ Asian ❏ Black ❏ Pacific Islander ❏ White ❏ Other ❏ Don't know
*42b. Are you of Hispanic origin, such as Mexican-American, Puerto Rican, or Cuban?	❏ Yes ❏ No
*43. What is the highest grade you completed in school?	❏ Grade school or less ❏ Some high school ❏ High school graduate ❏ Some college ❏ College graduate ❏ Postgraduate or professional degree
*44. What is your job or occupation? (Check only one)	❏ Health professional ❏ Manager, educator, professional ❏ Technical, sales, or administrative support ❏ Operator, fabricator, laborer ❏ Student ❏ Retired ❏ Homemaker ❏ Service ❏ Skilled crafts ❏ Unemployed ❏ Other

Continued

Healthier People Health Risk Appraisal—cont'd

*45. In what industry do you work (or did you last work)?

(Check only one)

- ❏ Electric, gas, sanitation
- ❏ Transportation, communication
- ❏ Agriculture, forestry, fishing
- ❏ Wholesale or retail trade
- ❏ Financial and service industries
- ❏ Mining
- ❏ Government
- ❏ Manufacturing
- ❏ Construction
- ❏ Other

User's Guide to Interpreting the Health Risk Appraisal Report Form

Unhealthy habits lead to early death or chronic illness. Every year, 1.3 million people die prematurely in the United States from conditions which could have been prevented or delayed. This Health Risk Appraisal (HRA) may help you avoid becoming one of these statistics by giving you a prediction of your health risks related to your particular characteristics and habits.

Risk factors

Most chronic diseases develop slowly in the presence of certain risk factors. Risk factors are either controllable or uncontrollable. Uncontrollable risk factors include factors such as your age, sex, and the health history of your family. Controllable risk factors include lifestyle habits that you can change, such as blood pressure, exercise, smoking, weight, cholesterol, and stress. You should focus on controllable risk factors.

Uncontrollable risk factors

1. Age
2. Sex
3. Heredity

Controllable risk factors

1. Blood pressure
2. Exercise
3. Smoking
4. Weight
5. Cholesterol
6. Stress

Choosing a habit to work on

Your Health Risk Appraisal is intended to encourage you to work on the habits you can change—to be the best that you can be. You don't have to change your entire lifestyle overnight—in fact, trying to change too many habits at once is probably the quickest way to discouragement and failure.

Health risk appraisal limits

Your Health Risk Appraisal does have limits. It is not a predictor, but rather an educational tool. It does not take into consideration whether or not you already have a medical condition and it does not consider more rare diseases and other health problems which are not fatal but can limit your enjoyment of life (such as arthritis).

What it does consider are the lifestyle factors over which you have a great degree of control and which account for a large number of premature deaths. Now that you are familiar with your particular health risks, it's time to do something about them!

Make a plan

Make a plan of how to change the habit you chose to work on. Write the plan down and keep it in sight. Be prepared for temptation! Observe the time, situation, or place that most often triggers your unhealthy habit and be ready to combat the urge when it appears. Let family and friends know of your goals, and ask for their encouragement.

Reward yourself

Rewards are an important part of changing behavior. Give yourself a reasonable reward when you accomplish your goal. Don't eat half a gallon of ice cream after losing 10 lbs! Choose a healthy and enjoyable reward. You've worked hard and are on the road to good health!

Lifestyle Questionnaire for School-Age Children

This tool increases children's and parents' awareness of activities that promote health and prevent injury. It also provides data that allow the nurse or health educator to assess the health education needs of children.

From Antwerp CV, Spaido AM: *MCN* 16 (3): 144, 1991.

Lifestyle Questionnaire for School-Age Children—cont'd

Activities that promote health	Yes	No	Sometimes
1. I sleep at least 8 hours every night.			
2. I brush my teeth twice a day.			
3. I visit the dentist every year.			
4. I watch less than 2 hours of TV every day.			
5. I exercise (running, biking, swimming, active sports) 1 hour every day.			
6. I eat fruits.			
7. I eat vegetables.			
8. I limit my intake of salty snacks and high-sugar snacks.			
9. I have a physical examination every 2 or 3 years.			
10. I stay away from cigarettes.			
11. I stay away from alcohol.			

Injury prevention	Yes	No	Sometimes
12. I wear a seat belt in an automobile.			
13. I look both ways when crossing streets.			
14. I follow bike safety rules.			
15. I stay away from lighters or matches.			
16. I never ride ATVs (all-terrain vehicles.)*			
17. I wear a helmet when I go on bike trips.			
18. I swim with a buddy.			
19. I wear a life jacket when I ride in a boat.			
20. I take medicine only with my parent's permission.			
21. I stay away from real guns.			
22. I tell my parents where I am going.			
23. I say "no" to drugs.			
24. Our home has a smoke detector that works.			

*The American Academy of Pediatrics recommends children not ride on these vehicles.

Continued

Lifestyle Questionnaire for School-Age Children—cont'd

	Yes	No	Sometimes
25. Our home has a fire extinguisher.			
26. If there is a fire, I know a safe way out of my house.			

Feelings	Yes	No	Sometimes
27. I think it is okay to cry.			
28. I enjoy my family.			
29. It is easy for me to fall asleep at night.			
30. My appetite is good.			
31. I like myself just the way I am.			

Lifestyle Assessment Questionnaire (National Wellness Institute)

Purpose

This assessment tool and the analysis it provides are designed to help you discover how the choices you make each day affect your overall health.

By participating in this assessment process, you will also learn how you can make positive changes in your lifestyle, enabling you to reach a higher level of wellness.

Some of the questions are personal. While you may leave them blank, the more information you provide about your current lifestyle, the more accurately the LAQ [Lifestyle Assessment Questionnaire] can assess your current level of wellness and risk areas.

Confidentiality

The National Wellness Institute, Inc. subscribes to the guidelines established by the Society of Prospective Medicine concerning confidentiality in the use of health risk appraisals and risk reduction systems. These guidelines specifically state that only the participant and health professionals authorized by the participant should receive copies of his/her own health risk appraisal results.

The National Wellness Institute, Inc. strongly encourages all users of the LAQ to strictly follow these guidelines and maintain the confidentiality of all answers.

What is Wellness?

Wellness is an active process of becoming aware of and making choices toward a higher level of well-being. **Remember,** leading a wellness lifestyle requires your **active involvement.** As you gain more knowledge about what enhances your well-being, you are encouraged to use this information to make informed choices which lead to a healthier life.

General Instructions

If you would like to have your test evaluated, **please write to the National Wellness Institute for the answer sheet.** Please make certain that you complete all of the information at the top of the answer sheet, including your zip code, group code, and social security number. If a group code has not been provided for you, leave this item blank.

Your questionnaire will be scored by an optical mark reading instrument; therefore, please use only a No. 2 (soft) pencil for marking your responses. To assure the most accurate results, follow the instructions shown on the answer sheet. If you do not wish to have your answers scored, please mark your answers on the following pages.

Section 1: Personal Data

Instructions

Please complete the following general information about yourself by marking your answers in the appropriate places on the LAQ answer sheet or circle the correct answer. Please take your time and read each question carefully.

1. Sex
   a) male
   b) female
2. Race
   a) White
   b) Black
   c) Hispanic
   d) Asian
   e) American Indian
   f) other

3. Age

4. Height (feet and inches)

5. Weight (pounds)

6. Body frame size
   a) small
   b) medium
   c) large

7. Marital status
   a) married
   b) widowed
   c) separated
   d) divorced
   e) single
   f) cohabiting

8. What was the total gross income of your household last year?
   a) under $12,000
   b) $12,000-$20,000
   c) $20,001-$30,000
   d) $30,001-$40,000
   e) $40,001-$50,000
   f) $50,001-$60,000
   g) over $60,000

9. What is the highest level of education you have completed?
   a) grade school or less
   b) some high school
   c) high school graduate
   d) some college or technical school
   e) college graduate
   f) postgraduate or professional degree

10. On the average day, how many hours do you watch television?
   a) 0 hours
   b) 1-3 hours
   c) 4-7 hours
   d) more than 8 hours

11. Where do you live?
   a) in the country
   b) in a city
   c) suburb
   d) small town

12. If you live in a city, suburb, or small town, what is the population?
   a) under 20,000
   b) 20,000-50,000
   c) 50,001-100,000

d) 100,001-500,000
e) over 500,000

Section 2: Lifestyle
Instructions
This section will help determine your level of wellness. It will also give you ideas for areas in which you might improve. Some questions touch on very personal subjects. Therefore, if you prefer to skip certain questions, you may. However, the more questions you answer, the more you will learn about your health and how to improve it.

Please respond to these statements using the following responses. If an item does not apply to you, do not mark it.

A *Almost always (90% or more of the time)*
B *Very often (approximately 75% of the time)*
C *Often (approximately 50% of the time)*
D *Occasionally (approximately 25% of the time)*
E *Almost never (less than 10% of the time)*

Physical exercise
Measures one's commitment to maintaining physical fitness.

1. I exercise vigorously for at least 20 minutes three or more times per week.
2. I determine my activity level by monitoring my heart rate.
3. I stop exercising before I feel exhausted.
4. I exercise in a relaxed, calm, and joyful manner.
5. I stretch before exercising.
6. I stretch after exercising.
7. I walk or bike whenever possible.
8. I participate in a strenuous activity (tennis, running, brisk walking, water exercise, swimming, handball, basketball, etc.).
9. If I am not in shape, I avoid sporadic (once a week or less often), strenuous exercise.
10. After vigorous exercise, I "cool down" (very light exercise such as walking) for at least five minutes before sitting or lying down.

Nutrition
Measures the degree to which one chooses foods that are consistent with the dietary goals of the United States as published by the Senate Select Committee on Nutrition and Human Needs.

11. When choosing nonvegetable protein, I select lean cuts of meat, poultry, fish, and low-fat dairy products.
12. I maintain an appropriate weight for my height and frame.

13. I minimize salt intake.
14. I eat fruits and vegetables, fresh and uncooked.
15. I eat breakfast.
16. I intentionally include fiber in my diet on a daily basis.
17. I drink enough fluid to keep my urine light yellow.
18. I plan my diet to insure an adequate amount of vitamins and minerals.
19. I minimize foods in my diet that contain large amounts of refined flour (bleached white flour, typical store bread, cakes, etc.).
20. I minimize my intake of fats and oils including margarine and animal fats.
21. I include items from all four basic food groups in my diet each day (fruits and vegetables; milk group; breads and cereals; meat, fowl, fish or vegetable proteins).
22. To avoid unnecessary calories, I choose water as one of the beverages I drink.
23. I avoid adding sugar to my foods. I minimize my intake of presweetened foods (sugarcoated cereals, syrups, chocolate milk, and most processed and fast foods).

Self-care

Measures the behaviors which help one prevent or detect early illnesses.

24. I use footgear of good quality designed for the activity or the job in which I participate.
25. I record immunizations to maintain up-to-date immunization records.
26. I examine my breasts or testes on a monthly basis.
27. I have my breasts or testes examined yearly by a physician.
28. I balance the type and amount of food I eat with exercise to maintain a healthy percent of body fat.
29. I take action to minimize my exposure to tobacco smoke.
30. When I experience illness or injury, I take necessary steps to correct the problem.
31. I engage in activities which keep my blood pressure in a range which minimizes my chances of disease (e.g., stroke, heart attack, and kidney disease).
32. I brush my teeth after eating.
33. I floss my teeth after eating.
34. My resting pulse is 60 or less.
35. I get an adequate amount of sleep.
36. If I were to have sex, I would take action to prevent unplanned pregnancy.

37. If I were to have sex, I would take action to prevent giving and/or getting sexually transmitted disease.

Vehicle safety
Measures one's ability to minimize chances of injury or death in a vehicle accident.

38. I do not operate vehicles while I am under the influence of alcohol or other drugs.
39. I do not ride with drivers who are under the influence of alcohol or other drugs.
40. I stay within the speed limit.
41. I practice defensive driving techniques.
42. When traffic lights change from green to yellow, I prepare to stop.
43. I maintain a safe driving distance between cars based on speed and road conditions.
44. Vehicles which I drive are maintained to assure safety.
45. Because they are safer, I use radial tires on cars that I drive.
46. When I ride a bicycle or motorcycle, I wear a helmet and have adequate lights/reflectors.
47. Children riding in my car are secured in an approved car seat or seat belt.
48. I use my seat belt while driving or riding in a vehicle.

Drug usage and awareness
Measures the degree to which one functions without the unnecessary use of chemicals.

49. I use prescription drugs and over-the-counter medications only when necessary.
50. If I consume alcohol, I limit my consumption to not more than one drink per hour and no more than two drinks per day.
51. I avoid the use of tobacco.
52. Because of the potentially harmful effects of caffeine (e.g., coffee, tea, cola, etc.), I limit my consumption.
53. I avoid the use of marijuana.
54. I avoid the use of hallucinogens (LSD, PCP, MDA, etc.).
55. I avoid the use of stimulants ("uppers"—e.g., cocaine, amphetamines, "pep pills," etc.).
56. I avoid the use of nonmedically prescribed depressants ("downers"—e.g., barbiturates, Quaaludes, minor tranquilizers, etc.).

57. I avoid using a combination of drugs unless under medical supervision.

58. I follow the instructions provided with any drug I take.

59. I avoid using drugs obtained from illegal sources.

60. I understand the expected effect of drugs I take.

61. I consider alternatives to drugs.

62. If I experience discomfort from stress or tension, I use relaxation techniques, exercise, and meditation instead of taking drugs.

63. I get clear directions for taking my medicine from my doctor or pharmacist.

Social/environmental

Measures the degree to which one contributes to the common welfare of the community. This emphasizes interdependence with others and nature.

64. I conserve energy at home.

65. I consider energy conservation when choosing a mode of transportation.

66. My social ties with family are strong.

67. I contribute to the feeling of acceptance within my family.

68. I develop and maintain strong friendships.

69. I do my part to promote a clean environment (i.e., air, water, noise, etc.).

70. When I see a safety hazard, I take action (warn others or correct the problem).

71. I avoid unnecessary radiation.

72. I report criminal acts I observe.

73. I contribute time and/or money to community projects.

74. I actively seek to become acquainted with individuals in my community.

75. I use my creativity in constructive ways.

76. My behavior reflects fairness and justice.

77. When possible, I choose an environment which is free of **noise** pollution.

78. When possible, I choose an environment which is free of **air** pollution.

79. I participate in volunteer activities benefiting others.

80. I help others in need.

81. I beautify those parts of my environment under my control.

82. Because of limited resources, I do my part to conserve.

83. I recycle aluminum, glass, and paper products.

84. I involve myself with people who support a positive lifestyle.

Emotional awareness and acceptance

Measures the degree to which one has an awareness and acceptance of one's feelings. This includes the degree to which one feels positive and enthusiastic about oneself and life.

85. I have a good sense of humor.
86. I feel positive about myself.
87. I feel there is a satisfying amount of excitement in my life.
88. My emotional life is stable.
89. I am aware of my needs.
90. I trust and value my own judgment.
91. When I make mistakes, I learn from them.
92. I feel comfortable when complimented for jobs well done.
93. It is okay for me to cry.
94. I have feelings of sensitivity for others.
95. I feel enthusiastic about life.
96. I find it easy to laugh.
97. I am able to give love.
98. I am able to receive love.
99. I enjoy my life.
100. I have plenty of energy.
101. My sleep is restful.
102. I trust others.
103. I feel others trust me.
104. I accept my sexual desires.
105. I understand how I create my feelings.
106. At times, I can be both strong and sensitive.
107. I am aware when I feel angry.
108. I accept my anger.
109. I am aware when I feel sad.
110. I accept my sadness.
111. I am aware when I feel happy.
112. I accept my happiness.
113. I am aware when I feel frightened.
114. I accept my feelings of fear.
115. I am aware of my feelings about death.
116. I accept my feelings about death.

Emotional management

Measures the degree to which one controls and expresses feelings and engages in effective, related behaviors.

117. I share my feelings with those with whom I am close.
118. I express my feelings of anger in appropriate ways.

119. I express my feelings of sadness in healthy ways.
120. I express my feelings of happiness in desirable ways.
121. I express my feelings of fear in appropriate ways.
122. I compliment myself for a job well done.
123. I accept constructive criticism without reacting defensively.
124. I set appropriate limits for myself.
125. I stay within the limits that I have set.
126. I recognize that I can have wide variations of feelings about the same person (such as loving someone even though you are angry with her/him at the moment).
127. I am able to develop close, intimate relationships.
128. I say "no" without feeling guilty.
129. I would feel comfortable seeking professional help to better understand and cope with my feelings.
130. I reduce feelings of failure by setting achievable goals.
131. I relax my body and mind without using drugs.
132. I can be alone without feeling lonely.
133. I am able to be spontaneous in expressing my feelings.
134. I accept responsibility for my actions.
135. I am willing to take the risks that come with making change.
136. I manage my feelings to avoid unnecessary suffering.
137. I make decisions with a minimum of stress and worry.
138. I accept the responsibility for creating my own feelings.
139. I can express my feelings about death.
140. I recognize grieving as a healthy response to loss.

Intellectual

Measures the degree to which one engages her/his mind in creative, stimulating mental activities, expanding knowledge, and improving skills.

141. I read a newspaper daily.
142. I read twelve or more books yearly.
143. On the average, I read one or more national magazines per week.
144. When I watch TV, I choose programs with informational/educational value.
145. I visit a museum or art show at least three times yearly.
146. I attend lectures, workshops, and demonstrations at least three times yearly.
147. I regularly use some of my time participating in hobbies such as photography, gardening, woodworking, sewing, painting, baking, art, music, writing, pottery, etc.

148. I read about local, state, national, and international political/public issues.

149. I learn the meaning of new words.

150. I engage in some type of writing activity such as a regular journal, letter writing, preparation of papers or manuscripts, etc.

151. I am interested in understanding the views of others.

152. I share ideas, concepts, thoughts, or procedures with others.

153. I gather information to enable me to make decisions.

154. I listen to radio and/or TV news.

155. I think about ideas different than my own.

Occupational

Measures the satisfaction gained from one's work and the degree to which one is enriched by that work. Please answer these items from your primary frame of reference, (e.g., your job, student, homemaker, etc.).

156. I enjoy my work.

157. My work contributes to my personal needs.

158. I feel that my job in some way contributes to my well-being.

159. I cooperate with others in my work.

160. I take advantage of opportunities to learn new work-related skills.

161. My work is challenging.

162. I feel my job responsibilities are consistent with my values.

163. I find satisfaction from the work I do.

164. I find healthy ways of reducing excessive job-related stress.

165. I use recommended health and safety precautions.

166. I make recommendations for improving worksite health and safety.

167. I am satisfied with the degree of freedom I have in my job to exercise independent judgments.

168. I am satisfied with the amount of variety in my work.

169. I believe I am competent in my job.

170. My co-workers and supervisors respect me as a competent individual.

171. My communication with others in my workplace is enriching for me.

Spiritual

Measures one's ongoing involvement in seeking meaning and purpose in human existence. It includes an appreciation for the depth and expanse of life and natural forces that exist in the universe.

172. I feel good about my spiritual life.
173. Prayer, meditation, and/or quiet personal reflection is/are important part(s) of my life.
174. I contemplate my purpose in life.
175. I reflect on the meaning of events in my life.
176. My values guide my daily life.
177. My values and beliefs help me to meet daily challenges.
178. I recognize that my spiritual growth is a lifelong process.
179. I am concerned about humanitarian issues.
180. I enjoy participating in discussions about spiritual values.
181. I feel a sense of compassion for others in need.
182. I seek spiritual knowledge.
183. My spiritual awareness occurs other than at times of crisis.
184. I believe in something greater or that I am part of something greater than myself.
185. I share my spiritual values.

Section 3: Health Risk Appraisal

Instructions

This section is intended to help you identify the problems most likely to interfere with the quality of your life. It will also show you choices you can make to stay healthy and avoid the most common causes of death for a person your age and sex.

This Health Risk Appraisal is not a substitute for a checkup or physical exam that you get from a doctor or nurse. It only gives you some ideas for lowering your risk of getting sick or injured in the future. It is NOT designed for people who already have HEART DISEASE, CANCER, KIDNEY DISEASE, OR OTHER SERIOUS CONDITIONS. If you have any of these problems and you want a Health Risk Appraisal anyway, ask your doctor or nurse to read this section (of the printout, if scored) with you.

If you don't know or are unsure of an answer, please leave that item blank.

1. Have you ever been told that you have diabetes?
   a. yes
   b. no

2. Does your natural mother, father, sister, or brother have diabetes?
   a. yes
   b. no
   c. not sure

3. Did either of your natural parents die of a heart attack before age 60? (If your parents are younger than 60, mark no).
   a. yes, one of them
   b. yes, both of them
   c. no
   d. not sure

4. Are you now taking medicine for high blood pressure?
   a. yes
   b. no

5. What is your blood pressure now?
   a. _____ systolic (high number)
   b. _____ diastolic (low number)

6. If you *do not* know the number, select the answer that describes your blood pressure.
   a. high
   b. normal or low
   c. don't know

7. What is your TOTAL cholesterol level (based on a blood test)?
   _____ (mg/dL)

8. What is your high-density lipoprotein (HDL) cholesterol level (based on a blood test)?   _____ (mg/dL)

9. How many cigars do you usually smoke per day?
   _____

10. How many pipes of tobacco do you usually smoke per day?
    _____

11. How many times per day do you usually use smokeless tobacco (chewing tobacco, snuff, pouches, etc)? _____

12. How would you describe your cigarette smoking habits?
    a. never smoked **Go to 15**
    b. used to smoke **Go to 14**
    c. still smoke **Go to 13**

13. How many cigarettes a day do you smoke?
    _____ cigarettes per day **Go to 15**

14. a. How many years has it been since you smoked cigarettes regularly?
       _____ years
    b. What was the average number of cigarettes per day that you smoked in the 2 years before you quit?
       _____ cigarettes per day

15. In the next 12 months, how many thousands of miles will you probably travel by each of the following?
(NOTE: US average = 10,000 miles)
  a. car, truck, or van: _____,000 miles
  b. motorcycle: _____,000 miles

16. On a typical day how do you USUALLY travel?
(Check one only)
  a. walk
  b. bicycle
  c. motorcycle
  d. subcompact or compact car
  e. midsize or full-size car
  f. truck or van
  g. bus, subway, or train
  h. mostly stay home

17. What percent of the time do you usually buckle your safety belt when driving or riding?
  _____ %

18. On the average, how close to the speed limit do you usually drive?
  a. within 5 mph of limit
  b. 6-10 mph over limit
  c. 11-15 mph over limit
  d. more than 15 mph over limit

19. How many times in the last month did you drive or ride when the driver had perhaps too much alcohol to drink?
  _____ times last month

20. When you drink alcoholic beverages, how many drinks do you consume in an average day? (If you *never* drink alcoholic beverages, write 0.)
  _____ alcoholic beverages/average day

21. On the average, how many days per week do you consume alcohol?
  _____ days/week

(MEN GO TO QUESTION 31)
WOMEN ONLY (QUESTIONS 22-30)

22. At what age did you have your first menstrual period?
  _____ years old
23. How old were you when your first child was born (if no children, write 0)?
  _____ years old

24. How long has it been since your last breast x-ray (mammogram)?

    a. less than 1 year ago

    b. 1 year ago

    c. 2 years ago

    d. 3 or more years ago

    e. never

25. How many women in your natural family (mother and sisters only) have had breast cancer?

    _____ women

26. Have you had a hysterectomy?

    a. yes

    b. no

    c. not sure

27. How long has it been since you had a Pap smear?

    a. less than 1 year ago

    b. 1 year ago

    c. 2 years ago

    d. 3 or more years ago

    e. never

28. How often do you examine your breasts for lumps?

    a. monthly

    b. once every few months

    c. rarely or never

29. About how long has it been since you had your breasts examined by a physician or nurse?

    a. less than 1 year ago

    b. 1 year ago

    c. 2 years ago

    d. 3 or more years ago

    e. never

30. About how long has it been since you had a rectal exam?

    a. less than 1 year ago

    b. 1 year ago

    c. 2 years ago

    d. 3 or more years ago

    e. never

WOMEN GO TO QUESTION 35
MEN ONLY (QUESTIONS 31-34)

31. About how long has it been since you had a rectal or prostate exam?

    a. less than 1 year ago

    b. 1 year ago

    c. 2 years ago

    d. 3 or more years ago

    e. never

32. Do you know how to properly examine your testes for lumps?

    a. yes

    b. no

    c. not sure

33. How often do you examine your testes for lumps?

    a. monthly

    b. once every few months

    c. rarely or never

34. About how long has it been since you had your testes examined by a physician or nurse?

    a. less than 1 year ago

    b. 1 year ago

    c. 2 years ago

    d. 3 or more years ago

    e. never

35. How many times in the last year did you witness or become involved in a violent fight or attack where there was a good chance of a serious injury to someone?

    a. 4 or more times

    b. 2 or 3 times

    c. 1 time or never

    d. not sure

36. Considering your age, how would you describe your overall physical health?

    a. excellent

    b. good

    c. fair

    d. poor

37. In an average week, how many times do you engage in physical activity (exercise or work which lasts at least 20 minutes without stopping and which is hard enough to make you breathe heavier and your heart beat faster)?

    a. less than 1 time per week

    b. 1 or 2 times per week

    c. at least 3 times per week

38. If you ride a motorcycle or all-terrain vehicle (ATV), what percent of the time do you wear a helmet?

    a. 75% to 100%

    b. 25% to 74%

c. less than 25%

d. does not apply to me

39. Do you eat some food every day that is high in fiber, such as whole grain bread, cereal, fresh fruits, or vegetables?

a. yes

b. no

40. Do you eat foods every day that are high in cholesterol or fat, such as fatty meat, cheese, fried foods, or eggs?

a. yes

b. no

41. In general, how satisfied are you with your life?

a. mostly satisfied

b. partly satisfied

c. not satisfied

42. Have you suffered a personal loss or misfortune in the past year that had a serious impact on your life? (For example, a job loss, disability, separation, jail term, or the death of someone close to you.)

a. yes, 1 serious loss or misfortune

b. yes, 2 or more

c. no

Section 4: Topics for Personal Growth

This section will help you identify areas in which you would like more information. In response to your selection from the following topics, we will provide you with resources or services to meet your requests.

Select topics on which you would like information. (Maximum of 4 topics.)

1. Responsible alcohol use
2. Stop-smoking programs
3. Sexuality
4. Gay issues
5. Depression
6. Loneliness
7. Exercise programs
8. Weight reduction
9. Self-breast exam
10. Medical emergencies
11. Nutrition
12. Relaxation
13. Stress reduction
14. Parenting skills

15. Marital or couples problems
16. Assertiveness training (how to say "no" without feeling guilty)
17. Biofeedback for tension headache and pain
18. Overcoming fears (i.e., high places, crowded rooms, etc.)
19. Educational career goal setting/planning
20. Spiritual or philosophical values
21. Communication skills
22. Automobile safety
23. Suicide thoughts or attempts
24. Substance abuse
25. Anxiety associated with public speaking, tests, writing, etc.
26. Enhancing relationships
27. Time-management skills
28. Death and dying
29. Learning skills (i.e., speed-reading, comprehension, etc.)
30. Financial management
31. Divorce
32. Alcoholism
33. Men's issues
34. Women's issues
35. Medical self-care
36. Dental self-care
37. Self-testes exam
38. Aging
39. Self-esteem
40. Premenstrual syndrome (PMS)
41. Osteoporosis
42. Recreation and leisure
43. Environmental issues

IMPORTANT—If you have finished completing all sections of the LAQ, please make sure you have answered the questions in Section 1 requesting your sex, race, age, height, and weight. Results cannot be evaluated for the Health Risk Appraisal section without this information.

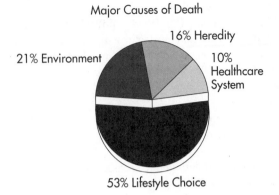

Major Causes of Death

21% Environment

16% Heredity

10% Healthcare System

53% Lifestyle Choice

You and Your Lifestyle Are the Major Determinants for Joyful Living

The circle graph above indicates the factors which contribute to your enjoyment and quality of life. While medical professionals contribute to the quality of your life, this graph clearly shows that the majority of those factors which contribute to your well-being are controlled by you. As you make responsible, informed choices, your chances of improving your health and well-being increase.

The LAQ's Role . . .

We believe this instrument is useful in helping individuals identify the most likely causes of death and disability. More important, it identifies those areas of self-improvement which will lead to higher levels of health and well-being.

The areas assessed in the LAQ emphasize the importance of creating a balance among the many different aspects of your lifestyle. Each of these areas affects one another and determines your overall wellness' status. Also, each provides an opportunity for learning, making responsible decisions, and personal growth.

We invite you to use the information provided by the LAQ to your best advantage to increase your level of wellness.

Words From the Past

Wellness is a term that has enjoyed growing popularity during the past several decades. Although the term was introduced relatively recently, the concept of prevention has been present for centuries. The following passages provide a brief glimpse of the wellness philosophy through the years. Wellness is a movement which has become a major part of modern culture and is the most important weapon available to combat lifestyle illnesses.

"For many years, while engaged in the practice of medicine, the author of this volume has been more and more impressed with the idea that the causes of suffering, diseases, and premature deaths, which we witness around us on every hand, lie near our own doors . . . and that the men and women of today, are, at least, equally as responsible for existing suffering, as those who have gone before them, and often much more so. In fact, he feels satisfied that by far the greatest portion of all the suffering, disease, deformity, and premature deaths which occur are the direct result of either the violation of, or the want of compliance with the laws of our being; calamities, which, were the requisite knowledge possessed by the community, can and should be avoided."

—JOHN ELLIS, M.D., 1859

"It is universally admitted at the present time that preventive medicine is of far greater importance than curative medication, and many of the most eminent members of the profession are devoting themselves exclusively to this branch."

—J. H. KELLOGG, M.D., 1902

"To ward off disease or recover health, men as a rule find it easier to depend on the healers than to attempt the more difficult task of living wisely."

—RENE DUBOS, Ph.D., 1959

"It's what you do hour by hour, day by day, that largely determines the state of your health; whether you get sick, what you get sick with, and perhaps when you die."

—LESTER BRESLOW, M.D., 1969

Therapeutic Exercise: Focus on Walking

What Exactly Is Meant by "Therapeutic Exercise"?

Therapeutic exercise is the motion of the body or its parts to achieve symptom-free movement and function. It is used to develop and retrain deficient muscles; to restore as much normal movement as possible to prevent deformity; to stimulate the functions of various organs and body systems; to build strength and endurance; and to promote relaxation.

Various theories and methods have been proposed to improve health through exercise and movement. Decreased physical activity, which may be the result of illness or treatment, can lead to anxiety, depression, weakness, fatigue, and nausea. Regular, moderate exercise can prevent these feelings and help a person feel energetic.

Aerobic exercise (the sustained rhythmic activity of large muscle groups, which entails using large amounts of oxygen) increases heart rate, stroke volume, respiratory rate, and relaxation of blood vessels. Cardiovascular fitness and increased stamina are the goals. Body fat is also reduced. Aerobic exercises include running, jogging, brisk walking, swimming, aquadynamics, and aerobic dance.

Always check with your doctor before beginning any exercise program and for help in choosing the type of exercise that is best for you. Whatever type you choose, the goal should be to maintain a regular, moderate exercise program to enhance physical and emotional health. The exercise should involve large muscle groups in dynamic movement for about 20 minutes 3 or more days a week. The exertion should be within limits appropriate to your physical status and needs. At the end of exercise you should feel replenished rather than bored, burned out, or excessively fatigued.

What Makes Walking a Good Form of Regular Exercise?

Walking allows for psychomotor expression without the hazards of contact sports and is adaptable to a wide range of weather or geographic conditions, schedules, personalities, and body types. It can be social or asocial, organized or unorganized as an activity. The long-term effects on joints and organs of regular, sustained, vigorous walking currently are unknown; physicians do report a lower incidence of the type of musculoskeletal damage resulting from the "pounding" effects of jogging.

Making Time for Exercising Regularly Is Hard. What Can I Do to Make It Easier?

There are two major obstacles to overcome in undertaking and maintaining an exercise program: making exercise part of a lifestyle and avoiding injury. Suggestions for making exercise a safe part of a lifestyle include the following:

1. Start in small increments, and keep it fun.
2. Avoid exercising for 2 hours after a large meal, and do not eat for 1 hour after exercising.

3. Include at least 10 minutes of warm-up and cool-down exercises.
4. Use proper equipment and clothing.
5. Post goals, pictures of the ideal self, and notes of encouragement in a readily seen place for self-encouragement.
6. Use visualization daily to picture successful attainment of exercise benefit (e.g., looking toned or graceful or achieving an ideal weight).
7. Keep records of weekly measures of weight, blood pressure, and pulse.
8. Focus on the rewards of exercise; keep a record of feelings, and compare differences in relaxation, energy, concentration, and sleep patterns.
9. Work with a peer or join a structured exercise class, running club, or fitness center. Spend more time with people dedicated to wellness.
10. Stop exercising or at least slow down and consult with a practitioner if any unusual, unexplainable symptoms occur.
11. Reward yourself for working toward exercise goals as well as attaining them. For example, after a month in an exercise program, buy a new pair of running shoes or treat yourself to a special wish.

What Does a Walking (or "Rhythmic Walking") Program Entail?

Rhythmic walking consists of walking briskly, arms swinging, so your whole body is involved in the rhythm of your movement and your heart rate is increased. It is a regular program to benefit every system of your body.

A good exercise plan starts slowly, allowing your body time to adjust. It is important that you do something to exercise the whole body on a regular basis. *Regular* means every day, or at least every other day; build up to about 20 minutes 3 or more days a week. The right kind of exercise never makes you feel sore, stiff, or exhausted.

We repeat: *first check with your physician.* Before starting a program, it is important to know if there are precautions you need to take. This is especially important if you have high blood pressure, diabetes, joint or bone problems, or heart disease. People with these conditions can exercise, but they must follow certain guidelines to do it safely.

Rhythmic walking is inexpensive. It requires no special equipment or uniforms. Wear comfortable clothes in which you can move freely. You must have the right kind of shoes. Running or jogging shoes or the shoes specially designed for walking are good. The wrong shoes can cause painful damage, such as tendinitis. Select shoes designed for walking, jogging, or running; look for a shock-absorbent cushioning midsole. A watch with a second hand to measure your heart rate is also important.

Everyone who exercises outside the home should carry identification and change for a telephone call and money for a taxi. Some people like to carry a small water bottle such as a plastic soda bottle. To carry these items, a small backpack or hip pack leaves your hands free to swing.

If it is wet, slippery, or hot, or if you feel unsafe walking in your neighborhood, enclosed shopping malls can be great places for walking. Some malls open early, before the shopping crowds arrive, especially for people who want to walk.

How Hard Should I Exercise?

Your heart rate is the best indicator of how hard your body is working. As you work harder, your heart rate increases; as you slow down, your heart rate decreases. You can take your pulse to measure your heart rate. To experience the benefits of exercise, you need to work hard enough to get your heart rate up to a certain point, called the *training heart rate,* and keep it there. Your nurse or doctor can tell you what your training heart rate should be and how to take your own pulse. Find these two things out before beginning your exercise regimen.

How Long Should I Exercise?

It is important to start exercising slowly and build up gradually. If you have been very ill or have not been exercising on a regular basis, start with a 5- or 10-minute walk and add 2 minutes each week. If you are able to build up endurance without problems, work up to 45 minutes daily or every other day. More than 60 minutes of rhythmic walking daily is not necessary.

A good workout consists of three phases: warm-up, training period, and cool-down. The warm-up is necessary to prepare the body for exercise. Warm up by walking slowly. Next, begin rhythmic walking. This is your training period. Work up to your target heart rate, and walk steadily for your set period of time. Finally, walk slowly to cool off. The cool-down is necessary to help your body recover and to prevent soreness or stiffness.

If you are exercising correctly, you should never feel exhausted after the cool-down. If you do, slow down and take it easier next time. If you feel fatigued for hours after exercise or if you feel sore and stiff, you have done too much or exercised incorrectly.

Starting to Exercise for a Healthy Heart

If you are recovering from heart surgery or a heart attack, your doctor has probably prescribed a daily graduated walking program to help your recovery. This program is also good if you have not exercised in a long time and your doctor recommends walking to help control your blood pressure or reduce your chances of cardiovascular disease.

Daily exercise may be one of the best gifts you can give yourself. It improves circulation, lowers blood pressure, helps in a weight control program, and strengthens your muscles. It can also help you sleep better, feel more energetic, and increase your sense of well-being.

General guidelines

1. If you are recovering from heart surgery or a heart attack, have someone with you for the first several weeks.
2. Wait at least 2 hours after eating.
3. Wear comfortable rubber-soled walking shoes and loose clothing.
4. Avoid extreme heat or cold. Don't exercise if the temperature is over 85° F (particularly if the humidity is over 75%) or under 20° F. During bad weather, walk in a covered shopping mall or gym.
5. Always begin with a 5-minute warm-up of stretching and slow walking.
6. Adopt a steady, rhythmic pace and keep it up. If you have attacks of leg cramps (claudication), you may need to alternate walking with rest periods.
7. Watch for signs of overexertion. Stop walking if any of these symptoms occurs: chest pain (angina), palpitations, irregular heartbeat, dizziness or light-headedness, shortness of breath for more than 10 minutes, nausea or vomiting, extreme fatigue, pale or splotchy skin, or "cold sweat." Call your doctor if these symptoms persist.
8. Cool down with light activity for 5 minutes; for example, if you are walking fast, slow down to a stroll.

Graduated walking program

Graduated walking programs are designed to slowly increase the time, distance, and walking pace. Because they begin very slowly, you may be tempted to skip ahead if you feel the schedule is "too easy." Don't. The graduated schedule allows your heart time to adjust to increasing amounts of work. Skipping ahead may overwork your heart. Carry out the program just as your doctor orders. If you develop symptoms of overexertion, return to the previous week's schedule until you are ready to progress.

You must know the exact distance to determine how fast you should walk. You can measure the distance on your car odometer. If you find you walk the distance in less time than the schedule specifies, slow your pace down next time. If it takes longer, you need to walk a little faster.

As soon as you stop walking, take your pulse. Your heart rate should not exceed the upper limit of the target heart rate set by your doctor. For many people, this is less than 115 beats per minute.

FIRST 9 WEEKS

Week	Walking Time	Distance
1	5 minutes	¼ mile
2	5 minutes	¼ mile
3	10 minutes	½ mile
4	10 minutes	½ mile
5	15 minutes	¾ mile
6	15 minutes	¾ mile
7	20 minutes	1 mile
8	20 minutes	1½ miles
9	30 minutes	2 miles

At this point, you are ready to extend your walking time. Because the exercise will be sustained for a longer time, your pace will need to be a little slower the first few weeks. By week 12, your walking speed will increase to a brisk walk.

WEEKS 10 TO 12

Week	Walking Time	Distance
10	40 minutes	2 miles
11	40 minutes	2 miles
12	60 minutes	3 miles

You must continue with an exercise program after week 12. You should continue your walking program, join a medically supervised walk-jog program, or add another form of exercise to your program such as bicycling. Follow your doctor's advice about the best program for you.

POISONS

Signs that Suggest the Presence of Certain Toxins

Sign	Inference
Abdominal colic	black widow spider bite
	heavy metals
	withdrawal from narcotic depressant
Ataxia	alcohol
	barbiturates
	bromides
	carbon monoxide
	hallucinogens
	heavy metals
	organic solvents
	phenytoin (Dilantin)
	tranquilizers
Coma and drowsiness	alcohol (ethyl)
	antihistamines
	barbiturates, other hypnotics
	carbon monoxide
	opiates
	salicylates
	tranquilizers
Convulsions or muscle twitching	alcohol
	amphetamines
	antihistamines
	boric acid
	camphor
	chlorinated hydrocarbon insecticides (DDT)
	cyanide
	lead
	organophosphate insecticides
	plants (azalea, iris, lily-of-the-valley, water hemlock)
	salicylates
	strychnine
	withdrawal from drugs: barbiturates, benzodiazepines (Valium, Librium), meprobamate
Paralysis	botulism
	heavy metals
	plants (poison hemlock, etc.)
	triorthocresyl phosphate (plasticizer)

From McKenry L, Salerno E: *Mosby's pharmacology in nursing,* ed 20, St Louis, 1998, Mosby.

Continued

Signs that Suggest the Presence of Certain Toxins—cont'd

Sign	Inference
Oliguria/anuria	carbon tetrachloride
	ethylene glycol (antifreeze)
	heavy metals
	hemolysis caused by naphthalene, plants, etc.
	methanol
	mushrooms
	oxylates
	petroleum distillates
	solvents
Oral signs	
Breath odors	
Acetone	acetone
	alcohol (methyl or isopropyl)
	phenol
	salicylates
Alcohol	ethyl alcohol
Bitter almonds	cyanide
Coal gas	carbon monoxide
Garlic	arsenic
	dimethyl sulfoxide (DMSO)
	phosphorus
	organophosphate insecticides
	thallium
Salivation	arsenic
	corrosive substances
	mercury
	mushrooms
	organophosphate insecticides
	thallium
Pupillary changes	
Dilated	amphetamines
	antihistamines
	atropine
	barbiturates (when combined with coma)
	cocaine
	ephedrine
	LSD (occasionally)
	methanol
	withdrawal from narcotic depressants (occasionally)
Constricted, pinpoint pupils	mushrooms (muscarinic)
	opiates
	organophosphate insecticides

Signs that Suggest the Presence of Certain Toxins—cont'd

Sign	Inference
Nystagmus on lateral gaze	barbiturates minor tranquilizers (meprobamate, benzo-diazepines), phenytoin (Dilantin)
Respiratory alterations Increased	amphetamines barbiturates (early sign) carbon monoxide methanol petroleum distillates salicylates
Paralysis/convulsing	botulism organophosphate insecticides
Slowed or depressed	alcohol (late sign) barbiturates (late sign) opiates tranquilizers
Wheezing/pulmonary edema	mushrooms (muscarinic) opiates organophosphate insecticides petroleum distillates
Skin color changes Jaundice	aniline dyes/coal tar colors arsenic carbon tetrachloride castor bean fava bean mushroom naphthalene (moth repellent/insecticide) yellow phosphorus
Red flush	alcohol antihistamines atropine boric acid carbon monoxide nitrites tricyclic antidepressants
Cyanosis	aniline dyes carbon monoxide cyanide nitrites strychnine

Continued

Signs that Suggest the Presence of Certain Toxins—cont'd

Sign	Inference
Violent emesis (with or without hematemesis)	aminophylline bacterial food poisoning boric acid corrosives fluoride heavy metals phenol salicylates

Lead Poisoning

Long-term effects of lead poisoning

Neurocognitive effects	Behavioral effects
Developmental delays Lowered IQ scores (2-8 points) Speech and language problems Reading skill deficits Visual-spatial problems Visual-motor problems Learning disabilities Lowered academic success	Aggression Hyperactivity Impulsivity Delinquency Disinterest Withdrawal

Sources of Lead*

Lead-based paint in deteriorating condition

Lead solder

Lead crystal

Battery casings

Lead fishing sinkers

Lead curtain weights

Lead bullets

Some of these may contain lead

    Ceramics ware

    Water

---

*The US Consumer Product Safety Commission issues alerts and recalls for products that contain lead and may unexpectedly pose a hazard to young children.

Pottery
Pewter
Dyes
Industrial factories (see below)
Vinyl miniblinds
Playground equipment
Collectible toys
Artists' paints
Pool cue chalk
Occupations and hobbies involving lead
Battery and aircraft manufacturing
Lead smelting
Brass foundry work
Radiator repair
Construction work
Bridge repair work
Painting contracting
Mining
Ceramics work
Stained glass making
Jewelry making

From Wong D, et al: *Whaley & Wong's nursing care of infants and children,* ed 6, St Louis, 1999, Mosby.

Reducing blood lead levels

Make sure child does not have access to peeling paint or chewable surfaces painted with lead-based paint, especially window sills and wells.

If a house was built before 1960 (possibly before 1980) and has hard-surface floors, wet mop them at least once a week. Wipe other hard surfaces (e.g., window sills, baseboards). If there are loose paint chips in an area, such as a window well, use a wet disposable cloth to pick up and discard them. Do not vacuum hard-surfaced floors or window sills or wells, because this spreads dust. Use vacuum cleaners with agitators to remove dust from rugs rather than vacuum cleaners with suction only. If a rug is known to contain lead dust and cannot be washed, it should be discarded.

Wash and dry child's hands and face frequently, especially before eating.

Wash toys and pacifiers frequently.

If soil around home is or is likely to be contaminated with lead (e.g., if home was built before 1960 or is near a major highway), plant grass or other ground cover; plant bushes around outside of house so that child cannot play there.

During remodeling of older homes, be sure to follow correct procedures. Be certain children and pregnant women are not in the home, day or night, until process is completed. After deleading, thoroughly clean house using cleaning solution to damp mop and dust before inhabitants return.

In areas where lead content of water exceeds the drinking water standard and a particular faucet has not been used for 6 hours or more, "flush" the cold-water pipes by running the water until it becomes as cold as it will get (30 seconds to greater than 2 minutes). The more time water has been sitting in pipes, the more lead it may contain.

Use only cold water for consumption (drinking, cooking, and especially for making infant formula). Hot water dissolves lead more quickly than cold water and thus contains higher levels of lead. May use first-flush water for nonconsumption uses.

Have water tested by a competent laboratory. This action is especially important for apartment dwellers; flushing may not be effective in high-rise buildings or in other buildings with lead-soldered central piping (Environmental Protection Agency, 1995).

Do not store food in open cans, particularly if cans are imported.

Do not use pottery or ceramic ware that was inadequately fired or is meant for decorative use for food storage or service. Do not store drinks or food in lead crystal.

Avoid folk remedies or cosmetics that contain lead.

Make sure that home exposure is not occurring from parental occupations or hobbies. Household members employed in occupations such as lead smelting should shower and change into clean clothing before leaving work. Construction and lead abatement workers may also bring home lead contaminants.

Make sure child eats regular meals, because more lead is absorbed on an empty stomach.

Make sure child's diet contains sufficient iron and calcium and not excessive fat.

Steps for prevention

Be alert for chipping and flaking paint.

Make sure child puts only safe, clean items in mouth.

Feed well-balanced meals that are low in fat and high in iron, calcium, and zinc.

Don't allow child to eat snow or icicles.

Use safe interior paints on toys, walls, furniture, etc.

Use pottery only for display if you're unsure about the glaze.

Store food in glass, plastic, or stainless steel containers, not in open cans.

Have your water tested, and draw drinking water only from the cold tap after allowing water to run for a few minutes (if you suspect lead danger).

Have children wash hands before eating.

Ask your local public health or housing/building official about an evaluation of lead hazards in your residence.

If you work with lead, shower and change before coming home.

Wash clothes separately from those of other family members.

Testing

Every child between the ages of 6 months and 6 years should be tested for lead at least once a year with a simple blood test. This may be done with a fingerstick or by venipuncture. If anyone in the household is diagnosed with lead poisoning, all other household members should be tested.

Screening for Lead Poisoning

Lead poisoning is one of the most common and preventable childhood environmental health problems in the United States. Although low-income, inner-city children have higher rates of lead poisoning, no socioeconomic group, geographic area, or racial or ethnic population is spared. In 1990, up to 3 million children under 6 years of age, 15% of all children in this age group, had blood lead levels greater than 10 $\mu g/dL$. Studies have shown associations between diminished intelligence, impaired neurobehavioral development, decreased hearing acuity, and growth inhibition and lead levels as low as 10 to 15 $\mu g/dL$.

Basics of lead screening

1. Risk assessment and counseling should begin during prenatal visits and continue after birth during regular office visits until at least the age of 6 years.

From Clinician's Handbook of Preventive Services: *Put prevention into practice: screening for lead,* 1994.

2. Each child's risk of lead toxicity should be evaluated. For this purpose, a structured set of questions such as that developed by the Centers for Disease Control and Prevention (CDC) (below) can be very helpful. If the answer to any of these questions is positive, the child is considered at high risk for exposure.

Recommended questions for assessing exposure risk

Does your child live in or regularly visit a house with peeling or chipping paint built before 1960? (This includes day care centers, preschools, homes of baby-sitters or relatives, etc.)

Does your child live in or regularly visit a house built before 1960 with recent, ongoing, or planned renovation or remodeling?

Does your child have a brother or sister, housemate, or playmate being followed or treated for lead poisoning (blood lead level ≥15 μg/dL)?

Does your child live with an adult whose job or hobby involves exposure to lead? (Such hobbies include ceramics, furniture refinishing, and stained glass work.)

Does your child live near an active lead smelter, battery recycling plant, or other industry likely to release lead?

Adapted from Centers for Disease Control and Prevention: *Preventing lead poisoning in young children: a statement by the Centers for Disease Control and Prevention,* Atlanta, 1991, Centers for Disease Control and Prevention.

3. Screening by measurement of the blood lead level is more sensitive and specific than measurement of the erythrocyte protoporphyrin (EP) level. Blood lead levels <25 μg/dL cannot be reliably detected by EP testing. Elevated EP levels (≥35 μg/dL) require confirmation with blood lead testing.

4. Because of possible contamination of capillary specimens from environmental sources, venous blood samples are preferable to capillary sampling for blood lead levels. If capillary samples must be used, the precautions listed below should be followed to minimize the chance of contamination. Elevated blood lead results (≥15 μg/dL) obtained on capillary specimens must be confirmed using venous blood. A child with a capillary lead level ≥70 μg/dL should be considered a medical emergency and retested with a venous sample immediately.

Recommendations for minimizing the contamination of capillary blood samples obtained by finger stick

Personnel who collect specimens should be well trained in and completely familiar with the collection procedure.

Puncturing the fingers of infants less than 1 year of age is not recommended. The heel is a more suitable site for these children.

If examination gloves are coated with powder, they should be rinsed with tap water.

The child's hand should be thoroughly washed with soap and water and then dried with a clean, low-lint towel.

Once washed, the finger or heel to be punctured should be cleansed with alcohol and not allowed to come into contact with any surface, including the child's other fingers.

Although its effectiveness in reducing contamination is under study, silicone spray can be used to form a protective layer between the skin and blood droplets.

The first droplet of blood, which contains tissue fluids, should be wiped off with sterile gauze or a cotton ball.

Do not collect blood that has run down the finger or onto the fingernail.

Contact between the skin and the collection container should be avoided.

Adapted from Centers for Disease Control and Prevention: *Preventing lead poisoning in young children: a statement by the Centers for Disease Control and Prevention,* Atlanta, 1991, Centers for Disease Control and Prevention.

5. Blood lead test results can be interpreted and managed according to the CDC recommendations following on pages 482-483.

CDC recommendations for follow-up of blood lead measurements

Class	Blood lead concentration (μg/dL)	Action	
I	≤9	Low risk:	6-35 months of age—Retest at 24 months of age (when blood levels peak), if resources allow. ≥36 and <72 months of age—Retesting not necessary unless history suggests exposure has increased.
		High risk:	6-35 months of age—Retest every 6 months. After two subsequent consecutive measurements are <10 μg/dL, or three are <15 μg/dL, retest once a year. ≥36 to 72 months of age—Retest once a year until sixth birthday.
IIA	10-14	Low risk:	6-35 months of age—Retest every 3-4 months. After two consecutive measurements are <10 μg/dL or three are <15 μg/dL, retest once a year. ≥36 and <72 months of age—Retesting not necessary if all previous test results are <15 μg/dL, unless history suggests exposure has increased.
		High risk:	6-35 months of age—Retest every 3-4 months. After two consecutive measurements are <10 μg/dL or three are <15 μg/dL, retest once a year. ≥36 and <72 months of age—Retest once a year until sixth birthday.
IIB	15-19	Retest every 3-4 months. The family should be given education and nutritional counseling and a detailed environmental history should be taken to identify any obvious sources or pathways of lead exposure. If venous blood level is in this range in two consecutive tests 3-4 months apart, environmental investigation and abatement should be conducted, if resources permit.	

Adapted from Centers for Disease Control and Prevention: *Preventing lead poisoning in young children: a statement by the Centers for Disease Control and Prevention,* Atlanta, 1997, Centers for Disease Control and Prevention.

Class	Blood lead concentration (μg/dL)	Action
III	20-44*	Retest every 3-4 months. Conduct a complete medical evaluation, including iron deficiency testing. Environmental lead sources should be identified and eliminated. Pharmacologic treatment may be necessary.
IV	45-69*	Begin medical treatment and environmental assessment and remediation within 48 hours.
V	≥70*	Begin medical treatment and environmental assessment and remediation immediately.

*Based on confirmatory blood lead level.

6. Laboratories where blood is tested for lead levels should participate in a blood-lead proficiency testing program, such as the collaborative program between the Health Resources and Services Administration and CDC.

7. Because iron deficiency can enhance lead absorption and toxicity, all children with blood lead levels ≥20 μg/dL should be tested for iron deficiency.

8. In addition to screening, it is important to provide guidance to parents about creating an environment safe from lead exposure for their children. Counseling should include advice on eliminating peeling or chipping paint, decreasing the lead content of water, preventing contact via hobbies or contaminated work clothing, remaining alert for pica behavior, and ensuring good hygiene. See Family Resources for publications to aid in counseling.

Family resources

Getting the Lead Out. Food and Drug Administration. Superintendent of Documents, Consumer Information Center-3C, PO Box 100, Pueblo, CO 81002.

Home Buyer's Guide to Environmental Hazards. Environmental Protection Agency. Superintendent of Documents, Consumer Information Center-3C, PO Box 100, Pueblo, CO 81002.

Important Facts about Childhood Lead Poisoning Prevention. Centers for Disease Control and Prevention, Lead Poisoning Prevention Program, 1600 Clifton Rd., Atlanta, GA 30333; (404) 639-7230.

What Everyone Should Know about Lead Poisoning. Alliance to End Childhood Lead Poisoning, 600 Pennsylvania Ave. SE, Suite 100, Washington, DC 20003 (individual copies); Channing L. Bete Co., Inc., 200 State Rd., South Deerfield, MA 01373; 1-800-628-7733 (bulk copies).

What You Should Know About Lead-Based Paint in Your Home. U.S. Consumer Product Safety Commission, Washington, DC 20207; 1-800-638-2666.

Provider resources

Case Studies in Environmental Medicine: Lead Toxicity. Agency for Toxic Substances and Disease Registry, Division of Health Education, Mailstop E33, 1600 Clifton Rd., Atlanta, GA 30333; (707) 639-6205.

Preventing Lead Poisoning in Young Children: A Statement by the Centers for Disease Control. Centers for Disease Control and Prevention, Lead Poisoning Prevention Program, 1600 Clifton Rd., Atlanta, GA 30333; (707) 488-4880.

Blood-Lead Proficiency Testing Program. Centers for Disease Control and Prevention. (707) 488-4880.

Lead Poisoning and Prevention

Your child has an unhealthy amount of lead in his or her body. Children get lead into their bodies in the following ways:

Eating paint chips that have lead
Eating paper with lead print
Drinking water from lead pipes
Breathing in lead dust

Testing for lead poisoning must be done by taking blood from your child's vein. The lead level will tell the health care provider what needs to be done for your child.

- Blood level of 10 to 19 μg/dL — No medicine needed*
- Blood level of 20 to 44 μg/dL — The child may need medicine to treat the lead*
- Blood level of 45 μg/dL or more — The child *must* be treated with medicine*

Lead can hurt your child because it causes many problems in the blood, brain, and kidneys. Some of the mild signs and symptoms of lead poisoning are stomach pain, nausea, vomiting, and loose or hard bowel movements. Other symptoms may include trouble sleeping, trouble thinking, headaches, seizures, sleepiness, a slow heart beat,

---

*The family needs to learn about lead poisoning and what they can do to prevent it. The child will need blood tests from time to time.

From Ball J: *Mosby's Pediatric Patient Teaching Guides,* ed. 1, St Louis, 1998, Mosby.

and developmental delays. All children with lead in their blood must be prevented from getting more. This means you must find out where your child gets the lead and make sure he or she does not get it again. Your healthcare provider and nurse will talk to you about this, and someone may also check your home.

Children with symptoms of lead poisoning and high amounts of lead also need treatment. They will receive medicine given by mouth or by an injection (shot) into the muscle or into the vein. To decrease your child's exposure to lead, you should do the following:

Watch your child closely to be sure that he or she eats only food items. Children who have a lot of lead in their blood often eat things that are not food, such as crayons, ashes, dirt, and cigarette butts.

Keep your child away from places or things with lead paint or chipping paint or plaster. Check other places where your child spends time for lead, such as the day care facility or the home of a relative.

Use a cleaner with phosphate (5% to 8%) to damp dust and mop floors, doors, and window sills. Do this two times a week to get rid of lead dust. (You can ask about brand names and buy this at a hardware store.) Do not dry sweep or vacuum, since this just spreads the dust more.

Give foods with a lot of calcium and iron, such as the following:

High calcium

Milk
Yogurt
Cheese
Ice cream

High iron

Cream of wheat, raisin bran, some oatmeals
Peanut butter
Beef, chicken, and tuna
Dried beans
Eggs

Keep toys and pacifiers that are put in the mouth clean and dry. Be sure to wash them if they fall on the floor.

Wash and dry your child's hands often, since children put them in their mouths.

If you have not used the water for more than 6 hours, turn the water on and let it run for 2 to 3 minutes before using it to drink or cook. (Water that sits in the pipes has more lead.)

Do not store food in open metal cans.

Wash fruits and vegetables before eating them.

Follow-up care

Your healthcare provider will tell you how often your child needs to have a blood test for lead and if your child needs treatment. Blood-work for the follow-up lead tests will be taken from your child's finger or heel. The tests should be quick and should not hurt very much. It is very important that you get these tests done. Please let your healthcare provider know if you have other children in your home. They will also need to be tested for lead.

Priority Groups for Screening Lead

Children ages 6 to 72 months who live in or are frequent visitors to de-teriorated housing built before 1960

Children ages 6 to 72 months who live in housing built before 1960 with recent, ongoing, or planned renovation or remodeling

Children ages 6 to 72 months who are siblings, housemates, or play-mates of children with known lead poisoning

Children ages 6 to 72 months whose parents or other household members participate in a lead-related occupation or hobby

Children ages 6 to 72 months who live near active lead smelters, battery recycling plants, or other industries likely to result in at-mospheric lead release

Poisonous Plants

A list of common house and garden plants is presented below. This is only a partial list, and some plants are known by more than one name. If you have questions about any plants not listed, call your local poison control center. There are many varieties of harmless plants that are possible to enjoy and still keep your children safe.

Nonpoisonous plants*

Abelia	Aster
African Violet	Begonia species
Airplane Plant	Carnation
Aloe	Cast Iron Plant
Aluminum Plant	China Doll Plant (not Evergreen)

*Reprinted with permission from Kentucky Regional Poison Control Center of Kosair Children's Hospital, 1999.

Chinese Evergreen
Christmas Cactus
Coleus species
Corn Plant
Croton
Dahlia
Daisy
Dandelion
Day Lily
Dracaena species
Easter Cactus
Fern species
  (except Asparagus)
Fig, Ficus
Gardenia
Geranium
Hens and Chickens
Honeysuckle
Impatiens
Jade Plant
Juniper Berries

Kalanchoe
Lipstick Plant
Magnolia
Marigold
Nasturtium
Norfolk Island Pine
Palm species
Petunia
Poinsettia
Prayer Plant
Pyracantha
Rubber Tree
Sansevieria, Snake Plant,
  Mother-in-Law's Tongue
Schefflera
Spider Plant
Swedish Ivy
Wandering Jew
Wild, Indian or Mock Strawberry
Yucca Plant
Zebra Plant

Poisonous Plants*

Acorns
Amaryllis
Apple (seeds)
Arrowhead Vine
Asparagus Fern
Apricot (pits)
Azalea
Black Locust
Buckeye, Horsechestnut
Burning Bush
Buttercup, Daffodil,
  Jonquil
Cactus (spines)
Caladium
Castor Bean
Cherry
  (leaves, pits, twigs)

Chrysanthemum
Crocus, Autumn
Dieffenbachia
  Dumb Cane
Dusty Miller
Elderberry
Elephant Ear
Eucalyptus
Hedge Apple
Hemlock (water, poison)
Holly
Hydrangea
Iris
Ivy species
Jack-in-the-Pulpit
Jequirity Bean
Jerusalem Cherry

Continued

Jimson Weed, Thornapple
Kentucky Coffee Tree
Lily of the Valley
Marijuana
Mistletoe
Morning Glory
Mushrooms (lawn, wild)
Nightshade
Oleander
Peace Lily
Peach (pits)
Philodendron

Poison Ivy, Oak, Sumac
Poke (root)
Pothos
Potato (sprouts, green)
Privet Berries
Rhododendron
Rhubarb (leaf blades)
Tobacco
Tulip (bulb)
Wisteria
Yew/Taxus

What to do if a plant poisoning occurs

If you suspect that someone has ingested any amount of a plant that you believe is toxic or that you are unsure of, follow these guidelines:

1. Remove any plant parts from the person's mouth.
2. Give the person a small amount of water to drink.
3. Call the nearest Poison Control Center immediately. Don't wait for symptoms to develop.

Steps for prevention

1. **Identify** all plants in your home and yard. This may be done by consulting a nursery, greenhouse, or florist. Show the plant to them.
2. **Label** the plants with proper names. You may want to write the name on tape and attach it to the pot. For the yard, you may want to make a map of the area indicating the name and location of each tree, plant, or bush. Keep this information handy in case of an emergency.
3. **Determine** which plants are safe and which are poisonous. Harmful plants should be kept well out of children's reach.
4. **Teach** children not to eat leaves, berries, buds, or flowers. Remind them to "look but don't lick—admire but don't pick."
5. **Store** all seeds and bulbs in a safe place.

Poisonous Parts of Common House and Garden Plants

Plant	Toxic part	Symptoms
Apple	Seeds	Releases cyanide when ingested in large quantities; may be fatal
Azalea	All parts	Nausea, vomiting, dyspnea, paralysis; may be fatal
Buttercup	All parts	Inflammation around mouth, stomach pains, vomiting, diarrhea, convulsions
Castor bean	Seeds	Burning of mouth and throat, excessive thirst, convulsions; one or two seeds are near the lethal dose for adults
Croton	Plant juice	Gastroenteritis
Daffodil	Bulb	Nausea, vomiting, diarrhea; may be fatal
Dieffenbachia	All parts	Intense burning and irritation of the mouth and tongue; death can occur if base of tongue swells enough to occlude air passages
English holly	Berries	Nausea, vomiting, diarrhea, central nervous system depression; may be fatal
English ivy	Leaves and berries	Dyspnea, vomiting, diarrhea, coma, and death
Hyacinth	Bulb	Nausea, vomiting, diarrhea; may be fatal
Iris	Underground stems	Digestive upset
Jasmine	All parts	Hallucinations, elevated temperature, tachycardia, paralysis
Lily-of-the-valley	All parts	Arrhythmia, mental confusion, weakness, shock, and death
Mistletoe	Berries	Acute stomach and intestinal irritations with diarrhea; may be fatal
Oak tree	Acorns	Kidney failure, gastritis
Oleander	All parts	Digestive upset, bloody diarrhea, respiratory depression, arrhythmia, blurred vision, coma, and death
Philodendron	All parts	Burning of lips, mouth, and tongue; swelling of tongue; dyspnea, kidney failure, and death

From Edelman CL, Mandle CL: *Health promotion throughout the lifespan,* ed 4, St Louis, 1998, Mosby.
Continued

Poisonous Parts of Common House and Garden Plants—cont'd

Plant	Toxic part	Symptoms
Poinsettia	Leaves	Severe irritation to mouth, throat, and stomach; may be fatal
Potato	All green parts	Cardiac depression; may be fatal
Tomato	Green parts	Cardiac depression; may be fatal
Violet	Seeds	Taken in quantity, cathartic effects can be serious to infants
Yew	Foliage, seeds, bark	Nausea, vomiting, diarrhea, dyspnea, dilated pupils; death is sudden

Nursing Interventions to Prevent Plant Poisoning in Infants

Keep plants out of reach of infants and young children.

Never eat any part of a plant except those parts grown or sold as food.

Keep jewelry made from unknown seeds or beans away from exploring infants.

Learn to identify poisonous plants around your house and garden.

Do not use unknown plants as medicines or teas.

Pay close attention to infants at play inside and outside.

Seek help whenever anyone chews or swallows a poisonous plant.

Be aware that infants are more susceptible than adults to the effects of poisonous plants.

From Edelman CL, Mandle CL: *Health promotion throughout the lifespan,* ed 4, St Louis, 1998, Mosby.

Common Household Poisons

A checklist of poisonous products found in the home follows. Experience has shown that the products in *italic* type are the most dangerous poisons.

Kitchen
Aspirin
Drain cleaners (lye)
Furniture polish
Oven cleaner
Automatic dishwasher detergent
Ammonia
Powder and liquid detergents
Cleanser and scouring powders
Metal cleaners
Rust remover
Pills
Carpet and upholstery cleaners
Bleach
Vitamins

General
Plants
Flaking paint
Repainted toys
Broken plaster

Bedroom
Sleeping drugs
Tranquilizers
Other drugs
Jewelry cleaner
Cosmetics
Perfume
After-shave
Cologne

Closets, attic, storage places
Rat poison, ant poison, and insecticides
Mothballs

Laundry room
Bleaches
Soap and detergents
Disinfectant
Bluing, dyes
Carbon tetrachloride

Bathroom, garage, basement
Aspirin
All drugs and pills
Drain cleaners (lye)
Iron pills
Toilet bowl cleaners
Shampoo, wave lotion, and sprays
Hand lotion
Creams
Nail polish and remover
Suntan lotions
Deodorants
Shaving lotions
Hair remover
Lye
Kerosene
Pesticides
Gasoline
Lighter fluid

Reprinted, with permission, from *Poison primer*, Galveston, Southeast Texas Poison Center. *Continued*

Common Household Poisons—cont'd

Turpentine	Paint
Paint remover and thinner	Weed killers
Antifreeze	Fertilizers
Lime	

INJURIES

Causes of Falls

Accidents
  True accidents (trips, slips, etc.)
  Interactions between environmental hazards and factors increasing
    susceptibility
Syncope (sudden loss of consciousness)
Drop attacks (sudden leg weaknesses, without loss of consciousness)
Dizziness or vertigo
  Vestibular disease
  Central nervous system (CNS) disease
Orthostatic hypotension
  Hypovolemia or low cardiac output
  Autonomic dysfunction
  Impaired venous return
  Prolonged bed rest
  Drug-induced hypotension
  Postprandial hypotension
Drug-related causes
  Diuretics
  Antihypertensives
  Tricyclic antidepressants
  Sedatives
  Antipsychotics
  Hypoglycemics
  Alcohol
Specific disease processes
  Acute illness of any kind ("premonitory fall")

From Kane R, Ouslander J, Abrass I: *Essentials of clinical geriatrics,* ed 4, New York, 1999, McGraw-Hill.

Causes of Falls—cont'd

Cardiovascular
 Arrhythmias
 Valvular heart disease (aortic stenosis)
 Carotid sinus syncope
Neurologic causes
 Transient ischemic attack (TIA)
 Stroke (acute)
 Seizure disorder
 Parkinson's disease
 Cervical or lumbar spondylosis (with spinal cord or nerve root compression)
 Cerebellar disease
 Normal-pressure hydrocephalus (gait disorder)
 CNS lesions (e.g., tumor, subdural hematoma)
Idiopathic (no specific cause identifiable)

Assessment for Clients Who Fall

1. Current medical problems _____
_____
_____

2. Medications _____
_____
_____

3. Is there a previous history of falls?
____ Yes ____ No
If yes:
Number of previous falls ____
Is there a pattern?
____ Yes ____ No
Frequency
_____

Time of day
_____

Position
_____
_____

From Kane R, Ouslander J, Abrass I: *Essentials of clinical geriatrics,* ed 4, New York, 1999, McGraw-Hill. *Continued*

Assessment for Clients Who Fall—cont'd

Activity

_____

_____

Circumstances

_____

_____

4. Circumstances surrounding current fall
   Time of day

   _____

   Location

   _____

   Relationship to specific activities (e.g., toileting, climbing or descending stairs, exercise, turning head)

   _____

   _____

   _____

   Witness(es)

   _____

   _____

   _____

   Environmental hazards (e.g., poor lighting, loose rug, uneven floor, other obstacles)

   _____

   _____

   _____

5. Client's description of and reasons for the fall (in client's words)

   _____

   _____

   _____

   _____

6. Questions to the client (or witness)
   a. Did you know you were going to fall?
      ____ Yes   ____ No
   b. After you fell, did you know what happened?
      ____ Yes   ____ No
   c. Did you lose consciousness (pass out)?
      ____ Yes   ____ No
      If yes, how long were you unconscious? ____ minutes.
      Were you aware of what happened after you awoke?
      ____ Yes   ____ No

Assessment for Clients Who Fall—cont'd

Had you lost control of your bowel or bladder?
____ Yes ____ No
d. Were you able to get up right away?
____ Yes ____ No
e. Did you have any pain or injury after the fall?
____ Yes ____ No
f. Did you do any of the following just before the fall?
____ Trip
____ Slip
____ Stand up quickly
____ Turn your head suddenly
____ Cough
____ Urinate
____ Have a bowel movement
____ Eat a large meal
g. Did you have any of the following symptoms just before you fell?
____ Light-headedness
____ Vertigo (spinning around the room or vice versa)
____ Palpitations
____ Shortness of breath
____ Weakness or numbness on one side of the body
____ Sudden weakness of both legs
____ Slurred speech
____ Difficulty saying what you wanted to say
____ Strange smells
____ Flashing lights (scotomata)

7. Physical assessment
a. Postural vital signs

	Supine	Sitting	Standing
Blood pressure	___ / ___	___ / ___	___ / ___
Pulse	_____	_____	_____
Blood pressure other arm		___ / ___	

b. Skin
____ Bruises
____ Diminished turgor
c. Vision
____ Adequate for independent ambulation
____ Limits mobility, but still independent
____ Inadequate for independent ambulation

Continued

Assessment for Clients Who Fall—cont'd

   d. Neck
- ____ Supple
- ____ Full range of motion
- ____ Symptoms with rotation

   e. Cardiovascular
- ____ Arrhythmia
- ____ Murmur suggestive of aortic stenosis
- ____ Signs of heart failure (Describe: _____)
- ____ Carotid bruit(s)

   f. Musculoskeletal
- ____ Trauma or suspected fracture
- ____ Deformity
- ____ Limited range of motion
- ____ Joint inflammation

   g. Podiatric
- ____ Are any of the following impairing ambulation?
- ____ Callouses
- ____ Bunions
- ____ Nail deformity
- ____ Ulceration
- ____ Poorly fitted or otherwise inadequate shoes

   h. Neurologic
- ____ Abnormal mental status
- ____ Focal neurologic sign(s)
- ____ Muscular weakness
- ____ Muscular rigidity/spasticity
- ____ Bradykinesia
- ____ Resting tremor
- ____ Peripheral neuropathy
- ____ Ataxia, finger to nose
- ____ Ataxia, heel to shin

Describe positive findings: _____

_____

   i. Mobility
- ____ Ambulates independently
- ____ Uses aid
  - ____ Cane
  - ____ Quad-cane
  - ____ Walker

Assessment for Clients Who Fall—cont'd

_____ Wheelchair, able to transfer independently
_____ Wheelchair, needs help to transfer

j. Stability and gait

	Normal	Abnormal
Sitting balance	_____	_____
Rising from sitting to standing	_____	_____
Standing balance with eyes open	_____	_____
Standing balance with eyes closed (Romberg's test)	_____	_____
Initiation of walking	_____	_____
Length of stride	_____	_____
Distance feet apart	_____	_____
Turning	_____	_____
Sitting down	_____	_____
Describe positive findings:		

_____

_____

_____

8. Diagnostic studies

Test/procedure   Result

_____   _____

_____   _____

_____   _____

_____   _____

_____   _____

_____   _____

_____   _____

_____   _____

_____   _____

Fall Risk Factors for Elders

Conditions

Female or single (incidence increases with age)

    Sedative and alcohol use, psychoactive medications

    Previous falls, unsteadiness, dizziness

    Acute and recent illness

    Pathologic conditions, drop attacks

    Cognitive impairment, disorientation

    Disability of lower extremities

    Abnormalities of balance and gait

    Foot problems

    Depression, anxiety

    Decreased vision or hearing

    Fear of falling

    Terminal drop (dies in following year to 2 years)

    Skeletal and neuromuscular changes that predispose to weakness and postural imbalance

    Acute and severe chronic illness, debilitation

    Functional limitations in self-care activities

Women (75 years and older)

    Multiple disorders and medications

    Wheelchair-bound

    Sensory deficits

    Impaired locomotion

    Predisposing physiologic and psychologic conditions

    Preoccupation with stressors

    Anxiety related to previous falls

    Confusion, dementia

Situations

Urinary urgency, particularly nocturia

Environmental hazards

Recent relocation

Assistive devices needed for walking

Inadequate or missing safety rails, particularly in bathroom

Poorly designed or unstable furniture

Low stools

High chairs and beds

From Ebersole P, Hess P: *Toward healthy aging: human needs and nursing response,* ed 5, St Louis, 1998, Mosby.

Fall Risk Factors for Elders—cont'd

Floor surfaces
Glossy, highly waxed floors
Wet, greasy, icy surfaces
Inadequate lighting
General clutter
Pets that inadvertently trip an individual
Electrical cords
Loose or uneven stair treads

Tinetti Evaluation Tool

Balance

Instructions: Subject is seated in a hard, armless chair. The following maneuvers are tested:

1. Sitting balance
   0 = Leans or slides in chair
   1 = Steady, safe
2. Arise
   0 = Unable without help
   1 = Able but uses arm to help
   2 = Able without use of arms
3. Attempts to arise
   0 = Unable without help
   1 = Able, but requires more than one attempt
   2 = Able to arise with one attempt
4. Immediate standing balance (first 5 seconds)
   0 = Unsteady (staggers, moves feet, marked trunk sway)
   1 = Steady but uses walker/cane or grabs other object for support
   2 = Steady without walker or cane or other support
5. Standing balance
   0 = Unsteady
   1 = Steady, but wide stance (medial heels >4″ apart) or uses cane/walker or other support
   2 = Narrow stance without support

From Ebersole P, Hess P: *Toward healthy aging: human needs and nursing response,* ed 5, St Louis, 1998, Mosby.

Tinetti Evaluation Tool—cont'd

6. Nudge (subject at maximum position with feet as close together as possible. Examiner pushes lightly on subject's sternum with palm of hand 3 times.)

    0 = Begins to fall

    1 = Staggers, grabs, but catches self

    2 = Steady

7. Eyes closed (at maximum position #6)

    0 = Unsteady

    1 = Steady

8. Turn 360°

    0 = Discontinuous steps

    1 = Continuous steps

    0 = Unsteady (grabs, staggers)

    1 = Steady

9. Sit down

    0 = Unsafe (misjudged distance; falls into chair)

    1 = Uses arms or not a smooth motion

    2 = Safe, smooth motion

___/16___ BALANCE SCORE

Gait

Instructions: Subject stands with examiner. Walks down hallway or across room, first at his/her usual pace, then back at a "rapid but safe" pace (using usual walking aid such as cane/walker).

10. Initiation of gait (immediately after told "go")

    0 = Any hesitancy or multiple attempts to start

    1 = No hesitancy

11. Step length and height (right foot swing)

    0 = Does not pass L. stance foot with step

    1 = Passes L. stance foot

    0 = R. foot does not clear floor completely with step

    1 = R. foot completely clears floor

12. Step length and height (left foot swing)

    0 = Does not pass R. stance foot with step

    1 = Passes R. stance foot

    0 = L. foot does not clear floor completely with step

    1 = L. foot completely clears floor

13. Step symmetry

    0 = R. and L. step length not equal (estimate)

    1 = R. and L. step length appear equal

Tinetti Evaluation Tool—cont'd

14. Step continuity
  0 = Stopping or discontinuity between steps
  1 = Steps appear continuous
15. Path (estimated in relation to floor tiles, 12″ wide. Observe excursion of one foot over about 10 feet of course.)
  0 = Marked deviation
  1 = Mild/moderate deviation or uses a walking aid
  2 = Straight without walking aid
16. Trunk
  0 = Marked sway or uses walking aid
  1 = No sway but flexion of knees or back or spreads arms out while walking
  2 = No sway, no flexion, no use of arms and no walking aid
17. Walk stance
  0 = Heels apart
  1 = Heels almost touching while walking

____**/12**____ GAIT SCORE

____**/28**____ TOTAL MOBILITY SCORE (BALANCE AND GAIT)

Home Safety Checklist

Place a check mark next to each question if the answer is yes. Use this checklist to correct all hazards in the home.

Housekeeping
____ Do you clean up spills as soon as they occur?
____ Do you keep floors and stairways clean and free of clutter?
____ Do you put away books, magazines, sewing supplies, and other objects as soon as you are through with them and never leave them on floors or stairways?
____ Do you store frequently used items on shelves that are within easy reach?

Adapted from National Safety Council: *Falling—the unexpected trip: a safety program for older adults* (Program Leader's Guide), Chicago, 1982, National Safety Council. Used with permission of the National Safety Council; copyright © 1982. In Kennedy-Malone L, Fletcher K, Plank L: *Management guidelines for gerontological nurse practitioners,* Philadelphia, 2000, FA Davis.

Home Safety Checklist—cont'd

Floors

____ Do you keep everyone from walking on freshly washed floors before they are dry?

____ If you wax floors, do you apply 2 thin coats and buff each thoroughly or use self-polishing wax?

____ Do all area rugs have nonslip backings?

____ Have you eliminated small rugs at the tops and bottoms of stairways?

____ Are all carpet edges tacked down?

____ Are rugs and carpets free of curled edges, worn spots, and rips?

____ Have you chosen rugs and carpets with short, dense pile?

____ Are rugs and carpets installed over good-quality, medium-thick pads?

Lighting

____ Do you have light switches near every doorway?

____ Do you have enough good lighting to eliminate shadowy areas?

____ Do you have a lamp or light switch within easy reach of every bed?

____ Do you have night lights in your bathrooms and in hallways leading from bedrooms to bathrooms?

____ Are all stairways well lit with light switches at both top and bottom?

Bathrooms

____ Do you use a rubber mat or nonslip decals in tubs and showers?

____ Do you have a grab bar securely anchored over each tub and shower?

____ Do you have a nonslip rug on all bathroom floors?

____ Do you keep soap in easy-to-reach receptacles?

Traffic lanes

____ Can you walk across every room in your home, and from one room to another, without detouring around furniture?

____ Is the traffic lane from your bedroom to the bathroom free of obstacles?

____ Are telephone and appliance cords kept away from areas where people walk?

Home Safety Checklist—cont'd

Stairways

——— Do securely fastened handrails extend the full length of the stairs on each side of the stairways?

——— Do the handrails stand out from the walls so you can get a good grip?

——— Are handrails distinctly shaped so you are alerted when you reach the end of a stairway?

——— Are all stairways in good condition, with no broken, sagging, or sloping steps?

——— Are all stairway carpeting and metal edges securely fastened and in good condition?

——— Have you replaced any single-level steps with gradually rising ramps or made sure such steps are well lighted?

Ladders and step stools

——— Do you always use a step stool or ladder that is tall enough for the job?

——— Do you always set up your ladder or step stool on a firm, level base that is free of clutter?

——— Before you climb a ladder or step stool, do you always make sure it is fully open and that the stepladder spreaders are locked?

——— When you use a ladder or step stool, do you face the steps and keep your body between the side rails?

——— Do you avoid standing on the top step of a step stool or climbing beyond the second step from the top on a stepladder?

Outdoor areas

——— Are walks and driveways in your yard and other areas free of breaks?

——— Are lawns and gardens free of holes?

——— Do you put away garden tools and hoses when they are not in use?

——— Are outdoor areas kept free of rocks, loose boards, and other tripping hazards?

——— Do you keep outdoor walkways, steps, and porches free of wet leaves and snow?

——— Do you sprinkle icy outdoor areas with de-icers as soon as possible after a snowfall or freeze?

——— Do you have mats at doorways for people to wipe their feet on?

——— Do you know the safest way of walking when you can't avoid walking on a slippery surface?

Home Safety Checklist—cont'd

Footwear

____ Do your shoes have soles and heels that provide good traction?

____ Do you avoid walking in stocking feet and wear house slippers that fit well and don't fall off?

____ Do you wear low-heeled oxfords, loafers, or good-quality sneakers when you work in your house or yard?

____ Do you replace boots or galoshes when their soles or heels are worn too smooth to keep you from slipping on wet or ice surfaces?

Personal precautions

____ Are you always alert for unexpected hazards, such as out-of-place furniture?

____ If young children visit or live in your home, are you alert for children playing on the floor and toys left in your path?

____ If you have pets, are you alert for sudden movements across your path and pets getting underfoot?

____ When you carry packages, do you divide them into smaller loads and make sure they do not obstruct your vision?

____ When you reach or bend, do you hold onto a firm support and avoid throwing your head back or turning it too far?

____ Do you always move deliberately and avoid rushing to answer the phone or doorbell?

____ Do you take time to get your balance when you change position from lying down to sitting and from sitting to standing?

____ Do you keep yourself in good condition with moderate exercise, good diet, adequate rest, and regular medical checkups?

____ If you wear glasses, is your prescription up-to-date?

____ Do you know how to reduce injury in a fall?

____ If you live alone, do you have daily contact with a friend or neighbor?

Types of Falls

1. Slips and trips: the patient may falsely attribute the fall to these causes when in reality it is due to a physical deficit.
2. Falls while attempting a difficult maneuver (such as climbing over a bed rail).
3. Syncope: the loss of consciousness immediately precedes the fall and may itself be preceded by a brief interval of giddiness or unsteadiness.
4. Seizure: the loss of consciousness accompanies the fall. It may be preceded by an aura. It may or may not be accompanied by clonic movements and incontinence.
5. Drop attack: sudden loss of muscular tone without loss of consciousness.
6. Vertigo: the patient experiences true dizziness (the room seems to spin) and falls to one side or the other.
7. Sliding off furniture: caused by weakness or somnolence.

From Wieman H, Calkins E: Falls. In Calkins E, Davis P, Ford M, editors: *The practice of geriatrics,* Philadelphia, 1986, WB Saunders.

Measures to Prevent Falls

Factor	Preventive measures
Footwear	Shoes with firm, nonskid, nonfriction soles; low heels; avoid walking in loose slippers or in stocking feet
Entrances, yards	Repair cracks in pavement; fill holes in lawn; remove all tripping hazards; well-lit walkways
Lighting	Light up shadowy areas; reduce glare with evenly distributed light; have light switches at room entrances; night light in bedroom, hall, bathroom
Floors	Carpet edges tacked down; carpets with shallow pile; nonskid wax on floors; nonskid backing for throw rugs; cords out of walking path; removal of all small objects from floor
Stairs	Lighting adequate, with switches at top and bottom of stairs; securely fastened and well-placed handrails on both sides of stairway; top and bottom steps marked with bright-colored adhesive strips; stair risers of no more than 6 inches; steps in good repair; no object on steps

Han R, Sloane P: *Primary care geriatrics: a case-based approach,* ed 3, St Louis, 1997, Mosby.

Continued

Measures to Prevent Falls—cont'd

Factor	Preventive measures
Bathroom	Raised toilet seat; grab bars for tub, shower, and toilet; nonskid rubber mat or strips in tub or shower; shower chair with handheld shower
Kitchen	Firm, nonmoveable kitchen table; rubber mat on floor in sink area; secure step stool if climbing is necessary; shelf and cupboard items at accessible height
Bedroom, living room	Bed at proper height; spills on floor cleaned up promptly; remove unstable tables and chairs; remove clutter in hallways and on floors

Measures to Prevent Fire and Burns

- Do not smoke in bed or when sleepy.
- When cooking, do not wear loose-fitting clothing (robes, nightgowns, pajamas).
- Set hot water thermostat at 120° F.
- Install a portable, handheld fire extinguisher in the kitchen.
- Keep access to outside doors unobstructed.
- Identify emergency exits in public buildings.
- If considering moving to a boarding home or foster home, check to see that it has smoke detectors, a sprinkler system, and fire extinguishers.
- Wear clothing that is nonflammable or treated with a flame-retardant finish. Wear less flammable materials of animal hair, wool, or silk.
- Avoid the use of electrical extension cords and do not overload electrical outlets.
- Install and maintain smoke detectors.
- Do not store flammable materials in the home.
- Call in an alarm before attempting to extinguish a fire, regardless of its size.

From Burke M, Walsh M: *Gerontologic nursing: wholistic care of the older adult,* ed 2, St Louis, 1997, Mosby.

General Safety Precautions

More deaths in the United States are caused by accidents than most people realize. In fact, accidents are the leading cause of death for children in this country. Yet about 90% of all accidents are preventable. Most households would reduce their annual need for emergency medical treatment if they would simply observe general safety precautions in a few key lifestyle areas.

Take time to check your own surroundings for potential hazards, and reduce or eliminate them. Below are some general guidelines for preventing common accidents. These guidelines encompass motor vehicles, sports and recreation, electrical and mechanical equipment, preventing falls, poisonings and ingestions, fire, and swimming pools. Use this as a checklist to evaluate your safety standards.

Motor vehicles
Naturally all automobiles should be maintained in good mechanical condition. Seat belts should be worn at all times; never start the car until everyone has buckled up. You'll be surprised at how little time it takes for your friends and family to start buckling up automatically whenever they ride with you! Look carefully in front and in back of the car before accelerating, and make sure all car doors are locked when a child travels in your car. Young children should never be left alone in a car, and heavy or sharp objects should not be placed on the same seat with a child. Small children should ride in a car seat appropriate for their age.

Sports and recreation
Many accidents in sports and recreation could be prevented by keeping equipment in good condition and proper working order.

We live in a rushed age. We often go directly from work to recreation or sports programs. Still, train yourself always to stop by the locker room first: always wear appropriate clothing and shoes (if needed) for the activity. You'll prevent a lot of injuries over the years by simply taking a few minutes before you play. Once involved in the sport or activity of your choice, do not attempt activities beyond your physical endurance. Injuring yourself will simply put you further back on the fitness scale.

Finally, keep all firearms and ammunition locked up.

Electrical and mechanical equipment

Only devices approved by Underwriters' Laboratories should be installed, and they should be inspected periodically. Dry your hands before touching appliances, and keep radios, fans, portable heaters, and hair dryers out of the bathroom. Discourage children from playing with or being in an area where appliances or power tools (e.g., washing machine, clothes dryer, saw, or lawn mower) are being used. Disconnect appliances after using them and before attempting minor repairs. Avoid overloading electrical circuits.

Keep garden equipment and machinery in a restricted area. As soon as each child in your household is old enough, teach him or her how to use the equipment properly.

Preventing falls

You might be surprised at the number of broken bones that are a result of falls in or around the house each year. These are not only painful, time consuming, and expensive to fix—they can also be pretty embarrassing! Here are a few quick tips for saving bones, medical bills, and face: Keep stairs well lighted and free of clutter; provide sturdy railings. Anchor small rugs securely, and use rubber mats in the bathtub and shower. Use only sturdy ladders for climbing.

Poisonings and ingestions

Poisonings and ingestions are the most common type of household accident among children and the elderly, but they can happen to anyone. Here are a few general guidelines: When cleaning, never mix bleaches with ammonia, vinegar, and other household cleaners. Label all medications clearly, and childproof your home by placing medications out of reach of children. But, just in case, keep emergency medical numbers clear, up-to-date, and easy to find.

Fire

Figure out an adequate fire escape plan, and routinely conduct home fire drills. Teach each child the escape routes as soon as he or she is old enough.

Keep a pressure-type hand fire extinguisher on each floor of your household. Instruct all family members who are old enough in its use. In addition, teach children about the danger of smoke inhalation. Use such slogans as "Stop, drop, and roll."

COMMUNICABLE AND INFECTIOUS DISEASES

Immunization Schedule

Immunization Protects Children

Regular checkups at your pediatrician's office or local health clinic are an important way to keep children healthy.

By making sure that your child gets immunized on time, you can provide the best available defense against many dangerous childhood diseases. Immunizations protect children against: hepatitis B, polio, measles, mumps, rubella (German measles), pertussis (whooping cough), diphtheria, tetanus (lockjaw), *Haemophilius influenzae* type b, chickenpox, and rotavirus. All of these immunizations need to be given before children are 2 years old in order for them to be protected during their most vulnerable period. Are your child's immunizations up-to-date?

The chart following includes immunization recommendations from the American Academy of Pediatrics. Remember to keep track of your child's immunizations—it's the only way you can be sure your child is up-to-date. Also, check with your pediatrician or health clinic at each visit to find out if your child needs any booster shots or if any new vaccines have been recommended since this schedule was prepared.

If you don't have a pediatrician, call your local health department. Public health clinics usually have supplies of vaccine and may give shots free.

From the American Academy of Pediatrics. The information contained here should not be used as a substitute for the medical care and advice of your pediatrician. There may be variations in treatment that your pediatrician may recommend based on individual facts and circumstances.

Recommended Childhood Immunization Schedule, United States, January-December 2000

Vaccines[1] are listed under routinely recommended ages. Bars indicate range of recommended ages for immunization. Any dose not given at the recommended age should be given as a "catch-up" immunization at any subsequent visit when indicated and feasible. Ovals indicate vaccines to be given if previously recommended doses were missed or given earlier than the recommended minimum age.

Age ▶ Vaccine ▼	Birth	1 mo	2 mos	4 mos	6 mos	12 mos	15 mos	18 mos	24 mos	4-6 yrs	11-12 yrs	14-16 yrs
Hepatitis B[2]	Hep B	Hep B			Hep B						(Hep B)	
Diphtheria, Tetanus, Pertussis[3]			DTaP	DTaP	DTaP		DTaP[3]			DTaP	Td	
H. influenzae type b[4]			Hib	Hib	Hib	Hib						
Polio[5]			IPV	IPV	IPV[5]					IPV[5]		
Measles, Mumps, Rubella[6]						MMR				MMR[6]	(MMR)[6]	
Varicella[7]						Var					(Var)[7]	
Hepatitis A[8]									Hep A[8]—In selected areas			

Approved by the Advisory Committee on Immunization Practices (ACIP), the American Academy of Pediatrics (AAP), and the American Academy of Family Physicians (AAFP). Licensed childhood vaccines as of 11/1/99. Additional vaccines may be licensed and recommended during the year. Licensed combination vaccines may be used whenever any components of the combination are indicated and its other components are not contraindicated. Providers should consult the manufacturer's package inserts for detailed recommendations.

[1] This schedule indicates the recommended ages for routine administration of currently

On October 22, 1999, the Advisory Committee on Immunization Practices (ACIP) recommended that Rotashield (RRV-TV), the only US-licensed rotavirus vaccine, no longer be used in the United States (MMWR Nov 3, 1999, 48[43]:1007). Parents should be reassured that their children who received rotavirus vaccine before July are not at increased risk for intussusception now.

[2] *Infants born to HBsAg-negative mothers should receive the 1st dose of hepatitis B (Hep*

B) vaccine by age 2 months. The 2nd dose should be at least 1 month after the 1st dose. The 3rd dose should be administered at least 4 months after the 1st dose and at least 2 months after the 2nd dose, but not before 6 months of age for infants.

Infants born to HBsAg-positive mothers should receive hepatitis B vaccine and 0.5 mL hepatitis B immune globulin (HBIG) within 12 hours of birth at separate sites. The 2nd dose is recommended at 1 month of age and the 3rd dose at 6 months of age.

Infants born to mothers whose HBsAg status is unknown should receive hepatitis B vaccine within 12 hours of birth. Maternal blood should be drawn at the time of delivery to determine the mother's HBsAg status; if the HBsAg test is positive, the infant should receive HBIG as soon as possible (no later than 1 week of age).

All children and adolescents (through 18 years of age) who have not been immunized against hepatitis B may begin the series during any visit. Special efforts should be made to immunize children who were born in or whose parents were born in areas of the world with moderate or high endemicity of hepatitis B virus infection.

3. The 4th dose of DTaP (diphtheria and tetanus toxoids and acellular pertussis vaccine) may be administered as early as 12 months of age, provided 6 months have elapsed since the 3rd dose and the child is unlikely to return at age 15 to 18 months. Td (tetanus and diphtheria toxoids) is recommended at 11 to 12 years of age if at least 5 years have elapsed since the last dose of DTP, DTaP, or DT. Subsequent routine Td boosters are recommended every 10 years.

4. Three *Haemophilus influenzae* type b (Hib) conjugate vaccines are licensed for infant use. If PRP-OMP (PedvaxHIB or ComVax [Merck]) is administered at 2 and 4 months of age, a dose at 6 months is not required. Because clinical studies in infants have demonstrated that using some combination products may induce a lower immune response to the Hib vaccine component, DTaP/Hib combination products should not be used for primary immunization in infants at 2, 4, or 6 months of age unless FDA-approved for these ages.

5. To eliminate the risk of vaccine-associated paralytic polio (VAPP), an alt-IPV schedule is now recommended for routine childhood polio vaccination in the United States. All children should receive four doses of IPV at 2 months, 4 months, 6 to 18 months, and 4 to 6 years. OPV (if available) may be used only for the following special circumstances:

1. Mass vaccination campaigns to control outbreaks of paralytic polio.
2. Unvaccinated children who will be traveling in <4 weeks to areas where polio is endemic or epidemic.
3. Children of parents who do not accept the recommended number of vaccine injections. These children may receive OPV only for the third or fourth dose or both; in this situation, health care professionals should administer OPV only after discussing the risk for VAPP with parents or caregivers.
4. During the transition to an all-IPV schedule, recommendations for the use of remaining OPV supplies in physicians' offices and clinics have been issued by the American Academy of Pediatrics (see *Pediatrics*, December 1999).

6. The 2nd dose of measles, mumps, and rubella (MMR) vaccine is recommended routinely at 4 to 6 years of age but may be administered during any visit, provided at least 4 weeks have elapsed since receipt of the 1st dose and that both doses are administered beginning at or after 12 months of age. Those who have not previously received the second dose should complete the schedule by the 11- to 12-year-old visit.

7. Varicella (Var) vaccine is recommended at any visit on or after the first birthday for susceptible children, ie, those who lack a reliable history of chickenpox (as judged by a health care professional) and who have not been immunized. Susceptible persons 13 years of age or older should receive 2 doses, given at least 4 weeks apart.

8. Hepatitis A (Hep A) is shaded to indicate its recommended use in selected states and/or regions; consult your local public health authority. (Also see *MMWR Morb Mortal Wkly Rep.* Oct 01, 1999;48(RR-12):1-37).

Recommended Schedule of Vaccinations for Adolescents Ages 11 to 12 Years

Immunobiologic	Indications	Name	Dose	Frequency	Route
Hepatitis A vaccine	Adolescents who are at increased risk of hepatitis A infection or its complications	HAVRIX ®*	720 EL.U. +/ 0.5 mL‡	A total of two doses at 0,§ 6-12 mo	IM‖
		VAQTA ®*	25 U/0.5 mL	A total of two doses at 0, 6-18 mo	IM
Hepatitis B vaccine	Adolescents not vaccinated previously for hepatitis B	Recombivax HB(R)*	5 µg/0.5 mL	A total of three doses at 0, 1-2, 4-6 mo	IM
		Engerix-B ®*	10 µg/0.5 mL	A total of three doses at 0, 1-2, 4-6 mo	IM
Influenza vaccine	Adolescents who are at increased risk for complication caused by influenza or who have contact with persons at increased risk for these complications	Influenza virus vaccine‖	0.5 mL	Annually (September-December)	IM
Measles, mumps, and rubella vaccine (MMR)	Adolescents not vaccinated previously with two doses of measles vaccine at ≥12 mo of age	MMR II ®*	0.5 mL	One dose	SC#
Pneumococcal polysaccharide vaccine	Adolescents who are at increased risk for pneumococcal disease or its complications	Pneumococcal vaccine polyvalent¶	0.5 mL	One dose	IM or SC

Tetanus and diphtheria toxoids (Td)	Tetanus and diphtheria toxoids, absorbed (for adult use)¶	Adolescents not vaccinated within the previous 5 yr	0.5 mL	Every 10 yr	IM
Varicella virus vaccine	VARIVAX ®*	Adolescents not vaccinated previously and who have no reliable history of chickenpox	0.5 mL	One dose**	SC

*Manufacturer's product name.

†Enzyme-limned immunosorbent assay (ELISA) unit.

‡Alternative dosage and schedule of 360 EL.U./0.5 mL and a total of three doses administered at 0, 1, and 6-12 months.

§0 months represents timing of the initial dose, and subsequent numbers represent months after the initial dose.

‖Intramuscular injection.

¶Generic name.

**Subcutaneous injection.

#Adolescents ≥13 years of age should be administered a total of two doses (0.5 ml/dose) subcutaneously at 0 and 4-8 weeks.

Immunizing Agents and Immunization Schedules for Healthcare Workers*

Generic name	Primary schedule and boosters	Indications	Major precautions and contraindications	Special considerations
Immunizing agents strongly recommended for healthcare workers				
Hepatitis B (HB) recombinant vaccine	Two doses IM 4 weeks apart; third dose 5 months after second; booster doses not necessary.	Preexposure: HCWs at risk for exposure to blood or body fluids.	On the basis of limited data, no risk of adverse effects to developing fetuses is apparent. Pregnancy should not be considered a contraindication to vaccination.	The vaccine produces neither therapeutic nor adverse effects on HBV-infected persons. Prevaccination serologic screening is not indicated for persons being vaccinated because of occupational risk. HCWs who have contact with patients or blood should be tested 1 to 2 months after vaccination to determine serologic response.
Hepatitis B immunoglobulin (HBIG)	0.06 mL/kg IM as soon as possible after exposure. A second dose of HBIG should be administered 1 month later if the HB	Postexposure prophylaxis: For persons exposed to blood or body fluids containing HbsAg and who are not immune to		

Immunobiologic	Schedule	Indications	Contraindications	Special considerations
	vaccine series has not been started.	HBV infection—0.06 mL/kg IM as soon as possible (but no later than 7 days after exposure).		
Influenza vaccine (inactivated whole-virus and split-virus vaccines)	Annual vaccination with current vaccine. Administered IM.	HCWs who have contact with patients at high risk for influenza or its complications; HCWs who work in chronic care facilities; HCWs with high-risk medical conditions or who are aged ≥65 years.	History of anaphylactic hypersensitivity to egg ingestion.	No evidence exists of risk to mother or fetus when the vaccine is administered to a pregnant woman with an underlying high-risk condition. Influenza vaccination is recommended during second and third trimesters of pregnancy because of increased risk for hospitalization.
Measles live-virus vaccine	One dose SC; second dose at least 1 month later.	HCWs born during or after 1957 who do not have documentation of having received 2 doses of live vaccine	Pregnancy; immunocompromised persons including HIV-infected persons who have evidence of severe	MMR is the vaccine of choice if recipients are likely to be susceptible to rubella and/or mumps as well as to measles. Per-

*Persons who provide healthcare to patients or work in institutions that provide patient care, e.g., physicians, nurses, emergency medical personnel, dental professionals and students, medical and nursing students, laboratory technicians, hospital volunteers, and administrative and support staff in healthcare institutions. *HAV,* Hepatitis A virus; *HBV,* hepatitis B virus; *HbsAg,* hepatitis B surface antigen; *HCW,* healthcare worker; *HIV,* human immunodeficiency virus; *IgA,* immunoglobulin A; *ID,* intradermal; *IM,* intramuscular; *MMR,* measles, mumps, rubella vaccine; *SC,* subcutaneous; *TB,* tuberculosis.

Continued

From Stanhope M, Lancaster J: *Community public health nursing,* ed 6, St Louis, 2000, Mosby.

Immunizing Agents and Immunization Schedules for Healthcare Workers*—cont'd

Generic name	Primary schedule and boosters (s)	Indications	Major precautions and contraindications	Special considerations
		on or after the first birthday or a history of physician-diagnosed measles or serologic evidence of immunity.† Vaccination should be considered for all HCWs who lack proof of immunity, including those born before 1957.	immunosuppression;‡ anaphylaxis after gelatin ingestion or administration of neomycin; recent administration of immune globulin.	sons vaccinated during 1963 to 1967 with a killed measles vaccine alone, killed vaccine followed by live vaccine, or with a vaccine of unknown type should be revaccinated with 2 doses of live measles virus vaccine.
Mumps live-virus vaccine	One dose SC; no booster.	HCWs believed to be susceptible can be vaccinated.† Adults born before 1957 can be considered immune.	Pregnancy; immunocompromised persons‡; history of anaphylactic reaction after gelatin ingestion or administration of neomycin.	MMR is the vaccine of choice if recipients are likely to be susceptible to measles and rubella as well as to mumps.
Rubella live-virus vaccine	One dose SC; no booster.	Indicated for HCWs, both men and women, who do not have documentation	Pregnancy; immunocompromised persons‡; history of anaphylactic reaction	The risk for rubella vaccine-associated malformations in the offspring of women pregnant when

		of having received live vaccine on or after their first birthday or laboratory evidence of immunity. Adults born before 1957, except women who can become pregnant, can be considered immune.†	after administration of neomycin.	vaccinated or who become pregnant within 3 months after vaccination is negligible. Such women should be counseled regarding the theoretical basis of concern for the fetus. MMR is the vaccine of choice if recipients are likely to be susceptible to measles or mumps as well as to rubella.
Varicella zoster live-virus vaccine	Two 0.5-mL doses SC 4 to 8 weeks apart if ≥13 years of age.	Indicated for HCWs who do not have either a reliable history of varicella or serologic evidence of immunity.†	Pregnancy, immunocompromised persons‡; history of anaphylactic reaction following receipt of neomycin or gelatin. Avoid salicylate use for 6 weeks after vaccination.	Vaccine is available from the manufacturer for certain patients with acute lymphocytic leukemia (ALL) in remission. Because 71% to 93% of persons without a history of varicella are immune, serologic testing before

†All HCWs (medical or nonmedical, paid or volunteer, full-time or part-time, student or nonstudent, with or without patient-care responsibilities) who work in healthcare institutions (e.g., inpatient and outpatient, public and private) should be immune to measles, rubella, and varicella.

‡Persons immunocompromised because of immunodeficiency disease, HIV infection (who should primarily not receive BCG, OPV, and yellow fever vaccines), leukemia, lymphoma or generalized malignancy, or immunosuppressed as a result of therapy with corticosteroids, alkylating drugs, antimetabolites, or radiation.

Continued

Immunizing Agents and Immunization Schedules for Healthcare Workers*—cont'd

Generic name	Primary schedule and boosters (s)	Indications	Major precautions and contraindications	Special considerations
				vaccination is likely to be cost-effective.
Varicella-zoster (VZIG)	Persons <50 kg: 125 U/10 kg IM, persons ≥50 kg: 625 U§	Persons known or likely to be susceptible (particularly assessing whether to those at high risk for complications, e.g., pregnant women) who have close and prolonged exposure to a contact case or to an infectious hospital staff worker or patient.	Serologic testing may help in immunoglobulin, administer VZIG. If use of VZIG prevents varicella disease, patient should be vaccinated subsequently.	
Bacille Calmette-Guérin (BCG) vaccine (tuberculosis)	One percutaneous dose of 0.3 mL; no booster dose recommended.	Should be considered only for HCWs in areas where multidrug tuberculosis is prevalent, a strong likelihood of infection exists, and where	Should not be administered to immunocompromised persons‡ and pregnant women.	In the United States, tuberculosis-control efforts are directed toward early identification, treatment of cases, and preventive therapy with isoniazid.

Other immunobiologics that are or may be indicated for healthcare workers

		comprehensive infection control precautions have failed to prevent TB transmission to HCWs.		
Immunoglobulin (Hepatitis A)	Postexposure—One IM dose of 0.02 mL/kg administered ≥2 weeks.	Indicated for HCWs exposed to feces of infectious patients.	Contraindicated in persons with IgA deficiency; do not administer within 2 weeks after exposure, after MMR vaccine, or 3 weeks after varicella vaccine. Delay administration of MMR vaccine for ≥3 months and varicella vaccine ≥5 months after administration of IG.	Administer in large muscle mass (deltoid, gluteal).
Hepatitis A vaccine	Two doses of vaccine either 6 to 12 months apart (HAVRIX [R]), or	Not routinely indicated for HCWs in the United States. Persons	History of anaphylactic hypersensitivity to alum or, for HAVRIX	

‡Persons immunocompromised because of immune deficiency disease, HIV infection (who should primarily not receive BCG, OPV, and yellow fever vaccines), leukemia, lymphoma or generalized malignancy, or immunosuppressed as a result of therapy with corticosteroids, alkylating drugs, antimetabolites, or radiation.

§Some experts recommend 125 U/10 kg regardless of total body weight.

Continued

Immunizing Agents and Immunization Schedules for Healthcare Workers*—cont'd

Generic name	Primary schedule and boosters (s)	Indications	Major precautions and contraindications	Special considerations
	6 months apart (VAQTA [R]).	who work with HAV-infected primates or with HAV in a research laboratory setting should be vaccinated.	(R), the preservative 2-phenoxyethanol. The safety of the vaccine in pregnant women has not been determined; the risk associated with vaccination should be weighed against the risk for hepatitis A in women who may be at high risk for exposure to HAV.	
Meningococcal polysaccharide vaccine (tetravalent A, C, W135, and Y)	One dose in volume and by route specified by manufacturer; need for boosters unknown.	Not routinely indicated for HCWs in the United States.	The safety of the vaccine in pregnant women has not been evaluated; it should not be administered during pregnancy unless the risk for infection is high.	

| Typhoid vaccine, IM, SC, and oral | IM vaccine: One 0.5 mL dose, booster 0.5 mL every 2 years. SC vaccine: two 0.5 mL doses, ≥4 weeks apart, booster 0.5 mL SC or 0.1 ID every 3 years if exposure continues. Oral vaccine: Four doses on alternate days. The manufacturer recommends revaccination with the entire four-dose series every 5 years. | Workers in microbiology laboratories who frequently work with *Salmonella typhi* | Severe local or systemic reaction to a previous dose. Ty21a (oral) vaccine should not be administered to immunocompromised persons‡ or to persons receiving antimicrobial agents. | Vaccination should not be considered an alternative to the use of proper procedures when handling specimens and cultures in the laboratory. |
| Vaccinia vaccine (smallpox) | One dose administered with a bifurcated needle; boosters administered every 10 years. | Laboratory workers who directly handle cultures with vaccinia, recombinant vaccinia viruses, or orthopox viruses that infect humans. | The vaccine is contraindicated in pregnancy, in persons with eczema or a history of eczema, and in immunocompromised persons‡ and their household contacts. | Vaccination may be considered for HCWs who have direct contact with contaminated dressings or other infectious material from volunteers in clinical studies involving recombinant vaccinia virus. |

Continued

Immunizing Agents and Immunization Schedules for Healthcare Workers*—cont'd

Generic name	Primary schedule and boosters (s)	Indications	Major precautions and contraindications	Special considerations
Other vaccine-preventable diseases				
Tetanus and diphtheria (toxoids [Td])	Two IM doses 4 weeks apart; third dose 6 to 12 months after second dose; booster every 10 years.	All adults.	Except in the first trimester, pregnancy is not a precaution. History of a neurologic reaction or immediate hypersensitivity reaction after a previous dose. History of severe local (Arthus-type) reaction after a previous dose. Such persons should not receive further routine or emergency doses of Td for 10 years.	Tetanus prophylaxis in wound management‖.
Pneumococcal polysaccharide vaccine (23 valent)	One dose, 0.5 mL, IM or SC; revaccination recommended for those at highest risk	Adults who are at increased risk of pneumococcal disease and its complications	The safety of vaccine in pregnant women has not been evaluated; it should not be admin-	

>5 years after the first dose.	because of underlying health conditions; older adults, especially those age ≥65 who are healthy.	istered during pregnancy unless the risk for infection is high. Previous recipients of any type of pneumococcal polysaccharide vaccine who are at highest risk for fatal infection or antibody loss may be revaccinated ≥5 years after the first dose.

‖See Centers for Disease Control and Prevention: Update on adult immunization: recommendations of the Advisory Committee on Immunization Practices (ACIP), *MMWR* 1991:40(No. RR-12):1-94.

Summary of Sexually Transmitted Diseases

Disease (causative agent)	Symptoms	Mode of transmission	Complications/ community health concerns	Treatment/nursing management
Herpes (herpes simplex virus; HSV 1, oral; HSV 2, genital)	*s/s:* 2-12 days after exposure or may be no symptoms. *1st s/s:* Burning or "prickly" sensation. *2nd:* Clusters of small blisters that rupture and cause painful ulcers. HSV 2 symptoms may include fever and other flulike symptoms. In women, vaginal discharge, painful intercourse, painful urination, and swollen and tender groin glands may be present. *Fetal effects:* Abortion, preterm labor. Birth canal exposure—blindness, brain damage, or death.	Direct contact with oral and genital secretions. Mother → infant transmission at birth. *Communicable:* Most contagious from time sores are present until they heal and scabs fall off; some are contagious without s/s. HSV 1 and HSV 2 viruses have recently been found in genital and oral sites previously thought to be exclusive of one or the other.	*Complications:* Increased risk of cervical cancer (Pap smear every year is recommended). Virus stays dormant in body and successive eruptions occur commonly as a result of stress or other illnesses. Recurrence in infected individuals (usually less severe) places new sexual partners at risk. Recurrence tends to become fewer over the years and stops recurring in some. Protection of sexual partners during infectious periods should be stressed; condom use is important.	Incurable; acyclovir is given to treat existing cases and suppress recurrent episodes. Treatment: Cold compresses (avoid heat as ↑ inflammation). Shorten time between episodes with keeping areas clean (Burow's solution) and dry (well-ventilated clothing). *Prevention:* Cesarean section birth for maternal active herpes. Avoid touching active blisters. Barrier contraceptives (latex condoms).
Cytomegalovirus (CMV)	Usually asymptomatic. If symptomatic, resembles	Transmitted through blood transfusions, organ	Immunosuppressed individuals are at risk for	Vaccine development is experimental and

	mononucleosis. *Fetal effects:* Low IQ, developmental delays, congenital anomalies, mental retardation, deafness, jaundice, hydrocephaly, epilepsy, stillbirth. Symptoms in newborns may not be immediately evident at birth but usually present during the first 6 months.	transplants, breast milk, from children's urine/feces/respiratory tract, and through sexual contact with semen and vaginal secretions. Transplacental transmission.	frequent infectious episodes (i.e., HIV). Transmission is so common that 60% of children in daycare centers have CMV in urine or saliva (usually spread by not washing hands). Virus remains in body for life.	minimally useful to date. *Prevention:* Not practical and not desirable as early infection provides immunity and, in girls, eliminates the risk of acquiring the virus for the first time during pregnancy.
Venereal warts or HPV (human papillomavirus)	Condylomata warts, "cauliflower appearance" in moist areas around sex organs, which may or may not be painful, may or may not be visible. Infants may develop respiratory symptoms.	Close contact with warts; may also be sexually transmitted, which is usual transmission. Passed to infants through the birth canal and found in child's throat or mouth. Usually shows 1-3 months after contact. *Communicable:* As long as the warts are evident.	*Complications:* Most serious complication is the link between the disease and malignancies of the cervix (Pap smear every year recommended) and genital tract. Can block opening to the vagina, urethra, rectum, or throat.	No cure. Cryotherapy, laser therapy, surgical removal, or podophyllin in tincture of benzoin compound to remove or destroy warts. *Prevention:* Abstain from sexual contact, use condoms, wash after contact.

Continued

HIV, human immunodeficiency virus; *s/s*, signs and symptoms.
Compiled by Frances A. Maurer and Gayle Hofland.
Smith C, Maurer F: *Community health nursing: theory and practice*, ed 2, Philadelphia, 2000, WB Saunders.

Summary of Sexually Transmitted Diseases—cont'd

Disease (causative agent)	Symptoms	Mode of transmission	Complications/ community health concerns	Treatment/nursing management
Gonorrhea (*Neisseria gonorrhoea*) (bacteria) Slang: clap, drip, strain	Frequently asymptomatic, 80% women, 10% men. Symptoms: *Women*—Pain, heavy purulent greenish vaginal discharge, pain in the genital and pelvic areas. *Men*—Thick whitish discharge from the penis, pain on urination, urinary frequency. *Rectal site*: Mucous discharge, intense irritation. *Throat site*: s/s sore throat. *Fetal effects*: Premature labor, stillbirth.	Primarily sexual contact. Can be transmitted to mucous membranes other than genitals (throat, rectum, eyes). Mother to infant via passage through birth canal. Signs and symptoms usually in 2 days → 3 weeks after sexual contact.	*Complications*: Include arthritis; blood, meningeal, and heart infections; and sterility. *Women*—Pelvic inflammatory disease (PID), ectopic pregnancy, sterility, premature labor, still birth. *Men*—Narrowing of the urethra and swelling of the testicles. Children born during an active case may contract ophthalmia neonatorum leading to blindness. Incidence is alarmingly high and most prevalent in young adults (15-35 years of age). *Chlamydia* is frequently present with gonorrhea.	One time dose of ceftriaxone, cefixime, ciprofloxacin, or ofloxacin. Antibiotics appropriate to treat for *Chlamydia* and trichomoniasis are often prescribed simultaneously. Test of cure in 4-7 days after treatment ends to ensure treatment effectiveness is especially important because drugresistant strains are becoming more frequent. *Prevention*: Abstain from sexual activity. Use condoms.

Chlamydia (bacteria)	*s/s:* In 5 days or longer, many times asymptomatic. Symptoms consist of other infections such as nongonococcal urethritis, PID, inflammation of cervix, abnormal discharge from penis or vagina, burning with urination, and bleeding between periods. *Fetal effects:* Stillbirth. *Infant effects:* As a result of vaginal delivery; eye/ear infections and pneumonia.	Primarily sexual contact, but infections can occur in other areas of the body if contact is made with the bacteria. Passage through the birth canal.	*Complications:* Women—PID, ectopic pregnancy, sterility, and cervical dysplasia. Men—Prostatitis, epididymitis, and sterility. Frequently occurs with other sexually transmitted diseases, especially gonorrhea. This is the most common, fastest spreading sexually transmitted disease, especially at ages 15-25 years.	Doxycycline, azithromycin, tetracycline, or erythromycin. Test of cure in 4-7 days after treatment is completed. *Prevention:* Abstain from sexual contact, use condoms.
Syphilis *(Treponema pallidum)* (bacteria)	Disease has three stages if left untreated. *First stage:* Chancre at site of infection (genital, rectum, lips); usually painless with contagious fluid. *Second stage:* Occurs 3-6 weeks later; generalized flulike	Sexual contact with chancre. Mother to baby during pregnancy (after 18th week). *Blood testing:* VDRL, RPR.	Incidence is increasing, especially among young adults. *Complications:* blindness, deafness, brain damage/insanity, paralysis, heart disease, and death.	Large-dose IM penicillin; if individual is allergic to penicillin, oral tetracycline or doxycycline is given. Patients must be rescreened at 3, 6, and 12 months because some infections are resistant to treatment.

Continued

Summary of Sexually Transmitted Diseases—cont'd

Disease (causative agent)	Symptoms	Mode of transmission	Complications/ community health concerns	Treatment/nursing management
	symptoms, and may have body rash (esp. soles of feet and palms of hands), sores (mucous patches that are highly infectious), inflamed eyes, and patchy hair loss. *Latent stage:* Signs and symptoms disappear, noninfectious at this point except can pass to baby. *Third stage:* Destruction of body organs (brain, skeleton, heart, and large blood vessels) via lesions called gummas. *Infants infected:* "Congenital syphillis": stillbirth, skeletal deformities, organ defects, can be treated in this stage.			Drug-resistant strains are becoming problematic. *Prevention:* Abstain from sexual activity, use condoms.

Universal Precautions

Instruments
To prevent infection through cuts, punctures, and nonintact skin:

- Needles: Do not recap. Do not bend, break, or remove needle.
- Sharps/instruments: Take care when *using, cleaning,* and *disposing.*
- Disposal: Place disposable needle-syringe unit and sharps into puncture-resistant container *immediately after use.*

Barriers
To prevent infection through eyes, nose, mouth, and nonintact skin:

- Gloves: Use when likely to ***touch*** the body fluids. Gloves are available for phlebotomy. Change after *each* patient contact. Do not reuse exam/surgical gloves. Housekeeping gloves can be reused if intact and properly cleaned.
- Protective eyewear, mask: Use if body fluid ***droplets in the air.***
- Gown: Use if body fluids are likely to ***splash on clothing.***
- Resuscitation bag (or other ventilation device): Use to avoid mouth-to-mouth contact. The barriers you use will require some judgment for exposure risk in each clinical situation.
- Infectious waste-linen: Before transport, bag and label for disposal or decontamination per your local procedures.

Disinfecting

- Hand washing must be immediate and thorough: Before and after *each* contact. After removal of gloves and barriers. After exposure to contamination. Wash other skin surfaces after contact or contamination.
- Spills: Clean and disinfect immediately—per policy.

Training will emphasize how *you* can work safely with hazards on your job to protect yourself, co-workers, and patients.

Adapted from OSHA: *Occupational exposure to bloodborne pathogens* (29 CFR 1910. 1030) Washington, DC, 2000, OSHA.

Universal Blood and Body Fluid Precautions

Because medical history and examination cannot reliably identify all clients infected with HIV or other blood-borne pathogens, blood and body-fluid precautions should be used consistently for *all* clients. This approach, previously recommended by the Centers for Disease Control and Prevention (CDC), referred to as *universal blood and body-fluid precautions* or *universal precautions,* should be used in the care of *all* clients, especially including those in emergency-care settings in which the risk of blood exposure is increased and the client's infection status usually is unknown.

1. All healthcare workers should routinely use appropriate barrier precautions to prevent skin and mucous membrane exposure when contact with blood or other body fluids of any client is anticipated. Gloves should be worn for touching blood and body fluids, mucous membranes, or nonintact skin of all clients; for handling items or surfaces soiled with blood or body fluids; and for performing venipuncture and other vascular access procedures. Gloves should be changed after contact with each client. To prevent exposure of mucous membranes of the mouth, nose, and eyes, masks and protective eye wear or face shields should be worn during procedures that are likely to generate droplets of blood or other body fluids. Gowns or aprons should be worn during procedures that are likely to generate splashes of blood or other body fluids.

2. Hands and other skin surfaces should be washed immediately and thoroughly if contaminated with blood or other body fluids. Hands should be washed immediately after gloves are removed.

3. All healthcare workers should take precautions to prevent injuries caused by needles, scalpels, and other sharp instruments or devices during procedures; when cleaning used instruments; during disposal of used needles; and when handling sharp instruments after procedures. To prevent needle-stick injuries, needles should not be recapped, purposely bent, or broken by hand, removed from disposable syringes, or otherwise manipulated by hand. After they are used, disposable syringes and needles, scalpel blades, and other sharp items should be placed in puncture-resistant containers for disposal; the puncture-

Modified from Centers for Disease Control: Recommendations for prevention of HIV transmission in health-care settings, *MMWR* 36(suppl 2S):35-185, 1987.

resistant containers should be located as close as practical to the use area. Large-bore reusable needles should be placed in a puncture-resistant container for transport to the reprocessing area.

4. Although saliva has not been implicated in HIV transmission, to minimize the need for emergency mouth-to-mouth resuscitation, bags or other ventilation devices should be available for use in areas where the need for resuscitation is likely.

5. Healthcare workers who have exudative lesions or weeping dermatitis should refrain from all direct patient care and from handling equipment for patient care until the condition resolves.

6. Pregnant healthcare workers are not known to be at greater risk for contracting HIV infection than are nonpregnant healthcare workers; however, if HIV infection develops during pregnancy, the infant is at risk of infection as a result of perinatal transmission. Because of this risk, pregnant healthcare workers should be especially familiar with and should strictly adhere to precautions to minimize the risk of HIV transmission.

Implementation of universal blood and body-fluid precautions for *all* clients eliminates the need for use of the isolation category of "blood and body fluid precautions" previously recommended by the CDC for clients known or suspected to be infected with blood-borne pathogens. Isolation precautions (e.g., for enteric and upper respiratory infections) should be used as necessary if associated conditions, such as infectious diarrhea or tuberculosis, are diagnosed or suspected.

These precautions should be used (1) in emergency departments and outpatient settings, including both physicians' and dentists' offices; (2) during cardiac catheterization and angiographic procedures; (3) during a vaginal or cesarean delivery or other invasive obstetric procedure in which bleeding may occur; and (4) during the manipulation, cutting, or removal of any oral or perioral tissues, including tooth structure, in which bleeding occurs or the potential for bleeding exists. The universal blood and body-fluid precautions listed here should be the minimum precautions for *all* invasive procedures.

Transmission of Infectious Agents

Transmission of infectious agents—Any mechanism by which an infectious agent is spread from a source or reservoir to a person. These mechanisms are as follows:

1) **Direct transmission:** Direct and essentially immediate transfer of infectious agents to a receptive portal of entry through which human or animal infection may take place. This may be by direct contact such as touching, biting, kissing, or sexual intercourse, or by the direct projection (droplet spread) of droplet spray onto the conjunctiva or onto the mucous membranes of the eye, nose, or mouth during sneezing, coughing, spitting, singing, or talking (usually limited to a distance of about 1 m or less).

2) **Indirect transmission:**
   a) Vehicle-borne—Contaminated inanimate materials or objects (fomites) such as toys, handkerchiefs, soiled clothes, bedding, cooking or eating utensils, surgical instruments or dressings; water, food, milk, and biological products including blood, serum, plasma, tissues, or organs; or any substance serving as an intermediate means by which an infectious agent is transported and introduced into a susceptible host through a suitable portal of entry. The agent may or may not have multiplied or developed in or on the vehicle before being transmitted.
   b) Vector-borne—(i) Mechanical: Includes simple mechanical carriage by a crawling or flying insect through soiling of its feet or proboscis or by passage of organisms through its gastrointestinal tract. This does not require multiplication or development of the organism. (ii) Biological: Propagation (multiplication), cyclic development, or a combination of these (cyclopropagative) is required before the arthropod can transmit the infective form of the agent to humans. An incubation period (extrinsic) is required following infection before the arthropod becomes **infective.** The infectious agent may be passed vertically to succeeding generations **(transovarian transmission); transstadial transmission** indicates its passage from one stage of life cycle to another, as nymph to adult. Transmission may be by injection of salivary gland fluid during biting, or by regurgitation or deposition on the skin of feces or other material capable of penetrating through the bite wound or through an area of

From Chin J, editor: *Control of communicable diseases manual,* ed 17, Washington, 2000, American Public Health Association.

trauma from scratching or rubbing. This transmission is by an infected nonvertebrate host and not a simple mechanical carriage by a vector as a vehicle. However, an arthropod in either role is termed a *vector.*

3) **Airborne:** The dissemination of microbial aerosols to a suitable portal of entry, usually the respiratory tract. Microbial aerosols are suspensions of particles in the air consisting partially or wholly of microorganisms. They may remain suspended in the air for long periods of time, some retaining and others losing infectivity or virulence. Particles in the 1 to 5 μm range are easily drawn into the alveoli of the lungs and may be retained there. Not considered as airborne are droplets and other large particles that promptly settle out (see Direct transmission, above).

a) Droplet nuclei—Usually the small residues that result from evaporation of fluid from droplets emitted by an infected host (see above). They may also be created purposely by a variety of atomizing devices, or accidentally as in microbiology laboratories or in abattoirs, rendering plants, or autopsy rooms. They usually remain suspended in the air for long periods of time.

b) Dust—The small particles of widely varying size that may arise from soil (as, e.g., fungus spores separated from dry soil by wind or mechanical agitation), clothes, bedding, or contaminated floors.

Insect Vectors of Disease

Mosquitos: malaria, yellow fever, dengue, filariasis, and equine and human encephalitis. Many mosquitos are also fierce biters, even if they do not carry diseases.

Biting flies: sandfly fever, leishmaniasis, bartonellosis, tularemia, African sleeping sickness, and onchocerciasis.

Lice: rickettsial diseases (epidemic typhus and trench fever) and relapsing fever.

Fleas: plague and rickettsial disease (endemic typhus) and some worm diseases.

Ticks: rickettsial diseases (Rocky Mountain spotted fever, Sao Paulo typhus, South African tick fever), tularemia, relapsing fever, tick typhus, Lyme disease, and some forms of encephalitis.

Mites: tsutsugamushi disease and related forms of scrub typhus.

From Edelman CL, Mandle CL: *Health promotion throughout the lifespan,* ed 4, St. Louis, 1998, Mosby.

Insect Vectors of Disease—cont'd

Cone-headed bugs: Chagas' disease.

Miscellaneous nuisance biters: horseflies, stable flies, and bedbugs are fierce biters but are not associated with any diseases.

Houseflies and other non–blood-sucking flies: intestinal infections such as diarrheas, dysenteries, typhoid fever, cholera, yaws, and possibly poliomyelitis. These flies mechanically transmit diseases by contamination of the food supply with human and animal feces or other filth. Cockroaches also have a similar role in the transmission of enteric diseases.

Lyme Disease—Important Facts

What is Lyme disease?

Lyme disease is an illness that is spread to humans by the bite of a tick carrying the infectious agent. This illness will cause a round, red area around the bite within a few days. Many times the victim will also complain of flulike symptoms including headache, fatigue, chills, and fever. If untreated, the illness will become a chronic illness causing problems in the joints, nervous system, and heart.

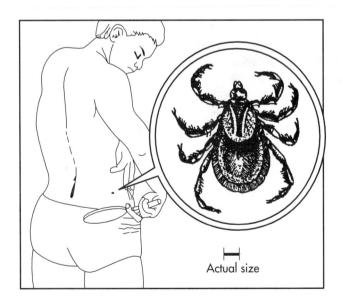

Actual size

From *Mosby's patient teaching guides,* St Louis, 1996, Mosby.

Although this disease has been reported throughout the United States, it is most common in the United States along the northeastern coast, northwestern coast, and in Minnesota and Wisconsin. The ticks that cause Lyme disease are most commonly carried by deer and rats usually found in these locations.

How can I prevent becoming infected with Lyme disease?

- Avoid tick-infested areas. Avoid walking in tall grass or in low brush. Mow grass and remove brush along paths, buildings, and campsites.
- If hiking, wear long pants and long-sleeved shirts tucked into the pants. Wear socks and closed-toe shoes.
- If traveling through brush and tall grass is unavoidable, check your body surfaces every 3 to 4 hours to check for attached ticks.

How should I remove a tick if I find one on my body?

If an attached tick is found, it should be removed promptly.

- To properly remove a tick, use tweezers (not fingers). Grasp the tick as close to your skin as possible, and gently pull the tick straight out. Twisting or jerking the tick body may cause it to break apart before all of it is removed.
- Dispose of the tick in alcohol or flush down a toilet. Do not crush the tick with your fingers.
- After you have removed the tick, wash the area of your body that was bitten with soap and water, and swab the area with an antiseptic.

How can I tell if I have Lyme disease?

If you have been bitten by a tick, especially in the areas of the United States where Lyme disease is most common, you should watch for early symptoms. Within a few days of being bitten, you will notice a red circle around the bite site. Many times the victim of a tick bite will also complain of flulike symptoms including headache, tiredness, chills, and fever. If you develop these symptoms, you should see your healthcare provider for evaluation and, if necessary, treatment. It is important that you do not delay treatment because treatment is most effective in the early stage of the disease.

Lyme Disease—Important Facts—cont'd

What is the treatment for Lyme disease?

If you do contract Lyme disease, you will be given antibiotics. It is very important that you take all of the medication, even if you do not feel ill. Relapses of this disease may occur even after the medication has been taken. Contact your healthcare provider if the symptoms come back after you have finished your medication.

GUIDELINES FOR SELECTED COMMON COMMUNICABLE DISEASES

Lyme Disease

Name:	Lyme borreliosis (Lyme disease). Tickborne disease commonly occurs in the summer in forested areas.
Method of diagnosis:	Diagnosis is based on clinical findings and serologic tests. Typical initial lesion looks like a bull's eye (erythema migrans) that expands in an annular manner. Can lead to neurologic or cardiac symptoms and may be accompanied by fatigue, fever, and stiff neck.
Reservoir:	Wild rodents, deer, and other animals maintain the cycle, with larval and nymphal ticks feeding on small mammals and adult ticks on deer.
Mode of transmission:	Tick-borne. Transmission does not occur until the tick has fed for 24 hours or more.
Incubation:	From 3 to 32 days after tick exposure.
Preventive measures:	Educate the public in mode of transmission by ticks and the means of personal protection. Avoid tick-infested areas. Apply tick repellant (DEET or autan) to pant legs and sleeves. Examine and remove any ticks promptly without crushing.
Control of client:	Isolation—none. Remove all ticks carefully. Early stage can be treated with antibiotics.

Adapted from Chin J, editor: *Control of communicable diseases manual,* ed 17, Washington, 2000, APHA.

Candidiasis (Thrush)

Name:	Candidiasis (Moniliasis, Thrush, Candidosis) A mycosis usually confined to the superficial layers of skin or mucous membranes, that presents clinically as oral thrush, intertrigo, vulvovaginitis, paronychia or onychomycosis. Ulcers or pseudo-membranes may be formed in the esophagus, stomach or intestine.
Method of diagnosis:	Evaluation of both laboratory and clinical evidence of candidiasis. The single most valuable laboratory test is microscopic demonstration of pseudohyphae and/or yeast cells in infected tissue or body fluids. Culture confirmation is important. Severe or recurrent oropharyngeal infection in an adult with no obvious underlying cause should suggest the possibility of HIV infection.
Infectious agents:	*Candida albicans, C. tropicalis, C. dubliniensis* and occasionally other species of *Candida.*
Reservoir:	People.
Mode of transmission:	By contact with secretions or excretions of mouth, skin, vagina, and feces from patients or carriers; by passage from mother to neonate during childbirth; and by endogenous spread.
Incubation:	Variable, 2-5 days for thrush in infants.
Preventive measures:	Detect early and treat locally any infection in the mouth, esophagus or urinary bladder of those with predisposing systemic factors to prevent systemic spread. Fluconazole chemo-prophylaxis decreases the incidence of deep candidiasis during the first 2 months follow-ing allogeneic bone marrow transplantation.
Control of client:	Isolation—None. Concurrent disinfection—Of secretions and contaminated articles
Specific treatment:	Topical nystatin or an azole (miconazole, clotri-mazole, ketoconazole, fluconazole) is useful in many forms of superficial candidiasis. Oral clotrimazole (Mycelex®) troches or nystatin suspension is effective for treatment of oral thrush. Itraconazole suspension (Sporanox®)

Candidiasis (Thrush)—cont'd

or fluconazole (Diflucan®) is effective in oral and esophageal candidiasis. Vaginal infection may be treated with oral fluconazole or topical clotrimazole, miconazole, butoconazole, terconazole, tioconazole, or nystatin.

Chickenpox

Name:	Chickenpox (varicella). This viral disease is rarely fatal; the most common cause of death in adults is primary viral pneumonia, and in children it is septic complications and encephalitis.
Method of diagnosis:	Diagnosis is based on clinical findings and laboratory microscopic examination of virus by electron microscope when required.
Reservoir:	People.
Mode of transmission:	A high rate of transmission from person to person by direct contact, droplet, or airborne spread of respiratory secretions.
Incubation:	From 2 to 3 weeks; commonly 14-16 days.
Preventive measures:	Protect high-risk individuals from exposure.
Control of client:	Isolation—exclude from school for 1 week after eruption first appears. Concurrent disinfection—articles soiled by discharges from nose, throat, and lesions.
	Specific treatment—While both vidarabine (adenine arabinoside, Ara-A®) and acyclovir (Zovirax®) are effective in treating varicella-zoster infections, the latter is generally considered the antiviral agent of choice for treatment of varicella. For herpes zoster, newer analogues with improved absorption after oral administration are available (valacyclovir and famcyclovir). These medications may shorten the duration of symptoms and pain of zoster in the normal older patient, especially if administered within 24 hours of rash onset.

Acute Conjunctivitis

Name: Conjunctivitis (pink eye). A common nonfatal bacterial infection of the eye.

Method of diagnosis: Confirmation of clinical diagnosis by microscopic examination of a stained smear or culture of the discharge is required to differentiate bacterial from viral or allergic conjunctivitis, or infection by adenovirus or enterovirus.

Reservoir: People.

Mode of transmission: Contact with discharges from eye or upper respiratory tract of infected person. Contaminated fingers. Clothing or other articles including shared eye makeup applicators, multiple-dose eye medication droppers.

Incubation: Usually 24 to 72 hours.

Preventive measures: Personal hygiene and treatment of affected eyes

Control of client: Isolation—exclude children from school during acute stage. Drainage and secretion precautions. Concurrent disinfection of discharge and soiled articles.
Immunization—none.

Specific treatment: Local application of an ointment or drops containing a sulfonamide, such as sodium sulfacetamide, gentamicin or combination antibiotics, such as polymyxin B with neomycin or trimethoprim is generally effective.

Tinea (Ringworm)

Name: Dermatophytosis (tinea, ringworm). Common fungal infection that can occur on the scalp, under nails, on the body, groin or perianal area, and the feet.

Method of diagnosis: Clinical observation of lesions. Scalp—mousy odor and yellow crusts on scalp. Nails—nail thickens, discolors, and is brittle with

Tinea (Ringworm)—cont'd

	buildup of caseous material under nail. Nail becomes chalky and disintegrates. Feet—scaling, cracking of skin between toes and blisters containing a thin, watery fluid. Laboratory examination of scalp under ultraviolet lamp (Wood's lamp) for yellow-green fluorescence. For nails, body, and feet, scrapings in potassium hydroxide preparation and microscopic examination for hyaline fungal elements.
Reservoir:	Scalp—people, animals (especially dogs, cats, cattle). Nails—people. Body—people, animals, soil. Feet—people.
Mode of transmission:	Scalp—direct skin-to-skin contact or indirectly from contaminated barber's clippers, combs. Nails, body, feet—direct contact from infected person or indirectly from contaminated shower stalls or floors. Also body infection may be caused from lesions of animals.
Incubation:	Scalp—10 to 14 days. Nails—unknown. Body—4 to 10 days. Feet—unknown.
Preventive measures:	Educate people not to use combs or brushes of others, strict personal hygiene. Launder clothes and towels with hot water or fungicidal agent. Clean shower floors with cresol.
Control of client:	Griseofulvin by mouth is treatment choice for scalp. Topical antifungal powders or ointments is treatment of choice for body/groin and feet, although griseofulvin is effective. For nails the treatment of choice is oral itraconazole and terbinafine for 3-18 months.

Enterobiasis (Pinworm)

Name:	Enterobiasis (pinworm disease). Pinworms are a common intestinal infection, usually benign and highly contagious.

Method of diagnosis: Diagnosis is made by applying transparent adhesive tape to the perianal region and examining the tape microscopically for eggs.

Reservoir: People. Pinworms in animals are not transmissible to people.

Mode of transmission: Direct transfer of infective eggs by hand from anus to mouth or indirectly through clothing, bedding, food, or other articles contaminated with eggs.

Incubation: Life cycle is 4 to 6 weeks. Eggs become infective within a few hours after being deposited at the anus and survive less than 2 weeks outside the host.

Preventive measures: Remove sources of infection by treatment. Daily morning showering preferred to tub baths. Frequent change to clean underclothing, night clothes, and bed sheets. Clean/vacuum house daily for several days after treatment. Education in personal hygiene, especially the need to wash hands before eating or preparing food. Avoid scratching bare anal area and nail biting. Reduce overcrowding in living arrangements. Keep toilets clean.

Control of client: Isolation—none. Concurrent disinfection— change bed linens and underwear carefully to avoid dispersing eggs into the air. Eggs killed at temperatures of 131° F for a few seconds; vacuum sleeping and living area daily for several days.

Specific treatment—Pyrantel pamoate (Antiminth®, Combantrin®), mebendazole (Vermox®) or albendazole (Zentel®). Treatment should be repeated after 2 weeks; concurrent treatment of the whole family may be advisable if several members are infected.

Ascarias (Roundworm)

Name:	Ascarias (roundworm infection). A common infection of the small intestine with few or no symptoms.
Method of diagnosis:	Microscopic examination of eggs in feces or observation of adult if worms passed from anus, nose, or mouth.
Reservoir:	People or soil infected with roundworm eggs.
Mode of transmission:	Ingestion of infective eggs from soil contaminated with feces. Not from person to person. Contaminated soil may be carried on feet or footwear.
Incubation:	Life cycle requires 4 to 8 weeks to complete.
Preventive measures:	Educate the public to use toilet facilities. Provide proper disposal of feces, and prevent soil contamination in areas near homes or where children play. Good hand washing before eating or handling food.
Control of client:	Isolation—none. Specific antihelminthic medications.

Foodborne Intoxications and Inspections

Foodborne diseases, including foodborne intoxications and foodborne infections, are terms applied to illnesses acquired by consumption of contaminated food; they are frequently and inaccurately referred to as food poisoning. Frequent causes of foodborne illnesses are: (1) toxins elaborated by bacterial growth in the food before consumption (*Clostridium botulinum, Staphylococcus aureus, Bacillus cereus,* scombroid fish poisoning) or in the intestines (*Clostridium perfringens*); (2) bacterial, viral, or parasitic infections, Rotavirus and salmonellosis; and (3) toxins produced by harmful algae species (ciguatera fish poisoning).

Foodborne disease outbreaks are recognized by the occurrence of illness within a usually short but variable period of time (from a few hours to a few weeks) after a meal, among individuals who have consumed foods in common. Prompt and thorough laboratory evaluation of cases and implicated foods is essential. Single cases of foodborne disease are difficult to identify unless, as in botulism, there is a distinctive clinical syndrome. Foodborne disease may be one of the most common causes of acute illness; many cases and outbreaks are unrecognized and unreported.

Prevention and control of these diseases, regardless of the specific cause, are based on the same principles: avoidance of food contamination, destruction or denaturation of the contaminants, and prevention of further spread or multiplication of contaminants. Ultimately, prevention depends on educating food handlers about proper practices in cooking and storage of food and personal hygiene. Toward this end, World Health Organization (WHO) has developed "Ten Golden Rules for Safe Food Preparation." These are as follows:

1. Choose foods processed for safety.
2. Cook food thoroughly.
3. Eat cooked foods immediately.
4. Store cooked foods carefully.
5. Reheat cooked foods thoroughly.
6. Avoid contact between raw food and cooked food.
7. Wash hands repeatedly.
8. Keep all kitchen surfaces meticulously clean.
9. Protect food from insects, rodents and other animals.
10. Use safe water.

Name:	**Staphylococcal food intoxication** *(Staphylococcus aureus).* An intoxication (not an infection) of abrupt and sometimes violent onset, with severe nausea, cramps, vomiting and prostration, often accompanied by diarrhea, and sometimes with subnormal temperature and lowered blood pressure.
Method of diagnosis:	Diagnosis is easier when a group of cases is seen with the characteristic acute, predominantly upper gastrointestinal (GI) symptoms and the short interval between eating a common food item and the onset of symptoms.
Reservoir:	People in most instances; occasionally cows with infected udders, as well as dogs and fowl.
Mode of transmission:	By ingestion of a food product containing staphylococcal enterotoxin. Foods involved are particularly those that come in contact with food handlers' hands, either without subsequent cooking or with inadequate heating or refrigeration, such as pastries,

custards, salad dressings, sandwiches, sliced meat and meat products.

Incubation period: Interval between eating food and onset of symptoms is 30 minutes to 8 hours, usually 2-4 hours.

Preventive measures:
1) Educate food handlers about: (a) strict food hygiene, sanitation and cleanliness of kitchens, proper temperature control, hand-washing, cleaning of fingernails; and (b) the danger of working with exposed skin, nose or eye infections and uncovered wounds.
2) Reduce food handling time (initial prepa-ration to service) to an absolute minimum, with no more than 4 hours at ambient temperature. Keep perishable foods **hot** (greater than 60° C/140° F) or **cold** (below 10° C/50° F; best is less than 4° C/39° F).
3) Temporarily exclude people with boils, abscesses and other purulent lesions of hands, face or nose from food handling.

Control of client, contacts, and the immediate environment:
1) Report to local health authority: Obligatory report of outbreaks of suspected or confirmed cases.
2) Specific treatment—Fluid replacement when indicated.

Epidemic measures:
1) By quick review of reported cases, determine time and place of exposure and the population at risk; obtain a complete listing of the foods served and embargo, under refrigeration, all foods still available. The prominent clinical features, coupled with an estimate of the incubation period, provide useful leads to the most probable etiologic agent. Collect specimens of feces and vomitus for laboratory examination; alert the laboratory to suspected etiologic agents. Interview a random sample of those exposed. Compare the attack rates for specific food items eaten and not eaten; the implicated food item(s) will usually have the greatest difference in attack rates. Most of the sick will have eaten the contaminated food.

2) Inquire about the origin of the incriminated food and the manner of its preparation and storage before serving. Look for possible sources of contamination and periods of inadequate refrigeration and heating that would permit growth of staphylococci. Submit any leftover suspected foods promptly for laboratory examination; failure to isolate staphylococci does not exclude the presence of the heat-resistant enterotoxin if the food had been heated.

3) Search for food handlers with skin infections, particularly of the hands. Culture all purulent lesions and collect nasal swabs from all foodhandlers. Antibiograms and/or phage typing of representative strains of enterotoxin producing staphylococci isolated from foods and food handlers and from vomitus or feces of patients may be helpful.

Disaster implications: A potential hazard in situations involving mass feeding and lack of refrigeration facilities. A particular problem of air travel.

International measures: WHO Collaborating Centres.

Name: ***Clostridium Perfringens* food intoxication** (*C. welchii* food poisoning, Enteritis necroticans, Pigbel). An intestinal disorder characterized by sudden onset of colic followed by diarrhea; nausea is common, but vomiting and fever are usually absent. Generally a mild disease of short duration, 1 day or less, and rarely fatal in healthy people.

Methods of diagnosis: When necessary, demonstration of *C. perfringens* in semiquantitative anaerobic cultures of food (10^5/g or greater) or patients' stool (10^6/g or greater) in addition to clinical and epidemiologic evidence. Detection of enterotoxin in the stool of ill persons also confirms the diagnosis.

Reservoir: Soil; also the GI tract of healthy people and animals (cattle, pigs, poultry and fish).

Mode of transmission: Ingestion of food that was contaminated by soil or feces and then held under conditions that permit multiplication of the organism. Almost all outbreaks are associated with inadequately heated or reheated meats, usually stews, meat pies, and gravies made of beef, turkey or chicken. Spores survive normal cooking temperatures. Outbreaks are usually traced to food catering firms, restaurants, cafeterias and schools that have inadequate cooling and refrigeration facilities for large-scale service.

Incubation period: From 6 to 24 hours, usually 10-12 hours.

Preventive measures: 1) Educate food handlers about the risks inherent in large scale cooking, especially of meat dishes. Where possible, encourage serving hot dishes while still hot from initial cooking.

2) Serve meat dishes hot, as soon as they are cooked, or cool them rapidly in a properly designed chiller and refrigerate until serving time; reheating, if necessary, should be thorough (internal temperature of at least 70° C/158° F, preferably 75° C/167° F or higher) and rapid.

Control of client: See *Control of Staphylococcal Intoxication.*

Name: ***Bacillus cereus* food intoxication**
An intoxication characterized in some cases by sudden onset of nausea and vomiting, and in others by colic and diarrhea. Illness generally persists no longer than 24 hours and is rarely fatal.

Method of diagnosis: When necessary, it is confirmed by performing quantitative cultures with selective media to estimate the number of organisms present in the suspected food (generally more than 10^5 organisms per gram of the incriminated food are required).

Reservoir: A ubiquitous organism in soil and the environment commonly found at low levels in raw, dried, and processed foods.

Mode of transmission: Ingestion of food that has been kept at ambient temperatures after cooking, permitting multiplication of the organisms. Most commonly associated with cooked rice that had subsequently been held at ambient room temperatures before reheating.

Incubation period: From 1 to 6 hours in cases where vomiting is the predominant symptom; from 6 to 24 hours where diarrhea is predominant.

Preventive measures: Foods should not remain at ambient temperature after cooking. Refrigerate leftover food promptly; reheat thoroughly and rapidly to avoid multiplication of microorganisms.

Control of client: See *Staphylococcal Food Intoxication.*

Name: **Scombroid fish poisoning** (Histamine poisoning). A syndrome of tingling and burning sensations around the mouth, facial flushing and sweating, nausea and vomiting, headache, palpitations, dizziness and rash that occur within a few hours after eating fish containing high levels of free histamine (more than 20 mg/100 g of fish); this occurs when the fish has undergone bacterial decomposition after capture. Risks appear to be greatest for fish imported from tropical or semitropical areas and fish caught by recreational fishermen, who may lack appropriate storage facilities for large fish.

Method of diagnosis: Confirmed by detection of histamine in epidemiologically implicated fish.

Control of client: Symptoms usually resolve spontaneously. In severe cases, antihistamines may be effective in relieving symptoms. There are no long-term sequelae.

Preventive measures: Adequate refrigeration of caught fish.

Name: **Ciguatera fish poisoning**
A syndrome of characteristic GI and neurologic symptoms may occur within 1 hour after eating tropical reef fish. This syndrome is caused by the presence in the fish of toxins elaborated by the dino-flagellate *Gambierdiscus toxicus* and other algae that grow on reefs under the sea.

Ciguatera is a significant cause of morbidity in areas in which consumption of reef fish is common—the Caribbean, southern Florida, Hawaii, the South Pacific, and Australia.

Preventive measures: The consumption of large predatory fish should be avoided, especially in the reef area. If available, "high-risk" fish should be screened before their consumption. The occurrence of toxic fish is sporadic and not all fish of a given species or from a given locale will be toxic.

Control of client: Intravenous infusion of mannitol (1 g/kg of a 20% solution, infused over 45 minutes) may have a dramatic effect on acute symptoms of ciguatera fish poisoning, particularly in severe cases.

Name: **Foodborne and intestinal botulism**
(Foodborne [the classic form] and intestinal [infant and adult] botulism.)
Foodborne botulism is a severe intoxication resulting from ingestion of contaminated food. The illness is characterized by acute bilateral cranial nerve impairment and descending weakness or paralysis.
Intestinal botulism is the most common form of botulism in the US; it results from ingestion of *Clostridium botulinum* spores with subsequent outgrowth. It affects infants under 1 year of age almost exclusively, but can affect adults who have altered GI anatomy and microflora. The illness typically begins with constipation, followed by lethargy, listlessness, poor feeding, ptosis, difficulty swallowing, loss of head control, hypotonia extending to generalized weakness ("floppy baby").

Method of diagnosis: Foodborne botulism made by demonstration of *C. botulinum* toxin in serum, stool, gastric aspirate or incriminated food; or by culture of *C. botulinum* from gastric aspirate or stool in a clinical case. Intestinal botulism established by identification of *C. botulinum*

	organisms and/or toxin in patient's feces or in autopsy specimens.
Reservoir:	Spores are ubiquitous in soil worldwide; they are frequently recovered from agricultural products, including honey. Spores are also found in marine sediments and in the intestinal tract of animals, including fish.
Mode of transmission:	Foodborne botulism is acquired by ingestion of food in which toxin has been formed, predominantly after inadequate heating during preservation and without subsequent adequate cooking. Most poisonings in the US are due to home-canned vegetables and fruits; meat is an infrequent vehicle. Intestinal botulism arises from ingestion of botulinum spores that then germinate in the colon, rather than by ingestion of preformed toxin. Possible sources of spores for infants are multiple, and include foods and dust. Honey, fed on occasion to infants, can contain *C. botulinum* spores.
Incubation period:	Neurologic symptoms of foodborne botulism usually appear within 12-36 hours, sometimes several days, after eating contaminated food. In general, the shorter the incubation period, the more severe the disease and the higher the case-fatality rate. The incubation period of intestinal botulism in infants is unknown, since the precise time that the infant ingested the causal botulinum spores cannot be determined.
Preventive measures:	Ensure effective control of processing and preparation of commercially canned and preserved foods. Educate those concerned with home canning and other food preservation techniques regarding the proper time, pressure, and temperature required to destroy spores, the need for adequately refrigerated storage of incompletely processed foods, and the effectiveness of boiling, with stirring, home canned vegetables for at least 10 minutes to destroy botulinum toxins.

Bulging containers should not be opened, and foods with off-odors should not be eaten or "taste tested." Commercial cans with bulging lids should be returned unopened to the vendor. Although *C. botulinum* spores are ubiquitous, identified sources such as honey, should not be fed to infants.

Control of client:

1) Report to local health authority: Immediate telephone report indicated.

2) Isolation: Not required, but handwashing is indicated after handling soiled diapers.

3) Concurrent disinfection: The implicated food(s) should be detoxified by boiling before discarding, or the containers broken and buried deeply in soil to prevent ingestion by animals. Contaminated utensils should be sterilized by boiling.

3) Specific treatment: Intravenous administration as soon as possible of 1 vial of polyvalent (AB or ABE) botulinum antitoxin, available from CDC, Atlanta, through state health departments is considered a part of routine treatment (the emergency telephone number at CDC for botulism calls during regular office hours is 404-639-2206; and after hours and on weekends is 404-639-2888). Serum should be collected to identify the specific toxin before antitoxin is administered, but antitoxin should not be withheld pending test results. Most important is immediate access to an intensive care unit so that respiratory failure, the usual cause of death, can be anticipated and managed promptly.

In intestinal botulism, meticulous supportive care is essential. Equine botulinum antitoxin is not used because of the hazard of sensitization and anaphylaxis. An investigational human derived botulinal immunoglobulin (BIg) is currently available for the treatment only of infant botulism patients under an FDA-approved open-label Treatment Investigational New Drug protocol from the California Department of Health Services. Antibiotics do not improve the course of the disease, and aminoglycoside antibiotics in particular may worsen it by causing a synergistic neuromuscular blockade. Thus, antibiotics should be used only to treat secondary infections. Assisted respiration may be required.

Name: **Rotaviral enteritis** (Sporadic viral gastroenteritis, severe viral gastroenteritis of infants and children).

A sporadic, seasonal, often severe gastroenteritis of infants and young children, characterized by vomiting, fever, and watery diarrhea. Rotaviral enteritis is occasionally associated with severe dehydration and death in young children.

Method of diagnosis: Rotavirus can be identified in stool specimens or rectal swabs by EM, ELISA, LA, and other immunologic techniques for which commercial kits are available.

Reservoir: Probably humans. The animal viruses do not produce disease in humans.

Mode of transmission: Probably fecal-oral with possible contact or respiratory spread. Although rotaviruses do not effectively multiply in the respiratory tract, they may be encountered in respiratory secretions. There is some evidence that rotavirus may be present in contaminated water.

Incubation period: Approximately 24-72 hours.

Preventive measures: In August 1998, an oral, live, tetravalent, rhesus-based rotavirus vaccine (RRV-TV) was licensed for use among infants in the US. This vaccine should be administered to infants between the ages of 6 weeks and 1 year. The recommended schedule is a three-dose series, with doses to be administered at ages 2, 4 and 6 months.

Intussusception (a bowel obstruction in which one segment of bowel becomes enfolded within another segment) was identified in prelicensure trials as a potential problem associated with RRV-TV. The most current vaccine recommendations will be posted on the CDC immunization website and on the CCDM website (see the Community Resources list in Part 1 for information on how to access these websites). The effectiveness of other preventive measures is undetermined. Hygienic measures applicable to diseases transmitted via the fecal-oral route may not be effective in preventing transmission. The virus survives for long periods on hard surfaces, in contaminated water, and on hands. It is relatively resistant to commonly used disinfectants but is inactivated by chlorine.

In day care, dressing infants with overalls to cover diapers has been demonstrated to decrease transmission of the infection.

Prevent exposure of infants and young children to individuals with acute gastroenteritis in family and institutional (day care or hospital) settings by a high level of sanitary practices; exclusion from day care centers is not necessary.

Passive immunization by oral administration of Ig has been shown to protect low birthweight neonates and immunocompromised children. Breast-feeding does not affect infection rates, but may reduce the severity of the gastroenteritis.

Control of client: Isolation: Enteric precautions, with frequent handwashing by caretakers of infants.

Concurrent disinfection: Sanitary disposal of diapers; place overalls over diapers to prevent leakage.

Quarantine: None.

Specific treatment: None. Oral rehydration therapy with oral glucose-electrolyte solution is adequate in most cases. Parenteral fluids are needed in cases with vascular collapse or uncontrolled vomiting. Antibiotics and antimotility drugs are contraindicated.

Name: **Salmonellosis**

A bacterial disease commonly manifested by an acute enterocolitis, with sudden onset of headache, abdominal pain, diarrhea, nausea, and sometimes vomiting. Dehydration, especially among infants or in the elderly, may be severe. Fever is almost always present. However, morbidity and associated costs of salmonellosis may be high.

Method of diagnosis: *Salmonella* may be isolated on enteric media from feces and blood. Specimens should be collected over several days, because excretion of the organisms may be intermittent. Serologic tests are not useful in diagnosis.

Reservoir: A wide range of domestic and wild animals, including poultry, swine, cattle, rodents, and pets such as iguanas, tortoises, turtles, terrapins, chicks, dogs, and cats.

Mode of transmission: By ingestion of the organisms in food derived from infected animals or contaminated by feces of an infected animal or person. This includes raw and undercooked (inadequate time for a given temperature) eggs and egg products, raw milk and raw milk products, contaminated water, meat and meat products, poultry and poultry products. In addition, pet turtles, iguanas, and chicks, and unsterilized pharmaceuticals of animal origin are potential sources of these bacteria.

Incubation period: From 6 to 72 hours, usually about 12-36 hours.

Preventive measures: 1) Educate food handlers and preparers about the importance of

    a) hand-washing before, during and after food preparation;

    b) refrigerating prepared foods in small containers;

    c) thoroughly cooking all foodstuffs derived from animal sources, particularly poultry, pork, egg products and meat dishes;

    d) avoiding recontamination within the kitchen after cooking is completed; and

e) maintaining a sanitary kitchen and protecting prepared foods against rodent and insect contamination.

2) Educate the public to avoid consuming raw or incompletely cooked eggs, as in eggs cooked "over easy" or "sunny side up," in eggnogs or homemade ice cream, and using dirty or cracked eggs.

3) Recognize the risk of *Salmonella* infections in pets. Chicks, ducklings, and turtles are particularly dangerous pets for small children.

Control of client:

1) Report to local health authority.

2) Isolation: Exclude symptomatic individuals from food handling and from direct care of infants, elderly, immunocompromised, and institutionalized patients. Proper handwashing should be stressed.

3) Concurrent disinfection: Of feces and articles soiled therewith.

4) Quarantine: None.

5) Specific treatment: For uncomplicated enterocolitis, none generally indicated except rehydration and electrolyte replacement with oral rehydration solution. Antibiotics may not eliminate the carrier state and may lead to resistant strains or more severe infections. However, infants under 2 months of age, the elderly, the debilitated, those with sickle cell disease, persons infected with HIV, or patients with continued or high fever or manifestations of extraintestinal infection should be given antibiotic therapy. In adults, ciprofloxacin is highly effective but its use is not approved for children; ampicillin or amoxicillin may also be used. TMP-SMX and chloramphenicol are alternatives when antimicrobial resistant strains are involved. Patients infected with HIV may require life-long therapy to prevent *Salmonella* septicemia.

Scabies

Name:	Scabies. A parasitic infection of the skin caused by a mite.
Method of diagnosis:	Recover the mite from its burrows and examine with microscope.
Reservoir:	People.
Mode of transmission:	Transfer of parasite is direct skin-to-skin contact. Can be transmitted through sexual contact.
Incubation:	2 to 6 weeks before onset of itching in persons without previous exposure, 1 to 4 days after reexposure.
Preventive measures:	Isolation—exclude infested individuals from school or work until the day after treatment. Educate the public for good hygiene. Launder underwear, clothing, and bed sheets used in the 48 hours before treatment.
Control of client:	Specific treatment: The treatment of choice for children is 5% permethrin. Alternatively, apply 1% gamma benzene hexachloride (lindane and Kwell® are contraindicated in premature neonates and used with caution in infants less than 1 year of age and in pregnant women); crotamiton (Eurax®). On the next day, a cleansing bath is taken and a change made to fresh clothing and bed-clothes. Itching may persist for 1-2 weeks; during this period it should not be regarded as a sign of drug failure or reinfestation. Overtreatment is common and should be avoided because of toxicity of some of these agents, especially gamma benzene hexachloride. In about 5% of cases, a second course of treatment may be necessary after an interval of 7-10 days if eggs survived the first treatment. Close supervision of treatment, including bathing, is necessary.

Roseola

Name:	Exanthema subitum (roseola—sixth disease). An acute viral infection characterized by fever and rash, usually in children under 4 years of age; nonthreatening.
Method of diagnosis:	Clinical observation of a maculopapular rash and high fever.
Reservoir:	People.
Mode of transmission:	Not well delineated.
Incubation:	About 10 days.
Control of client:	Educate the public to use good hygiene and hand-washing techniques to reduce infections. No specific treatment.

Rubella

Name:	Rubella (German measles). A mild febrile, viral infectious disease with a diffuse maculopapular rash sometimes resembling that of measles or scarlet fever.
Method of diagnosis:	Clinical observation and laboratory testing.
Reservoir:	People.
Mode of transmission:	Airborne droplet spread of nasopharyngeal secretions.
Incubation:	14-18 days; can range 14-21 days.
Preventive measures:	Vaccinated with live attenuated vaccine. Educate public to encourage immunizations. Avoid contact with respiratory secretions of infected individual.
Control of client:	Report to local health authority. Keep children out of school at least 7 days after appearance of rash.

Measles (Rubeola)

Name:	Measles. Hard measles or red measles.
Method of diagnosis:	Clinical observation and epidemiologic grounds, although blood test for antibody level is preferred.

Reservoir:	People.
Mode of transmission:	Airborne by droplet spread, direct contact with nasal or throat secretion of infected persons.
Incubation:	About 10 days but may be 7-18 days from exposure to onset of fever, usually 14 days until rash appears.
Preventive measures:	Vaccinate with live attenuated vaccine. Avoid respiratory secretions of infected individual. Educate the public to encourage immunization.
Control of client:	Report to health authority. Children should be kept out of school for at least 4 days after rash appears.

Giardiasis

Name:	Giardiasis. A protozoa infection of the upper small intestine often asymptomatic but may result in a variety of intestinal symptoms. Highly associated with drinking water.
Method of diagnosis:	Diagnosed by identifying cysts or trophozoites in feces under a microscope.
Reservoir:	People and possibly beaver and other wild or domestic animals.
Mode of transmission:	Ingestion of cysts in fecally contaminated water. Person-to-person transmission occurs by hand-to-mouth transfer of cysts from feces of an infected person.
Incubation:	3 to 25 days or longer, median 7 to 10 days.
Preventive measures:	Protect public water supplies at risk of human or animal fecal contamination. Sanitary disposal of feces. Boil water or treat with bleach or iodine before drinking. Educate the public about good hand washing, especially child care personnel.
Control of client:	Isolation—enteric precautions. Concurrent disinfection—sewage disposal system for feces. Treatment with flagyl or quinacrine.

Herpes Varicella

Name: Herpes varicella (shingles). Local evidence of inflammation and blistering along sensory nerve. Not life threatening, but lesions are painful. Occurs mostly in older adults. The same virus that causes chickenpox.

Method of diagnosis: Clinical presentation and laboratory microscopic visualization of virus or isolation of virus in tissue culture.

Reservoir: People.

Mode of transmission: A low rate of transmission from vesicle fluid.

Incubation: From 2 to 3 weeks.

Preventive measures: Protect high-risk individuals from exposure.

Control of client: Isolation—none. Concurrent disinfection—articles soiled by discharges from lesions.

Immunization—none. Specific treatment—vidarabine and acyclovir are effective in the treatment of varicella with the latter being the treatment of choice.

Mumps

Name: Mumps. An acute viral infection of the salivary glands.

Method of diagnosis: Clinical observation. Occasionally blood test may be used.

Reservoir: People.

Mode of transmission: By droplet spread and direct contact with saliva of an infected person.

Incubation: Range 14-25 days—usually 15-18 days.

Preventive measures: Administer live attenuated vaccine anytime after 1 year of age. Avoid contact with nose and throat secretions of infected individuals. Educate the public to encourage immunization.

Control of client: Respiratory isolation for 9 days from onset of swelling. Concurrent disinfection of articles soiled with nose and throat secretions.

Tuberculosis

Name:	Tuberculosis (TB). A mycobacterial disease usually affecting the lungs but will infect other organs. The initial infection often goes unnoticed.
Method of diagnosis:	Acid-fast bacilli from sputum observed under microscope.
Reservoir:	People, occasionally cattle, badgers, and other mammals.
Mode of transmission:	Exposure to tubercle bacilli in airborne droplets from nasopharyngeal secretions of infected person.
Incubation:	From infection to a primary lesion in 2 to 10 weeks. Can remain latent for years.
Preventive measures:	1) Promptly identify, diagnose and treat potentially infectious patients with TB. Establish case finding and treatment facilities for infectious cases to reduce transmission.
	2) Make available medical, laboratory, and x-ray facilities for prompt examination of patients, contacts, and suspects; facilities for early treatment of cases and people at high risk for infection; and beds for those needing hospitalization.
Control of client:	1) Report to local health authority when diagnosis is suspected. Case report should indicate if it is bacteriologically positive or based on positive tuberculin reaction and clinical and/or x-ray findings.
	2) Isolation: For pulmonary tuberculosis, control of infectivity is best achieved by prompt specific drug therapy, which usually produces sputum conversion within 4-8 weeks. Patient should be taught to cover both mouth and nose when coughing or sneezing. The need to adhere to the prescribed chemotherapeutic regimen must be emphasized repeatedly to all patients. Directly observed therapy should be used when logistically and financially feasible and in particular for persons with suspected drug resistance, a previous history of poor

compliance to therapy, or who live in conditions in which relapse would result in exposure of many other persons.

3) Concurrent disinfection: Handwashing and good housekeeping practices should be maintained according to routine.

4) Quarantine: None.

5) Management of contacts: In the US, preventive treatment for 3 months is recommended for skin test negative close contacts; the skin test should then be repeated to determine the need for additional preventive therapy.

Specific treatment: Directly observed therapy is highly effective and is recommended for treatment of TB. Treatment is a 6 month regimen consisting of isoniazid (INH), rifampin (RIF), and pyrazinamide (PZA) is recommended for the first 2 months followed by INH and PZA for 4 months. A four-drug initial therapy (including ethambutol (EMB) or streptomycin (SM)) is recommended if the infection was acquired in areas where an increased prevalence of INH resistance has been reported. After drug susceptibility results are available, a specific drug regimen can be selected.

Pediculosis

Name:	Pediculosis (lice). A common infestation of the head, pubic area, or clothing seams.
Method of diagnosis:	Clinical observation. Nit egg can be seen and verified under a microscope.
Reservoir:	Infested people.
Mode of transmission:	Direct contact with an infested person.
Incubation:	Eggs of lice hatch in 7-10 days. The egg to egg life cycle of lice is about 3 weeks. Nits can remain viable for about 1 month but must feed from human host within 24 hours of hatching.

Preventive measures:
1) Educate the public on the value of destroying eggs and lice by early detection, safe and thorough treatment of the hair, laundering clothing and bedding in hot water (55°C or 131°F for 20 min), dry cleaning or setting dryers at hot cycle.
2) Avoid physical contact with infested individuals and their belongings, especially clothing and bedding.
3) Perform regular, direct inspection of children in a group setting for head lice and, when indicated, of body and clothing for body lice.
4) In high-risk situations, use appropriate repellents on hair, skin and clothing.

Control of client: Isolation—physical contact isolation for 24 hours after application of effective insecticide. Examination of household and other close contacts. Laundering of infected clothes, bedding, cosmetic articles. Use Kwell, Pyrinate, RID, or similar agent, and repeat in 10 days.

Pertussis

Name: Pertussis (whooping cough). An acute bacterial respiratory illness resulting in paroxysmal coughing.

Method of diagnosis: Diagnosis based on microscopic examination of secretions swabbed from the nasopharynx.

Reservoir: Infected people.

Mode of transmission: Usually from direct contact with discharges from respiratory mucous membranes of infected person by airborne droplets.

Incubation: Commonly 6-20 days.

Preventive measures: Active immunization series and education of public and especially parents for immunization of children.

Control of client: Report to local health authority. Isolation for known cases. Terminal cleaning. Erythromycin therapy may shorten communicability.

Definitions of Positive Tuberculin Skin Test (TST) Results in Infants, Children, and Adolescents

TSTs should be read at 48 to 72 hours after placement

Induration ≥5 mm

Children in close contact with known or suspected contagious cases of tuberculosis disease:

- Households with active or previously active cases if treatment cannot be verified as adequate before exposure, treatment was initiated after the child's contact, or reactivation of latent tuberculosis infection is suspected

Children suspected to have tuberculosis disease:

- Chest radiograph consistent with active or previously active tuberculosis
- Clinical evidence of tuberculosis disease*

Children receiving immunosuppressive therapy[†] or with immunosuppressive conditions, including HIV infection

Induration ≥10 mm

Children at increased risk of disseminated disease:

- Young age: younger than 4 years of age
- Other medical conditions, including Hodgkin disease, lymphoma, diabetes mellitus, chronic renal failure, or malnutrition

Children with increased exposure to tuberculosis disease:

- Born or whose parents were born in high-prevalence regions of the world
- Frequently exposed to adults who are HIV-infected, homeless,

---

These definitions apply regardless of previous bacille Calmette-Guérin (BCG) immunization (see also interpretation of TST results in prior recipients of BCG); erythema at TST site does not indicate a positive test. HIV indicates human immunodeficiency virus.

*Evidence by physical examination or laboratory assessment that would include tuberculosis in the working differential diagnosis (e.g., meningitis).

†Including immunosuppressive doses of corticosteroids.

users of illicit drugs, residents of nursing homes, incarcerated or institutionalized persons, and migrant farm workers

• Travel and exposure to high-prevalence regions of the world

Induration ≥15 mm

Children 4 years of age or older without any risk factors

DISABILITIES

Case Management Process and Roles

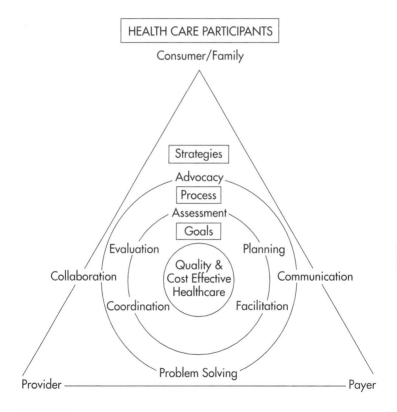

From Hoeman S: *Rehabilitation nursing: process and application,* ed 2, St Louis, 1996, Mosby.

Case management: a process directed at coordinating resources and creating flexible, cost-effective healthcare options in collaboration with the treatment team for individuals and their families to facilitate optimum healthcare outcomes.

The specific activities of the case manager blend with the stages of the nursing process or clinical reasoning process to form a framework for nursing case management. Referring to the case management model developed by the National Task Force on Case Management, the process involves assessment, planning, facilitation, coordination, and evaluation.

Nurse Case Management in Rehabilitation

Escalating healthcare costs have given rise to the development of new and more effective approaches to the delivery of healthcare services. One such approach, that of case management, has emerged as a significant trend in managed healthcare. Nurses, with their specialized knowledge and skills in caring for persons with disabilities, are in a unique position to serve as case managers for clients in acute, rehabilitation, and community settings.

Case management is the process of planning, organizing, coordinating, and monitoring the services and resources needed to respond to a client's healthcare needs. Case management does not usually involve hands-on nursing care of clients. By assessing, planning, implementing, coordinating, and evaluating, the rehabilitation nurse case manager ensures the delivery of cost-effective, quality healthcare services that helps the client move toward optimal health following a disabling illness or injury.

I. **Case management goals**
   A. The nurse case manager uses a goal-oriented approach emphasizing both quality and cost-effectiveness of services; goals include the following
      1. Outcomes of care
         a. Optimal functioning and independence in the least restrictive environment
         b. Prevention of complications

From McCourt A, editor: *The specialty practice of rehabilitation nursing: a core curriculum,* ed 3, Skokie, Ill, 1993, The Rehabilitation Nursing Foundation of the Association of Rehabilitation Nurses.

      c. Effective coping with the disability

      d. A successful return to work, school, and community

  2. System outcomes: Provision of timely, appropriate services by qualified service providers

  3. Minimization of healthcare costs

B. The rehabilitation nurse case manager facilitates outcomes of case management

  1. As a *coordinator,* the case manager facilitates client access to healthcare services and coordinates and monitors all health care provided to the client; timely provision and continuity of services are essential to effective coordination

  2. As a *collaborator,* the nurse case manager collaborates with the facility-based and community-based rehabilitation teams through ongoing communication

  3. As an *educator,* the case manager promotes or provides the education of clients regarding their health status and prevention of complications or further disability; emphasis is placed on self-management and responsibility for health care needs

  4. As an *advocate,* the nurse case manager strives to promote the client's optimal functioning and independence in the community

II. Client characteristics and referral considerations

A. Early identification of clients is essential to successful case management and subsequent achievement of outcomes; ideally, this should occur at the onset of disability

  1. Internal, or facility-based, case managers typically serve all clients receiving care and initiate services on a client's admission

  2. External case managers receive referrals primarily from insurance carriers and other third-party payers

    a. These referrals are usually based on predetermined criteria used by the referral source and encompass clients with catastrophic illnesses or injuries, those at high risk for the long-term consequences of disability, and those with work-related illnesses or injuries

    b. External case managers often can facilitate early identification of clients needing case management through ongoing education of referral sources and reviews of claim files

B. Clients of all ages are served by nurse case managers; those who provide services to children and older adult client populations need additional specialized knowledge

1. Children served by case managers include those with disabilities at birth, those with developmental disabilities, and those with acquired catastrophic illness or injury

2. Community reintegration of children, with an emphasis on education, is a major focus of the rehabilitation team and case manager

3. Older adult clients include those who, through the case manager's coordination of appropriate services, can continue to function independently in their community

4. The case manager facilitates placement when a client's remaining at home is no longer feasible

C. Considerations in referring clients for case management

1 The nature and severity of the illness or injury

a. Catastrophic illness or injuries: Multiple trauma, burns, head injury, spinal cord injury, stroke, cancer, and AIDS

b. Workers' compensation cases: Back injury, chronic pain, soft tissue or joint injury, or repetitive motion disorder

c. Presence of secondary disability

2. Type of treatment received or recommended

3. Emotional and behavioral status

4. Age

5. Available social support systems

III. **Role functions of the nurse case manager: correspond to the phases of the nursing process**

A. Assessment

1. A comprehensive assessment is completed on referral to the case manager; authorization, if necessary, is obtained before the assessment, which is performed in the client's home whenever possible

2. Assessment data are collected from a variety of sources

a. Interview with client and client's family

b. Attending physician and other healthcare disciplines involved in client's care

c. Review of medical records and school reports

d. Employer contact in workers' compensation cases

3. Areas of emphasis during assessment
    a. Present illness or injury as well as health status
        1) Diagnosis, prognosis, current treatment, and future treatment recommendations
        2) Functional abilities and activities of daily living
    b. Psychosocial status
        1) Emotional and behavioral response to illness or injury
        2) Roles, relationships, and family functioning
    c. Financial status
        1) Income sources
        2) Eligibility for additional funding sources
    d. Home environment
        1) Accessibility
        2) Safety
    e. Educational and vocational assessment
        1) Educational
            a) Current ability to read and write
            b) Level of education completed; degrees held
            c) Specialized training obtained in military service
            d) Eligibility for Department of Veterans' Affairs training benefits
        2) Vocational
            a) Past employment
                (1) Jobs held
                (2) Duration of employment
                (3) Reason(s) for leaving job(s)
                (4) Special skills attained
                (5) Union involvement
                (6) Client's verbalized or demonstrated attitude toward employer, co-workers, union
            b) Transferable skills
                (1) Help determine client's vocational potential
                (2) Are determined by analyzing client's past work history
                (3) Can be determined by using various resources
                    (a) Vocational Diagnosis and Assessment of Residual Employability (VDARE) worksheet
                    (b) *Dictionary of Occupational Titles* (US Department of Labor, Employment and Training Administration, 1991)

    c) Job analysis
      (1) Formalized process for observing a job as it is performed and describing its characteristics, including its physical demands, working conditions, prerequisite general education, training time, and required aptitudes
      (2) A means to compare job characteristics with postinjury abilities
      (3) A method for observing or measuring a job's physical demands
        (a) Lifting
        (b) Carrying
        (c) Bending
        (d) Reaching
        (e) Grasping
        (f) Standing
        (g) Walking
        (h) Talking
        (i) Hearing
        (j) Seeing
      (4) Classifying physical demands as described in the *Dictionary of Occupational Titles* (US Department of Labor, Employment and Training Administration, 1991.)
        (a) Sedentary (0 to 10 lb lifted frequently)
        (b) Light (10 lb lifted frequently; 20 lb lifted occasionally)
        (c) Medium (20 lb lifted frequently; 50 lb lifted occasionally)
        (d) Heavy (50 lb lifted frequently; 100 lb lifted occasionally)
        (e) Very heavy (more than 100 lb lifted frequently)

B. Planning
  1. Problems or nursing diagnoses are formulated from assessment data

2. Rehabilitation plan is developed in partnership with the client, family, and facility-based or community-based rehabilitation team members
   a. Rehabilitation plan has several features
      1) Short- and long-term goals or expected outcomes that are patient centered
      2) Recommendations for care, treatment, and services
      3) Target dates for achievement of goals or outcomes
      4) Costs of services
      5) Treatment alternatives and associated costs
      6) Available community resources or alternate funding sources
      7) Discharge plans, when appropriate
   b. Community-based rehabilitation team members include
      1) Nurse case manager
      2) Rehabilitation counselor
      3) Claims representative for client's insurance carrier, third-party payer, or private funding source
      4) Employer or volunteer supervisor for noncompetitive placement
      5) School personnel
      6) Client's attorney
      7) Discharge planner
      8) Community health nurse
3. Service providers are evaluated according to whether they offer quality services at reasonable cost
4. Authorization for services usually is obtained through client's insurance carrier or third-party payer
5. Long-term planning for catastrophic cases is done through development of life care plans
   a. Life care plans involve projection of comprehensive needs and costs over the course of the lifetime of the person with a catastrophic illness or injury
   b. Life care plans are often used in litigation of catastrophic cases; however, most important, they serve to provide a framework for the long-term care needs of clients and families
   c. Life care plans include projections of future rehabilitation interventions and costs as the client ages, experiences a change in medical status, or requires periodic reinitiation of health care services

6. In workers' compensation cases, the primary goal is return to work
   a. A return-to-work hierarchy is used to determine an appropriate vocational goal
   b. Hierarchy includes return-to-work alternatives
      1) Same job and same employer
      2) Same job (modified) and same employer
      3) Different job and same employer
      4) Same job but different employer
      5) Same job (modified) but different employer
      6) Different job and different employer
      7) Different job involving retraining; employer could be either same or different
      8) Self-employment

C. Implementation
   1. Involves procurement and coordination of monitoring of the care, treatment, and services provided to the client
   2. Services can include various options
      a. Medical or surgical treatment
      b. Inpatient, outpatient, day treatment, or community reintegration rehabilitation programs
      c. Specialized rehabilitation programs for persons with head injuries, spinal cord injuries, burns, chronic pain
      d. Skilled, intermediate, or long-term nursing care
      e. Home health care
      f. Attendant care or providing assistance with behavioral management
      g. Home evaluation services and home modification
      h. Orthotic and prosthetic devices
      i. Durable medical equipment and supplies
      j. Psychologic services
      k. Outpatient or home-based physical, occupational, speech, or cognitive therapy; community skills or life skills training
      l. Independent or transitional living centers
      m. Hospice care
      n. Transportation services
      o. Meal programs
      p. Support groups

    q. Vocational services
       1) Work hardening
       2) Vocational evaluation
       3) Vocational counseling
       4) Job placement or supported employment
       5) Job modifications
       6) Work adjustment
       7) On-the-job training or job coaching
       8) Formal training
       9) Volunteer or noncompetitive placement
       10) Referral to vocational rehabilitation office

3. Community reintegration is addressed
    a. Access to community agencies is obtained
    b. Reentry to the home or an alternative living site is facilitated

4. Costs of services are negotiated, whenever possible, taking into account preferred provider organization (PPO) networks and mandated fee schedules

5. Services are coordinated through ongoing communication and collaboration among rehabilitation team members
    a. Case manager attends team staff meetings, whenever possible, in all settings
    b. Client progress is communicated by and to rehabilitation team members

D. Evaluation

1. Outcomes are evaluated and progress toward goal achievement is identified

2. Goals are modified when necessary

3. Successful goal achievement ideally determines the discontinuation of case management services or case closure; cases can be closed for various other reasons as well
    a. Client is unwilling to participate in services
    b. Attending physician is not receptive to case management
    c. Client's attorney is not receptive to case management
    d. Closure is requested by insurance carrier or third-party payer
    e. Funding has been exhausted

4. If goals are unable to be met or funding is exhausted, case manager must refer client to community agencies

5. Case closure in external case management includes a cost-benefit analysis
6. Case closure should also identify circumstances under which the case will be reopened
   a. Change in medical status
   b. Impact of aging
   c. Progression of illness
   d. Change in family structure
   e. Change in placement
   f. Reinitiation of rehabilitation services

IV. Legislative and regulatory influences on case management

A. The nurse case manager must have knowledge of federal, state, and local governmental regulations and legislation and their impact on healthcare services
B. The nurse case manager will encounter regulatory and service systems that require knowledge of the benefits provided
   1. Medicare
   2. Medicaid
   3. Private healthcare insurance
   4. Social Security disability
   5. Veterans' Affairs disability
   6. Workers' compensation
   7. State vocational rehabilitation programs
   8. Other federal, state, and local agencies
   9. Community groups
C. Much legislation at the federal, state, and local levels affects case management practice
   1. Economic Opportunity Acts of 1964 and 1974: Initiated Head Start program; included children with disabilities in 1974
   2. Rehabilitation Act of 1973 and the amendments of 1978: Provided funding for variety of efforts
      a. Vocational rehabilitation
      b. Affirmative action efforts to employ qualified persons with disabilities
      c. Accessibility of federally funded building and transportation systems
      d. Funding for independent living
   3. Education for All Handicapped Children Act of 1975 and the amendments of 1986: Provided funding for educational assistance and early intervention programs for children with disabilities

4. Americans with Disabilities Act of 1990: Mandated nondiscrimination in the employment of persons with disabilities and barrier-free transportation systems and buildings

V. Current issues in case management

A. Quality assurance for case management practice

1. Essential component of rehabilitation case management services

2. Provides a mechanism for the case manager to evaluate the case management provided; aspects to be evaluated include the following

   a. Client outcomes

   b. System outcomes based on accepted standards of practice

   c. Client satisfaction

3. Quality assurance data are used to strengthen ongoing provision of case management services

B. Governmental regulation of practice that includes scope of nurse case managers, state nurse practice acts, educational preparation, and referral or funding source guidelines

C. Legal and ethical issues influencing practice

1. Many insurance claims involve litigation and thus attorneys are often actively involved in cases; attorneys are considered members of the rehabilitation team and should be kept informed of services provided to clients as well as the benefits of each service

2. Complete and accurate documentation of all case management services provided is essential, because these records are admissible as evidence in a court of law

3. When funding for case management services is terminated, referrals to community and government-supported agencies should be initiated

D. Accountability to clients

1. In external case management (services are provided on a fee-for-service basis): Nurse case manager's services usually are retained by the insurance carrier or third-party payer, but may be retained by the family directly or by the attorney, trustee, or court-appointed guardian

   a. Case manager's primary responsibility is to the client

   b. Case manager's level of responsibility to the referral source should be defined before initiation of case management services; goals and outcomes of the case management services expected by the referral source and case manager should be identified in measurable terms

2. In internal case management: Nurse case manager has a responsibility to all rehabilitation team members to ensure that all services provided are in the best interest of the client and directed toward discharge goals

E. Funding

1. Claim dollars available for services to the client are often limited due to parameters of the policy

2. The rehabilitation nurse case manager should be aware of a client's insurance policy limits, because insurance carriers set aside reserves to pay claim costs

3. Often the case manager is required to provide funding of services within the policy limits and thus must be proactive and creative in developing a rehabilitation plan for the client

4. When funding is from a reinsurance source, the case manager must be familiar with monies available (e.g., trusts, annuities, estate funds) and recommend services accordingly throughout the client's lifespan

F. Regulation of case management practice

1. Federal and state governments are beginning to determine some aspects of case management practice

2. Credentialing of case managers: Professional bodies are also attempting to determine recommended education, experience, and certification

a. A baccalaureate education

b. A minimum of 2 years of clinical experience in rehabilitation or a related specialty

c. Certification in rehabilitation nursing (Certified Rehabilitation Registered Nurse [CRRN] credential)

3. Nurse case managers must take a strong leadership role in influencing future regulatory efforts

Access to Healthcare Services

Access to healthcare historically has been a challenge to those with disabilities. Healthcare providers must be able to define strategies for obtaining healthcare services, identify the available financial resources, be knowledgeable regarding public laws governing access to healthcare services, and assist those with disabilities in securing and using healthcare services.

I. **Access to healthcare for people with disabilities**
   A. Obstacles to healthcare services
      1. Geographic location
         a. Availability and transportation issues related to access to health care facilities and community resources
         b. Access to home-based care services
         c. Prohibitive cost of transportation services
         d. Limited public funds for assistance with obtaining vehicle modifications or purchasing a vehicle (e.g., a van with hand controls), which decreases access to healthcare services, especially in rural areas
      2. Architectural issues related to accessibility (including buildings and grounds)
         a. Parking lot accessibility and design
         b. Sidewalk accessibility
         c. Office building accessibility and design
         d. Healthcare facility accessibility and design
      3. Attitudes: Discrimination by healthcare providers toward older clients
         a. Age can impose additional limits on healthcare access secondary to payer source limits (e.g., Medicare coverage for home care services, equipment, and outpatient services)
         b. Elderly people often have additional and more complex health problems
         c. Discrimination can lead to poor self-esteem due to increased physical, social, and psychologic stressors
         d. Ageism may bring about job discrimination or loss of a job, with a subsequent loss of medical benefits
      4. Lack of information about care needs of those with disabilities

From McCourt A, editor: *The specialty practice of rehabilitation nursing: a core curriculum,* ed 3, Skokie, Ill, 1993, The Rehabilitation Nursing Foundation of the Association of Rehabilitation Nurses.

5. Economic constraints
   a. Personal finances
      1) Loss of medical benefits, Supplemental Security Income (SSI), or Social Security Disability Insurance (SSDI) if a disabled person is employed and earns more than the allowable amount
      2) Possible reduction in Social Security benefits and medical benefits if a person with a disability marries
      3) Medical benefits that are now tied to income criteria and encourage disabled persons to be dependent on the system
   b. Unavailability of medical benefits for people with disabilities under Medicare until 2 years after the onset of the disability
      1) Discourages persons with disabilities from seeking healthcare services
      2) Raises possibility of disabled persons being without any medical benefits if they do not qualify for state assistance or Medicaid and thus contributes to increased numbers of indigent persons seeking healthcare services
      3) Raises possibility that people with disabilities will seek healthcare services only when healthcare needs are well advanced and require hospitalization
      4) Begins a cycle that increases the burden on healthcare providers to supply free care and contributes to an increase in the overall cost of healthcare services
   c. Limited eligibility for funding for attendant care
      1) Funding that is usually tied to eligibility for income assistance
      2) Long waiting periods that frequently last for 1 or 2 years
      3) Minimal reimbursement for attendants, which makes it difficult to recruit and retain qualified attendants
      4) Programs that require the clients to be able to manage their own workers independently and to handle training and payroll, which may not be possible for persons with severe disabilities or the elderly
      5) Strict definitions of what constitutes a disability that may disqualify many of those who need the services

      d. Ability to obtain needed equipment, supplies, and medications
  1) Dependence on insurance coverage
  2) Possible requirement of a down payment (in cash)
  3) Frequent limits on additional equipment covered by insurance
  4) Possible inability to obtain the necessary equipment (e.g., a padded commode chair with removable arms for a person with a spinal cord injury)
6. Limited funding for independent living arrangements (residential and nonresidential models)
  a. Continued limitation of funds for independent living centers (ILCs) despite their having been mandated by the Rehabilitation, Comprehensive Services and Developmental Disabilities Amendments of 1978 (Public Law 95-602)
  b. Some support through Medicaid Title XIX (state) funding for attendant assistance and community support services
  c. The rarity of ILC programs in rural areas
7. Issues in attendant training
  a. On-the-job training
  b. Lack of regulations regarding worker qualifications
  c. No supervision of work performance
  d. Lack of public funding that would allow control over worker qualifications and performance
  e. Lack of availability of attendants able to meet the specialized needs of the pediatric population
B. Limited healthcare services: Limits might arise due to attitudes, architectural designs, or reimbursement limits
  1. Limited counseling services
    a. Medical social worker services are usually available only through home care agencies
    b. Few psychiatrists and psychologists make home visits
    c. Reimbursement for counseling is limited
  2. Special healthcare needs of people with disabilities
    a. Obstetric and gynecologic services
      1) Exam tables that are accessible to women with disabilities
      2) Healthcare providers knowledgeable in obstetric and gynecologic areas

3) Specialized training for personnel (e.g., how to care for a spinal cord injured person who has had a baby)

b. Dental services

1) Offices that are architecturally accessible

2) Accessible, comfortable office chairs

3) Elimination of financial obstacles to preventive care (e.g., insurance such as Medicare or Medicaid that does not cover preventive care)

II. Obtaining access to community resources and healthcare services (Figure 3-1)

A. Contact local governmental disability office, city commission, or city departments to determine public services available to persons with disabilities

1. Accessible housing

a. Established referral system in place

b. Technical assistance

c. Development, design, and building assistance

d. Home mortgage loans

e. Availability of accessible public housing

f. Funding for adaptations in private residences

2. Transportation

a. Designated parking

b. Private transportation services

c. Public transportation (e.g., availability, accessibility)

d. Reduced bus passes

e. Paratransit

f. Parking stickers

3. Advocacy

a. Established advisory council

b. Involvement of advocacy groups with community agencies

c. Funding for programs

d. Information exchange regarding disability issues (e.g., legislation)

e. Appointment of persons with disabilities to governmental boards and commissions

f. Legal assistance

g. Public education regarding disability issues

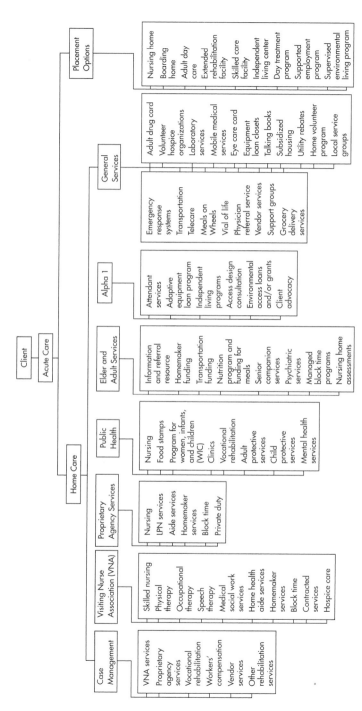

Figure 3-1 Gaining access to community resources.

4. Employment
   a. Affirmative action for hiring the disabled
   b. Training and placement assistance; supported employment services
   c. Funding for environmental modifications
5. Recreation
   a. Accessible community centers and leisure programs
   b. Special events focused on population with disabilities (e.g., wheelchair division of marathon races)
6. Supportive services
   a. Information and referral
   b. Counseling
   c. Personal care assistance programs
   d. Telecommunication devices for the deaf; sign language interpreters (e.g., at public hearings)
   e. Homemaker services
   f. Augmentative communication aids, adaptive toys, assistive technology
   g. Health screening services
   h. Funding for rehabilitation technology services and adaptive equipment
   i. Access to electronic bulletin-board systems
7. Education
   a. Availability of educational opportunities
   b. Funding
   c. Building accessibility
   d. Programs for disadvantaged children
   e. Therapy services available in school systems (e.g., occupational therapy, speech and language therapy, physical therapy)
   f. Head Start program; early intervention programs
   g. Bilingual education
   h. Acquisition of equipment to supplement special education and related services; training in computer technology
   i. Self-help groups
   j. Playground accessibility; school environment modifications
   k. Specialized buses, cars, vans to meet the needs of school children

B. Contact other local agencies or healthcare professionals
   1. Social workers in hospitals, rehabilitation centers, extended-care facilities, government bureaus
   2. Department of health and human services
   3. Visiting nurse associations (VNAs)
   4. Case managers at private insurance companies
   5. Physicians' referral services
   6. Local bureau of elder and adult services
   7. Vendors
   8. Mental health departments
   9. American Association of Retired Persons
   10. Department of Veterans' Affairs
C. Contact public affairs departments of local media

III. **Funding sources for gaining access to rehabilitation and supportive services in the community**
   A. Agencies and sectors receiving state funding through appropriation of monies or grants or through direct reimbursement
      1. VNAs and private not-for-profit home care agencies
      2. Alpha I (member of National Council on Independent Living)
         a. Is funded through state and federal monies
         b. Provides services to people with disabilities
            1) Peer support, attendant services, client advocacy
            2) Access to design consultation
               a) Education of design professionals and the public regarding legal requirements for creating accessible environments
               b) Building product information
               c) Design review
               d) Assessments of home after occupancy
            3) Environmental access grants and loans
            4) Loan program for adaptive equipment
               a) Low-interest loans
               b) Loans available to citizens and businesses to purchase technological aids that enhance independence in the home, workplace, or other environment
            5) Independent living programs: Provide instruction on and hands-on experience in transitional living skills
            6) Adapted vehicle driving evaluation and education

      7) Monitoring of access issues
         a) Watchdog project to correct building code violations and publicize standards for accessible design
         b) Statewide network of grassroots advocacy
         c) Group that informs the design and construction industries about legal requirements for building or remodeling public buildings and public housing
         d) Group that files complaints or litigation if corrective action is not taken

3. Proprietary (for-profit) agencies
4. Public health services
   a. Nursing services
      1) Home visits for health teaching and screening
      2) Clinics for blood pressure, screening, child immunizations, and flu vaccines
   b. Vocational rehabilitation
   c. Adult and child protective services
5. Elder and adult services
6. Transportation resources
   a. Public transportation
   b. Private organizations receiving state funds to purchase vans with lifts and to serve the elderly, those with disabilities, and those who have state benefits (e.g., Medicaid, paratransit)
7. Independent living programs
   a. Services vary according to locality and program
      1) Referral to housing and training in independent living skills
      2) Permanent residential, transitional residential, or temporary housing
      3) Attendant referral, training, or management training
      4) Client and system advocacy
      5) Disability awareness among community
      6) Equipment repair and referral
      7) Reduction of environmental barriers
      8) Promotion of consumer involvement in community activities and information and referral services
   b. Program components vary with each independent living program

    8. Extended rehabilitation facilities, skilled nursing facilities, boarding homes

    9. Vendor services

      a. Durable medical equipment

      b. Intravenous therapy: Hydration, total parenteral nutrition, antibiotics, blood and blood products, pain management

      c. Chemotherapy

      d. Medical supplies

      e. Oxygen or ventilator services

      f. Nutrition-related services

      g. Enteral feedings

  10. Selective professional services

      a. Physicians' visits (office and home)

      b. Inpatient and outpatient hospital services

      c. Counseling services

      d. Outpatient phlebotomy services

      e. Mobile medical services (e.g., x-rays, electrocardiographs in the home)

      f. Eye care cards (e.g., funding for eye exams, eyeglasses)

  11. Programs

      a. Adult day care

      b. Day treatment programs (e.g., for those with a head injury or with Alzheimer's disease)

      c. Supervised environmental living program

      d. Hospice

      e. Prosthetic and orthotic devices

B. Agencies and sectors receiving federal funding through appropriation of monies, grants, or direct reimbursement to agencies for services that they provide

    1. VNAs and private not-for-profit agencies providing home care services

    2. Vendor services

    3. Some independent living programs

    4. Outpatient phlebotomy services

    5. Physicians' visits (office and home)

    6. Extended rehabilitation facilities

    7. Hospice care

    8. Prosthetic and orthotic devices

    9. Mobile medical services

    10. Inpatient and outpatient hospital services (acute and reha-
        bilitation)
    11. Outpatient rehabilitation services (e.g., hospital-based,
        VNA, private)
  C. Department of Veterans' Affairs services
    1. Inpatient and outpatient hospital services
    2. Pharmacy services
    3. Vocational rehabilitation services
    4. Nursing home care
    5. Home health care
    6. Orthotic and prosthetic devices
    7. Durable medical and adaptive equipment
    8. Services for the visually impaired
    9. Home modifications for people with disabilities
    10. Mortgage loans
  D. Federal or state-subsidized assistance based on income, age,
     or disability
    1. Adult drug cards
    2. Subsidized housing
    3. Utility and telephone rebates
    4. Eye care cards
        a. Provide reimbursement for eye examinations and
           glasses
        b. Are unavailable for those holding state medical cards
           because they would duplicate some coverage
    5. Health care services at public clinics (e.g., immunizations,
       flu vaccines)
    6. Meals on Wheels program
    7. Talking books
  E. Elder and adult services
    1. Services funded primarily for those over age 62
    2. Age and income are the two main criteria for determining
       eligibility for programs
    3. Services provided by typical senior companion program
        a. Respite care
        b. Running errands
        c. Taking clients out to do errands
        d. Light housekeeping

IV. Nursing interventions to help clients gain access to healthcare resources
  A. Coordinating referrals to not-for-profit and private home care agencies
  B. Identifying agencies that provide free care or sliding scale fees for services based on income and the duration of needed services
  C. Arranging for social work services to assist with access to community systems for obtaining subsidized housing, Medicaid applications, SSI, SSDI, counseling services, advocacy assistance, equipment needs, and transportation and to find organizations that provide community services
  D. Contacting the local department of human services regarding services available for rehabilitation care needs
  E. Contacting legislators to support funding for transferring client to an ILC and for attendant training, as well as for supplemental funding that allows those with disabilities to work without a drastic reduction in or termination of medical benefits
  F. Attending public hearings on issues affecting people with disabilities
  G. Acting as a community advocate to promote increased environmental accessibility, decreased architectural barriers, increased access to public transportation, decreased cost of services to elderly clients on fixed incomes, and increased access to health care services
  H. Making referrals to rehabilitation counselors, peer counselors, and those providing psychologic services
  I. Contacting state disability office, commission(s), or department(s) for assistance
  J. Promoting the education of healthcare providers and caregivers within facilities and the community
     1. Providing in-service education
     2. Consulting one-on-one with providers regarding healthcare issues, ways to manage individual clients' healthcare needs, and ways to promote access to healthcare services
     3. Encouraging family involvement early in the rehabilitation process and teaching about equipment, procedures, medications, and ways to manage emergencies

4. Coordinating a home visit by the rehabilitation team to evaluate the need for home modifications, equipment, and ways to improve safety

5. Making referrals to appropriate community resources

6. Promoting interagency communication regarding rehabilitation needs, follow-up teaching needs, and previous nursing interventions in the event of a transfer to a different environment

7. Periodically reassessing and evaluating the client's ability to perform ADLs, changes in level of independence, health care needs, and barriers to gaining access to required services

8. Contacting healthcare providers in the community to determine access to buildings, cost of services, insurance coverage, ways to modify the office environment, and the availability of transportation

K. Speaking at service club meetings

L. Actively participating in professional organizations that support legislation and advocacy activities for people with disabilities (see Figure 3-2 for a list of laws governing access to rehabilitation services)

M. Promoting appointment of people with disabilities to public offices and commissions, and to private-sector industry and business boards

N. Helping clients with disabilities prepare testimony for legislative hearings

O. Participating in health planning endeavors and advocating for services that meet the needs of children and adults

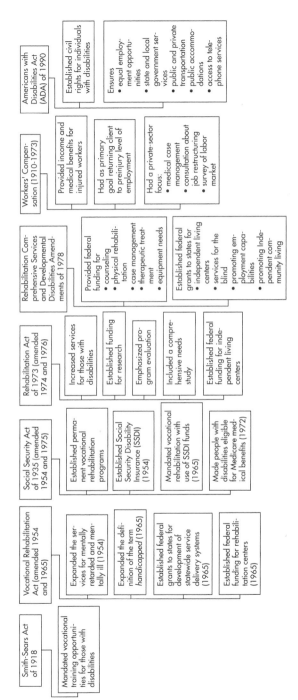

Figure 3-2 Laws governing access to rehabilitation services.

Preserving Self: From Victim, to Client, to Disabled Person

The basic social psychologic process of "preserving self" explains the strategies used in each stage and requires deliberate action, focused energy, and tremendous effort and will. The strategies used to preserve self change in each stage of the model. At the beginning, when physical survival is in jeopardy, the strategies were primarily physical. Protecting self is a process of "taking time out" and of shutting down, in the stage of disruption. In the stage of enduring the self, it is passively learning to "take it" and to bear the treatments. Finally, in the stage of striving to regain the self, preserving the self is the work of regaining and redefining the self as a disabled person.

The stages of preserving self

Stage I Vigilance: becoming engulfed	Stage II Disruption: taking time out	Stage III Enduring the self: confronting and regrouping	Stage IV Striving to regain self: merging the old and the new reality
Being vigilant Experiencing clarity of thought Experiencing the expansion of time	Being in a shattered reality Experiencing memory gaps, "fog" Dreaming vividly, frequently bizarre, confused with reality	Learning to endure Living through pain and treatments Grasping the implications of the injury	Making sense Seeking information about the accident Recognizing it "could be worse"
Being directive, protecting the living, breathing self	Vacillating sleep/wake cycles	Trying to "bear it," learning to "take it"	

Distancing subjective from objective body	Perceiving the world as changing and hostile	Learning to accept dependence	Getting to know and trust the altered body
Observing dispassionately	Anchoring onto the significant other	Latching onto the significant other	Learning limitations
Becoming two-personned	Trying to "keep myself together"	Not tolerating being left alone	Viewing life beyond self
		Seeking distraction	Revising/modifying life goals
		Seeking encouragement	
		Seeking entertainment	
		Learning physical limitations	
Relinquishing to caregivers	Recognizing reality	Doing the work of healing	Accepting the consequences of the experience
Surrendering	Beginning the struggle	Living with setbacks and discouragement	Realizing they can "hack it"
Becoming calm		Keeping a score card	Evaluating meaning
		Refusing to accept the damage	Redefining self

Assessment of Equipment Needs for the Disabled Client

Activity	Problem	Equipment	Comments
Transfers	One-sided impairment	Sliding board	A smooth-surfaced wooden board with a center hole placed between client and transfer object. The board is placed under client's upper thigh.
	Lower extremity impairment	Sliding board, trapeze	
	All extremities impaired	Sliding board with one-person assist	
		Hoyer lift	The Hoyer lift is a hydraulic lift using a sling to hold client. It may also be useful with an overweight dependent client.
	Low endurance	Sliding board	
	Visual impairment	Not applicable*	Orientation to environment
	Auditory impairment	Not applicable	
Mobility	One-sided impairment	Manual wheelchair with one-hand drive, ambulatory with walker, cane (straight, narrow-base or wide-base quad), or crutches	
	Lower extremity impairment	Manual wheelchair (standard or sports model), ambulatory with braces and assistive devices	
	All extremities impaired		

Low endurance	Motorized wheelchair with specific drive control (hand, breath, chin)	The various drive controls are specific to patient's functional ability. Breath and chin controls are used for clients who have no function in upper extremities, but who have good head and neck control. The hand control can be adapted with differently shaped devices.
	Manual wheelchair, motorized wheelchair, motorized scooter	Client must have good balance to operate motorized scooter.
Visual impairment	Seeing eye dog; cane	Orientation to environment. If a person leads the client, client must hold onto the person's upper arm and be given verbal cues.
Auditory impairment	Not applicable	
Toileting One-sided impairment	Toilet bars, raised toilet seat, bedpan, bedside commode, shower commode chair, toileting stick	The shower commode chair can be placed directly over toilet. The toileting stick is used by clients who have limited reach. It holds toilet paper and assists with cleaning.
Lower extremity impairment	Toilet bars, bedside commode, shower commode chair, suppository insertor, digital stimulator	These are used to assist client with limited mobility/grasp.
All extremities impaired	Bedside commode, toileting stick, shower commode chair, suppository insertor, digital stimulator	
Low endurance	Bedside commode	
Visual impairment	Not applicable	Orientation to environment; consistency maintained with placement of objects

Continued

*No specific equipment recommendations are required.

Adapted from Pedretti L: *Occupational theory: practice skills for physical dysfunction*, ed 4, St Louis, 1996, Mosby.

Assessment of Equipment Needs for the Disabled Client—cont'd

Activity	Problem	Equipment	Comments
Toileting—cont'd			
	Auditory impairment	Not applicable	
	Bedridden	Bedpan or urinal, absorbent pads	
Feeding	One-sided impairment	Nonskid pad	Prevents objects from skidding. It is placed beneath the object.
		Rocker knife	Rocker knife is a curved-blade knife that allows patient to cut food with one hand by using a rocking motion
		Scoop dish, plate guard	Both devices have high sides so patient can push food against the sides, preventing food from sliding off plate.
	Lower extremity impairment	Not applicable	
	All extremities impaired	Electric self-feeder	Electrically brings utensil to client's mouth.
		Utensils with built-up handles	Used for clients with decreased grasp.
		ADL/universal cuff, C-clip holder	Both devices wrap around palm of hand to hold utensils. They are used by clients who have limited or no grasp.
		Swivel spoon or spoon-fork combination	Can compensate for limited supination.
		Long plastic straws and straw chips on glasses/cups	
	Low endurance	Not applicable	Pace activity level.

Activity	Impairment	Equipment	Comments
	Visual impairment	Not applicable	Consistency in organization; verbal cuing exploration of dish; memory training. When cuing the individual, you must describe position of food, utensils, and beverage by associating the positions with the numbers on a clock.
	Auditory impairment	Not applicable	
Hygiene			
Brushing/combing hair	One-sided impairment	Not applicable	
	Lower extremity impairment	Not applicable	
	All extremities impaired	Long-handled brush or comb, built-up handle, C-clip holder	
	Low endurance	Not applicable	Pace activity level.
	Visual impairment	Not applicable	
	Auditory impairment	Not applicable	
Brushing teeth	One-sided impairment	Suction denture brush	Client needs to place toothbrush on counter to stabilize. Open toothpaste tube with one hand and squeeze onto toothbrush.
	Lower extremity impairment	Not applicable	
	All extremities impaired	Suction denture brush, built-up handle, C-clip holder, toothbrush	
	Low endurance	Electric toothbrush	
	Visual impairment	Use Braille labels on items	
	Auditory impairment	Not applicable	
Bathing	One-sided impairment	Long-handled sponge, suction nail brush, soap on a rope, wash mitt	

Continued

Assessment of Equipment Needs for the Disabled Client—cont'd

Activity	Problem	Equipment	Comments
Hygiene— cont'd			
Bathing— cont'd	Lower extremity impairment	Long-handled sponge, handheld shower, transfer tub bench	
	All extremities impaired	Long-handled sponge, suction nail brush, wash mitt, soap on a rope, digital read-out temperature faucets, safety rails	Water temperature must be checked on *full* sensation areas. Nonskid surface is recommended in tub.
	Low endurance	Long-handled sponge	Consistency in organization of supplies helpful.
	Visual impairment	Raised letters on faucets	
	Auditory impairment	Not applicable	
Shaving	One-sided impairment	Electric shaver	
	Lower extremity impairment	Not applicable	
	All extremities impaired	Electric razor, C-clip holder for razor (manual or electric), shaving cream dispenser handle	The shaving cream dispenser handle is lever apparatus attached to spray nozzle to assist in pressing down. This is for clients with limited hand control.
		Built-up handle for manual razor	
	Low endurance	Electric razor	Decreases chance of cutting oneself
	Visual impairment	Electric razor	
	Auditory impairment	Not applicable	

Dressing

Putting on lower-extremity clothing	One-sided impairment	Dressing stick	Wooden stick with hook on the end to aid in reaching and hooking clothing
		Stocking aid	Oval-shaped plastic device with loops on top. Stocking is fitted over plastic, foot is placed into stocking, and loops are pulled upward.
	Lower extremity impairment	Dressing stick, reacher, trouser and sock pulls	The pulls are loops that are attached to clothing. Client places hand or wrist through loop. The wrist is used for pulling by clients who lack grasp.
		Leg lifter	The leg lifter may be either webbing or a strap to assist client in lifting leg for positioning to dress.
	All extremities impaired	Dressing stick, reacher, trouser pull, stocking aid, zipper pull	The zipper pull is a small loop or ring attached to the zipper for a client with limited hand control.
	Low endurance	Reacher	
	Visual impairment	Not applicable	Client sets up own system for identifying colors and styles; for example, by using a different knot on the label to distinguish clothing of different colors (e.g., red = 2 knots).
Putting on upper-extremity clothing	Auditory impairment	Not applicable	
	One-sided impairment	Velcro closure for bras or shirts, front closing bra, button hook	
	Lower extremity impairment	Not applicable	

Continued

Assessment of Equipment Needs for the Disabled Client—cont'd

Activity	Problem	Equipment	Comments
Dressing Putting on upper-extremity clothing—cont'd	All extremities impaired	Hook-and-logo closure for bras, button hook, dressing stick	Pace activity level.
	Low endurance	Not applicable	
	Visual impairment	Not applicable	
	Auditory impairment	Not applicable	
Dressing Putting on shoes	One-sided impairment	Elastic laces, Hook-and-logo closure, long shoe horn, slip-on shoes	
	Lower extremity impairment	Not applicable	
	All extremities impaired	Elastic laces, Hook-and-logo closure, long shoe horn, slip-on shoes	
	Low endurance	Long shoe horn, Hook-and-logo closure, slip-on shoes	
	Visual impairment	Not applicable	
	Auditory impairment	Not applicable	

Activity	Impairment	Device	Description
Communication	One-sided impairment	Low mounted telephone, portable telephones, shoulder rest for telephone, intercom systems, personal alarm systems	
	Lower extremity impairment	Low mounted telephone, portable telephone	
		Dialing stick	Stick is placed in a hand splint or in the mouth to assist with dialing telephone.
	All extremities impaired	Push-button telephone, automatic dialer, speaker telephone, alternate telephone devices, various electronic and/or computerized devices are available	The alternate telephone devices are used to gain access to telephone. The specific type of control depends on patient's upper extremity function.
	Low endurance	Portable telephone	Place within easy access.
	Visual impairment	Large number outlays for telephone with raised numbers or braille; automatic dialer	
	Auditory impairment	Telecommunicator (teletype or telecommunication device)	This provides a visual display or printout of incoming messages when attached to the telephone. Telephone may also be installed with a light system to indicate incoming calls.
		Volume control on hand set	
Meal preparation	One-sided impairment	Rocker knife; rehabilitation cutting board	The rehabilitation cutting board is a wooden board with two stainless steel nails projecting to secure food for cutting.
		Nonskid pad	
		Cart	To transport food

Continued

Assessment of Equipment Needs for the Disabled Client—cont'd

Activity	Problem	Equipment	Comments
Meal preparation— cont'd	All extremities impaired	Cane holder	Holder clips onto cane to balance on the countertop.
			Joint protection techniques for arthritics
		Adapted utensils	Utensils are adapted with built-up handles or clips to secure onto hand if client has poor control.
		Nonskid pad	
		Rehabilitation cutting board	
		Zim jar opener	
		Electric can opener	
		Lapboard	To transport items
		Reacher	
		Bag attached to wheelchair	Modification for the wheelchair-bound patient.
		Lower countertops	
	Lower extremity impairment	Reacher, lapboard, bag attached to walker, lower countertops	
	Low endurance	High stool	Pace activity level.
			A high stool enables patient to sit while working, thereby decreasing energy expenditure.
	Visual impairment	Not applicable	Consistent organization, labeling, using touch, verbal cuing, marking dials, long oven mitts, memory training, orient to environment
	Auditory impairment	Not applicable	

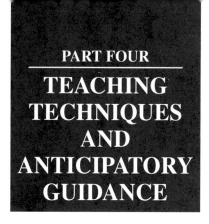

PART FOUR

TEACHING TECHNIQUES AND ANTICIPATORY GUIDANCE

Anticipatory guidance and client teaching are central to public and community health nursing practice. The nurse draws from numerous sources for appropriate information to share with the client. The following items will assist in this endeavor.

EDUCATIONAL TECHNIQUES

Fundamentals of Teaching

General approach
1. Convey respect; be genuine.
2. Reduce social distance between self and others as much as possible.
3. Promote sense of trust and an open interaction; a trusting relationship fosters self-understanding and motivation to follow a teaching plan.
4. Elicit description of feelings from the client about the subject matter or situation to relieve tension and meet the learner's needs.
5. Be organized in presentation.
6. Use a comfortable setting and audiovisual aids as indicated.
7. Encourage questions, disagreement, and comments to ensure that your presentation stays focused on client needs and meets teaching goals.
8. Encourage, support, and reinforce as you present content.

Teaching specific content
1. Begin at knowledge level of client; consider readiness to learn.
2. Determine what client wants to know and already knows.
3. Answer the client's questions first; the client will then be more receptive to the information presented.

Murray R, Zentner J: *Health assessment and promotion strategies through the lifespan,* ed 6, Stamford, CT, 1997, Appleton & Lange. *Continued*

Fundamentals of Teaching—cont'd

4. Build on what the client knows. Gently refute myths or misunderstandings.
5. Relate information to behavior patterns, lifestyle, and sociocultural background to increase likelihood of their being followed by the client.
6. Assist client in reworking your ideas to fit cultural, religious, or family values and customs to ensure that the material to be learned will be practiced.
7. Be logical in sequence of content.
8. Present more basic or simpler content prior to more advanced or complex information.
9. Present one idea, or a group of related ideas, at a time, rather than many diverse ideas together.
10. Demonstrate as you describe directions, suggestions, or ideas, if possible.
11. Break content into units and a series of sessions, if necessary. Do not present too many ideas at one time.
12. Teach the family as thoroughly as the client to ensure that suggestions on interpersonal relationships and other concerns will be followed.
13. Present the same information to friends, employer, occupational health nurse, schoolteacher, clergyman, or significant community leader, if possible and relevant.
14. Provide written instructions in addition to oral presentations.
15. Provide feedback and reinforcement to the client as you provide opportunity for practice and review.

Individual teaching
Programmed learning
Material is presented in carefully planned sequential steps through program instruction books or a teaching machine, a simple manually operated machine or a complex computer. One frame of information is presented at a time. The learner then tests his or her grasp of the information in the frame by writing, or in the case of a computer, keying, a response to a question, usually a multiple-choice type. The book or machine then gives the correct response. If the learner's response was incorrect, the program presents (or, in the case of a book, directs him or her to turn to) a repetition of the information or a more detailed explanation.

Literature
Pamphlets and *brochures* describe preventive measures, signs and symptoms of disease, and major steps of intervention. These are published by many healthcare organizations and agencies, often for specific diseases or groups.
Autobiographies of persons with certain disease processes and "how-to" books by persons who have experienced certain health problems directly or indirectly pass along suggestions to others.

Audiovisual material
A recorder and cassettes explaining preventive measures, disease processes, or specific instructions can be loaned to the client. He or she can stop the

cassette at any point and replay necessary portions until satisfied with the learning. "Talking Books" is a program that records information for the visually impaired. Closed-circuit television or videotape setups allow the person to hear and view material.

Note that these methods of individual instruction are only individual to a certain point. Only when the client can check learning with a *resource* person, ask further questions as necessary, and have help in making personal applications will learning become more significant. That process involves you. The person does not learn from a machine alone.

Computer

Instructions for prevention and healthcare for any condition, information related to growth and development and care of the child, adolescent, and adult of any age is available through computer-assisted instruction formats. Computer programs for client teaching are available for home and healthcare agencies. For example, a graph along with instructions can teach a patient about bypass surgery. A parent can be shown exactly how tubes will be placed in a child's ear.

Group teaching

Client groups provide a channel through which feelings and needs can be expressed and met, especially if the people have similar problems, such as colostomy and diabetes. Thus, you can use the group process to enhance health teaching or for therapy to aid coping with problems. You may work with a group that has formed to accomplish some specific goal such as losing weight, promoting research to find a cure for cancer, or providing guidance to parents with mentally retarded children. In some cases, information is not enough. Social support is also necessary, especially when engaging in a lesser-valued activity—such as not eating excessive sweet foods.

Evaluation of teaching

1. Check frequently to determine if content is of interest or being understood.
2. Have client repeat content or give examples of application of content.
3. Have client review previously covered content, and its application, at each teaching session.
4. Determine the amount of learning that has occurred.

Tips on Teaching Clients

The following are four steps you can use in planning your teaching strategy:

1. Teach the **smallest amount** possible to do the job.
2. Make your point as **vivid** as you can.
3. Have the client **restate** and demonstrate the information.
4. **Review** repeatedly.

The following are important principles:

- Don't overstuff. Limit yourself to the essentials.
- Give a little—get a little. Feedback and practice are the methods by which the learning takes place.
- Three or four items of instruction are enough at any one time for clients.
- Space the learning. Understanding takes time and practice.
- Anxiety is the enemy. Do everything you can to help your clients overcome it.
- Reward every possible step with encouraging words. Clients need all the help they can get!

From Doak C, Doak L, Root J: *Teaching patients with low literacy skills,* Philadelphia, 1985, JB Lippincott.

Levels of Application of Preventive Measures

The chart below, developed by H.R. Leavell and E.G. Clark, shows the natural history of a disease as it relates to the three levels of prevention, then identifies specific activities that can be used for each level of prevention.

Natural history of a disease

Prepathogenesis period	Pathogenesis period		
Interrelations among agent, host, and environmental factors →Stimulus	Early pathogenesis →Discernible early lesions	→Advanced disease	→Convalescence

Levels of prevention

Primary prevention		Secondary prevention		Tertiary prevention
Health promotion	*Specific protection*	*Early diagnosis and prompt treatment*	*Disability limitation*	*Rehabilitation*
Health education	Use of specific immunizations	Case-finding measures, individual and mass	Adequate treatment to arrest disease process and prevent further complications and sequelae	Provision of hospital and community facilities for retraining and education for maximum use of remaining capacities
Good standard of nutrition adjusted to developmental phase of life	Attention to personal hygiene	Screening surveys		

Adapted from Leavell HR, Clark EG: *Preventive medicine for the doctor in his community,* ed 3, New York, 1965, McGraw-Hill.

Continued

Levels of Application of Preventive Measures—cont'd

Primary prevention		Secondary prevention		Tertiary prevention
Attention to personality development	Use of environmental sanitation	Selective examinations	Provision of facilities to limit disability and prevent death	Education of the public and industry to employ the rehabilitated
Provision of adequate housing, recreation, and agreeable working conditions	Protection against occupational hazards	Cure and prevention of disease processes		As full employment as possible
	Use of specific nutrients	Prevention of the spread of communicable diseases		Selective placement
Marriage counseling and sex education	Protection from carcinogens	Prevention of complications and sequelae		Work therapy in hospitals
Genetics	Avoidance of allergens	Shortened period of disability		Use of sheltered colony
Periodic selective examinations				

Criteria to Differentiate and Discriminate Among Preventive Approaches

Criteria	Types of approaches		
	Primary Proactive pretherapeutic	**Secondary** Para-active paratherapeutic	**Tertiary** Reactive therapeutic
1. Risk	Low to minimal	High: in need but not critical	Very high: critical
2. Reversibility	High: 100% to 66%	Medium: 66% to 33%	Low to very low: 33% to 0%
3. Probability of breakdown	Low but potential	Medium but probable	High and real (actual)
4. Population	Nonclinical: labeled but not diagnosable	Preclinical and diagnosable	Clinical: critical and diagnosed
5. Ability to learn	High	Medium	Low
6. Goals	Increase competence and resistance to breakdown	Decrease stress and chance of crisis	Restore to minimum functioning
7. Type of involvement	Voluntary: many choices	Obligatory: decrease in choices	Mandatory: no other choices available
8. Recommendations	"Could benefit by it." "It would be nice."	"You need it before it's too late." "Recommend strongly that you do it."	"It is necessary." "Nothing else will work." "Other choices would be more expensive" (i.e., hospitalization, incarceration)
9. Cost	Low	Medium	High
10. Effectiveness	High(?)	Questionable yet to be found	Relatively low
11. Personnel	Lay volunteers and pre- and paraprofessionals	Middle-level professionals	Professionals
12. Types of intervention	General, learning, strengthening, enrichment	More specific to behavior, that is, programmed materials	Specialized therapy
13. Degree of structure	High	Medium	Low
14. Degree of specificity	General and topical	Individualized	Specific to the symptom

From L'Abate L: *Building family competence*, Newbury Park, Calif, 1990, Sage Publications.

CERTAIN POPULATIONS

Physiologic Changes from Aging and Alterations in Teaching Techniques

Aging changes	Teaching techniques
Reaction time	
Lengthens	• Slow pace of presentations; do not rush response; provide liberal practice time • Give smaller amounts of information at each session • Repeat information frequently • Use analogies relevant to individual • Give reinforcement to verbal instructions with handouts, videos, practice
Manual dexterity	
Decreases	• Use tape-recorded instructions • Select precut appliances • Use anatomic models
Vision	
Lens yellows and thickens	• Avoid blue and green paper or print for teaching materials • Use nonglossy paper • Use large print for instructions • Make sure eyeglasses are worn • Make handouts of most important points
Lens accommodation decreases	• Make sure eyeglasses are worn • Use magnifying mirror • Use large graphic representations and hand gestures
Pupils are smaller; decreased amount of light to retina Decreased depth perception	• Use soft white light to reduce glare • Focus light directly on objects • Have light source behind client • Mark pump sprayer with bright nail polish toward direction of spray • Draw line with felt-tip pen to designate area of clamp placement and fill line of pouch • Use stoma guide strips • Allow for slightly larger pouch opening
Hearing	
Ability to discriminate sounds is reduced	• Speak more slowly • Use short sentences • Use *slightly* louder tone • Do not shout • Face client when speaking; do not cover mouth • Speak into client's ear

Continued

Hearing—cont'd

Ability to hear high frequencies and to distinguish consonant sounds (such as *c, ch, f, s, sh,* and *z*) is reduced	• Check whether hearing aid is worn • Determine whether client hears better with one ear • Maintain eye contact when speaking; make sure eyeglasses are being worn • Eliminate background noise • Allow time for client to repeat information

Adapted from Blaylock B: Enhancing self-care of the elderly client: practical tips for ostomy care, *J ET Nurs* 18:120, 1991. Used with permission. Added information from Welch-McCaffrey D: To teach or not to teach? Overcoming barriers to patient education in geriatric oncology, *Oncol Nurs Forum* 13:25-31, 1986. Also from Wilson CM et al: Educating the older cancer patient: obstacles and opportunities, *Health Educ Q* 10(suppl):76-87, 1984. From Boyle D: The elderly patient with cancer: teaching/learning considerations for ostomy, wound and continence management, *Progressions* 6(1):19, 1994.

Elderly Clients' Special Learning Needs

- Make sure the client is ready to learn before trying to teach. Watch for clues that would indicate that the client is preoccupied or too anxious to comprehend the material.
- Sit facing the client so that he or she can watch your lip movements and facial expressions.
- Speak slowly.
- Keep your tone of voice low; elderly persons can hear low sounds better than high-frequency sounds.
- Present one idea at a time.
- Emphasize concrete rather than abstract material.
- Give the client enough time in which to respond, because elderly persons' reaction times are longer than those of younger persons.
- Focus on a single topic to help the client concentrate.
- Keep environmental distractions to a minimum.
- Defer teaching if the client becomes distracted or tired or cannot concentrate for other reasons.
- Invite another member of the household to join the discussion.
- Use audio, visual, and tactile cues to enhance learning and help the client remember information.
- Ask for feedback to ensure that the information has been understood.

Modified from Fielo S, Rizzolo M: Handle with caring: meeting elderly clients' special learning needs, *Nurs Health Care* 9(4):193, 1988.

- Use past experience; connect new learning to that already learned.
- Compensate for physical discomfort and sensory decrements.
- Support a positive self-image in the learner.
- Use creative teaching strategies.
- Respond to identified interests of learners.
- Emphasize and integrate emotional and personal values in the acquisition of skills and ideas.

Teaching Guidelines for the Elderly Client With Cancer

- Ask how much, who wants to know, and what is the priority learning need?
- Determine the amount of information that was useful in the past.
- Review the sociocultural mix of your client caseload; consider modifications needed in teaching materials.
- Consider environmental impediments before teaching.
- Teach in phases, not "all at once"; break topics down into manageable concepts.
- Anticipate possible adherence difficulties.
- Include the family in teaching sessions.
- Use peer educational approach when possible.
- Plan clear, concise, and repetitive instruction.
- Reinforce teaching, particularly if this diagnosis or current problem is a new one (within the last 6 months).

From Boyle D: The elderly patient with cancer: teaching/learning considerations for ostomy, wound and continence management, *Progressions* 6(1):19, 1994.

Health Learning Needs for Individuals of Different Health Status

Health content grouped by functional health patterns	Health status		
	Wellness	Acute illness	Chronic illness
Health perception–health management			
Health monitoring	Regular screening exams: physical, dental, eye Breast self-exam/testicular exam Risk factors Environmental sensitivity Immunizations Lifestyle appraisal BP monitoring Seven signs of cancer	Symptom monitoring Follow-up healthcare When to call a professional	Symptom monitoring Follow-up healthcare When to call a professional Risk factors Environmental sensitivity Immunizations
Illness care	Identification and treatment of minor illness When to call a professional How to enter the healthcare system Over-the-counter medications	Illness-related information: symptoms, treatment, tests, equipment, medications, potential outcomes Recuperation: resumption of normal ADLs—diet, activity, work/school	Home care regimen Signs and symptoms of crisis When to call a professional How to enter the healthcare system Adaptation of treating minor illness due to chronic disease Over-the-counter medications/implications with chronic disease

From Boyd M et al: *Health teaching in nursing practice: a professional model*, ed 3, Stamford, CT, 1998, Appleton & Lange.   *Continued*

Health Learning Needs for Individuals of Different Health Status—cont'd

Health content grouped by functional health patterns	Health status		
	Wellness	Acute illness	Chronic illness
Safety	Home, work, auto Hygiene Smoking Avoiding carcinogens Alcohol and other drug use/abuse	Ambulation Hygiene Smoking Dangers of equipment	Home, work, auto Hygiene Smoking Avoiding carcinogens Alcohol and other drug use/abuse
Nutritional-Metabolic	Balancing nutrients Weight control Understanding nutrition labels	Adjustment for illness Equipment and feeding aids	Balancing nutrients to meet needs Weight control Adaptive devices
Elimination	Normal elimination Methods to promote	Changes in elimination Equipment to assist	Changes in elimination Adaptive equipment Importance of regular habits
Activity-Exercise	Regularity Amounts Methods to promote Incorporation into lifestyle	Hazards of immobility Adjustment for disease Energy conservation	Hazards of immobility Adjustment for disease Energy conservation Incorporation into lifestyle Assistive devices

Sleep-Rest	Amounts Natural induction	Adjustments for illness	Adjustments for illness Sleep aids Adaptive equipment
Cognitive-Perceptual			
Self-perception	Normal body functions Building self-esteem	Pain management Body changes from illness	Pain management Body changes from illness Building self-esteem
Role-Relationship	Parenting Developmental crises	Family roles during illness	Developmental crises Managing social situations Managing caregiver role strain
Sexuality	Sexual function and identity Contraception/family planning Safe sex Menopause	Changes associated with illness	Changes associated with illness Adaptations for illness Managing effects of medications
Coping-Stress	Self-responsibility Diversions Relaxation techniques Use of support systems	Self-responsibility Diversions Meeting physiologic needs Use of support systems	Self-responsibility Diversions Personal space Use of support systems Relaxation techniques

Client Teaching at Different Developmental Stages

Physical maturation
How well developed are the client's fine motor skills?
Does the client have good hand-eye coordination?
How does the client rate his or her own manual dexterity?
How much practice does the client usually need to learn a new psychomotor skill?
Can the client write?

Cognitive development
Formal educational experience?
How does the client use verbal language?
What is the level of reading ability?
Level of cognition:
  Does the client use experiences and perceptions or symbols when explaining the surrounding world?
  What is the client's understanding of past, present, future relationships?
Memory:
  How good is immediate recall? Recall after 15 minutes to an hour? Recall after longer periods of time?
  What improves the client's ability to remember?
How responsible is the client for self-care?

Psychosocial development
Life-stage tasks:
  What are the client's goals?
  What are the health-related aspects?
Role-relationships:
  What is the family composition?
  What roles do family members play? Who makes decisions?
  What are the communication patterns?
  What level of support do family members provide one another? Resources available (financial and other)?
  What is the involvement in the community?

From Boyd M et al: *Health teaching in nursing practice: a professional model,* ed 3, Stamford, CT, 1998, Appleton & Lange.

Implications for the Toddler's Health Learning

Key developmental factors	Implications for health learning
Physical maturation	
Motor: Upright mobility grossly coordinated	Able to learn simple activities: Dressing, washing, "exercise," tooth brushing
Hand-eye coordination: Manipulation of large objects	
Cognitive development	
Sensorimotor (Piaget)	Learns from actual experiences and use of senses; incorporate learning in play activities
Distractible	
Communication:	Short—2-5 minutes—sessions work best
Vocabulatory 500-1000 words	Use concrete, nonthreatening terms relative to sensory experiences
Expression mainly through motor channels	Approach honestly
Active fantasy life	For events, teach just prior to experience
Recognizes simple concrete objects	Able to learn to pick out good "snacks" and body parts
Psychosocial development	
Autonomy vs. shame and doubt (Erikson)	Involve parents and encourage pleasant tactile or visual reinforcement of behaviors
Separation anxiety	
Need for security, parental approval	Provide safety and comfort in learning environment
Utilizes mobility for coping	Incorporate activity during learning or as part of what is to be learned
Learning occurs largely through social interaction and modeling	Demonstrate, encourage parental modeling

From Boyd M et al: *Health teaching in nursing practice: a professional model,* ed 3, Stamford, CT, 1998, Appleton & Lange.

Implications for the Preschooler's Health Learning

Key developmental factors	Implications for health learning
Physical maturation	
Motor: Runs easily, beginning ability to balance	Help be independent with basic self-care; provide needed reminders
Expands environment	
Well-developed bowel and bladder control	
Hand-eye coordination	
Manipulation of large pencils and crayons still results in a degree of imprecision	
Able to build fairly complicated block structures	
Cognitive development	
Preoperational (Piaget)	Provide experiences for learning safety rules, rationale, body functions, address, phone number
Communication:	
Vocabulary 1000-2000 words	Use simple, concrete, non-threatening terms
Still relies heavily on symbolism and mobility of play	Use actual situations, visual symbols (drawings, dolls, pictures, puppets), and sensory experiences
Vague understanding about bodily functions, interested in conception and childbirth	Provide role play with actual or simulated equipment
Reality still not discriminated from fantasy	Elicit feedback through child's terms and play experiences
Curious	Give opportunity for practice, repetition
Limited attention span	
Egocentric	
Relates time to common events in daily life	Answer questions honestly and in an accepting manner without embarrassment
	Focus on the positive in relation to the child
	Plan brief—15 minutes maximum—learning sessions
	Relate events to known daily habits
Psychosocial development	
Initiative vs. guilt (Erikson)	Involve parents, remind of the role of parental modeling
Family remains of primary importance, although other persons may be significant	Specify body parts and sensory experiences involved in procedures
Imitation of same-sex parent role	
Fear of body injury	

From Boyd M et al: *Health teaching in nursing practice: a professional model,* ed 3, Stamford, CT, 1998, Appleton & Lange.

Implications for the School-Age Child's Health Learning

Key developmental factors	Implications for health learning
Physical maturation	
Motor: Moves energetically but with increasing grace and balance	Teach simple psychomotor tasks to young school-ager and more complex, such as insulin injections, after age 8-9
Able to participate in skilled sports	
Hand-eye coordination: Control and timing of motor movements well developed by age 8-9	
Cognitive development	
Concrete operations (Piaget)	Provide experiences learning about healthful eating, injury control, sexuality, basic first aid, exercise regimens, symptom control
Communication:	
Extensive vocabulary	
Understands cause and effect	
Attention span expands to allow 2-3 hours' work at a time	Use language—verbal and some written—using known terms, diagrams, and models
Decision-making skills develop	Clarify misconceptions
Develops orientation to past, present, and some future time	Give explanations of purpose and role in activities or procedures
	Plan lessons of 15-30 minutes
	Allow to make simple decisions related to own health and illness
	Give time to think through and sort out new things
Psychosocial development	
Industry vs. inferiority (Erikson)	Praise is a good reinforcer
Expanding interaction with peers	May learn well in group setting
Competition, compromise, and cooperation develop	Privacy is important
Increased awareness of sexual self and own uniqueness	Allow control through some help in planning
Fears disability, loss of status, loss of control	

From Boyd M et al: *Health teaching in nursing practice: a professional model,* ed 3, Stamford, CT, 1998, Appleton & Lange.

Implications for the Adolescent's Health Learning

Key developmental factors	Implications for health learning
Physical maturation	
Motor: near adult capacity	Provide experiences with self-care
Physical growth spurts may produce temporary clumsiness	skills
Hand-eye coordination: very discrete	Provide practice manipulating equipment for own medical treatments
Cognitive development	
Formal operations (Piaget)	Determine interest in accident
Communication:	prevention, environmental safety,
Interprets language	sexuality, health promotion
Understands satire and nuance	activities, substance abuse, illness
Understands complexities	regimens
Orientated to past, present, and future	Use verbal and written language, diagrams, and models
	Focus on both present health state and implications of health state on future outcomes
Psychosocial development	
Identity vs. identity diffusion (Erikson)	Promote own decisions related to health
Struggles for independence and self-control	Allow control through help with planning and goal setting
Group acceptance very important	Work with adolescent and parents separately
Compares own appearance and function with an ideal image	Provide privacy and confidentiality
Exploring ideas for future life	Involve in appropriate group activities

From Boyd M et al: *Health teaching in nursing practice: a professional model,* ed 3, Stamford, CT, 1998, Appleton & Lange.

Implications for Young and Middle Adult's Health Learning

Key developmental factors	Implications for health learning
Physical maturation	
Motor: During young adulthood, systems function at peak	Promote independence in all aspects of self-care and health decision-making
Some decrease in muscle tone during middle adulthood; outcome varies	Recognize that actions may be influenced by past experiences, economics, sociocultural practices, personal values
Hand-eye coordination: at best during young adulthood, declines not seen until late adulthood	
Energy: more quickly expended and more slowly recovered	
Cognitive development	
Full cognitive capacity	Recognize learners identify own readiness to learn
Flexibility, past experience, and confidence help with learning	Provide content relevant to existing life
Learning motivated when it is meaningful and applicable to needs	Use experiential as well as written and verbal methods
	Use past knowledge and experience as reference points
	Use analogies to illustrate more complex ideas
Psychosocial development	
Intimacy vs. self-isolation (Erikson—young adult)	Involve with planning and goal setting
Generativity vs. self-absorption and stagnation (Erikson—mature adult)	Determine learning needs to help cope with role changes, developmental changes in career, lifestyle alternatives to prevent and manage illness
Lifestyle choices—career, family important	
Self-sufficiency of early adulthood expands to include social and civic responsibilities	

From Boyd M et al: *Health teaching in nursing practice: a professional model,* ed 3, Stamford, CT, 1998, Appleton & Lange.

Implications for the Older Adult's Health Learning

Key developmental factors	Implications for health learning
Physical maturation	
Sensory changes:	Use distinct, large configurations in visual aids, clean glasses; good lighting; eliminate glare; use high-contrast colors
Decreased acuity and accommodation of vision	
Loss of perception of high tone sounds and some sound discrimination	Speak clearly, at a normal rate, close to learner. Increase loudness and deepen pitch as needed
More easily fatigued, less able to sit for lengthy periods	Provide short learning sessions
	Teach when most alert and rested
Cognitive development	
Affected by motivation, interest, sensory alteration	Present content at a slow pace or foster self-pacing
Decreased speed of response	Allow adequate response time
Less efficient short-term memory	Provide repetition, opportunities for recall
Simultaneous activities disruptive	Present smaller amounts of information at one time
	Eliminate distracting sights and sounds
Psychosocial development	
Ego integrity vs. despair (Erikson)	Mutually establish reachable short-term goals
Well-developed lifestyle habits	
Changes in roles occur through retirement, loss of spouse (others) through death	Encourage participation in decision-making and planning for learning
	Integrate new behaviors with previously established ones
Changes in body image due to effects of aging	Encourage family members to participate
	Apply to current situation

From Boyd M et al: *Health teaching in nursing practice: a professional model,* ed 3, Stamford, CT, 1998, Appleton & Lange.

SPEECH AND LANGUAGE CONDITIONS

Sign Language for Common Health Situations

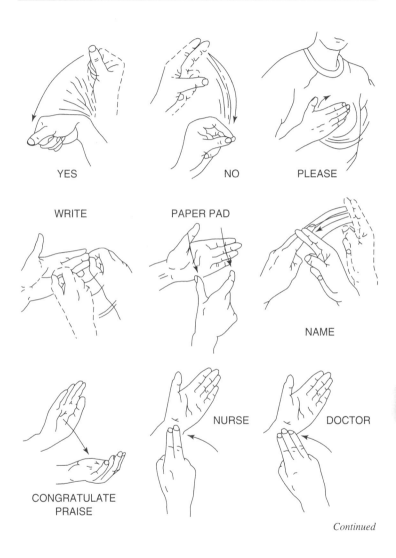

YES

NO

PLEASE

WRITE

PAPER PAD

NAME

CONGRATULATE
PRAISE

NURSE

DOCTOR

Continued

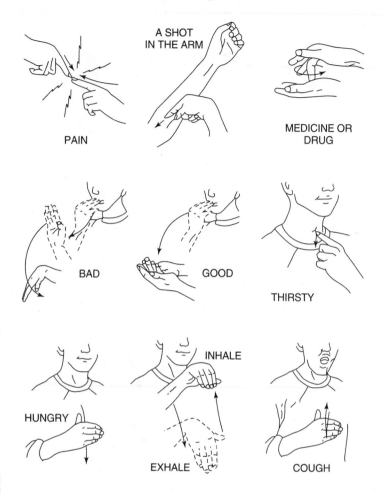

PAIN

A SHOT
IN THE ARM

MEDICINE OR
DRUG

BAD

GOOD

THIRSTY

HUNGRY

INHALE

EXHALE

COUGH

Manual Sign Language Alphabet

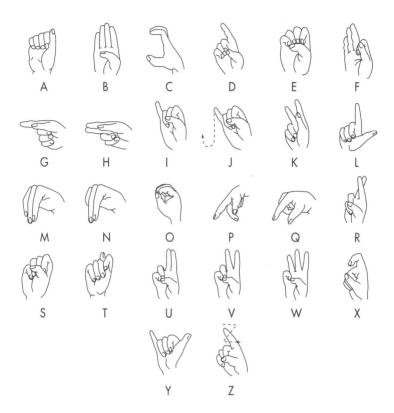

Tips for Communicating With a Hearing Impaired Person

The person who is hard of hearing must be made aware that someone is speaking to them. A hearing impaired person addressed from behind or at their side often cannot hear the speaker. Always get their attention first by touching the shoulder or arm gently and by approaching from the front. If the person has a "good" ear, move to that side before speaking.

Some practical hints for speaking to a hearing-impaired person include the following:

- The speaker should position himself or herself directly in front of the person.
- The speaker should ensure good lighting so their face can be easily seen.
- Communication is visual; thus, body language is essential.
- The speaker should use simple words and sentences.
- The speaker should not cover his or her mouth, chew gum, or eat when speaking.
- The speaker should have a paper to write out key words.
- When a hearing aid is used, the speaker should direct his or her speech to the battery unit of the listener's hearing aid (worn in the ear or as a body unit). The speaker should not shout, but should speak distinctly. A hearing aid is an amplifier, and it will distort sounds that are too loud.
- If a person uses sign language, the speaker should inquire which hand or arm is used for signing. This is especially important when planning for IV care.

Keep It Simple—Reading Skills Rules

Clients with poor reading skills are more likely to understand written information presented at the fifth-grade reading level. Readability formulas may be useful as screening tools because they're easy to use and give quantitative ratings. The SMOG Readability Index is one such formula that's most often used by educators. It uses the average number of sentences and syllables in three 100-word passages to determine grade-level readability estimates. Following are some general tips:

- Use a conversational style and an active voice in writing. For example, say, "Use a measuring cup for vegetables" instead of "A measuring cup should be used for vegetables."
- Use short words and sentences whenever possible.
- State the topic of the paragraph in the first sentence so the client will know immediately what the paragraph is about.
- Limit the number of ideas on one page.

From Fain J: When your patient can't read, *Am J Nurs* 6:160, 1994.

- Don't put words in all capital letters, handwriting, or a stylized type-face. Using 16- to 18-point type with uppercase and lowercase letters makes it easier to decode words.
- Break up long stretches of narrative with subtitles and captions.
- Write lists—don't bury sequential information or series of events or ideas in narrative form.
- Leave plenty of open white space on the printed page. This will help clients concentrate on the educational message by minimizing distracting elements.
- Use arrows, circles, and underlining to help focus attention on the message.
- Black print on white or yellow paper is the most easily read. In contrast, pale green, pink, and blue are difficult to read.
- Dull finishes are preferable to glossy paper.
- Illustrations (with enough detail to emphasize the intended message) and photographs add appeal.
- Be sure pictures portray only intended messages.

SMOG Testing to Check Literacy Skills

The SMOG formula was originally developed by G. Harry McLaughlin in 1969. It will predict the grade-level difficulty of a passage within 1.5 grades in 68% of the passages tested. That may be close enough for your purposes. It is simple to use and faster than most other measures. The procedure is presented below.

Instructions

1. You will need 30 sentences. Count out 10 consecutive sentences near the beginning, 10 consecutive from the middle, and 10 from the end. For this purpose, a sentence is any string of words punctuated by a period (.), an exclamation point (!), or a question mark (?).
2. From the entire 30 sentences, count the words containing **three or more syllables,** including repetitions.
3. Obtain the grade level from Table 4-1, or you may calculate the grade level as follows: Determine the nearest perfect square root of the total number of words of three or more syllables and then add a constant of 3 to the square root to obtain the grade level.

From Doak C, Doak L, Root J: *Teaching patients with low literacy skills,* Philadelphia, 1985, JB Lippincott.

Example:

Total number of multisyllabic (3 or more syllables) words	67	
Nearest perfect square	64	
Square root	8	
Add constant of 3	11	This is the grade level.

Table 4-1 SMOG conversion table

Word count	Grade level
0-2	4
3-6	5
7-12	6
13-20	7
21-30	8
31-42	9
43-56	10
57-72	11
73-90	12
91-110	13
111-132	14
133-156	15
157-182	16
183-210	17
211-240	18

Developed by Harold C. McGraw, Office of Educational Research, Baltimore County Public Schools, Towson, Maryland.

Special rules for SMOG testing

- Hyphenated words are **one** word.
- For numerals, pronounce them aloud and count the syllables pronounced for each numeral (e.g., for the number 573, five = 1, hundred = 2, seventy = 3, and three = 1, or 7 syllables).
- Proper nouns should be counted.
- If a long sentence has a colon, consider each part of it as a separate sentence. However, if possible, avoid selecting that segment of the passage.
- The words for which the abbreviations stand should be read aloud to determine their syllable count (e.g., Oct. = October = 3 syllables).

SMOG on shorter passages

Sometimes it may be necessary to assess the readability of a passage of less than 30 sentences. You can still use the SMOG formula to obtain an approximate grade level by using a conversion number from Table 4-2 and then using Table 4-1 to find the grade level.

First count the number of sentences in your material and the number of words with three or more syllables. In Table 4-2, in the left-hand column, locate the number of sentences, and locate the conversion number in the column opposite. Multiply the word count found earlier by the conversion number. Use this number in Table 4-2 to obtain the corresponding grade level.

Table 4-2 SMOG conversion for samples with fewer than 30 sentences

Number of sentences in sample material	Conversion number
29	1.03
28	1.07
27	1.1
26	1.15
25	1.2
24	1.25
23	1.3
22	1.36
21	1.43
20	1.5
19	1.58
18	1.67
17	1.76
16	1.87
15	2.0
14	2.14
13	2.3
12	2.5
11	2.7
10	3

From Doak C, Doak L, Root J: *Teaching patients with low literacy skills,* Philadelphia, 1985, JB Lippincott.

For example, suppose your material consisted of 15 sentences and you counted 12 words of three or more syllables in this material. Proceed as follows:

1. In Table 4-2, left-hand column, locate the number of sentences in your material. For your material, the number is 15.
2. Opposite 15 in the adjacent column, find the conversion number. The conversion number for 15 is 2.0.

3. Multiply your word count, 12, by 2 to get 24.
4. Now look at Table 4-2 to find the grade level. For a word count of 24, the grade level is 8.

Readability Graph

1. Select three 100-word passages from near the beginning, middle, and end of the book. Skip all proper nouns.
2. Count the total number of sentences in each 100-word passage (estimating to nearest tenth of a sentence). Average these three numbers.
3. Count the total number of syllables in each 100-word sample. There is a syllable for each vowel sound; for example: cat (1), blackbird (2), continental (4). Don't be fooled by word size; for example: polio (3), through (1). Endings such as -y, -ed, -el, or -le usually make a syllable, for example: ready (2), bottle (2). You may find it convenient to count every syllable over one in each word and add 100. Average the total number of syllables for the three samples.
4. Plot on the graph the average number of sentences per 100 words and the average number of syllables per 100 words. Most plot points fall near the heavy curved line. Perpendicular lines mark off approximate grade level areas.

EXAMPLE

	SENTENCES PER 100 WORDS	SYLLABLES PER 100 WORDS
100-word sample page 5	9.1	122
100-word sample page 89	8.5	140
100-word sample page 160	7.0	129
	3)24.6	3)391
Average	**8.2**	**130**

Plotting these averages on the graph, we find they fall in the fifth grade area; hence the book is about fifth grade difficulty level. If great variability is encountered either in sentence length or in the syllable count for the three selections, then randomly select several more passages and average them in before plotting.

From Fry E: *J Reading* 11:514, 1968.

Gunning FOG Index^{sm} Scale

1. Select a sample of writing 100 to 125 words long. If the piece is long, take several samples and average the results.
2. Calculate the average number of words per sentence. Treat independent clauses as separate sentences. "In school we studied; we learned; we improved" counts as three sentences.
3. Count the number of words of three syllables or more. In your count, omit capitalized words; combinations of short words like *bookkeeper* or *manpower;* or verbs made into three syllables by adding "*-es*" or "*-ed.*" Divide the count of long words by the passage length to get the percentage.
4. Add 2 (average sentence length) and 3 (percentage of long words). Multiply the sum by the factor 0.4, and ignore the digits following the decimal point.

The result is the years of schooling needed to read the passage with ease. Few readers have over 17 years of schooling, so any passage over 17 gets a FOG Index of "17-plus."

From Gunning R, Kallan R: *How to take the fog out of business writing,* Chicago, 1994, Dartnell. The Fog Index^{sm} Scale is a service mark licensed exclusively to RK Communication Consultants by D. and M. Mueller.

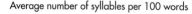

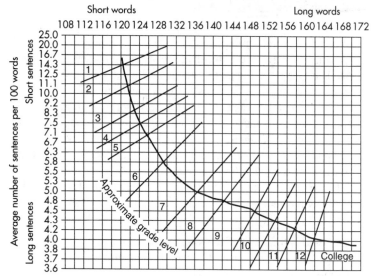

Graph for estimating readability. *Directions:* Randomly select three 100-word passages from a book or an article. Plot average number of syllables and average number of words per sentence on graph to determine area of readability level. Choose more passages per book if great variability is observed. *From Fry E:* J Reading *11:514, 1968.*

Nursing Suggestions to Encourage Language Development in Preschoolers

Read to the child. Encourage the child to be an active listener by pausing at times during the story to ask such questions as, "What do you think will happen next?"; "Why do you think the boy said that?"; and "What would you do now?"

Praise the child's storytelling.

Always respond to the child's questions. At times a response must be delayed; for example, if the parent is driving in heavy traffic and the child asks a question that requires a complex answer, the parent might say, "That's a very good question, let's talk about that as soon as we get home." The parent should remind the child later of the question and respond if the child still is interested.

Never tease or criticize a child about his verbalizations. If the child is excited and talking so fast that he is fumbling over words, the parent might say, "I can't listen that fast. Slow down a little for me." This is much more encouraging than, "You talk too fast. No one can understand you."

Play games that are language focused, such as naming the colors of houses or kinds of flowers as parent and child walk to the store.

From Edelman CL, Mandle CL: *Health promotion throughout the lifespan,* ed 4, St Louis, 1998, Mosby.

Administration and Scoring of the Preschool Readiness Experimental Screening Scale (PRESS)

NAME   BIRTH DATE

SCHOOL   DATE

1. a. What color is grass? _____
    b. What color is the sky if there are no clouds? _____
2. a. Repeat four numbers (one success in two tries): 4-1-7-3 or 3-8-6-4 _____
    b. Recognize four tongue blades. _____

3. a. Does Christmas come in the winter or the summer? _____
    b. Where is your heel? _____

4. Draw a square (best success in two tries). _____
5. a. Comprehension and performance _____
    b. Personal-social maturity _____
                            TOTAL _____

Comments:

PRESS General Outline and Record Form. The children were asked to reproduce a standard 1-inch square.

From Rogers WB Jr, Rogers RA: *Clin Pediatr* 11:10, 1972, and Rogers WB Jr, Rogers RA: *Clin Pediatr* 14, 253.

Introduction
As the child is placed on the examining table and the records and equipment are organized, the nurse says:

1. "Mrs. Smith, as I examine Johnny I will be asking him a few questions, so please don't talk to him for a few minutes." The nurse smiles and asks: "Ok?"
2. "Johnny, I hear you're going to start kindergarten soon. Do you think you'll like that?"

Knowledge of colors
These questions are asked during the eye, ear, nose, throat (EENT) examination:

1. "I hear your teacher will want you to know colors. Do you know any colors yet?"
2. "If she asks you to color a house, what color should you make the grass?"
3. "And what color should you make the sky if there are no clouds?"

Knowledge of numbers
These questions are asked during the heart and lung examination:

1. "If the teacher tells you some numbers, could you remember them and repeat them back to her?"
2. "I'm going to tell you some numbers. Now you remember them and say the same numbers right back to me." (4-1-7-3 and 3-8-6-4)
3. "If the teacher asks you to count, could you do that?"
4. "Tell me, how many tongue blades are there?" At this point place four tongue blades on the table beside the child.

Instructions for use of PRESS
Parents of preschoolers often ask how to tell if their child is ready for school or for a particular school program. School readiness can be

From Edelman CL, Mandle CL: *Health Promotion Throughout the Lifespan,* ed. 3, St Louis, 1994, Mosby.

thought of as the fit between the child's skill level, the child's and family's psychosocial status, and the characteristics of the particular school program. Any questions about an individual child's readiness should only be answered after all of these components are addressed. The developmental testing used during the toddler years is less accurate as the child approaches school age. Some appropriate tools can help to identify the child's skill level.

A widely used tool is *PRESS,* or *Preschool Readiness Experimental Screening Scale.* Determinations of its validity indicate that it is reliable in assessing school readiness. The nurse can administer it easily during a health assessment. The central concern is *not* measurement of intellectual level but rather screening for developmental lags or abnormalities that would interfere with the child's ability to succeed in the academic and social world of school. The tool was constructed for the average capabilities of 5-year-old children but may be useful in estimating readiness in children slightly older or younger.

When obtaining more specific scores of developmental age is necessary, the nurse may use one of the screening tools specific to the preschool child. Such screening tools provide only a rough estimate of ability but may be useful in identifying those children who need more extensive evaluation of intellectual capacity.

SUBSTANCE ABUSE

The Progression and Recovery of the Alcoholic in the Disease of Alcoholism

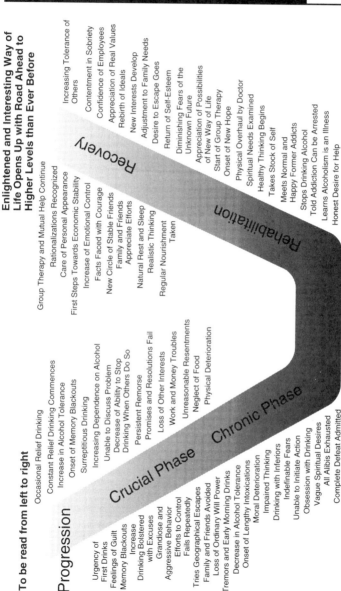

From Jellinek EM, QJ Stud Alcohol 13:672, 1952.

Stages of Chemical Dependence

Characteristics	Early stage	Middle stage	Late stage
Pattern of use	Regular	Daily	Continuous
Motives for use	To relax, sleep, achieve euphoria	To feel "normal"	To avoid uncomfortable psychologic or physiologic states (to avoid withdrawal symptoms)
Tolerance	Tolerant	Tolerant	Lower threshold of tolerance
Dependence	Psychologic dependence	Psychologic dependence and possible physiologic dependence	Psychologic and physiologic dependence
Job performance	May be somewhat diminished	Decreased productivity	Impaired performance
Social and community relations	Arguments over use	Increasing isolation	Withdrawal from community activities and social relationships

Adapted from Clark J, Queener S, Karb V: *Pharmacologic basis of nursing practice,* ed 6, St Louis, 2000, Mosby; Fortinash K, Holoday-Worret P: *Psychiatric mental health nursing,* ed 2, St Louis, 2000, Mosby.

Substance Use Prevention

Definition
Prevention of an alcoholic or drug use lifestyle

Activities
Assist patient to tolerate increased levels of stress, as appropriate
Prepare patient for difficult or painful events
Reduce irritating or frustrating environmental stress

From McCloskey JC, Bulechek GM: *Nursing interventions classification (NIC),* ed 2, St Louis, 1996, Mosby.

Reduce social isolation, as appropriate

Support measures to regulate the sale and distribution of alcohol to minors

Lobby for increased drinking age

Recommend responsible changes in the alcohol and drug curricula for primary grades

Conduct programs in schools on the avoidance of drugs and alcohol as recreational activities

Encourage responsible decision-making about lifestyle choices

Recommend media campaigns on substance use issues in the community

Instruct parents in the importance of example in substance use

Instruct parents and teachers in the identification of signs and symptoms of addiction

Assist patient to identify substitute tension-reducing strategies

Support or organize community groups to reduce injuries associated with alcohol, such as SADD and MADD

Survey students in grades 1 through 12 on the use of alcohol and drugs and alcohol-related behaviors

Instruct parents to support school policy that prohibits drug and alcohol consumption at extracurricular activities

Assist in the organization of post-activities for teenagers for such functions as prom and homecoming

Facilitate coordination of efforts between various community groups concerned with substance use

SPECIFIC CONDITIONS/ILLNESSES

Advantages and Disadvantages of Contraceptive Methods in the Adolescent

Method	Advantages	Disadvantages
Abstinence	100% effective in prevention of sexually transmitted diseases (STDs) and pregnancy No medical visit needed	Peer pressure for intercourse
Withdrawal Withdrawal of penis before ejaculation		High failure rate Some seminal fluid often released before ejaculation Ejaculate at vaginal orifice may enter vagina No STD protection
Rhythm Refrain from intercourse during fertile period	Encourages couple participation	Requires a predictable menstrual cycle, unusual in early and middle adolescence No STD protection High failure rates
Barrier methods Condom *Male:* Penile covering to trap sperm *Female:* Inserted into vagina with base covering part of perineum	No prescription needed Easy to use STD protection No medical complications	Interrupts intercourse May have decreased sensations Requires consistent use
Diaphragm Cervical covering to prevent sperm from reaching eggs Used with spermicidal jelly	May be inserted 4 to 6 hours before intercourse Effective when used correctly Few medical complications May be reused	Little STD protection Requires fitting by medical personnel Requires body awareness and comfort with touching oneself for insertion

Method/Description	Advantages	Disadvantages
Sponge Cervical covering	May be inserted up to 6 hours before intercourse	May increase incidence of urinary tract infection
Releases a spermicide	Can be obtained without prescription	Minimal STD protection
		Requires body awareness and comfort with touching self
		May be difficult to remove
		Decreased effectiveness in parous women
		High failure rate unless used with condom
Spermicides Foam, jelly, cream, suppositories	Available without prescription	Interrupts sexual experience
Inserted into vagina to kill sperm	Inexpensive	Messy
	Easy to use	Must use consistently
	No major health concerns	
Oral contraceptives Estrogen and progesterone-like compounds that inhibit ovulation	Few medical complications in teens	Requires prescription
	99% effective if used correctly	Expensive
	No interruption of intercourse	No STD protection
	Regulates menses, decreased dysmenorrhea and acne	Small weight gain
Norplant Levonorgestrel slowly released into vascular system for 5 years	No interruption of intercourse	No STD protection
Inhibits ovulation, thickens cervical mucosa; 6 small rods inserted into upper arm	Long-term, highly effective protection against pregnancy	Significant weight gain
	Pregnancy prevention begins 24 hours after insertion	Irregular menses
	Once removed, fertility returns immediately	Requires minor surgical procedure
		Expensive

From Wong DL, et al: *Whaley and Wong's nursing care of infants and children*, ed 6, St Louis, 1999, Mosby.

Advantages and Disadvantages of Contraceptive Methods in the Adolescent—cont'd

Method	Advantages	Disadvantages
Depo Provera Progestin that suppresses hormonal cycle and prevents ovulation Injection given every 3 months	No interruption of intercourse Invisible method	No STD protection Significant weight gain Irregular menses or amenorrhea Decreased libido Fertility may be delayed Must return to care provider every 3 months for injection
Postcoital contraception Combined estrogen–progestin pill containing ethinyl estradiol; given within 72 hours of unprotected sex and repeated 12 hours later; prevents implantation	Useful in unplanned sexual intercourse	No STD protection May experience nausea Effectiveness dependent on phase of menstrual cycle Not intended for repeated use

Pelvic Muscle Exercises

The pelvic floor is made up of muscles responsible for holding the body's lower organs, including the bladder. Because we walk upright, quite a bit of pressure is put on these organs as we walk, exercise, cough, or pick up something. When these muscles are weakened by childbirth or hormonal changes (such as those caused by menopause) or as a result of surgery or lower back injury, small amounts of urine may leak with physical activity. This condition is called stress incontinence, and it affects many women and some men.

Stress incontinence may be controlled without surgery in many cases. Exercising the pelvic muscles is a good way to strengthen them. Pelvic exercises (sometimes called Kegel exercises, after Dr. Arnold Kegel) are an excellent way to improve the fitness of the pelvic floor muscles.

Pelvic muscle exercises for women

First, it is important to locate and identify the correct muscles to exercise. The muscles you wish to exercise surround the urethra (the tube where urine leaves your body) and the vagina. You can find this muscle by practicing stopping your urine in midstream. Tighten (contract) the muscles to stop the urine; release the muscles to continue urination. Your nurse will help you locate the correct muscles. She may gently place a gloved finger in the vagina and ask you to contract the muscles around her finger, or she may use a special machine that helps you find and contract the correct muscles. The special machine uses sound or visual signals to help you understand how to contract and release the pelvic muscles. The nurse will also help you avoid tightening your abdominal or thigh muscles. Contracting these muscles will not help you strengthen the pelvic muscles.

It is helpful to practice Kegel exercises while urinating because correct muscle tightness will stop the flow of urine. During urination, tighten your muscles until the flow stops. The buttocks will be squeezed together. Hold back the flow for 3 to 5 seconds and then relax and start the flow of urine again. Repeat this stopping and starting of urinating flow 10 times, or until there is no more urine. Later you will be able to vary your muscle tightness from a rapid pace to a prolonged 10- to 30-second period.

As soon as you think you understand how to contract and release the pelvic muscles, here's how to proceed:

- Choose a time and place to exercise. You will need about 15 minutes to do your exercises.
- You will find the best position to do your exercises with practice. Some women prefer to sit or stand; others lie on the back with the head elevated on a pillow.
- Tighten the pelvic muscles as hard as you can.
- Hold the muscle tight for 10 seconds—you may find it helpful to count to 10—then relax the muscle for 10 seconds.
- Repeat this exercise 10 times.
- Ask your nurse or doctor how many times a day (repetitions) you need to perform the exercise (generally, it is best to begin with 10 repetitions and work up to 35 to 50 repetitions every other day). Remember that one repetition consists of 10 seconds of tightening and 10 seconds of relaxation.

You may wish to try a variation of this exercise.

- While sitting, standing, or lying with your head elevated, tighten and release the pelvic muscles in rapid succession. Repeat this 15 times.
- In the same position, tighten the pelvic muscles while you exhale. Hold the muscle for a count of 30. Repeat this exercise 10 times.

Nursing Counseling for Families about Enuresis

- Enuresis is a common problem.
- No serious physical problem is present, although the child may have a small or immature bladder.
- It is often inherited; other family members may have had the same problem. With time the child will be cured, usually by adolescence.
- The child is not wetting the bed intentionally; it is not a conscious act.
- The parents are not at fault.
- If a treatment is tried, the child needs to be responsible for dealing with both the problem and the treatment.
- Punishment when the child is wet should be replaced with praise when dry (positive reinforcement).

From Edelman CL, Mandle CL: *Health promotion throughout the lifespan,* ed 4, St Louis, 1998, Mosby.

- Parents may wake the child to urinate before they go to bed.
- A family plan for dealing with the wet bed and child can decrease family arguments. The plan may include who strips the bed and where the sheets go. The child should play a major role in this process to understand the impact of this behavior on the family and to learn responsibility for the act.

Suggestions for Content of Education Program for Diabetes

a) General facts

- Definition of diabetes mellitus
- Basic anatomy and physiology
- Basic metabolism of carbohydrates, protein, and fats
- Classification of diabetes (type 1, type 2, gestational, etc.)

b) Psychologic adjustment

- Client self-assessment
- What is "compliance?"
- Successful adjustment and coping (living with a chronic disease, work, travel, and vacation)
- Expressing feelings openly
- Collaboration between client and healthcare team

c) Family involvement

- Diabetes as a family challenge
- Coping with feelings (client and family)
- Learning to recognize and work with adverse family dynamics
- Coping with the healthcare system

d) Nutrition

- Learning to structure a daily diet
- Learning a dietary system: exchange system, flexible diet, menu plans, others
- Understanding dietary concepts: food content, food groups, glycemic indices, others

Adapted from Centers for Disease Control and Prevention, Department of Health and Human Services, Public Health Services, National Center for Chronic Disease Prevention and Health Promotion, Division of Diabetes Translation Publications. Available: http://www.cdc.gov/diabetes.

- Defining, achieving, and maintaining weight goals
- Special occasions—how to enjoy them
- Nutritional resources

e) Exercise

- Benefits
- Methods
- Precautions
- Food and insulin adjustment
- Heart rate

f) Medications

- Goal of treatment
- Oral agents:
  - Explanation of use
  - Action
  - Cautions
  - Drug interactions
- Insulin:
  - Explanation of use
  - Action
  - Cautions (especially Somogyi effect)
  - Strengths—purities
  - Injection techniques
  - Complications of treatment—hypoglycemia, antibodies, lipodystrophy
  - Dose and timing

g) Relationship between nutrition/exercise/medication

- Putting it all together
- How each relates to the other

h) Monitoring

- Goals
- Kinds of monitoring available
- Strengths and limitations of each kind
- How to use monitoring to achieve and maintain good glucose control

i) Hyperglycemia and hypoglycemia

- Definition of hyperglycemia and hypoglycemia
- What to do for each
- When to call the healthcare team

- Prevention of each
- Record keeping

j) Illness

- Effect of illness on diabetes
- Monitoring glucose/ketones
- Sick day guidelines (including diet)
- When to call the healthcare team

k) Complications (prevent, treat, rehabilitate)

- Kinds of complications
- Possible causes of complications
- Self-care for prevention of complications
- Referral and treatment
- Rehabilitation

l) Hygiene (skin, teeth, feet, genitals, etc.)

- Relationship to diabetes care
- Self-care measures to prevent complications

m) Benefits and responsibilities of care

- Maintaining short- and long-term life goals
- Client-professional care partnership
- Rights of the client
- Responsibilities of the client

n) Use of healthcare systems

- Ensuring prompt referral, coordinated care and continuing access to medical and educational services
- Identifying and using available resources

o) Community resources

- Agencies available
- Who, what, when, where to call
- Licensing and employment regulations
- Insurance considerations
- Use of local library

The Relaxation Response

Content	Instructional activities	Evaluation
Describe the characteristics and benefits of relaxation	Discuss physiologic changes associated with relaxation and contrast these with behaviors of anxiety	Client identifies own responses to anxiety Client describes elements of a relaxed state
Teach deep-muscle relaxation through a sequence of tension-relaxation exercises	Engage client in the progressive procedure of tensing and relaxing voluntary muscles until the body as a whole is relaxed	Client is able to tense and relax all muscle groups Client identifies those muscles that become particularly tense
Discuss the relaxation procedure of meditation and its components	Describe the elements of meditation and assist client in using this technique	Client selects a word or scene with pleasant connotations and engages in relaxed meditation
Assist in overcoming anxiety-provoking situations through systematic desensitization	With client, construct a hierarchy of anxiety-provoking situations or scenes Through imagination or reality, work through these scenes using relaxation techniques	Client identifies and ranks anxiety-provoking situations Client exposes self to these situations while remaining in a relaxed state
Allow the rehearsing and practical use of relaxation in a safe environment Encourage client to use relaxation techniques in life	Role-play stressful situations with the nurse or other clients Assign homework of using the relaxation response in everyday experiences Support success of client	Client becomes more comfortable with new behavior in a safe, supportive setting Client uses relaxation response in life situations Client is able to regulate anxiety response through use of relaxation techniques

From Stuart GW, Sundeen SJ: *Principles and practice of psychiatric nursing*, ed 5, St Louis, 1995, Mosby.

Managing Pain without Drugs

There are several techniques you can use to relieve pain without taking drugs or to enhance the effect of your pain medication—**relaxation, imagery, distraction,** and **skin stimulation.**

Relaxation

Relaxation relieves pain by easing muscle tension. Easing muscle tension can also help you feel less tired and anxious and help other pain-relieving methods work better.

How to relax.   Sit or lie down, preferably in a quiet place. Be sure you are comfortable. Do not cross your legs or arms.

Take a deep breath, and tense your muscles (you may tense up your whole body or concentrate on one set of muscles at a time, such as your facial muscles or those in your arms and hands).

Hold your breath, and keep your muscles tense.

Release your breath and your muscles at the same time. Let your body go limp (repeat for other muscle areas if you are concentrating on one set at a time).

You can add imagery (see below) or music to help you relax. Relaxation tapes are also available.

Don't be discouraged if relaxation doesn't help immediately. Practice the relaxation technique for 2 weeks before you give it up. If you find that it aggravates your pain, try another method.

Imagery

Imagery involves using your imagination to create mental scenes that use all your senses: sight, sound, touch, smell, and taste. You can imagine exotic locations or revisit one of your favorite places. You can create stories and characters to add to your scenes. Imagery can take your mind off your anxiety, boredom, and pain.

How to use imagery.   Close your eyes. A few moments of the relaxation technique (see above) will help your body and mind prepare for imagery.

Let your mind begin forming its image. The following is an example of imagery:

Imagine that you are at the seashore. You are sitting in the wet sand; the afternoon sun is warm on your shoulders. The ocean rolls into the shore in gentle waves, and the water laps teasingly at your toes. A hungry pair of seagulls cries overhead and take swift, darting dives at a dog that is scavenging along the shore. Your tension lessens with each wave that touches your toes and retreats. You close your eyes and take a deep, slow breath of salt-filled air. You are completely relaxed. Stay on the beach as long as you like.

To end the image, count to three and open your eyes. Resume your regular activities slowly.

Distraction

A distraction is any activity that takes your mind off your pain and focuses your attention elsewhere. Doing crafts, reading a book, watching television, or listening to music through headphones can all help distract your mind. Distraction works well when you are waiting for drugs to take effect or if you have brief bouts of pain. Sometimes people can take their minds off their pain for long periods, especially if the pain is mild.

Skin stimulation

Skin stimulation is used to block pain sensation in the nerves. Pressure, massage, hot and cold applications, rubbing, and mild electrical current are all ways to stimulate the skin. However, if you are undergoing radiation treatment, consult your doctor before applying any skin stimulation.

You can do skin stimulation at the site of the pain, near it, or on the opposite side of pain. For example, stimulating the left wrist when the right wrist is in pain can actually ease the pain in the right wrist.

Pressure.   Using your entire hand, the heel of your hand, your thumb, your knuckles, or both hands, apply at least 15 seconds of pressure at the point where you feel pain. Keep trying spots around the painful area if you find no relief the first time. You may extend the time you apply pressure to 1 minute.

Massage.   You or someone else can perform the slow, circular motions of massage. The feet, back, neck, and scalp can be massaged to relieve tension and pain anywhere in the body. Some people prefer to use oils or lotions during the massage. If deep massage is too uncomfortable, try light stroking. Do not massage red, raw, or broken skin.

Heat and cold.   Some people prefer cold; others prefer heat. Use whichever works best for you. A convenient way to use cold is to freeze gel-filled packs and wrap them in towels. Ice cubes can also be used. Heat can be applied with a heating pad; hot, moist towels; or a hot water bottle or by taking a hot bath. Be careful not to burn your skin with water that is too hot or to go to sleep with a heating pad on. Don't expose your skin to intense cold for very long.

Transcutaneous electrical nerve stimulation (TENS). TENS can be used to eliminate or ease pain. A TENS unit is a pocket-sized, battery-operated device that provides a mild, continuous electrical current through the skin by the use of two to four electrodes, which are taped onto the skin. Lead wires connect the electrodes to the device. It is this mild electrical current that blocks or modifies the pain messages and replaces them with a buzzing, tingling sensation. It is also thought that TENS may stimulate the body's production of endorphins, natural pain relievers.

Typical Characteristics of Codependence

- Over-involvement with a dysfunctional person.
- Obsessive attempts to control the dysfunctional person's behavior.
- A strong need for approval from others:
  –Low self esteem
  –Feels worthless when not productive
  –Pleases others and not self
- Constantly making personal sacrifices to help the dysfunctional person be "cured" of the problem behavior:
  –Overresponsibility to others
  –Feels trapped in the relationship

Adapted from Stuart G, Laraia M: *Stuart and Sundeen's principles and practice of psychiatric nursing,* ed 6, St Louis, 1998, Mosby.

Appropriate Expression of Anger

Content	Instructional activities	Evaluation
Help the patient identify anger.	Focus on nonverbal behavior. Role play nonverbal expression of anger. Label the feeling using the patient's preferred words.	Patient demonstrates an angry body posture and facial expression.
Give permission for angry feelings.	Describe situations in which it is normal to feel angry.	Patient describes a situation in which anger would be an appropriate response.
Practice the expression of anger.	Role play fantasized situations in which anger is an appropriate response.	Patient participates in role play and identifies behaviors associated with expression of anger.
Apply the expression of anger to a real situation.	Help identify a real situation that makes the patient angry. Role play a confrontation with the object of the anger. Provide positive feedback for successful expression of anger.	Patient identifies a real situation that results in anger. Patient is able to role play expression of anger.
Identify alternative ways to express anger.	List several ways to express anger, with and without direct confrontation. Role play alternative behaviors. Discuss situations in which alternatives would be appropriate.	Patient participates in identifying alternatives and plans when each might be useful.
Confrontation with a person who is a source of anger.	Provide support during confrontation if needed. Discuss experience after confrontation takes place.	Patient identifies the feeling of anger and appropriately confronts the object of the anger.

From Stuart G, Laraia M: *Stuart and Sundeen's principles and practice of psychiatric nursing*, ed 6, St Louis, 1998, Mosby.

Guide to Contraindications and Precautions to Immunizations, January 2000[a]

Vaccine	Contraindications	Precautions[b]	Not contraindications (vaccines may be given)
General for all vaccines (DTaP/ DTP[c], IPV, OPV, MMR, Hib, HBV, Var)	Anaphylactic reaction to a vaccine contraindicates further doses of that vaccine Anaphylactic reaction to a vaccine constituent contraindicates the use of vaccines containing that substance	Moderate or severe illnesses with or without a fever	Mild to moderate local reaction (soreness, redness, swelling) following a dose of an injectable antigen Low-grade or moderate fever following a prior vaccine dose Mild acute illness with or without low-grade fever Current antimicrobial therapy Convalescent phase of illnesses Prematurity (same dosage and indications as for healthy, full-term infants) Recent exposure to an infectious disease History of penicillin or other nonspecific allergies or fact that relatives have such allergies Pregnancy of mother or household contact Unimmunized household contact

This information is based on the recommendations of the Advisory Committee on Immunization Practices (ACIP) and of the Committee on Infectious Diseases of the American Academy of Pediatrics (AAP). Sometimes these recommendations vary from those in the manufacturers' product label. For more detailed information, providers should consult the published recommendations of the ACIP, AAP, and the manufacturers' package inserts. These guidelines, originally issued in 1993, have been updated to give current recommendations as of 2000 (based on information available as of December 1999).

See end of table (p. 652) for footnote legend.

Continued

Guide to Contraindications and Precautions to Immunizations, January 2000[a]—cont'd

Vaccine	Contraindications	Precautions[b]	Not contraindications (vaccines may be given)
DTaP/DTP[c]	Encephalopathy within 7 days of administration of previous dose of DTaP/DTP	Temperature of 40.5° C (104.8° F) within 48 hours after vaccination with a prior dose of DTaP/DTP Collapse or shock-like state (hypotonic-hyporesponsive episode) within 48 hours of receiving a prior dose of DTaP/DTP Seizures within 3 days of receiving a prior dose of DTaP/DTP[d] Persistent inconsolable crying lasting 3 hours, within 48 hours of receiving a prior dose of DTaP/DTP GBS within 6 weeks after a dose[e]	Family history of seizures[d] Family history of sudden infant death syndrome Family history of an adverse event after DTaP/DTP administration
IPV	Anaphylactic reactions to neomycin or streptomycin	Pregnancy	

Vaccine	Contraindications		
OPV[f,g]	Infection with HIV or a household contact with HIV Known altered immunodeficiency (hematologic and solid tumors, congenital immunodeficiency, and long-term immunosuppressive therapy) Immunodeficient household contact	Pregnancy	Breastfeeding Current antimicrobial therapy Mild diarrhea
MMR	Pregnancy Anaphylactic reaction to neomycin Anaphylactic reaction to gelatin Known altered immunodeficiency (hematologic and solid tumors, congenital immunodeficiency, severe HIV infection, and long-term immunosuppressive therapy)	Recent (within 3 to 11 months, depending on product and dose) immune globulin administration[h] Thrombocytopenia or history of thrombocytopenic purpura[h,j] ...	Tuberculosis or positive PPD Simultaneous tuberculin skin testing Breastfeeding Pregnancy of mother of recipient Immunodeficient family member or household contact Infection with HIV Nonanaphylactic reactions to eggs or neomycin
Hib	None		
Hepatitis B	Anaphylactic reaction to baker's yeast	...	...
Varicella	Pregnancy Anaphylactic reaction to neomycin Anaphylactic reaction to gelatin Infection with HIV Known altered immunodeficiency (hematologic and solid tumors, congenital immunodeficiency, and long-term immunosuppressive therapy)	Recent immune globulin administration Family history of immunodeficiency[k]	Pregnancy Pregnancy in the mother of the recipient Immunodeficiency in a household contact Household contact with HIV

Continued

Guide to Contraindications and Precautions to Immunizations, January 2000[a] —cont'd

[a]DTaP indicates diphtheria and tetanus toxoids and acellular pertussis; DTP, diphtheria and tetanus toxoids and pertussis; IPV, inactivated poliovirus; OPV, oral poliovirus; MMR, measles-mumps-rubella; Hib, *Haemophilus influenzae* type b; HBV, hepatitis B virus; Var, varicella; GBS, Guillain-Barré syndrome; HIV, human immunodeficiency virus; and PPD, purified protein derivative (tuberculin).

[b]The events or conditions listed as precautions, although not contraindications, should be considered. If the risks are believed to outweigh the benefits. The benefits and risks of administering a specific vaccine to a person under the circumstances should be considered. If the risks are believed to outweigh the benefits, the immunization should be withheld; if the benefits are believed to outweigh the risks (for example, during an outbreak or foreign travel), the immunization should be given. Whether and when to administer DTaP (or DTP) to children with proven or suspected underlying neurologic disorders should be decided on an individual basis.

[c]DTP is no longer recommended in the United States.

[d]Acetaminophen given before administering DTaP (or DTP) and thereafter every 4 hours for 24 hours should be considered for children with a personal or with a family (ie, siblings or parents) history of seizures.

[e]The decision to give additional doses of DTaP (or DTP) should be based on consideration of the benefit of further vaccination vs the risk of recurrence of GBS. For example, completion of the primary series in children is justified.

[f]A theoretical risk exists that the administration of multiple live virus vaccines within 30 days (4 weeks) of one another if not given on the same day will result in suboptimal immune response. No data substantiate this risk, however.

[g]OPV is no longer recommended for routine use in the United States.

[h]An anaphylactic reaction to egg ingestion previously was considered a contraindication unless skin testing and, if indicated, desensitization had been performed. However, skin testing no longer is recommended as of 1997.

[i]The decision to vaccinate should be based on consideration of the benefits of immunity to measles, mumps, and rubella vs the risk of recurrence or exacerbation of thrombocytopenia after vaccination, or from natural infections of measles or rubella. In most instances, the benefits of vaccination will be much greater than the potential risks and justify giving MMR, particularly in view of the even greater risk of thrombocytopenia after measles or rubella disease. However, if a prior episode of thrombocytopenia occurred in temporal proximity to vaccination, not giving a subsequent dose may be prudent.

[j]Measles vaccination may temporarily suppress tuberculin reactivity. MMR vaccine may be given after, or on the same day as, tuberculin testing. If MMR has been given recently, postpone the tuberculin test until 4 to 6 weeks after administration of MMR. If giving MMR simultaneously with the tuberculin skin test, use the Mantoux test and not multiple puncture tests, because the latter require confirmation if positive, which would have to be postponed for 4 to 6 weeks.

[k]Varicella vaccine should not be given to a member of a household with a family history of immunodeficiency until the immune status of the recipient and other children in the family is documented.

Quitting Smoking

Your doctor has told you to quit smoking. You want to, but you aren't sure of the best way. Perhaps you've tried before. Or you're afraid you'll gain weight.

What's the best way to quit?

There are many ways to quit smoking, but you need only one thing— *the desire to quit.* Once you have that all-important ingredient, you will succeed.

You can quit "cold turkey," or you can set a quit date and taper off gradually over a 2-week period. Some people find it helpful to have support from others who are quitting at the same time. Your local chapter of the American Lung Association, the American Cancer Society, or the American Heart Association or a hospital in your community can help you locate a smoking cessation class. Or you can use the "buddy system"—make a pact with a friend who wants to quit and provide support for each other.

Many people find chewing nicotine gum or using a nicotine patch helpful for the first few weeks. Talk to your doctor about prescribing one of these for you.

Adopt as many techniques as you think will work for you, and use them all.

What about withdrawal symptoms?

Keep in mind that most smokers actually have a double addiction: physical and psychological. You will need to deal with both aspects.

Physical withdrawal can be a problem for heavy smokers (more than one pack a day). The symptoms vary from one person to another, but common complaints are headaches, constipation, irritability, nervousness, trouble concentrating, and insomnia. You may even cough more for the first week after quitting as your cilia become active again. This is actually a sign that your body is healing itself.

You can do several things to ease the withdrawal symptoms. Although you may fear that you'll be craving a cigarette all the time, each urge actually lasts only 2 or 3 minutes. When it hits, do a minute or two of deep-breathing exercises to calm the urge; close your eyes, take a deep breath, and slowly let it out. If you still feel a craving, change your activity—walk around or do something that requires both hands, or do something that you especially enjoy.

Drink lots of water to help flush the toxins from your body. Eat a healthy, well-balanced diet. Many authorities say that eating less meat and more fresh vegetables and fruits helps reduce withdrawal symptoms. To combat aftermeal cravings, leave the table immediately and brush your teeth. Sugarless gum or hard candy, a toothpick, or unsalted, shelled sunflower seeds satisfy the oral craving without adding calories.

Daily exercise (unless your doctor advises you not to) will help relax you and hasten recovery from the effects of nicotine.

Try to avoid situations that you associate with smoking, such as a morning cup of coffee or a before-dinner drink. You may need to modify your habits for a while until the withdrawal period is over. This also means avoiding spending too much time around other smokers.

Write down all your reasons for quitting smoking to remind yourself whenever you're discouraged or tempted to smoke. Keep the list handy and look at it often. And feel proud of yourself for quitting.

Will I gain weight?

According to recent studies, only about one third of ex-smokers gain some weight; one third lose weight, and one third stay the same. The key to not gaining weight is not to eat every time you crave a smoke. As long as you maintain a well-balanced diet, don't snack between meals, and exercise, you shouldn't experience any weight problems.

What if I fail?

Many people who have successfully quit smoking failed the first time they tried. Often they describe these "failures" as valuable learning experiences that helped them succeed the next time. Whatever you do, don't give up. More than 36 million Americans have already quit. You can, too.

Blood Pressure Recommendations for Follow-Up and Classification—Adult

Blood Pressure Measurement and Clinical Evaluation

Classification of blood pressure for adults aged 18 years and older*

| Category | Blood pressure, mm Hg | | |
	Systolic (SBP)	Diastolic (DBP)	
Optimal†	<120 and	<80	
Normal	<130 and	<85	
High-normal	130-139 or	85-89	
Hypertension‡			
Stage 1	140-159 or	85-89	
Stage 2	160-179 or	100-109	
Stage 3	≥180 or	≥ 110	

*Not taking antihypertensive drugs and not acutely ill. When systolic and diastolic blood pressures fall into different categories, the high category should be selected to classify the individual's blood pressure status. In addition to classifying stages of hypertension on the basis of average blood pressure levels, clinicians should specify presence or absence of target organ disease and additional risk factors. This specificity is important for risk classification and treatment.

†Optimal blood pressure with respect to cardiovascular risk is less than 120/80 mm Hg. However, unusually low readings should be evaluated for clinical significance.

‡Based on the average of 2 or more readings taken at each of 2 or more visits after an initial screening.

From US Department of Health and Human Services; Public Health Service; National Institutes of Health; National Heart, Lung and Blood Institute; *Sixth Report of the Joint National Committee on Prevention, Detection, Evaluation, and Treatment of High Blood Pressure,* Nov 1997.

Detection and Confirmation

Hypertension detection begins with proper blood pressure measurements, which should be obtained at each healthcare encounter. The following techniques are recommended:

- Patients should be seated in a chair with their back supported and their arm bared and supported at heart level. Patients should refrain from smoking or ingesting caffeine during the 30 minutes preceding the measurement.
- Under special circumstances, measuring blood pressure in the supine and standing positions may be indicated.
- Measurement should begin after at least 5 minutes of rest.

The appropriate cuff size must be used to ensure accurate measurement. The bladder within the cuff should encircle at least 80% of the arm. Many adults will require a large adult cuff.

- Measurements should be taken preferably with a mercury sphygmomanometer; otherwise, a recently *calibrated* aneroid manometer or a *validated* electronic device can be used.
- Both SBP and DBP should be recorded. The first appearance of sound (phase 1) is used to define SBP. The disappearance of sound (phase 5) is used to define DBP.
- Two or more readings separated by 2 minutes should be averaged. If the first 2 readings differ by more than 5 mm Hg, additional readings should be obtained and averaged.
- Clinicians should explain to patients the meaning of their blood pressure readings and advise them of the need for periodic remeasurement. The following table provides follow-up recommendations based on the initial set of blood pressure measurements:

Recommendations for follow-up based on initial blood pressure measurements for adults

Initial blood pressure, mm Hg*		Follow-up recommended**
Systolic	**Diastolic**	
<130	<85	Recheck in 2 yr
130-139	85-89	Recheck in 1 yr***
140-159	90-99	Confirm within 2 mo***
160-179	100-109	Evaluate or refer to source of care within 1 mo
≥180	≥110	Evaluate or refer to source of care immediately or within 1 wk depending on clinical situation

*If systolic and diastolic are different, follow recommendations for shorter follow-up (e.g., 160/86 mm Hg should be evaluated or referred to source of care within 1 month).
**Modify the scheduling of follow-up according to reliable information about post–blood pressure measurement, other cardiovascular risk factors, or target organ.

Blood Pressure Measurement

Patient should:

- Rest for 5 minutes before measurement.
- Refrain from smoking or ingesting caffeine for 30 minutes prior to measurement.
- Be seated with feet flat on floor, back and arm supported, arm at heart level.

Clinician should:

- Use the appropriate size cuff for the patient; the bladder should encircle at least 80% of the upper arm.
- Use calibrated or mercury manometer.
- Average two or more readings, separated by at least 2 minutes.

Primary Prevention

Encourage patients to make healthy lifestyle choices:

- Quit smoking to reduce cardiovascular risk.
- Lose weight, if needed.
- Restrict sodium intake to no more than 100 mmol per day.
- Limit alcohol intake to no more than 1-2 drinks per day.
- Get at least 30-45 minutes of aerobic activity on most days.
- Maintain adequate potassium intake—about 90 mmol per day.
- Maintain adequate intakes of calcium and magnesium.

Goal

Set a clear goal of therapy based on patient's risk. Control blood pressure **to below:**

- 140/90 mm Hg for patients with uncomplicated hypertension; set a lower goal for those with target organ damage or clinical cardiovascular disease.
- 130/85 mm Hg for patients with diabetes.
- 125/75 mm Hg for patients with renal insufficiency with proteinuria greater than 1 g per 24 hours.

Treatment

Begin with lifestyle modifications (see *Primary prevention*) for all patients. Be supportive!

- Add pharmacologic therapy if blood pressure remains uncontrolled.
- Start with a diuretic or beta-blocker unless there are compelling indications to use other agents. Use a low dose and titrate upward. Consider low-dose combinations.
- If no response, try a drug from another class or add a second agent from a different class (diuretic if not already used).

Adherence

- Encourage lifestyle modifications. Be supportive!
- Educate patient and family about disease. Involve them in measurement and treatment.
- Maintain communications with patient.
- Discuss how to integrate treatment into daily activities.
- Keep care inexpensive and simple.
- Favor once-daily, long-acting formulations.
- Use combination tablets, when needed.
- Consider using generic formulas or larger tablets that can be divided. This may be less expensive.
- Be willing to stop unsuccessful therapy and try a different approach.
- Consider using nurse case management.

Risk Groups for Blood Pressure Readings

- Determine blood pressure stage.
- Determine risk group by major risk factors and TOD/CCD.
- Determine treatment recommendations (by using the table following).
- Determine goal blood pressure.
- Refer to specific treatment recommendations.

Major risk factors

- Smoking
- Dyslipidemia
- Diabetes mellitus
- Age >60 years
- Sex:
  - Men
  - Postmenopausal women
- Family history:
  - Women <age 65
  - Men <age 55

TOD/CCD

(Target Organ Damage/
Clinical Cardiovascular Disease)

Heart diseases
- Left ventricular hypertrophy
- Angina/prior myocardial infarction
- Prior coronary artery bypass graft
- Heart failure

Stroke or transient ischemic attack

Nephropathy

Peripheral arterial disease

Hypertensive retinopathy

Blood pressure stages (mm Hg)	Risk Group A No major risk factors No TOD/CCD	Risk Group B At least one major risk factor, not including diabetes No TOD/CCD	Risk Group C TOD/CCD and/or diabetes, with or without other risk factors
High-normal (130-139/85-89)	Lifestyle modification	Lifestyle modification	Drug therapy for those with heart failure, renal insufficiency, or diabetes Lifestyle modification
Stage 1 (140-159/90-99)	Lifestyle modification (up to 12 months)	Lifestyle modification (up to 6 months) For patients with multiple risk factors, clinicians should consider drugs as initial therapy, plus lifestyle modifications.	Drug therapy Lifestyle modification
Stages 2 and 3 (≥160/≥100)	Drug therapy Lifestyle modification	Drug therapy Lifestyle modification	Drug therapy Lifestyle modification

Example: A patient with diabetes and a blood pressure of 142/94 mm Hg plus left ventricular hypertrophy should be classified as having stage 1 hypertension with target organ disease (left ventricular hypertrophy) and with another major risk factor (diabetes). This patient would be categorized as **Stage 1, Risk Group C,** and recommended for immediate initiation of pharmacologic treatment.

Continued

Goal blood pressure

<140/90 mm Hg Uncomplicated hypertension, Risk Group A, Risk Group B, Risk Group C except for the following:

<130/85 mm Hg Diabetes; renal failure; heart failure

<125/75 mm Hg Renal failure with proteinuria >1 g/24 hours

Specific treatment recommendations

Lifestyle modification should be definitive therapy for some patients and adjunctive therapy for all patients recommended for pharmacologic therapy.

Initial drug choices

- Start with a low dose of a long-acting once-daily drug, and **titrate dose**
- Low-dose combinations may be appropriate

Uncomplicated hypertension	Compelling indications		Specific indications for the following drugs:
Diuretics Beta-blockers	Diabetes type 1	start with ACE inhibitor if proteinuria is present	ACE inhibitors Angiotension II receptor blockers Alpha-blockers Alpha-beta-blockers Beta-blockers Calcium channel blockers Diuretics
	Heart failure	start with ACE inhibitor or diuretic	
	Myocardial infarction	beta-blocker (non-ISA) after MI; ACE inhibitor for LV dysfunction after MI	
	Isolated systolic hypertension (older patients)	diuretics (preferred) or calcium channel blockers (long-acting DHP)	

Body Mass Index

Body mass is the figure you get by dividing your weight in kilograms by the square of your height in meters.

1. To convert weight to kilograms, divide pounds without clothes by 2.2: _____.
2. To convert to meters, divide your height in inches (without shoes) by 39.4 (   ) ___, then square it: _____.
3. Divide (1) by (2). Body mass index = _____.

For men, desirable body mass is 22-24. Above 28.5 is overweight; above 33 is seriously overweight.

For women, desirable body mass is 21-23. Overweight begins at 27.5, and seriously overweight is above 31.5.

From Williams S: *Essentials of nutrition and diet therapy,* ed 7, St Louis, 1999, Mosby.

Self-Help Devices

Grooming devices

A long-handled comb: curved handle or built-up handle to enlarge it.*
Built-up handle hair brush.*
Extension mirror to be fit around client's neck. These can also be purchased with a magnifying mirror. They are available in department stores.
Fingernail brush. Mounts with two suction cups to adhere to cabinet or sink top. Allows the client to clean fingernails with the use of only one hand. This model can also be used in the kitchen for a vegetable brush.

Dressing aids

Sock and stocking aids. These have long handles or straps, allowing the client to put on socks and stockings from a sitting position.
Long-handled shoe horn with built-up handle.* Put on shoes in a sitting position.

---

*All built-up handles can be made by applying foam rubber curlers or pipe insulation or by applying bicycle handles.

Adapted from Pedretti L: *Occupational therapy practice skills for physical dysfunction,* ed 4, St Louis, 1996, Mosby.

Elastic shoelaces. These permit shoes to be tied once. They come in various lengths and colors and allow lace shoes to be slipped on without tying.

Combination button aid and zipper pull. Built-up handle and wire loop on one end allow one-handed buttoning. Hook on the other end allows for zipper pull.

Dressing stick. This 24-inch stick with hooks on both ends assists in pulling up trousers, underclothing, and so on, for the client who is unable to bend.

Eating aids

Dishes. Dishes are available with one side built up to allow food to be pushed up and trapped on cutlery. Entire sets of dishes are available in Melamine in attractive designs. A homemade plate guard can also be attached to the plates used by the client.

Cutlery. Handles can be built up by use of plastic foam curlers or narrow foam rubber pipe insulation, or they can be purchased with wood built-up handles.

Securing of straws: A bulldog clip can be secured to the edge of the glass and a straw inserted through the hole on the clip handle and into the liquid.

Cutting board. The corner of a cutting board can be built up with small pieces of wood or other material. It can be used to anchor bread for buttering or other items needing to be anchored.

A jar opener can be mounted in the kitchen for ease of opening jars with one hand.

Drinking cups. Large-handled mugs can be purchased. In addition, cups are available with nonspill tops and with large handles and holders that can be shaped to fit tumblers, soft-drink cans, and so forth.

A nonslip material (similar to that used in bathtubs) applied under dishes can be used at the table to prevent their slipping.

An adjustable cuff can be purchased that can be applied to the hand and various sizes of handles can be secured in the cuff. This is appropriate for persons having little or no grip.

Tablecloth clamps, purchased at the dime store and applied to the dining table, secure the table cloth and prevent it from slipping.

Nonslip placemats are available in various colors.

Large-handled vegetable peeler, large-handled food grater, and one-handed slicing knife and frame for slicing bread are available commercially.

A two-sided suction holder (for holding soap; available in the dime store) can also be used under plates and other dishes to hold them in place.

Communication and security

Automatic night-lights are available.

Magnifiers of various magnitudes and sizes are commercially available.

Telephones can be amplified for adjustable volume control. Big-button telephones are available with hands-free speaker.

Wiring can be done in the home for hearing-impaired clients to allow a lamp to flash on and off when a doorbell or telephone rings.

Radio-controlled switches are available for remote control (up to 40 feet away) of lights, small appliances, and television.

Clothing

Regular gowns and pajama tops can be seamed down the back and attached with velcro or ties, for ease of application.

Large terrycloth and vinyl bibs with "gutters" to catch crumbs and spills are available or can be made.

Reachers

Simple long tongs (used for barbecue) often suffice to reach items beyond arm's length.

Other reachers have magnetic tips, easy gripping devices, and adjustable "jaws."

Wheelchair and walker accessories

A basket or bag can be applied to the front of a walker for carrying small items.

A small holder with a squeeze clamp to be applied to the front of the wheelchair, below the armrest, is available for carrying small items that fall easily.

A cup or soft-drink-can holder can be applied by putting a squeeze clamp on the front of the wheelchair below the armrest.

A lap board (available in dime stores) assists the wheelchair client to write and eat.

Assistive devices for ambulation. **A,** Straight canes. **B,** Pickup walker. **C,** Quad cane. **D,** Standard walker. *From Hoeman SP,* Rehabilitation nursing: process and application, *ed 2, St Louis, 1996, Mosby.*

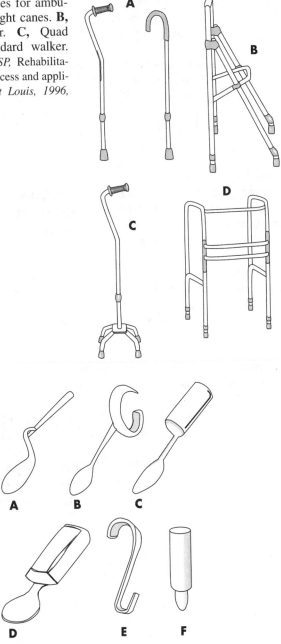

Hand manipulation aids. **A,** Swivel spoon. **B,** Vertical palm self-handle spoon. **C,** Built-up handle spoon. **D,** Universal cuff holds various utensils. **E,** Doorknob turner. **F,** Telephone dialing stick.

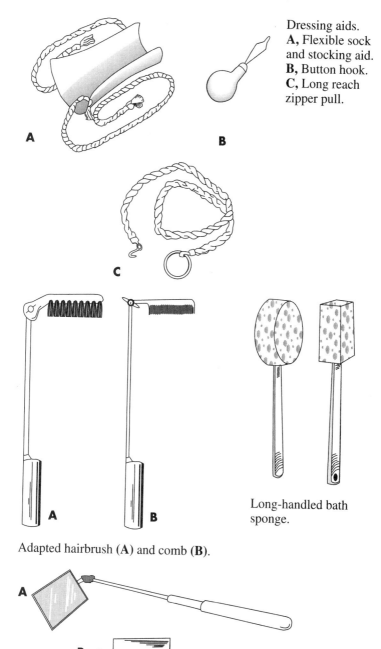

Dressing aids.
A, Flexible sock and stocking aid.
B, Button hook.
C, Long reach zipper pull.

Long-handled bath sponge.

Adapted hairbrush (**A**) and comb (**B**).

Long-handled skin inspection mirror (**A**) and reach zipper pull (**B**).

SCREENING TOOLS, TECHNIQUES, AND DIAGNOSTIC CRITERIA

SPEECH, VISION, HEARING, AND LANGUAGE

Vision, Hearing, and Language Screening Procedures

Method	Age	Procedure	Normal response
Vision*			
Following	Infancy	Shine light or hold bright object in front of infant's line of vision; move slowly side to side.	Follow light or bright object up to 180°.
Turn to light response	Infancy	Hold back of head to bright light source.	Eyes turn toward source of light.
Optokinetic drum	Infancy	Twirl drum stripes slowly in front of infant's eyes.	Nystagmus occurs.
Herschberg reflex (corneal light reflex)	Infancy through adolescence	Shine penlight into child's eyes; note where light reflex falls. For older children: Have child focus and stare at point 14 inches and then 20 inches away before shining light into eyes.	Light reflex falls in same position in eye.
Cover test	Toddler through adolescence	Have child focus on specified spot first 14 inches, then 20 inches away. While child is focusing, one eye is completely covered for 5 to 10 seconds. Cover is then removed and eye observed for movement. Procedure repeated for other eye.	No wandering or sharp, jerky movement of eyes noted, indicating ability to focus.

*From Stanhope M, Lancaster J: *Community and public health nursing,* ed 5, St Louis, 2000, Mosby.

Method	Age	Procedure	Normal response
Snellen E	Preschool	Child is instructed to point finger in direction that the E or table legs are pointing from a distance of 20 feet. Test each eye separately, then together. Test as far down on chart as child can go.	Visual acuity of 20/30 to 20/40.
Snellen alphabet	School age through adolescence	Child stands 20 feet from chart and reads letters. Each eye is tested separately and then together. Testing usually started at 20/30 or 20/40 line and child is allowed to test as far down chart as possible. Passing score consists of reading majority of letters (or Es) on each line.	Visual acuity of 20/20.
Hearing*			
Startle reflex	Newborn	Loud noise or bang made near infant's ears.	Jumps at noise, blinks, cries, or widens eyes.
Tracks sound	3 to 6 months	Make noise, call name, or sing.	Eyes shift toward sound; responds to mother's voice; coos to verbalization.
Recognizes sound	6 to 8 months	As preceding, from out of line of vision.	Turns head toward sound; responds to name, babbles to verbalization.

Continued

Vision, Hearing, and Language Screening Procedures—cont'd

Method	Age	Procedure	Normal response
Hearing*—cont'd			
Localization of sound	8 to 12 months	Call name or use tuning fork or say words.	Localizes source of sound; turns head (and body at times) toward sound, repeats words
Pure tone screening —play	Toddler to preschool	Demonstrate to child by putting headphones on and making believe you hear sound. As you say "I hear it," put a block in box or ring on holder. Put headphones on child and give block or ring to use. Sound a 50 dB tone at 1000 Hz and guide child's hand with block to box. When child can do this alone, begin screening. Set at 25 dB at 1000 Hz. If child responds, go to 2000, 4000, and 6000 Hz. Praise child and place new block in hand. Switch to other ear and test.	Should respond at 25 dB at any frequency.
Pure-tone audiometry	School age through adolescence	Explain procedure to child. Place headphones on ears. Test one ear at a time in sequence as preceding (i.e., 25 dB at 1000, 2000, 4000, and 6000 Hz). Have child raise hand to indicate sound is heard.	Should respond at 25 dB at any frequency.

Method	Age	Procedure	Normal response
Tuning fork test	Some preschoolers; school age to adolescence		
A. Weber's test		Strike tuning fork to make it vibrate and place the stem in midline of scalp. Ask child if sound is same in both ears or louder in either ear.	Sound heard equally well in both ears.
B. Rinne test		Strike tuning fork until it vibrates, place stem on child's mastoid until he or she no longer hears it. Then place vibrating fingers of fork 1 to 2 inches in front of concha. Ask child if he or she can still hear sound.	Sound from fork vibrating in air should be heard when child can no longer hear sound with stem against mastoid (air conduction is greater than bone conduction).
Language			
Assessment of child's language comprehension	3 to 6 years	Child points to picture named by examiner Assesses single word vocabulary and 2-word, 3-word, and 4-word phrases	Child able to name picture understandably
Peabody Picture Vocabulary Test	2½ to 18 years	Child looks at picture and points to one named by examiner	Child able to respond correctly/following directions
Preschool Language Scale	Birth to 3 years	Observation of child's performance	Depending on age level, child should be able to point to picture, follow direction, or manipulate objects
Expressive One Word Picture Vocabulary	2 to 12 years	Child looks at picture and names what is seen	Child able to follow directions and articulate response at age level

Major Developmental Characteristics of Hearing

Age (months)	Development
Birth	Responds to loud noise by startle reflex
	Responds to sound of human voice more readily than to any other sound
	Low-pitched sounds, such as lullaby, metronome, or heartbeat, have quieting effect
2-3	Turns head to side when sound is made at level of ear
3-4	Locates sound by turning head to side and looking in same direction
4-6	Can localize sounds made below ear, which is followed by localization of sound made above ear; will turn head to the side and then look up or down
	Begins to imitate sounds
6-8	Locates sounds by turning head in a curving arc
	Responds to own name
8-10	Localizes sounds by turning head diagonally and directly toward sound
10-12	Knows several words and their meaning, such as "no," and names of members of the family
	Learns to control and adjust own response to sound, such as listening for sound to occur again
18	Begins to discriminate between harshly dissimilar sounds, such as sound of doorbell and train
24	Refines gross discriminative skills
36	Begins to distinguish more subtle differences in speech sounds, such as between "e" and "er"
48	Begins to distinguish such similar sounds as "f" and "th" or between "f" and "s"
	Listening becomes considerably refined
	Able to be tested with an audiometer

From Wong DL, Hess, CS: *Wong and Whaley's clinical manual of pediatric nursing,* ed 5, St Louis, 2000, Mosby.

Major Developmental Characteristics of Language and Speech

Age (years)	Normal language development	Normal speech development	Intelligibility
1	Says two to three words with meaning Imitates sounds of animals	Omits most final/some initial consonants Substitutes consonants "m," "w," "p," "b," "k," "g," "n," "t," "d," and "h" for more difficult sounds Height of unintelligible jargon at 18 mo.	Usually no more than 25% intelligible to unfamiliar listener
2	Uses two- to three-word phrases Has vocabulary of about 300 words Uses "I," "me," "you"	Uses above consonants with vowels but inconsistently/with much substitution Omission of final consonants Articulation lags behind vocabulary	At age 2 years, 65% intelligible in context
3	Says four- to five-word sentences Has vocabulary of about 900 words Uses "who," "what," and "where" Uses plurals, pronouns, and prepositions	Masters "b," "t," "d," "k," and "g"; sounds "r," and "l" may still be unclear, omits or substitutes "w" Repetitions and hesitations common	At age 3 years, 70% to 80% intelligible
4 to 5	Has vocabulary of 1500 to 2100 words Able to use most grammatic forms correctly, such as past tense of verb with "yesterday" Uses complete sentences with nouns, verbs, prepositions, adjectives, etc.	Masters "f" and "v"; may still distort "r," "l," "s," "z," "sh," "ch," "y," and "th" Little or no omission of initial or last consonant	Speech is totally intelligible, although some sounds are still imperfect
5 to 6	Has vocabulary of 3000 words, comprehends "if," "because," and "why"	Masters "r," "l," and "th"; may still distort "s," "z," "sh," "ch," and "j" (usually mastered by age 7½ to 8)	

From Wong DL, Hess CS: *Wong and Whaley's clinical manual of pediatric nursing*, ed 5, St Louis, 2000, Mosby.

Landmarks of Speech, Language, and Hearing Ability During the Preschool Period

Age (months)	Receptive language	Expressive language	Related hearing ability
42	Up to 4200 words; knows words such as what, where, how, funny, we, surprise, secret; knows number concepts to 2, how to answer questions accurately, such as do you have a dog, which is the girl, what toys do you have.	Up to 1200 words in mostly complete sentences averaging four to five words per sentence; uses all 50 phonemes; 7% of sentences are compound or complex; averages 203 words per hour; rate of speech is faster; relates experiences and tells about activities in sequential order; uses words such as what, where, how, see, little, funny, they, we, he, she, several; can say a nursery rhyme; asks permission; 95% of speech is intelligible.	Begins to make the fine discriminations among similar speech sounds, such as the difference between *f* and *th* or *f* and *s*. Child has matured enough to be tested with an audiometer. At this age formal hearing testing usually can be carried out. Not only has hearing developed to its optimum level, but listening has also become considerably refined.
48	Up to 5600 words; carries out three-item commands consistently; knows why we have houses, books, umbrella, key; knows nearly all colors, words such as somebody, anybody, even, almost, now, something, like, bigger, too, full name, one or two songs, number concepts to 4; understands most preschool stories; can complete opposite analogies,	Up to 1500 words in sentences averaging five to six words per sentence; averages 400 words per hour; counts to 3, repeats four digits, names three objects, and repeats nine-word sentences from memory; names the primary colors, some coins; relates fanciful tales; enjoys rhyming nonsense words and using exaggerations; demands reasons	

such as brother is a boy, sister is a _____; in daytime it is light, at night it is _____.

why and how; questioning is at a peak, up to 500 a day; passes judgment on own activity; can recite a poem from memory or sing a song; uses words such as even, almost, something, like, but; typical expressions might include I'm so tired, you almost hit me, now I'll make something else.

54

Up to 6500 words; knows what a house, window, chair, and dress are made of and what we do with our eyes and ears; understands differences in texture and composition, such as hard, soft, rough, smooth; begins to name or point to penny, nickel, dime; understands if, because, why, when.

Up to 1800 words in sentences averaging five to six words; now averages only 230 words per hour—is satisfied with less verbalization; does little commanding or demanding; likes surprises; about 1 in 10 sentences is compound or complex, and only 8% of sentences are incomplete; can define 10 common words and count to 20; common expressions are I don't know, I said, tiny, funny, because; asks questions for information, and learns to manipulate and control persons and situations with language.

Adapted from Chinn PL: *Child health maintenance: concepts in family-centered care*, ed 2, St Louis, 1979, Mosby. In Edelman CL, Mandle CL: *Health promotion through the lifespan*, ed 4, St Louis, 1998, Mosby.

Continued

Landmarks of Speech, Language, and Hearing Ability During the Preschool Period—cont'd

Age (months)	Receptive language	Expressive language	Related hearing ability
60	Up to 9600 words; knows number concepts to 5; knows and names colors; defines words in terms of use such as a horse is to ride; also defines wind, ball, hat, stove; understands words such as if, because, when; knows what the following are for: horse, fork, legs; begins to understand right and left.	Up to 2200 words in sentences averaging six words; can define ball, hat, stove, policeman, wind, horse, fork; can count five objects and repeat four or five digits; definitions are in terms of use; can single out a word and ask its meaning; makes serious inquiries—what is this for, how does this work, who made those, what does it mean; language is now essentially complete in structure and form; uses all types of sentences, clauses, and parts of speech; reads by way of pictures, and prints simple words.	

Nurse's Interventions for Screening Vision and Hearing of Preschoolers

Be skilled in the use of the equipment.

Avoid the term *test,* because even some preschoolers have come to associate test with anxiety and possibly failure.

Allow the child to ask questions and examine the equipment.

Do vision and hearing screening early in the visit before anything intrusive or painful.

Do screening in a quiet, private area so the child is not distracted by people or noises.

Praise the child for cooperating.

If the child becomes distracted or tired, take a brief break before beginning again.

Discuss the results of the screening with the child using simple, positive terms.

From Edelman CL, Mandle CL: *Health promotion throughout the lifespan,* ed 4, St Louis, 1998, Mosby.

Clues for Detecting Visual Impairment

Cause	Behavior	Signs/symptoms
Congenital blindness	Does not follow a moving light; no orientation response to visual stimuli Does not initiate eye-to-eye contact with caregiver	Constant nystagmus Fixed pupils Marked strabismus Slow lateral movements
Refractive errors	Rubs eyes excessively Tilts head or thrusts head forward Has difficulty in reading or other close work Holds books close to eyes Writes or colors with head close to table Clumsy; walks into objects Blinks more than usual or is irritable when doing close work Is unable to see objects clearly Does poorly in school, especially in subjects that require demonstration, such as arithmetic	Dizziness Headache Nausea following close work
Strabismus	Squints eyelids together or frowns Has difficulty in focusing from one distance to another Inaccurate judgment in picking up objects	Diplopia Photophobia Dizziness

	Unable to see print or moving objects clearly Closes one eye to see Tilts head to one side If combined with refractive errors, may see any of the above	Headache Cross-eye
Glaucoma	Mostly seen in acquired types—loses peripheral vision; may bump into objects that are not directly in front of him; sees halos around objects; may complain of mild pain or discomfort (severe pain, nausea, and vomiting if sudden rise in pressure)	Redness Excessive tearing (epiphora) Photophobia Spasmodic winking (blepharospasm) Corneal haziness Enlargement of the eyeball (buphthalmos)
Cataract	Gradually less able to see objects clearly May lose peripheral vision	Nystagmus (with complete blindness) Gray opacities of lens Strabismus

From Wong DL, Hess CS: *Wong and Whaley's clinical manual of pediatric nursing*, ed 5, St Louis, 2000, Mosby.

Denver Eye Screening Test

The Denver Eye Screening Test (DEST) assesses visual acuity in children 3 years or older by using a single card for the letter E (20/30) from a distance of 15 feet. A complete instructional manual is available. General guidelines include the following:

1. Mark a distance of 15 feet for testing.
2. Use the large **E** (20/100) to explain and demonstrate the testing procedure to the child.
3. Use the small **E** for actual testing. Test each eye separately using the occluder.
4. Consider the results *abnormal* if the child fails to correctly identify the direction of the small **E** over three trials.
5. Test children from 2½ to 2¹¹⁄₁₂ years of age or those untestable with the letter **E** using the picture (Allen) cards. (Cooperative children as young as 2 years can also be tested.)
6. Show each card to the child at close range to make certain he can identify it.
7. Present the pictures at a distance of 15 feet for actual testing. Test each eye separately if possible.
8. Consider the results *abnormal* if the child fails to correctly name three of the seven cards in three to five trials.
9. Screen children from 6 to 30 months of age by testing for the following:
   a. Fixation (ability to follow a moving light source or spinning toy)
   b. Squinting (observation of the child's eyes or report by parent)
   c. Strabismus (report by parent and performance on cover and pupillary light reflex tests)
10. Consider the results *abnormal* if failure to fixate, presence of a squint, or failing two of the three procedures for strabismus.
11. Retest all children with abnormal findings. Refer those with a repeat failure.

From Wong DL, Hess CS: *Wong and Whaley's clinical manual of pediatric nursing,* ed 5, St Louis, 2000, Mosby.

Tuning Fork Tests

Test and steps	Rationale

Weber's test (lateralization of sound) (Figure 4-1)

Hold the fork at its base and tap it lightly against the heel of the palm.

Place the base of the vibrating fork on the top of the client's head or middle of forehead.

Ask the client where sound is heard (on one or both sides).

A client with normal hearing hears sound equally in both ears or in midline of head. In conduction deafness, sound is heard in the impaired ear. In unilateral sensorineural hearing loss, sound is identified in the good ear.

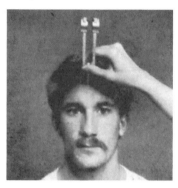

Rinne test (comparison of air and bone conduction)

Strike the tuning fork against the knuckle.

Place the vibrating fork on the mastoid process.

Ask the client to inform you when sound is no longer heard.

Immediately place the vibrating fork close to the external ear meatus.

Ask the client to inform you if sound can be heard.

Normally, sound can be heard longer through air than through bone (positive Rinne). In conduction deafness, sounds through bone conduction can be heard after air conduction sounds become inaudible (negative Rinne). In sensorineural deafness, sound is heard longer through air.

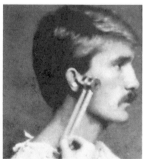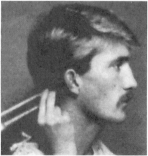

From Potter PA, Perry AG: *Fundamentals of nursing,* ed 4, St Louis, 1997, Mosby.

GROWTH AND DEVELOPMENT

Normal Tooth Formation in the Child

Teeth	Lower (mandibular) appear at age	Upper (maxillary) appear at age
Primary (Figure 4-2, A)		
Central incisors	5 to 7 months	6 to 8 months
Lateral incisors	12 to 15 months	8 to 11 months
Cuspids (canines)	16 to 20 months	16 to 20 months
First molars	10 to 16 months	10 to 16 months
Second molars	20 to 30 months	20 to 30 months
Total per jaw—10		
Total—20		
Permanent (Figure 4-2, B)		
Central incisors	6 to 7 years	6 to 7 years
Lateral incisors	7 to 9 years	8 to 9 years
Cuspids (canines)	8 to 11 years	11 to 12 years
First bicuspids	10 to 12 years	10 to 11 years
Second bicuspids	11 to 13 years	10 to 12 years
First molars (6-year molars)	6 to 7 years	6 to 7 years
Second molars (12-year molars)	12 to 13 years	12 to 13 years
Third molars (wisdom teeth)	17 to 22 years	17 to 22 years
Total set—32		

From Ingalls AJ, Salerno MC: *Maternal and child health nursing,* St Louis, 1991, Mosby.

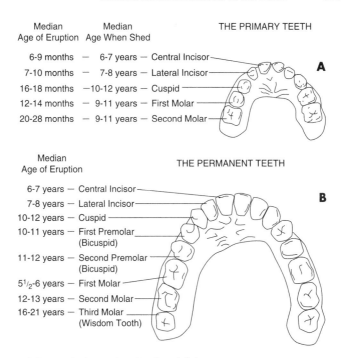

Median Age of Eruption	Median Age When Shed	THE PRIMARY TEETH
6-9 months	— 6-7 years —	Central Incisor
7-10 months	— 7-8 years —	Lateral Incisor
16-18 months	—10-12 years —	Cuspid
12-14 months	— 9-11 years —	First Molar
20-28 months	— 9-11 years —	Second Molar

A

Median Age of Eruption	THE PERMANENT TEETH
6-7 years —	Central Incisor
7-8 years —	Lateral Incisor
10-12 years —	Cuspid
10-11 years —	First Premolar (Bicuspid)
11-12 years —	Second Premolar (Bicuspid)
5½-6 years —	First Molar
12-13 years —	Second Molar
16-21 years —	Third Molar (Wisdom Tooth)

B

Figure 4-2 Tooth formation in the child. *From Wong DL, Whaley LF: Clinical manual of pediatric nursing, ed 4, St Louis, 1996, Mosby.*

Developmental Tools Used to Assess Children With Chronic Conditions

Types of screening tools	Test/source	Age level	Method	Comments
General development	Battelle Developmental Inventory (BDI) (1984) Authors: J Newborg, J Stock, L Wnek, J Guidubaldi, and J Svinicki Source: Riverside Publishing Co 8420 Bryn Mawr Ave Chicago, IL 60631	Birth–8 years	Structured test format Parent and teacher interview Observation	• Includes a screening test that can be used to identify areas of development in need of a complete comprehensive BDI • Full BDI consists of 341 test items in five domains: personal-social, adaptive, motor, communication, and cognitive 1-1½ hours to administer* • Screening test consists of 96 items taking 20-35 minutes to administer
	Bayley Scales of Infant Development-Second Edition (1993) Author: N Bayley Source: The Psychological Corp Harcourt, Brace, Jovanovich, Inc 6277 Sea Harbor Dr Orlando, FL 32887	1-42 months	Observation/ demonstration	• Evaluates motor, mental, and behavior of the infant and toddler • Diagnoses normal vs. delayed development • New scoring procedures allow the examiner to determine a child's developmental age equivalent for each ability domain • Requires a qualified practitioner to examine and evaluate the infant

Bender Visual Motor Gestalt Test	≥3 years	Demonstration	• Used as an evaluation tool for developmental problems in children: learning disabilities, retardation, psychosis, organic brain disorders • 10 minutes to administer
Author: L Bender Source: American Orthopsychiatric Association, Inc Seventh Ave, 18th Floor New York, NY 10001			
Brigance Diagnostic Inventory of Early Development (Revised) (1991)	1 month–7 years	Performance task by child	• Assesses skills in all areas required for P.L.101-476 eligibility • Criterion and normative referenced, curriculum based • May be administered by paraprofessional with supervision • Does not require special equipment for testing
Author: A Brigance Source: Curriculum Associates, Inc 5 Esquire Rd North Billerica, MA 01862-2589			
Developmental Profile II	Birth–9½ years	Parent or teacher report	• Screens children for delays in five domains: physical (motor and muscle development), self-help, social, academic, communication • 186 items takes 20-30 minutes to administer • Can be computer scored
Authors: G Alpern, T Boll, and M Shearer Source: Western Psychological Services 12031 Wilshire Blvd Los Angeles, CA 90025-1251			

*Can be administered by professional or nonprofessional. Some special training required. Needs to understand testing procedures and be capable of developing rapport with children.

From Jackson PL, Vessey JA: *Primary care of the child with a chronic condition*, ed 2, St Louis, 1996, Mosby.

Continued

Developmental Tools Used to Assess Children With Chronic Conditions—cont'd

Types of screening tools	Test/source	Age level	Method	Comments
	Hawaii Early Learning Profile (HELP) (1979) Authors: SF Furuno, KA O'Reilly, CM Hosaka, TT Inatsuka, TL Allman, B Zeisloft, and S Parks Source: Vort Corporation PO Box 60880 Palo Alto, CA 94306	Birth–36 months	Observation Parent interview	• 685 developmental tasks used to assess six domains: cognition, language, gross motor, fine motor, social-emotions, and self-help • Criterion referenced, curriculum based • Each domain takes 15-30 minutes to administer. Domains may be selected for individual use
	Minnesota Infant Development Inventory (1988) Minnesota Early Child Development Inventory (1988) Minnesota Preschool Development Inventory (1984) Author: H Ireton and E Thwing	Birth–15 months 1–3 years 3–6 years	Observation/interview Parent report True/False	• A first level screening tool • Measures the infant's development in five domains: gross motor, fine motor, language, comprehension, and personal-social • Provides a profile of the child's strengths and weaknesses • 60-80 items on each inventory

Source: Behavior Science Systems PO Box 1108 Minneapolis, MN 55458			
Rapid Developmental Screening Checklist Author: Committee on Children with Handicaps, American Academy of Pediatrics Source: MJ Giannini, MD Director, Mental Retardation Institute New York Medical College Valhalla, NY 10595	1 month– 5 years	Checklist	• Requires minimal time allotment
Riley Motor Problems Inventory (RMPI) Author: GD Riley Source: Western Psychological 12031 Wilshire Blvd Los Angeles, CA 90025	≥4 years	Performance tasks by the child	• Provides a quantified system for observation and measurement of neurologic signs that lead to problems in speech, language, learning, and behavior • Needs to be administered by a qualified clinician

Continued

Developmental Tools Used to Assess Children With Chronic Conditions—cont'd

Types of screening tools	Test/source	Age level	Method	Comments
General	Wheel Guide to Normal Milestones of Development Author: U Hayes Source: A Developmental Approach to Case Findings, ed. 2 US Dept of Health and Human Services Superintendent of Documents Washington, DC 20402	1–3 years	Observation	• Assesses basic reflexes and developmental milestones • Reinforces the normal growth and development patterns of children
Adaptive behavior	AAMR Adaptive Behavior Scale-School, ed. 2 ABS-S:2 (1981-1993) Authors: N Lambert, K Nihira, and H Leland Source: PRO-ED, Inc 8700 Shoal Creek Blvd Austin, TX 76758-6897	3–21 years	Performance tasks, observation, and parent report	• Used as a screening tool and for instructional planning • Can be an indicator in assessing children whose adaptive behavior indicates possible mental retardation, learning difficulties, or emotional disturbances. Provides 16 domain scores. • Previously called AAMD Adaptive Behavior Scale • Software for scoring available

	AAMR Adaptive Behavior Scale Residential and Community, ed. 2 ABS-RC:2 (1969–1993)
	Authors:
	  K Nihira, H Leland, and N Lambert
	Source:
	  PRO-ED, Inc
	  8700 Shoal Creek Blvd.
	  Austin, TX 78758-6897
		3–21 years	Performance task, observation, and parent report	• Similar to AAMR-School
				• Provides scores in 18 domains, including: independent functioning, language development, social behavior, and physical development
				• Software for scoring available

	Vineland Adaptive Behavior Scales
	Authors:
	  SS Sparrow, DA Balla, and
	    DV Cicchetti
	Source:
	  American Guidance Services, Inc
	  4201 Woodland Rd
	  Circle Pines, MN 55014-1796
		Birth–adult	Semi-structured interview with observation caregiver, observation	• Assesses adaptive behavior in four sectors: communication, daily living skills, socialization, and motor skills
				• Can be used with mentally retarded and disabled individuals
				• 20–40 minutes to administer

Temperament	Temperament Assessment Battery for Children (TABC) (1988)
	Author:
	  RP Martin
	Source:
	  Clinical Psychology Publishing Co, Inc
	  #4 Conant Square
	  Brandon, VT 05733
		3–7 years	Structured test format	• Measures basic personality-behavioral dimensions in the areas of: activity, adaptability, approach/withdrawal, intensity, distractibility, persistence
				• 10–20 minutes to administer

Continued

Developmental Tools Used to Assess Children With Chronic Conditions—cont'd

Types of screening tools	Test/source	Age level	Method	Comments
	Carey and McDevitt Revised Temperament Questionnaire: Toddler Temperament Scale Authors: W Fullard, SC McDevitt, and WB Carey Source: W Fullard, PhD Dept of Educational Psychology Temple University Philadelphia, PA 19122	1–3 years	Interview	• Provides an objective measure of the child's temperament profile • Fosters more effective interactions between parent and child • 95 items, 6-pt frequency scale
	Carey and McDevitt Revised Temperament Questionnaire: Behavior Style Questionnaire Authors: SC McDevitt and WB Carey	3–7 years	Interview	• Provides an objective measure of the child's temperament profile • Fosters more effective interactions between parent and child

	Source: SC McDevitt, PhD Dev Profile II Devereaux Center 6436 E Sweetwater Scottsdale, AZ 85254		
	Infant Temperament Questionnaire (ITQ) Authors: WB Carey and SC McDevitt Source: WB Carey, MD 319 W Front St Media, PA 19063	4–8 months	Interview Parent Report	• Provides an objective measure of the infant's temperament profile • Fosters more effective interactions between parent and infant
Vision	Allen Picture Card Test of Visual Acuity Author: HF Allen Source: LADOCA Project and Publishing Foundation E 51st Ave and Lincoln St Denver, CO 80216	3–6 years	Observation	• Preschooler screening test for visual acuity • Trained volunteers/screeners can conduct the testing • Teach child names of pictures before testing

Continued

Developmental Tools Used to Assess Children With Chronic Conditions—cont'd

Types of screening tools	Test/source	Age level	Method	Comments
	Denver Eye Screening Test (DEST) (1973) Authors: WK Frankenberg, AD Goldstein, and J Barker Source: LADOCA Project and Publishing Foundation E 51st Ave and Lincoln St Denver, CO 80216	3 years	Observation	• Identifies children with acuity problems • Good for preschool-age children unable to respond to the Snellen Illiterate E Test
	HOTV (Matching symbol test) Author: O Lippmann Source: Wilson Ophthalmic Corp PO Box 496 Mustang, OK 73064	>3 years	Flashcards	• Good for young children or those who don't like to verbalize • Children name the four letters H, O, T, and V on a chart for testing at 10-20 feet and match them to a demonstration card • Avoids the problem with image reversal and eye-hand coordination that can occur with the letter E

	Picture Card Test (Adaptation of the Pre-school Vision Test) Author: HF Allen Source: LADOCA Project and Publishing Foundation E 51st Ave and Lincoln St Denver, CO 80216	≥2½ years	Interview/"name the picture"	• Identifies children with acuity problems
	Snellen Illiterate E Test Author: H Snellen Source: National Society for Blindness 79 Madison Ave American Association of Ophthalmology 1100 17th St NW Washington, DC 20036	≥3 years	Observation using two persons as a team in screening	• Intended as a screening measure for central acuity of preschool-aged children and of other children who have not learned to read
Speech and language	The Bzoch-League Receptive Expressive Emergent Language Scale (REEL) Author: KR Bzoch and R League	Birth–3 years	Paper-pencil inventory Parent interview	• Identifies children needing further follow-up in language • 15-20 minutes to administer

Continued

Developmental Tools Used to Assess Children With Chronic Conditions—cont'd

Types of screening tools	Test/source	Age level	Method	Comments
	Source: University Park Press 360 N Charles St Baltimore, MD 21201			
	Denver Articulation Screening Exam (DASE) (1971-1973) Authors: AF Drumwright and WK Frankenburg Source: Denver Developmental Materials, Inc PO Box 6919 Denver, CO 80206-0919	2½–6 years	Observation	• Designed to identify significant developmental delay in the acquisition of speech sounds • Good for screening children who may be economically disadvantaged and have a potential speech problem with articulation—pronunciation • Administered by a qualified professional; special training required for the nonprofessional • 10-15 minutes to administer
	Emergent Language Milestone Scale (ELM) (1984) Source: Education Corporation PO Box 721 Tulsa, OK 74101	Birth–36 months	Interview/observation	• Screening instrument for auditory expressive, auditory receptive, and visual components of language

	Tool	Age	Method	Description

	Peabody Picture Vocabulary Test, Revised (PPVT-R) (1981)
	Authors:
	  LM Dunn and LM Dunn
	Source:
	  American Guidance Service
	  4201 Woodland Rd
	  Circle Plains, MN 55014-1796
		≥2½ years	Individual "Point to" response test	• IQ used to assess receptive vocabulary, not a measure of speech/language skills
				• Measures hearing vocabulary for standard American English
				• Used with non-English-speaking students to screen for mental retardation or giftedness
				• Requires a qualified practitioner to administer
				• 10-20 minutes to administer

	Riley Articulation and Language Test, Revised (RALT-R)
	Author:
	  GD Riley
	Source:
	  Western Psychological
	  12031 Wilshire Blvd
	  Los Angeles, CA 90025
		≥4 years	Performance tasks by the child	• 2-3 minute screening test, identifies children in need of speech therapy
				• Provides a quantified system for observation and measurement of neurologic signs that lead to problems in speech, language, learning, and behavior
				• Needs to be administered by a qualified clinician

Hearing	Noise Stik
	Author:
	  LH Eckstein
	Source:
	  Eckstein Bros, Inc
	  4807 W 118th Pl
	  Hawthorne, CA 90250
		Birth–3 years	Behavioral response to auditory stimulation	• Handheld free-field screener for use in the early detection of infant hearing loss

Continued

Developmental Tools Used to Assess Children With Chronic Conditions—cont'd

Types of screening tools	Test/source	Age level	Method	Comments
Child behavior and cognition	Kaufman Brief Intelligence Test (K-BIT) (1990) Authors: AS Kaufman and NL Kaufman Source: American Guidance Service 4201 Woodlawn Rd Circle Pines, MN 55014-1796	4–90 years	Structured test format	• Quick measure of intelligence, may not be substituted for comprehensive measure of intelligence • Assess expressive vocabulary, definitions, matrices • 15-30 minutes to administer
	Brazelton Neonatal Behavioral Assessment Scale Author: TB Brazelton Source: JB Lippincott, Co 227 Washington Square Philadelphia, PA 19106-3780	3 days–4 weeks		• Used as a predictive tool in clinical practice and research for behavioral and neurologic assessment • Tests 27 behavioral items in the areas of habitation, orientation, motor maturity, variation, self-quieting, and social • Requires a trained examiner and 20-30 minutes to administer
	Child Behavior Checklist Author: TM Achenbach	4–18 years	Observation/interview	• Provides an overview of the child's behavior • Parent and teacher forms available

			• Measures the skills needed to learn reading, spelling, and arithmetic • 15-30 minutes to administer
	Source: Center for Children, Youth, and Families University of Vermont 1 S Prospect St Burlington, VT 05401 Source: Jastak Associates, Wide Range, Inc PO Box 3410 Wilmington, DE 19804-0250		
Stress anxiety	State–Trait Anxiety Inventory for children (STAIC) (1970-1973) Authors: CD Spielberg, CD Edwards, RE Lushene, J Montuori, and D Platzek Source: Consulting Psychologists Press, Inc 3803 E Bayshore Rd Palo Alto, CA 94303	4–6 grades	Group or individual Self-administered	• Measures anxiety in elementary school children • Title on test is "How I Feel Questionnaire" • 20 minutes to administer
	State—Trait Anxiety Inventory (STAI) (1968-1984) Authors: CD Spielberger, RL Gorsuch, R Lushene, PR Vagg, and GA Jacobs	9–16 years and adults	Group administration, test booklet Spanish and English available	• Designed to assess anxiety as an emotional state (S-Anxiety) and individual differences in anxiety proneness as a personality trait (T-Anxiety)

Continued

Developmental Tools Used to Assess Children With Chronic Conditions—cont'd

Types of screening tools	Test/source	Age level	Method	Comments
	Consulting Psychologists Press, Inc 3803 E Bayshore Road Palo Alto, CA 94303			• 10-20 minutes to administer

	Stress Response Scale (SRS) (1979-1993)
	Author:
	  LA Chandler
	Source:
	  Psychological Assessment Resources, Inc
	  PO Box 998
	  Odessay, FL 33556
		5–14 years	Group or individual structured test	• Designed to identify behavior or emotional problems: Impulsive (acting out), passive-aggressive, impulsive (overactive), repressed, or dependent
				• Software available for scoring
				• 5 minutes to administer

Self-concept	Piers-Harris Children's Self-Concept Scale (The Way I Feel About Myself) (PHCSCS) (1969-1984) Authors: EV Piers and DB Harris	8–18 years	Descriptive statements Used by group or individual	• 80 questions requiring yes-no response • Assesses a raw self-concept score plus cluster scores for behavior, intellectual and school status, physical appearance and attributes, anxiety, popularity, happiness, and satisfaction

Category	Tool	Population	Method	Description
				• 15-20 minutes to administer
Family function	Feetham Family Functioning Survey (FFFS) (1982) Authors: Feetham and Humenick Source: Nursing Systems and Research Children's National Medical Center 111 Michigan Ave, NW Washington, DC 20010	Family	Self-reporting instrument	• 25 questions evaluating six areas of functioning: household tasks, child care, sexual and moral relations, interaction with family and friends, community involvement, and sources of support • 10 minutes to administer • Used for identifying specific areas of dysfunction in a stressed family
	Home Observation for Measurement of the Environment (HOME) (1984) Authors: R Bradley and B Caldwell Source: Center for Research on Teaching & Learning University of Arkansas at Little Rock 2801 S University Ave Little Rock, AR 72204-1099	Birth–3 years 3–6 years	Interview and direct observation of the interaction between the caretaker and the child	• Two separate instruments designed to assess the quantity and quality of social, emotional, and cognitive support available to a child within the home • The inventory for children birth to 3 yrs contains 45 items; the inventory for 3 to 6-year-old children contains 55 items • Each inventory takes about 1 hour

Continued

Developmental Tools Used to Assess Children With Chronic Conditions—cont'd

Types of screening tools	Test/source	Age level	Method	Comments
Child behavior and cognition	Pediatric Symptom Checklist Authors: M Murphy and M Jellinek Source: Dr. Mike Jellinek Child Psychology Service Mass General Hospital in Boston ACC725 Boston, MA 02114	6–18 years	Parent completed	• Used to screen for areas of weakness requiring more detailed diagnostic testing in scholastic achievement • Parent completed form • A child self-report version • Version for 2-5 years also available • 5 minutes to administer
	Peabody Individual Achievement Test: Revised (PIAT-R) (1970-1989) Authors: LM Dunn and FC Markwardt, Jr Source: American Guidance Service 4201 Woodland Rd Circle Pines, MN 55014-1796	K–12 grade	Interview and written test	• Used to screen for areas of weakness requiring more detailed diagnostic testing in scholastic achievement • Must be administered by a psychologist • 50-70 minutes to administer • Assesses reading recognition such as reading comprehension, total reading, mathematics, spelling, written expression

| Riley Preschool Developmental Screening Inventory (RPDSI)
Author:
  CMD Riley
Source:
  Western Psychological
  12031 Wilshire Blvd
  Los Angeles, CA 90025 | 3–5 years | Observation | • For children who have the tendency for academic problems
• Requires a qualified clinician to administer
• Used to screen for emotional, learning, and behavioral problems |
| Wide Range Achievement Test (WRAT)3(1940-1993)
Author:
  GS Wilkinson | 5–75 years | Paper-pencil subtests | • Used for education placement, vocational assessment, and job placement training
• Large print edition is available |

Denver Developmental Screening Test/Denver II

One of the most widely used screening tests for assessing a young child's development is the *Denver Developmental Screening Test* (DDST) which has been substantially revised and renamed the *Denver II.* It is composed of four major categories (personal-social, fine motor-adaptive, language, and gross motor) and is applicable for children from birth through 6 years of age. The age divisions are monthly until 24 months and then every 6 months until 6 years of age. Up to 24 months of age, allowances are made for infants who were born prematurely by subtracting the number of weeks of missed gestation from their present age and testing them at the adjusted age. For example, a 16-week-old infant who was born 4 weeks early is tested at a 12-week adjusted age level.

To determine relative areas of advancement and areas of delay, sufficient items should be administered to establish the baseline and ceiling levels in each sector. To identify cautions, all items intersected by the age line are administered. To screen solely for developmental delays, only the items located totally to the *left* of the child's age line are administered. Scoring methods and criteria for referral are under investigation.

Directions for administration

1. Try to get child to smile by smiling, talking, or waving. Do not touch him/her.
2. Child must stare at hand several seconds.
3. Parent may help guide toothbrush and put toothpaste on brush.
4. Child does not have to be able to tie shoes or button/zip in the back.
5. Move yarn slowly in an arc from one side to the other, about 8 inches above child's face.
6. Pass if child grasps rattle when it is touched to the backs or tips of fingers.
7. Pass if child tries to see where yarn went. Yarn should be dropped quickly from sight from tester's hand without arm movement.
8. Child must transfer cube from hand to hand without help of body, mouth, or table.
9. Pass if child picks up raisin with any part of thumb and finger.
10. Line can vary only 30° or less from tester's line.

Modified from Wong DL, et al: *Whaley and Wong's nursing care of infants and children,* ed 6, St Louis, 1999, Mosby.

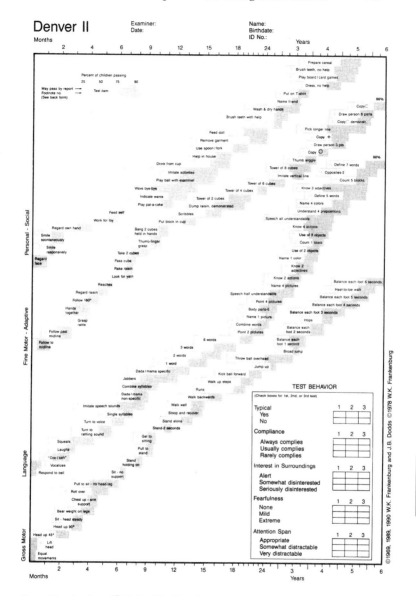

From Frankenburg WK, Dodds JB: The Denver II: a major revision and restandardization of the Denver developmental screening test, Pediatrics *89:91-97, 1992.*

11. Make a fist with thumb pointing upward and wiggle only the thumb. Pass if child imitates and does not move any fingers other than the thumb.

   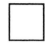

| **12.** Pass any enclosed form. Fail continuous round motions. | **13.** Which line is longer? (Not bigger.) Turn paper upside down and repeat. (pass 3 of 3 or 5 of 6). | **14.** Pass any lines crossing near midpoint. | **15.** Have child copy first. If failed, demonstrate. |

When giving items 12, 14, and 15, do not name the forms. Do not demonstrate 12 and 14.

16. When scoring, each pair (2 arms, 2 legs, etc.) counts as one part.
17. Place one cube in cup and shake gently near child's ear, but out of sight. Repeat for other ear.
18. Point to picture and have child name it. (No credit is given for sounds only.) If less than four pictures are named correctly, have child point to picture as each is named by tester.

19. Using doll, tell child: Show me the nose, eyes, ears, mouth, hands, feet, tummy, hair. Pass 6 of 8.
20. Using pictures, ask child: Which one flies? . . . says "meow"? . . . talks? . . . barks? . . . gallops? Pass 2 of 5, 4 of 5.
21. Ask child: What do you do when you are cold? . . . tired? . . . hungry? Pass 2 of 3, 3 of 3.
22. Ask child: What do you do with a cup? What is a chair used for? What is a pencil used for? Action words must be included in answers.
23. Pass if child correctly places *and* says how many blocks are on paper. (1, 5).

24. Tell child: Put block **on** table: **under** table: **in front of** me, **behind** me. Pass 4 of 4. (Do not help child by pointing, moving head or eyes.)

25. Ask child: What is a ball? . . . lake? . . . desk? . . . house? . . . banana? . . . curtain? . . . fence? . . . ceiling? Pass if defined in terms of use, shape, what it is made of, or general category (such as banana is fruit, not just yellow). Pass 5 of 8, 7 of 8.

26. Ask child: If a horse is big, a mouse is ___? If fire is hot, ice is ___? If the sun shines during the day, the moon shines during the ___? Pass 2 of 3.

27. Child may use wall or rail only, not person. May not crawl.

28. Child must throw ball overhand 3 feet to within arm's reach of tester.

29. Child must perform standing broad jump over width of test sheet (8½ inches).

30. Tell child to walk forward heel-to-toe, heel within 1 inch of toe. Tester may demonstrate. Child must walk 4 consecutive steps.

31. In the second year, half of normal children are noncompliant. **OBSERVATIONS:**

Cultural Awareness: The Denver Developmental Screening Tests

When administering the DDST, the nurse must consider cultural variations that can erroneously label the child delayed. For example, Southeast Asian children have demonstrated delays in the areas of personal-social development because of lack of familiarity with games, such as pat-a-cake, and in language because of differences in word usage, such as absence of plurals. The more protective parental attitude of Southeast Asians toward the young child may also prevent early learning of self-help skills. Several of these variations were noted also in native African children. Further research is needed to determine if cultural variations affect screening results with the Denver II.

Modified from Wong DL, et al: *Whaley and Wong's nursing care of infants and children,* ed 6, St Louis, 1999, Mosby.

Denver II Scoring

Interpretation of the Test

(These are suggested guidelines.)
The DENVER II is interpreted as follows:

Normal:
- No Delays and a maximum of 1 Caution.
- Conduct routine rescreening at next well-child visit.

Suspect:
- Two or more Cautions and/or One or more Delays.
- Because communities' and programs' priorities differ in types or severity of problems they seek to identify in screening, it will be necessary to adjust Suspect criteria to most efficiently achieve their goals. Tables of percentages of Cautions and Delays that may be expected for different demographic groups are provided in the DENVER II Technical Manual, pages 20-22.
- Rescreen in 1–2 weeks to rule out temporary factors such as fatigue, fear, and illness.

Untestable:
- Refusal scores on one or more items completely to the left of the age line or on more than one item intersected by the age line in the 75%–90% area.
- Rescreen in 1–2 weeks.

Referral Considerations

If, upon rescreening, the test result is again Suspect or Untestable, whether or not to refer should be determined by the clinical judgement of the supervising professional based on:

- Profile of test results (which items are Cautions and Delays)
- Number of Cautions and Delays
- Rate of past development
- Other clinical considerations (clinical history, examination, etc.)
- Availability of referral resources

From Frankenburg WK, Dodds JB, et al: *The Denver II training manual,* ed 2, Denver, 1992, Denver Developmental Materials.

Monitoring the Screening program is discussed in the *DENVER II Technical Manual,* pages 20-22. The use of such monitoring is strongly recommended to assist the supervising professional in establishing and adjusting referral criteria.

Denver Articulation Screening Examination

Another widely used screening test is the *Denver Articulation Screening Examination* (DASE). The child repeats each word after the examiner. The examiner circles the underlined sounds that the child pronounces correctly. The total correctly pronounced sounds is the Raw Score.

DENVER ARTICULATION SCREENING EXAMINATION

for children 2½ to 6 years of age

Instructions: Have child repeat each word after you. Circle the underlined sounds that he pronounces correctly. Total correct sounds is the Raw Score. Use charts on reverse side to score results.

NAME

HOSP. NO.

ADDRESS

Date: _____ Child's Age: _____ Examiner: _____ Raw Score: _____

Percentile: _____ Intelligibility: _____ Result: _____

1. <u>t</u>able
2. <u>sh</u>irt
3. <u>d</u>oor
4. <u>tr</u>unk
5. <u>j</u>umping

6. <u>zipper</u>
7. <u>gr</u>apes
8. <u>fl</u>ag
9. <u>th</u>umb
10. <u>toothbr</u>ush

11. <u>s</u>ock
12. <u>v</u>acuum
13. <u>y</u>arn
14. <u>m</u>o<u>th</u>er
15. <u>tw</u>in<u>kl</u>e

16. <u>wagon</u>
17. <u>gum</u>
18. <u>h</u>ouse
19. <u>pen</u>c<u>il</u>
20. <u>fish</u>

21. <u>leaf</u>
22. <u>c</u>arro<u>t</u>

Intelligibility: (circle one)   1. Easy to understand
                                 2. Understandable ½ the time.

3. Not understandable
4. Can't evaluate

Comments:

Date: _____ Child's Age: _____ Examiner: _____ Raw Score: _____

Percentile: _____ Intelligibility: _____ Result: _____

1. table	6. zipper	11. sock	16. wagon	21. leaf
2. shirt	7. grapes	12. vacuum	17. gum	22. carrot
3. door	8. flag	13. yarn	18. house	
4. trunk	9. thumb	14. mother	19. pencil	
5. jumping	10. toothbrush	15. twinkle	20. fish	

Intelligibility: (circle one)

1. Easy to understand   3. Not understandable
2. Understandable ½ the time.   4. Can't evaluate

Comments:

Date: _____ Child's Age: _____ Examiner: _____ Raw Score: _____

Percentile: _____ Intelligibility: _____ Result: _____

1. table	6. zipper	11. sock	16. wagon	21. leaf
2. shirt	7. grapes	12. vacuum	17. gum	22. carrot
3. door	8. flag	13. yarn	18. house	
4. trunk	9. thumb	14. mother	19. pencil	
5. jumping	10. toothbrush	15. twinkle	20. fish	

Intelligibility: (circle one)

1. Easy to understand   3. Not understandable
2. Understandable ½ the time.   4. Can't evaluate

Comments:

To score DASE words: Note Raw Score for child's performance. Match raw score line (extreme left of chart) with column representing child's age (to the closest previous age group). Where raw score line and age column meet number in that square denotes percentile rank of child's performance when compared to other children that age. Percentiles above heavy line are ABNORMAL percentiles, below heavy line are NORMAL.

Percentile rank

Raw Score	2½ yr.	3.0	3½	4.0	4½	5.0	5½	6 yr
2	1							
3	2							
4	5							
5	9							
6	16							
7	23							
8	31	2						
9	37	4	1					
10	42	6	2					
11	48	7	4					
12	54	9	6	1	1			
13	58	12	9	2	3	1		
14	62	17	11	5	4	2	1	
15	68	23	15	9	5	3	2	
16	75	31	19	12	5	4	2	
17	79	38	25	15	6	6	3	
18	83	46	31	19	8	7	4	

19	86	51	38	24	10	9	5	1
20	89	58	45	30	12	11	7	3
21	92	65	52	36	15	15	9	4
22	94	72	58	43	18	19	12	5
23	96	77	63	50	22	24	15	7
24	97	82	70	58	29	29	20	15
25	99	87	78	66	36	34	26	17
26	99	91	84	75	46	43	34	24
27		94	89	82	57	54	44	34
28		96	94	88	70	68	59	47
29		98	98	94	84	84	77	68
30		100	100	100	100	100	100	100

To Score Intelligibility:

	Normal		**Abnormal**
2½ years	Understandable ½ the time, or, "easy"		Not understandable
3 years and older	Easy to understand		Understandable ½ time Not understandable

Test Results: 1. **Normal** on DASE and Intelligibility = **Normal**

2. **Abnormal** on DASE and/or Intelligibility = **Abnormal**

*If abnormal on initial screening, rescreen within 2 weeks. If abnormal again, child should be referred for complete speech evaluation.

Growth Measurements: Birth to 18 Years

Height and weight measurements for boys

	Height by percentiles						Weight by percentiles					
	5		50		95		5		50		95	
Age*	cm	inches	cm	inches	cm	inches	kg	lb	kg	lb	kg	lb
Height and weight measurements for boys												
Birth	46.4	18¼	50.5	20	54.4	21½	2.54	5½	3.27	7¼	4.15	9¼
3 months	56.7	22¼	61.1	24	65.4	25¾	4.43	9¾	5.98	13¼	7.37	16¼
6 months	63.4	25	67.8	26¾	72.3	28½	6.20	13¾	7.85	17¼	9.46	20¾
9 months	68.0	26¾	72.3	28½	77.1	30¼	7.52	16½	9.18	20¼	10.93	24
1 yrs.	71.7	28¼	76.1	30	81.2	32	8.43	18½	10.15	22½	11.99	26½
1½	77.5	30½	82.4	32½	88.1	34¾	9.59	21¼	11.47	25¼	13.44	29½
2†	82.5	32½	86.8	34¼	94.4	37¼	10.49	23¼	12.34	27¼	15.50	34¼
2½†	85.4	33½	90.4	35½	97.8	38½	11.27	24¾	13.52	29¾	16.61	36½
3	89.0	35	94.9	37¼	102.0	40¼	12.05	26½	14.62	32¼	17.77	39¼
3½	92.5	36½	99.1	39	106.1	41¾	12.84	28¼	15.68	34½	18.98	41¾

4	95.8	37¾	102.9	40½	109.9	43¼	13.64	30	16.69	36¾	20.27	44¾
4½	98.9	39	106.6	42	113.5	44¾	14.45	31¾	17.69	39	21.63	47¾
5	102.0	40¼	109.9	43¼	117.0	46	15.27	33¾	18.67	41¼	23.09	51
6	107.7	42½	116.1	45¾	123.5	48½	16.93	37¼	20.69	45½	26.34	58
7	113.0	44½	121.7	48	129.7	51	18.64	41	22.85	50¼	30.12	66½
8	118.1	46½	127.0	50	135.7	53½	20.40	45	25.30	55¾	34.51	76
9	122.9	48½	132.2	52	141.8	55¾	22.25	49	28.13	62	39.58	87¼
10	127.7	50¼	137.5	54¼	148.1	58¼	24.33	53¾	31.44	69¼	45.27	99¾
11	132.6	52¼	143.3	56½	154.9	61	26.80	59	35.30	77¾	51.47	113½
12	137.6	54¼	149.7	59	162.3	64	29.85	65¾	39.78	87¾	58.09	128
13	142.9	56¼	156.5	61½	169.8	66¾	33.64	74¼	44.95	99	65.02	143¼
14	148.8	58½	163.1	64¼	176.7	69½	38.22	84¼	50.77	112	72.13	159
15	155.2	61	169.0	66½	181.9	71½	43.11	95	56.71	125	79.12	174½
16	161.1	63½	173.5	68¼	185.4	73	47.74	105¼	62.10	137	85.62	188¾
17	164.9	65	176.2	69¼	187.3	73¾	51.50	113½	66.31	146¼	91.31	201¼
18	165.7	65¼	176.8	69½	187.6	73¾	53.97	119	68.88	151¾	95.76	211

*Years unless otherwise indicated.

†Height data include some recumbent length measurements, which make values slightly higher than if all measurements had been of stature (standing height).

From Wong DL, et al: *Whaley and Wong's nursing care of infants and children,* ed 6, St Louis, 1999, Mosby. As modified from National Center for Health Statistics, Health Resources Administration: Conversion of metric data to approximate inches and pounds by Ross Laboratories, Hyattsville, Md, Department of Health, Education and Welfare.

Continued

Growth Measurements: Birth to 18 Years—cont'd

Height and weight measurements for girls

Age*	Height by percentiles						Weight by percentiles					
	5		50		95		5		50		95	
	cm	inches	cm	inches	cm	inches	kg	lb	kg	lb	kg	lb
Height and weight measurements for girls												
Birth	45.4	17¾	49.9	19¾	52.9	20¾	2.36	5¼	3.23	7	3.81	8½
3 months	55.4	21¾	59.5	23½	63.4	25	4.18	9¼	5.4	12	6.74	14¾
6 months	61.8	24¼	65.9	26	70.2	27¾	5.79	12¾	7.21	16	8.73	19¼
9 months	66.1	26	70.4	27¾	75.0	29½	7.0	15½	8.56	18¾	10.17	22½
1 yrs.	69.8	27½	74.3	29¼	79.1	31¼	7.84	17¼	9.53	21	11.24	24¾
1½	76.0	30	80.9	31¾	86.1	34	8.92	19¾	10.82	23¾	12.76	28¼
2†	81.6	32¼	86.8	34¼	93.6	36¾	9.95	22	11.8	26	14.15	31¼
2½†	84.6	33¼	90.0	35½	96.6	38	10.8	23¾	13.03	28¾	15.76	34¾
3	88.3	34¾	94.1	37	100.6	39½	11.61	25½	14.1	31	17.22	38
3½	91.7	36	97.9	38½	104.5	41¼	12.37	27¼	15.07	33¼	18.59	41

4	95.0	37½	101.6	40	108.3	42¾	13.11	29	15.96	35¼	19.91	44
4½	98.1	38½	105.0	41¼	112.0	44	13.83	30½	16.81	37	21.24	46¾
5	101.1	39¾	108.4	42¾	115.6	45½	14.55	32	17.66	39	22.62	49¾
6	106.6	42	114.6	45	122.7	48¼	16.05	35½	19.52	43	25.75	56¾
7	111.8	44	120.6	47½	129.5	51	17.71	39	21.84	48¼	29.68	65½
8	116.9	46	126.4	49¾	136.2	53½	19.62	43¼	24.84	54¾	34.71	76½
9	122.1	48	132.2	52	142.9	56¼	21.82	48	28.46	62¾	40.64	89½
10	127.5	50¼	138.3	54½	149.5	58¾	24.36	53¾	32.55	71¾	47.17	104
11	133.5	52½	144.8	57	156.2	61½	27.24	60	36.95	81½	54.0	119
12	139.8	55	151.5	59¾	162.7	64	30.52	67¼	41.53	91½	60.81	134
13	145.2	57¼	157.1	61¾	168.1	66¼	34.14	75¼	46.1	101¾	67.3	148¼
14	148.7	58½	160.4	63¼	171.3	67½	37.76	83¼	50.28	110¾	73.08	161
15	150.5	59¼	161.8	63¾	172.8	68	40.99	90¼	53.68	118¼	77.78	171½
16	151.6	59¾	162.4	64	173.3	68¼	43.41	95¾	55.89	123¼	80.99	178½
17	152.7	60	163.1	64¼	173.5	68¼	44.74	98¾	56.69	125	82.46	181¾
18	153.6	60½	163.7	64½	173.6	68¼	45.26	99¾	56.62	124¾	82.47	181¾

*Years unless otherwise indicated.

†Height data include some recumbent length measurements, which make values slightly higher than if all measurements had been of stature (standing height).

Schedule of Clinical Preventive Services

Birth to 10 years

Interventions considered
  and recommended for the
  Periodic Health Examination

Leading causes of death
  Conditions originating in perinatal
    period
  Congenital anomalies
  Sudden infant death syndrome (SIDS)
  Unintentional injuries (non–motor
    vehicle)
  Motor vehicle injuries

Interventions for the general population

Screening

Height and weight
Blood pressure
Vision screen (age 3-4 yr)
Hemoglobinopathy screen (birth)[1]
Phenylalanine level (birth)[2]
T_4 and/or TSH (birth)[3]

Counseling

Injury prevention
Child safety car seats (age <5 yr)
Lap-shoulder belts (age ≥5 yr)
Bicycle helmet; avoid bicycling near traffic
Smoke detector, flame retardant sleepwear
Hot water heater temperature <120° F
Window/stair guards, pool fence
Safe storage of drugs, toxic substances, firearms and matches
Syrup of ipecac, Poison Control Center phone number
CPR training for parents/caretakers

Diet and exercise
Breast-feeding, iron-enriched formula and foods (infants and toddlers)
Limit fat and cholesterol; maintain caloric balance; emphasize grains, fruits,
  vegetables (age ≥2 yr)
Regular physical activity

Substance use
Effects of passive smoking*
Anti-tobacco message*

Dental health
Regular visits to dental care provider*
Floss, brush with fluoride toothpaste daily*
Advice about baby bottle tooth decay*

From *Guide to clinical preventive services: report of the US Preventive Services Task Force,* ed 2, Baltimore, 1996, Williams & Wilkins.

Immunizations

Diphtheria-tetanus-pertussis (DTP)[4]
Oral poliovirus (OPV)[5]
Measles-mumps-rubella (MMR)[6]
H. influenzae type b (Hib) conjugate[7]
Hepatitis B[8]
Varicella[9]

Chemoprophylaxis

Ocular prophylaxis (birth)

Interventions for high-risk populations

Population	Potential interventions
	(See detailed high-risk definitions)
Preterm or low birth weight	Hemoglobin/hematocrit (HR1)
Infants of mothers at risk for HIV	HIV testing (HR2)
Low income; immigrants	Hemoglobin/hematocrit (HR1); PPD (HR3)
Tuberculosis (TB) contacts	PPD (HR3)
Native American/Alaska Native	Hemoglobin/hematocrit (HR1); PPD (HR3); hepatitis A vaccine (HR4); pneumococcal vaccine (HR5)
Travelers to developing countries	Hepatitis A vaccine (HR4)
Residents of long-term care facilities	PPD (HR3); hepatitis A vaccine (HR4); influenza vaccine (HR6)
Certain chronic medical conditions	PPD (HR3); pneumococcal vaccine (HR5); influenza vaccine (HR6)
Increased individual or community lead exposure	Blood lead level (HR7)
Inadequate water fluoridation	Daily fluoride supplement (HR8)
Family history of skin cancer; nevi; fair skin, eyes, hair	Avoid excess/midday sun, use protective clothing* (HR9)

[1]Whether screening should be universal or targeted to high-risk groups will depend on the proportion of high-risk individuals in the screening area, and other considerations. [2]If done during first 24 hr of life, repeat by age 2 wk. [3]Optimally between day 2 and 6, but in all cases before newborn nursery discharge. [4]2, 4, 6, and 12-18 mo; once between ages 4-6 yr (DTaP may be used at 15 mo and older). [5]2, 4, 6-18 mo; once between ages 4-6 yr. [6]12-15 mo and 4-6 yr. [7]2, 4, 6 and 12-15 mo; no dose needed at 6 mo if PRP-OMP vaccine is used for first 2 doses. [8]Birth, 1 mo, 6 mo; or, 0-2 mo, 1-2 mo later, and 6-18 mo. If not done in infancy: current visit, and 1 and 6 mo later. [9]12-18 mo; or any child without hx of chickenpox or previous immunization. Include information on risk in adulthood, duration of immunity, and potential need for booster doses.
*The ability of clinician counseling to influence this behavior is unproven.

Overview

HR1 = Infants age 6-12 mo who are: living in poverty, black, Native American or Alaska Native, immigrants from developing countries, preterm and low birth weight infants, infants whose principal dietary intake is unfortified cow's milk.

HR2 = Infants born to high-risk mothers whose HIV status is unknown. Women at high risk include: past or present injection drug use; persons who exchange sex for money or drugs, and their sex partners; injection drug-using, bisexual, or HIV-positive sex partners currently or in past; persons seeking treatment for sexually transmitted diseases (STDs); blood transfusion during 1978-1985.

HR3 = Persons infected with HIV, close contacts of persons with known or suspected TB, persons with medical risk factors associated with TB, immigrants from countries with high TB prevalence, medically underserved low-income populations (including homeless), residents of long-term care facilities.

HR4 = Persons living ≥2 yr in or traveling to areas where the disease is endemic and where periodic outbreaks occur (e.g., countries with high or intermediate endemicity; certain Alaska Native, Pacific Island, Native American, and religious communities). Consider for institutionalized children aged ≥2 yr. Clinicians should also consider local epidemiology.

HR5 = Immunocompetent persons ≥2 yr with certain medical conditions, including chronic cardiac or pulmonary disease, diabetes mellitus, and anatomic asplenia. Immunocompetent persons ≥2 yr living in high-risk environments or social settings (e.g., certain Native American and Alaska Native populations).

HR6 = Annual vaccination of children ≥6 mo who are residents of chronic care facilities or who have chronic cardiopulmonary disorders, metabolic diseases (including diabetes mellitus), hemoglobinopathies, immunosuppression, or renal dysfunction.

HR7 = Children about age 12 mo who: 1) live in communities in which the prevalence of lead levels requiring individual intervention, including residential lead hazard control or chelation, is high or undefined; 2) live in or frequently visit a home built before 1950 with dilapidated paint or with recent or ongoing renovation or remodeling; 3) have close contact with a person who has an elevated lead level; 4) live near lead industry or heavy traffic; 5) live with someone whose job or hobby involves lead exposure; 6) use lead-based pottery; or 7) take traditional ethnic remedies that contain lead.

HR8 = Children living in areas with inadequate water fluoridation (<0.6 ppm).

HR9 = Persons with a family history of skin cancer, a large number of moles, atypical moles, poor tanning ability, or light skin, hair, and eye color.

Ages 11-24 years

Interventions considered and recommended for the Periodic Health Examination	Leading causes of death
	Motor vehicle/other unintentional injuries
	Homicide
	Suicide
	Malignant neoplasms
	Heart diseases

Interventions for the general population

Screening

Height & weight
Blood pressure[1]
Papanicolaou (Pap) test[2] (females)
Chlamydia screen[3] (females <20 yr)
Rubella serology or vaccination hx[4] (females >12 yr)
Assess for problem drinking

Counseling

Injury prevention
Lap/shoulder belts
Bicycle/motorcycle/ATV helmets*
Smoke detector*
Safe storage/removal of firearms*

Substance use
Avoid tobacco use
Avoid underage drinking and illicit drug use*
Avoid alcohol/drug use while driving, swimming, boating, etc.*

Sexual behavior
STD prevention: abstinence*; avoid high-risk behavior*; condoms/female barrier with spermicide*
Unintended pregnancy: contraception

Diet and exercise
Limit fat and cholesterol; maintain caloric balance; emphasize grains, fruits, vegetables
Adequate calcium intake (females)
Regular physical activity*

---

[1] Periodic BP for persons aged ≥21 yr. [2] If sexually active at present or in the past q ≤3 yr. If sexual history is unreliable, begin Pap tests at age 18 yr. [3] If sexually active. [4] Serologic testing, documented vaccination history, and routine vaccination against rubella (preferably with MMR) are equally acceptable alternatives. [5] If not previously immunized: current visit, 1 and 6 mo later. [6] If no previous second dose of MMR. [7] If susceptible to chickenpox.
*The ability of clinician counseling to influence this behavior is unproven.

Continued

Dental health
Regular visits to dental care provider*
Floss, brush with fluoride toothpaste daily*

Immunizations
Tetanus-diphtheria (Td) boosters (11-16 yr)
Hepatitis B[5]
MMR (11-12 yr)[6]
Varicella (11-12 yr)[7]
Rubella[4] (females >12 yr)

Chemoprophylaxis
Multivitamin with folic acid (females)

Interventions for high-risk populations

Population	Potential interventions (See detailed high-risk definitions)
High-risk sexual behavior	RPR/VDRL (HR1); screen for gonorrhea (female) (HR2), HIV (HR3), chlamydia (female) (HR4); hepatitis A vaccine (HR5)
Injection or street drug use	RPR/VDRL (HR1); HIV screen (HR3); hepatitis A vaccine (HR5); PPD (HR6); advice to reduce infection risk (HR7)
TB contacts; immigrants; low income	PPD (HR6)
Native Americans/Alaska Natives	Hepatitis A vaccine (HR5); PPD (HR6); pneumococcal vaccine (HR8)
Travelers to developing countries	Hepatitis A vaccine (HR5)
Certain chronic medical conditions	PPD (HR6); pneumococcal vaccine (HR8); influenza vaccine (HR9)
Settings where adolescents and young adults congregate	Second MMR (HR10)
Susceptible to varicella, measles, mumps	Varicella vaccine (HR11); MMR (HR12)
Blood transfusion between 1975-1985	HIV screen (HR3)
Institutionalized persons; health care/lab workers	Hepatitis A vaccine (HR5); PPD (HR6); influenza vaccine (HR9)
Family history of skin cancer; nevi; fair skin, eyes, hair	Avoid excess/midday sun, use protective clothing* (HR13)
Prior pregnancy with neural tube defect	Folic acid 4.0 mg (HR14)
Inadequate water fluoridation	Daily fluoride supplement (HR15)

Overview
HR1 = Persons who exchange sex for money or drugs, and their sex partners; persons with other STDs (including HIV); and sexual contacts of persons with active syphilis. Clinicians should also consider local epidemiology.

HR2 = Females who have: two or more sex partners in the last year; a sex partner with multiple sexual contacts; exchanged sex for money or drugs; or a history of repeated episodes of gonorrhea. Clinicians should also consider local epidemiology.

HR3 = Men who had sex with men after 1975; past or present injection drug use; persons who exchange sex for money or drugs, and their sex partners; injection drug-using, bisexual, or HIV-positive sex partner currently or in the past; blood transfusion during 1978-1985; persons seeking treatment for STDs. Clinicians should also consider local epidemiology.

HR4 = Sexually active females with multiple risk factors including: history of prior STD; new or multiple sex partners; age under 25; nonuse or inconsistent use of barrier contraceptives; cervical ectopy. Clinicians should consider local epidemiology of the disease in identifying other high-risk groups.

HR5 = Persons living in, traveling to, or working in areas where the disease is endemic and where periodic outbreaks occur (e.g., countries with high or intermediate endemicity; certain Alaska Native, Pacific Island, Native American, and religious communities); men who have sex with men; injection or street drug users. Vaccine may be considered for institutionalized persons and workers in these institutions, military personnel, and day-care, hospital, and laboratory workers. Clinicians should also consider local epidemiology.

HR6 = HIV positive, close contacts of persons with known or suspected TB, healthcare workers, persons with medical risk factors associated with TB, immigrants from countries with high TB prevalence, medically underserved low-income populations (including homeless), alcoholics, injection drug users, and residents of long-term facilities.

HR7 = Persons who continue to inject drugs.

HR8 = Immunocompetent persons with certain medical conditions, including chronic cardiac or pulmonary disease, diabetes mellitus, and anatomic asplenia. Immunocompetent persons who live in high-risk environments or social settings (e.g., certain Native American and Alaska Native populations).

HR9 = Annual vaccination of: residents of chronic care facilities; persons with chronic cardiopulmonary disorders, metabolic diseases (including diabetes mellitus), hemoglobinopathies, immunosuppression, or renal dysfunction; and healthcare providers for high-risk patients.

HR10 = Adolescents and young adults in settings where such individuals congregate (e.g., high schools and colleges), if they have not previously received a second dose.

HR11 = Healthy persons aged ≥ 13 yr without a history of chickenpox or previous immunization. Consider serologic testing for presumed susceptible persons aged ≥ 13 yr.

HR12 = Persons born after 1956 who lack evidence of immunity to measles or mumps (e.g., documented receipt of live vaccine on or after the first birthday, laboratory evidence of immunity, or a history of physician-diagnosed measles or mumps).

HR13 = Persons with a family or personal history of skin cancer, a large number of moles, atypical moles, poor tanning ability, or light skin, hair, and eye color.

HR14 = Women with prior pregnancy affected by neural tube defect who are planning pregnancy.

HR15 = Persons aged <17 yr living in areas with inadequate water fluoridation (<0.6 ppm).

Ages 25-64 years

Interventions considered and recommended for the Periodic Health Examination	Leading causes of death Malignant neoplasms Heart diseases Motor vehicle and other unintentional injuries Human immunodeficiency virus (HIV) infection Suicide and homicide

Interventions for the general population

Screening

Blood pressure
Height and weight
Total blood cholesterol (men age 35-64, women age 45-64)
Papanicolaou (Pap) test (women)[1]
Fecal occult blood test[2] and/or sigmoidoscopy (≥50 yr)
Mammogram ± clinical breast exam[3] (women 50-69 yr)
Assess for problem drinking
Rubella serology or vaccination hx[4]
    (women of childbearing age)

Counseling

Substance use
Tobacco cessation
Avoid alcohol/drug use while driving, swimming, boating, etc.*

Diet and exercise
Limit fat and cholesterol; maintain caloric balance; emphasize grains, fruits, vegetables
Adequate calcium intake (women)
Regular physical activity*

Injury prevention
Lap/shoulder belts
Motorcycle/bicycle/ATV helmets*
Smoke detector*
Safe storage/removal of firearms*

Sexual behavior
STD prevention: avoid high-risk behavior*; condoms/female barrier with
   spermicide*
Unintended pregnancy: contraception

Dental health
Regular visits to dental care provider*
Floss, brush with fluoride toothpaste daily*

Immunizations
Tetanus-diphtheria (Td) boosters
Rubella[4] (women of childbearing age)

Chemoprophylaxis
Multivitamin with folic acid (women planning or capable of pregnancy)
Discuss hormone prophylaxis (peri- and postmenopausal women)

Interventions for high-risk populations

Population	Potential interventions
	(See detailed high-risk definitions)
High-risk sexual behavior	RPR/VDRL (HR1); screen for gonorrhea (female) (HR2), HIV (HR3), chlamydia (female) (HR4); hepatitis B vaccine (HR5); hepatitis A vaccine (HR6)
Injection or street drug use	RPR/VDRL (HR1); HIV screen (HR3); hepatitis B vaccine (HR5); hepatitis A vaccine (HR6); PPD (HR7); advice to reduce infection risk (HR8)
Low income; TB contacts; immigrants, alcoholics	PPD (HR7)
Native Americans/Alaska Natives	Hepatitis A vaccine (HR6); PPD (HR7); pneumococcal vaccine (HR9)
Travelers to developing countries	Hepatitis B vaccine (HR5); hepatitis A vaccine (HR6)
Certain chronic medical conditions	PPD (HR7); pneumococcal vaccine (HR9); influenza vaccine (HR10)
Blood product recipients	HIV screen (HR3); hepatitis B vaccine (HR5)

[1]Women who are or have been sexually active and who have a cervix: q ≤ 3 yr. [2]Annually. [3]Mammogram q1-2 yr, or mammogram q1-2 yr with annual clinical breast examination. [4]Serologic testing, documented vaccination history, and routine vaccination (preferably with MMR) are equally acceptable.
*The ability of clinician counseling to influence this behavior is unproven.

Continued

Population	Potential interventions
Susceptible to measles, mumps, or varicella	MMR (HR11); varicella vaccine (HR12)
Institutionalized persons	Hepatitis A vaccine (HR6); PPD (HR7); pneumococcal vaccine (HR9); influenza vaccine (HR10)
Healthcare/lab workers	Hepatitis B vaccine (HR5); hepatitis A vaccine (HR6); PPD (HR7); influenza vaccine (HR10)
Family history of skin cancer; fair skin, eyes, hair	Avoid excess/midday sun, use protective clothing* (HR13)
Previous pregnancy with neural tube defect	Folic acid 4.0 mg (HR14)

Overview

HR1 = Persons who exchange sex for money or drugs, and their sex partners; persons with other STDs (including HIV); and sexual contacts of persons with active syphilis. Clinicians should also consider local epidemiology.

HR2 = Women who exchange sex for money or drugs, or who have had repeated episodes of gonorrhea. Clinicians should also consider local epidemiology.

HR3 = Men who had sex with men after 1975; past or present injection drug use; persons who exchange sex for money or drugs, and their sex partners; injection drug-using, bisexual, or HIV-positive sex partner currently or in the past; blood transfusion during 1978-1985; persons seeking treatment for STDs. Clinicians should also consider local epidemiology.

HR4 = Sexually active women with multiple risk factors including: history of STD; new or multiple sex partners; nonuse or inconsistent use of barrier contraceptives; cervical ectopy. Clinicians should also consider local epidemiology.

HR5 = Blood product recipients (including hemodialysis patients), persons with frequent occupational exposure to blood or blood products, men who have sex with men, injection drug users and their sex partners, persons with multiple recent sex partners, persons with other STDs (including HIV), travelers to countries with endemic hepatitis B.

HR6 = Persons living in, traveling to, or working in areas where the disease is endemic and where periodic outbreaks occur (e.g., countries with high or intermediate endemicity; certain Alaska Native, Pacific Island, Native American, and religious communities); men who have sex with men; injection or street drug users. Consider for institutionalized persons and workers in these institutions, military personnel, and day care, hospital, and laboratory workers. Clinicians should also consider local epidemiology.

HR7 = HIV positive, close contacts of persons with known or suspected TB, healthcare workers, persons with medical risk factors associated with TB, immigrants from countries with high TB prevalence, medically underserved low-income populations (including homeless), alcoholics, injection drug users, and residents of long-term care facilities.

HR8 = Persons who continue to inject drugs.

HR9 = Immunocompetent institutionalized persons aged ≥50 yr and immunocompetent persons with certain medical conditions, including chronic cardiac or pulmonary disease, diabetes mellitus, and anatomic asplenia. Immunocompetent persons who live in high-risk environments or social settings (e.g., certain Native American and Alaska Native populations).

HR10 = Annual vaccination of residents of chronic care facilities; persons with chronic cardiopulmonary disorders, metabolic diseases (including diabetes mellitus), hemoglobinopathies, immunosuppression or renal dysfunction; and healthcare providers for high-risk patients.

HR11 = Persons born after 1956 who lack evidence of immunity to measles or mumps (e.g., documented receipt of live vaccine on or after the first birthday, laboratory evidence of immunity, or a history of physician-diagnosed measles or mumps).

HR12 = Healthy adults without a history of chickenpox or previous immunization. Consider serologic testing for presumed susceptible adults.

HR13 = Persons with a family or personal history of skin cancer, a large number of moles, atypical moles, poor tanning ability, or light skin, hair, and eye color.

HR14 = Women with previous pregnancy affected by neural tube defect who are planning pregnancy.

Age 65 and older

Interventions considered and recommended for the Periodic Health Examination	Leading causes of death
	Heart diseases
	Malignant neoplasms (lung, colorectal, breast)
	Cerebrovascular disease
	Chronic obstructive pulmonary disease
	Pneumonia and influenza

Interventions for the general population

Screening

Blood pressure
Height and weight
Fecal occult blood test[1] and/or sigmoidoscopy
Mammogram ± clinical breast exam[2] (women ≤69 yr)
Papanicolaou (Pap) test (women)[3]
Vision screening
Assess for hearing impairment
Assess for problem drinking

Counseling

Substance use
Tobacco cessation
Avoid alcohol/drug use while driving, swimming, boating, etc.*

Diet and exercise
Limit fat and cholesterol; maintain caloric balance; emphasize grains, fruits, vegetables
Adequate calcium intake (women)
Regular physical activity*

Injury prevention
Lap/shoulder belts
Motorcycle and bicycle helmets*
Fall prevention*
Safe storage/removal of firearms*
Smoke detector*
Set hot water heater to <120° F*
CPR training for household members

Dental health
Regular visits to dental care provider*
Floss, brush with fluoride toothpaste daily*

Sexual behavior
STD prevention: avoid high-risk sexual behavior*; use condoms*

Immunizations

Pneumococcal vaccine
Influenza[1]
Tetanus-diphtheria (Td) boosters

Chemoprophylaxis

Discuss hormone prophylaxis (peri- and postmenopausal women)

Interventions for high-risk populations

Population	Potential interventions (See detailed high-risk definitions)
Institutionalized persons	PPD (HR1); hepatitis A vaccine (HR2); amantadine/rimantadine (HR4)
Chronic medical conditions; TB contacts; low income; immigrants; alcoholics	PPD (HR1)
Persons ≥75 yr; or ≥70 yr with risk factors for falls	Fall prevention intervention (HR5)
Cardiovascular disease risk factors	Consider cholesterol screening (HR6)
Family history of skin cancer; nevi; fair skin, eyes, hair	Avoid excess/midday sun, use protective clothing* (HR7)
Native Americans/Alaska Natives	PPD (HR1); hepatitis A vaccine (HR2)
Travelers to developing countries	Hepatitis A vaccine (HR2); hepatitis B vaccine (HR8)
Blood product recipients	HIV screen (HR3); hepatitis B vaccine (HR8)
High-risk sexual behavior	Hepatitis A vaccine (HR2); HIV screen (HR3); hepatitis B vaccine (HR8); RPR/VDRL (HR9)
Injection or street drug use	PPD (HR1); hepatitis A vaccine (HR2); HIV screen (HR3); hepatitis B vaccine (HR8); RPR/VDRL (HR9); advice to reduce infection risk (HR10)
Healthcare/lab workers	PPD (HR1); hepatitis A vaccine (HR2); amantadine/rimantadine (HR4); hepatitis B vaccine (HR8)
Persons susceptible to varicella	Varicella vaccine (HR11)

[1]Annually. [2]Mammogram q1-2 yr, or mammogram q1-2 yr with annual clinical breast exam. [3]All women who are or have been sexually active and who have a cervix. Consider discontinuation of testing after age 65 if previous regular screening with consistently normal results.

*The ability of clinician counseling to influence this behavior is unproven.

Overview

HR1 = HIV positive, close contacts of persons with known or suspected TB, healthcare workers, persons with medical risk factors associated with TB, immigrants from countries with high TB prevalence, medically underserved low-income populations (including homeless), alcoholics, injection drug users, and residents of long-term care facilities.

HR2 = Persons living in, traveling to, or working in areas where the disease is endemic and where periodic outbreaks occur (e.g., countries with high or intermediate endemicity; certain Alaska Native, Pacific Island, Native American, and religious communities); men who have sex with men; injection or street drug users. Consider for institutionalized persons and workers in these institutions, and day-care, hospital, and laboratory workers. Clinicians should also consider local epidemiology.

HR3 = Men who had sex with men after 1975; past or present injection drug use; persons who exchange sex for money or drugs, and their sex partners; injection drug-using, bisexual, or HIV-positive sex partner currently or in the past; blood transfusion during 1978-1985; persons seeking treatment for STDs. Clinicians should also consider local epidemiology.

HR4 = Consider for persons who have not received influenza vaccine or are vaccinated late; when the vaccine may be ineffective due to major antigenic changes in the virus; for unvaccinated persons who provide home care for high-risk persons; to supplement protection provided by vaccine in persons who are expected to have a poor antibody response; and for high-risk persons in whom the vaccine is contraindicated.

HR5 = Persons aged 75 years and older; or aged 70-74 with one or more additional risk factors including: use of certain psychoactive and cardiac medications (e.g., benzodiazepines, antihypertensives); use of ≥4 prescription medications; impaired cognition, strength, balance, or gait. Intensive individualized home-based multifactorial fall prevention intervention is recommended in settings where adequate resources are available to deliver such services.

HR6 = Although evidence is insufficient to recommend routine screening in elderly persons, clinicians should consider cholesterol screening on a case-by-case basis for persons ages 65-75 with additional risk factors (e.g., smoking, diabetes, or hypertension)

HR7 = Persons with a family or personal history of skin cancer, a large number of moles, atypical moles, poor tanning ability, or light skin, hair,

HR8 = Blood product recipients (including hemodialysis patients), persons with frequent occupational exposure to blood or blood products, men who have sex with men, injection drug users and their sex partners, persons with multiple recent sex partners, persons with other STDs (including HIV), travelers to countries with endemic hepatitis B.

HR9 = Persons who exchange sex for money or drugs and their sex partners; persons with other STDs (including HIV); and sexual contacts of persons with active syphilis. Clinicians should also consider local epidemiology.

HR10 = Persons who continue to inject drugs.

HR11 = Healthy adults without a history of chickenpox or previous immunization. Consider serologic testing for presumed susceptible adults.

Pregnant women**

Interventions considered and recommended for the Periodic Health Examination

Interventions for the general population

Screening

First visit
Blood pressure
Hemoglobin/hematocrit
Hepatitis B surface antigen (HBsAg)
RPR/VDRL
Chlamydia screen (<25 yr)
Rubella serology or vaccination history
D(Rh) typing, antibody screen
Offer CVS (<13 wk)[1] or amniocentesis (15–18 wk)[1] (age ≥35 yr)
Offer hemoglobinopathy screening
Assess for problem or risk drinking
Offer HIV screening[2]

Follow-up visits
Blood pressure
Urine culture (12–16 wk)
Offer amniocentesis (15–18 wk)[1] (age ≥35 yr)
Offer multiple marker testing[1] (15–18 wk)
Offer serum α-fetoprotein[1] (16–18 wk)

Counseling

Tobacco cessation; effects of passive smoking
Alcohol/other drug use
Nutrition, including adequate calcium intake
Encourage breast-feeding
Lap/shoulder belts
Infant safety car seats
STD prevention: avoid high-risk sexual behavior*; use condoms*

Chemoprophylaxis

Multivitamin with folic acid[3]

---

[1]Women with access to counseling and follow-up services, reliable standardized laboratories, skilled high-resolution ultrasound and, for those receiving serum marker testing, amniocentesis capabilities. [2]Universal screening is recommended for areas (states, counties, or cities) with an increased prevalence of HIV infection among pregnant women. In low-prevalence areas, the choice between universal and targeted screening may depend on other considerations. [3]Beginning at least 1 mo before conception and continuing through the first trimester.

*The ability of clinician counseling to influence this behavior is unproven.

**See ages 11-24 and 25-65 for other preventive services recommended for women of this age group.

Population	Potential interventions
	(See detailed high-risk definitions)
High-risk sexual behavior	Screen for *Chlamydia* (1st visit) (HR1), gonorrhea (1st visit) (HR2), HIV (1st visit) (HR3); HBsAg (3rd trimester) (HR4); RPR/VDRL (3rd trimester) (HR5)
Blood transfusion 1978–1985	HIV screen (1st visit) (HR3)
Injection drug use	HIV screen (HR3); HBsAg (3rd trimester) (HR4); advice to reduce infection risk (HR6)
Unsensitized D-negative women	D(Rh) antibody testing (24–28 wk) (HR7)
Risk factors for Down syndrome	Offer CVS[1] (1st trimester), amniocentesis[1] (15–18 wk) (HR8)
Prior pregnancy with neural tube defect	Offer amniocentesis[1] (15–18 wk), folic acid 4.0 mg[3] (HR9)

Overview

HR1 = Women with history of STD or new or multiple sex partners. Clinicians should also consider local epidemiology. Chlamydia screen should be repeated in 3rd trimester if at continued risk.

HR2 = Women under age 25 with two or more sex partners in the last year, or whose sex partner has had multiple sexual contacts; women who exchange sex for money or drugs; and women with a history of repeated episodes of gonorrhea. Clinicians should also consider local epidemiology. Gonorrhea screen should be repeated in the 3rd trimester if at continued risk.

HR3 = In areas where universal screening is not performed due to low prevalence of HIV infection, pregnant women with the following individual risk factors should be screened: past or present injection drug use; women who exchange sex for money or drugs; injection drug-using, bisexual, or HIV-positive sex partner currently or in the past; blood transfusion during 1978–1985; persons seeking treatment for STDs.

HR4 = Women who are initially HBsAg negative who are at high risk due to injection drug use, suspected exposure to hepatitis B during pregnancy, multiple sex partners.

HR5 = Women who exchange sex for money or drugs, women with other STDs (including HIV), and sexual contacts of persons with active syphilis. Clinicians should also consider local epidemiology.

HR6 = Women who continue to inject drugs.

HR7 = Unsensitized D-negative women.

HR8 = Prior pregnancy affected by Down syndrome, advanced maternal age (≥35 yr), known carriage of chromosome rearrangement.

HR9 = Women with previous pregnancy affected by neural tube defect.

Conditions for which clinicians should remain alert

Condition	Population
Symptoms of peripheral arterial disease	Older persons, smokers, diabetic persons
Skin lesions with malignant features	General population, particularly those with established risk factors
Symptoms and signs of oral cancer and premalignancy	Persons who use tobacco, older persons who drink alcohol regularly
Subtle or nonspecific symptoms and signs of thyroid dysfunction	Older persons, postpartum women, persons with Down syndrome
Signs of ocular misalignment	Infants and children
Symptoms and signs of hearing impairment	Infants and young children (<3 yr)
Large spinal curvatures	Adolescents
Changes in functional performance	Older persons
Depressive symptoms	Adolescents, young adults, persons at increased risk for depression
Evidence of suicidal ideation	Persons with established risk factors for suicide
Various presentations of family violence	General population
Symptoms and signs of drug abuse	General population
Obvious signs of untreated tooth decay or mottling, inflamed or cyanotic gingiva, loose teeth, and severe halitosis	General population
Evidence of early childhood caries, mismatching of upper and lower dental arches, dental crowding or malalignment, premature loss of primary posterior teeth (baby molars) and obvious mouth breathing	Children

SLEEP

Sleep Interview

General data

1. Statement of the sleep problem by client, bed partner, or family: obtain a quantifiable answer about sleep, such as never sleeps, dozes off for an hour several times a night, or has trouble sleeping 5 nights out of 7, every other night, or on weekends only
2. Initiation of sleep problem: when possible, elicit cause
3. Factors that make it worse or better
4. Previous occurrences to client or to other family member or friend
5. Modifications that need to be made for daytime activities or travel
6. Memories of frightening or upsetting incidences during sleep, such as sudden illness or death of a loved one or damage from storm, fire, or robbery
7. Occurrences of accidents or "near misses" as a result of sleep problems *(very important)*

Insomnia data

(Remember that a complaint of insomnia may be caused by sleep apnea or other difficulties with sleep.)

1. Time person gets into bed and time person falls asleep
2. Number and times of awakenings at night
3. Interval before returning to sleep after each awakening
4. Time of final awakening, time of arising from bed, and what wakes the person up, such as noises, alarm clock, or treatment
5. Daytime naps: number, when, and how long
6. Dozing off briefly (same question as napping, but some persons answer this question differently)
7. Lying down to rest on couch or "resting eyes for a moment" (this counts as napping because person may be falling asleep)
8. Practices used to assist with sleep: type and regularity of use
9. Changes in sleep patterns because of sleep deficit
10. Places where sleep occurs more readily, such as somewhere else in the house or on vacation
11. Concerns that delay getting into bed or falling asleep
12. Amount of and recent changes in caffeine intake (coffee, tea, colas, other caffeinated beverages, caffeinated gum) and alcohol

From Phipps WJ, Sands J, Lehman MK, et al: *Medical-surgical nursing: concepts and clinical practice,* ed 5, St Louis, 1995, Mosby.

13. Types of weekly exercise and recreational activities
14. Measures of coping with concerns
15. Recent illness or loss of relatives, friends, or pets
16. Activities of others in house or neighborhood that affect sleep, such as child who returns home late, spouse who leaves home early in morning, noise from a neighbor or dog, and noise from a nearby highway or airport

Sleep apnea data

1. Description or reenactment by bed partner of the person's breathing pattern, including sound and volume of snoring, length of time that no air passes, and how the person starts to breathe again
2. Description by bed partner of differences in client's breathing while on back, each side, and stomach and of changes in client's skin color while asleep
3. Presence of morning headaches
4. Difficulty in awakening for the day
5. Number of pillows used; preference of sleeping in a certain chair
6. Degree of sleepiness during day; falling asleep at a movie, during a conversation, or while driving

Narcolepsy-related data

1. Presence of sudden irresistible urges to sleep; falling asleep and then awakening a few minutes later feeling refreshed
2. Experiences of a sudden loss of muscle tone, leading to drooping of the head or slumping to the floor, that occur during episodes of strong emotions (surprise, laughter, anger)
3. Experiences on awakening of feeling paralyzed until touched by another
4. Presence of visual, auditory, or tactile hallucinations at time of sleep initiation or awakening
5. Family history of unusual experiences in sleep

Sleep schedule data

1. Working hours
2. Experience of going to bed later each night
3. Daily schedule activities, flexibility
4. Changes in sleep schedule as a result of changes in life schedule, such as retirement or hospitalization
5. Interruption of sleep because of family activities
6. Practice of sleeping through the day or staying up at night because of a specific purpose, such as fear that a calamity will befall during the night

Other sleep-related events

1. Uncomfortable feelings in legs when ready to fall asleep: location, type of sensations, duration, actions that make it better or worse, attempted remedies, and effect on sleep
2. Reports from bed partner of client kicking or moving legs in sleep
3. Bed-wetting: frequency, time of occurrence, actions that make it better or worse, and reports of any nights of dryness
4. Dreams: upsetting recurring dreams, frightening nightmares, or sleep terrors
5. Sleepwalking: initiation, frequency, ability to be awakened easily or guided back to bed, experience of injury while sleepwalking, actions that make it better or worse, and steps taken to keep the person safe
6. Teeth grinding during sleep
7. Dysfunctions associated with sleep, such as chest pain, shortness of breath, heartburn/ulcer pain, morning headache, asthmatic attacks, frequent awakenings to urinate, hot flashes in menopausal women, coughing, choking and gagging, and arthritic or other neuromuscular pain

External Factors Regulating Sleep

Sunrise, sunset, and length of day
Ambient temperature
Physical activity and rest
Timing and composition of meals
Timing of social/environmental cues, such as increased morning traffic noise

Modified from Association of Sleep Disorder Centers and the Association for the Psychophysiological Study of Sleep, *Sleep* 2(1):21, 1979. In Phipps WJ, Sands J, Lehman MK, et al: *Medical-surgical nursing: concepts and clinical practice,* ed 5, St Louis, 1995, Mosby.

Classification of Sleep and Arousal Disorders

Disorders of initiating and maintaining sleep (DIMS)

1. Psychophysiologic: transient and situational, persistent
2. Associated with:
   a. Psychiatric disorders: symptom and personality disorders, affective disorders, other functional psychoses
   b. Use of drugs and alcohol: tolerance to or withdrawal from central nervous system (CNS) depressants, sustained use of CNS stimulants, sustained use of or withdrawal from other drugs, chronic alcoholism
   c. Sleep-induced respiratory impairment: sleep apnea DIMS syndrome, alveolar hypoventilation DIMS syndrome
   d. Sleep-related (nocturnal) myoclonus DIMS syndrome and/or restless legs
   e. Other medical, toxic, and environmental conditions
   f. Child-onset DIMS
   g. Other DIMS conditions: repeated rapid eye movement (REM) interruptions, atypical polysomnographic features
   h. No DIMS abnormality: "short sleeper," subjective DIMS complaints without objective findings

Disorders of excessive somnolence (DOES)

1. Psychophysiologic: transient and situational, persistent
2. Associated with:
   a. Psychiatric disorders: symptom and personality disorders, affective disorders, other functional psychoses
   b. Use of drugs and alcohol: tolerance to or withdrawal from CNS stimulants, sustained use of CNS depressants
   c. Sleep-induced respiratory impairment: sleep apnea DOES syndrome, alveolar hypoventilation DOES syndrome
   d. Sleep-related (nocturnal) myoclonus DOES syndrome and/or restless legs
   e. Other medical, toxic, and environmental conditions
   f. Other DOES conditions
   g. Intermittent DOES (periodic) syndromes: Kleine-Levin syndrome, menstrual-associated syndrome
   h. Insufficient sleep
   i. Sleep drunkeness

From Phipps WJ, Sands J, Lehman MK, et al: *Medical-surgical nursing: concepts and clinical practice,* ed 5, St Louis, 1995, Mosby.

3. Narcolepsy
4. Idiopathic CNS hypersomnolence
5. No DOES abnormality: "short sleeper," subjective DOES complaints without objective findings

Disorders of the sleep-wake schedule

1. Transient: time-zone (jet lag) syndrome, work shift change in conventional sleep-wake schedule
2. Persistent: frequently changing sleep-wake schedule, delayed sleep phase syndrome, advanced sleep phase syndrome, non–24-hour sleep-wake syndrome, irregular sleep-wake pattern

Dysfunctions associated with sleep, sleep stages, or partial arousals—Parasomnias or disorders of arousal

1. Sleepwalking (somnambulism)
2. Sleep terror (pavor nocturnus, incubus)
3. Sleep-related enuresis
4. Other dysfunctions
   a. Dream anxiety attacks (nightmares)
   b. Familial sleep paralysis
   c. Impaired sleep-related penile tumescence
   d. Sleep-related epileptic seizures, bruxism, head banging (jactatio capitis nocturna), painful erections, cluster headaches and chronic paroxysmal hemicrania, abnormal swallowing syndrome, asthma, cardiovascular symptoms, gastroesophageal reflux, hemolysis (paroxysmal nocturnal hemoglobinuria)
   e. Asymptomatic polysomnographic findings

Parasomnias or Disorders of Arousal

Type of dysfunction	Comments
Sleepwalking	Walking while asleep
Sleep terror	Panic attack while asleep
Sleep-related enuresis	Bed-wetting; event begins in stage 3/4 sleep, and enuresis occurs as sleep lightens
Dream anxiety attacks	Nightmares; REM phenomenon
Sleep-related epileptic seizures	Seizures occur more often during sleep; explains why sleep encouraged during short routine electroencephalograms (EEGs)
Sleep-related bruxism	Teeth grinding; dental assistance may be needed to preserve teeth

From Phipps WJ, Sands J, Lehman MK, et al: *Medical-surgical nursing: concepts and clinical practice,* ed 5, St Louis, 1995, Mosby.

Type of dysfunction	Comments
Sleep-related head banging (jactatio capitis nocturna)	Rhythmic head rocking and banging common in young children under age 5 years; occurs in stage 1/2 sleep
Familial sleep paralysis	Inability to move when first awakening
Sleep-related cluster headaches	Associated with REM and relieved by indomethacin
Sleep-related abnormal swallowing syndrome	Inadequate swallowing of saliva during sleep
Sleep-related asthma	Early morning increase in bronchoconstriction; 46% of asthmatic attacks occur during last third of night
Sleep-related cardiovascular symptoms	Include paroxysmal nocturnal dyspnea, myocardial infarction (peak incidence 4 AM to 6 AM), nocturnal angina, and premature ventricular contrictions (more common in REM sleep)
Sleep-related gastroesophageal reflux	Caused more by posture than sleep
Sleep-related hemolysis	Probably related to combination of respiratory acidosis, change in acid-base balance, renal clearance of defective red blood cells
Morning headaches	May be related to sleeping longer on weekends and delaying usual morning dose of caffeine
Impairment in penile erections	Changes in normal incidence of erections; painful erections

CANCER

Warning Signs That May Indicate the Presence of Childhood Cancer

Cancer remains a leading cause of death (1 in 5) in children under 15 years of age, second only to accidents. In the United States each year, 12.5 of 100,000 children develop cancer.

General
- Documented weight loss without explanation, failure to thrive
- Persistent poor appetite
- Easy tiring or lack of energy

Leukemia or lymphomas: "liquid tumors" (cancer of the blood, blood-making system, lymph nodes)

- Persistent fever (more than 2 weeks)
- Bruising without injury and purple or red patches appearing on the skin
- Swollen glands (lymph nodes) unrelated to infection
- Persistent bone pain or limping
- Paleness of the lips, skin, nails, or lining of the eyes

Brain tumor

- Recurrent headaches, especially accompanied by vomiting, particularly in the morning
- Reflection in the pupil of the eye (eye tumor)
- Unexplained, persistent changes in behavior

Kidney tumors

- Lump in the abdomen or enlargement of the abdomen
- Blood in the urine
- Bulging of the eyes
- Unexplained persistent cough or chest pain
- A firm mass in the muscles

Make bath time examination time

- These complaints or physical findings should only be interpreted as *warnings* of possible serious disease. If present, you should consult your physician at once. Don't forget that your children should be examined by a physician every year. The earlier that cancer is detected, the better the chances are for a cure. With current treatment methods of surgery, radiation therapy, and chemotherapy (administration of anticancer drugs), the survival rate of children with certain forms of cancer has improved dramatically.

Cancer Prevention Tips

- On a daily basis, choose foods high in dietary fiber (fruits, vegetables, and whole-grain breads and cereals).
- Choose foods low in dietary fat.
- If you drink alcoholic beverages, do so only in moderation.

From National Institutes of Health, Cancer Information Services. Available: http://cis.nci.nih.gov/contact/screen.html.

- Avoid unnecessary x-rays.
- Know and follow health and safety rules of your workplace.
- Avoid too much sunlight: wear protective clothing; use effective sunscreens.
- Take estrogens only as long as necessary.
- Above all, don't smoke.

Nutrition and Dietary Recommendations for Cancer Prevention

Although no diet can guarantee full protection against any disease, the American Cancer Society believes that the following recommendations offer the best nutrition information currently available to help Americans reduce their risk of cancer.

Choose most of the foods you eat from plant sources

Eat five or more servings of fruits and vegetables each day; eat other foods from plant sources, such as breads, cereals, grain products, rice, pasta, or beans several times each day.

Limit your intake of high-fat foods, particularly from animal sources

Choose foods low in fat; limit consumption of meats, especially high-fat meats.

Be physically active: achieve and maintain a healthy weight

Physical activity can help protect against some cancers, either by balancing caloric intake with energy expenditure or by other mechanisms.

Limit consumption of alcoholic beverages, if you drink at all

Alcoholic beverages, along with cigarette smoking and use of snuff and chewing tobacco, cause cancers of the oral cavity, esophagus, and larynx.

From American Cancer Society: *Cancer facts and figures—2000*, Atlanta, 2000, The Society.

Summary of American Cancer Society Recommendations for the Early Detection of Cancer in Asymptomatic People

Site	Recommendation
Cancer-related Checkup	A cancer-related checkup is recommended every 3 years for people aged 20-40 and every year for people age 40 and older. This exam should include health counseling and, depending on a person's age, might include examinations for cancers of the thyroid, oral cavity, skin, lymph nodes, testes, and ovaries, and for some non-malignant diseases.
Breast	Women 40 and older should have an annual mammogram, an annual clinical breast examination (CBE) by a health care professional, and should perform monthly breast self-examination. The CBE should be conducted close to the scheduled mammogram. Women ages 20-39 should have a clinical breast examination by a health care professional every 3 years and should perform monthly breast self-examination.
Colon & Rectum	Beginning at age 50, men and women should follow one of the examination schedules below: • A fecal occult blood test every year and a flexible sigmoidoscopy every five years.* • A colonoscopy every 10 years.* • A double-contrast barium enema every 5 to 10 years.* *A digital rectal exam should be done at the same time as sigmoidoscopy, colonoscopy, or double-contrast barium enema. People who are at moderate or high risk for colorectal cancer should talk with a doctor about a different testing schedule.
Prostate	The ACS recommends that both the prostate-specific antigen (PSA) blood test and the digital rectal examination be offered annually, beginning at age 50, to men who have a life expectancy of at least 10 years and to younger men who are at high risk. Men in high-risk groups, such as those with a strong familial predisposition (i.e., two or more affected first-degree relatives), or blacks may begin at a younger age (i.e., 45 years).
Uterus	**Cervix:** All women who are or have been sexually active or who are 18 and older should have an annual Pap test and pelvic examination. After three or more consecutive satisfactory examinations with normal findings, the Pap test may be performed less frequently. Discuss the matter with your physician. **Endometrium:** Women at high risk for cancer of the uterus should have a sample of endometrial tissue examined when menopause begins.

From American Cancer Society, Inc, © 2000.

Prevention, Screening, and Early Detection of Cancer

The number of people who develop cancer is on the rise—it is estimated that one in three Americans will have some type of cancer. Some of these cancers can be cured in the early stages, but not when the disease is too advanced. Early detection and treatment are the keys to curing cancer; preventing cancer in the first place is even better.

General prevention guidelines

There is much you can do to help prevent cancer. Smoking has been scientifically proven to cause cancer, so if you smoke, stop. What you eat can also have an effect on whether you develop cancer. The following are dietary recommendations for preventing cancer:

Reduce the amount of fat in your diet to 30% of your total daily calorie intake.

Limit the amount of alcohol you drink to one or two drinks a day.

Limit the amount of charbroiled, smoked, and salted foods you eat.

Maintain your ideal weight.

Eat foods high in:

Vitamin A—apricots, peaches, carrots, spinach, asparagus, squash, and sweet potatoes.

Vitamin C—oranges, lemons, grapefruit, strawberries, tomatoes, cabbage, and walnuts

Vitamin E—lettuce, alfalfa, and vegetable oils

Fiber—fresh vegetables and fruits, whole grain breads and cereals, nuts, beans, and peas

Prevention, screening, and early detection guidelines for common cancers

Breast cancer.   Reduce the amount of fat in your diet. Any one or a combination of these signs may be a warning signal for cancer: a lump in the breast; dimpling of the skin; a sinking in of the nipple, or discharge from the nipple; swelling in the breast; or a change in the size or shape of the breast. Early detection includes breast self-examination once a month; a yearly breast examination by a healthcare provider; a baseline mammogram between the ages of 35 and 39; and a yearly mammogram after age 40. If you have a family history of breast cancer, you should start having mammograms at age 30.*

---

*American Cancer Society guidelines; National Cancer Institute recommends baseline mammogram at or about age 40 for women not at risk.

Cervical cancer. Avoid sex at an early age (especially before age 18), and don't have numerous partners. Use *condoms,* and practice good perineal hygiene. Cancer warning signs include abnormal vaginal bleeding and spotting after having sex. Early detection involves an annual Pap smear for women over age 18. After at least three normal examinations, the test can be done less often.

Colon/rectal cancer. Follow the dietary guidelines listed above. Have colorectal polyps removed. Cancer warning signs include rectal bleeding, a change in stools, pain in the abdomen, and pressure on the rectum. Early detection includes an annual digital rectal examination starting at age 40; an annual stool blood test starting at age 50; and an annual inspection of the colon with a special instrument (sigmoidoscopy) starting at age 50.

Endometrial cancer. Follow the dietary guidelines listed above. Discuss with your doctor the benefits and risks of estrogen therapy if you are past menopause. Cancer warning signs include abnormal vaginal bleeding and pain or a mass in the abdomen. Early detection includes pelvic examinations and endometrial biopsy at menopause and in high-risk women.

Head and neck cancer. Follow the dietary guidelines listed above. Avoid tobacco in all forms. Practice good oral hygiene. Cancer warning signs include difficulty chewing; a persistent sore throat; hoarseness; a color change in the mouth; earache; a lump in the neck; loss of sense of smell; and difficulty breathing. Early detection includes monthly oral self-examination and an annual physical exam.

Lung cancer. Do not smoke. Follow guidelines at work to reduce exposure to cancer-causing substances. Warning signs include a persistent cough or cold; pain in the chest; wheezing; difficulty breathing; and a change in the volume or odor of phlegm. No tests exist for early detection.

Prostate cancer. There are no prevention guidelines for prostate cancer. Warning signs include difficulty urinating, painful and frequent urination, and blood in the urine. Early detection includes an annual digital rectal exam starting at age 40; measurement of PSA is controversial.

Skin cancer. Use a sunscreen with a sun protection factor (SPF) of at least 15 (the SPF is shown on the bottle) and wear protective clothing when in the sun. Avoid tanning booths. Cancer warning signs include a change in a wart or mole, and a sore that does not heal. Early detection includes an annual physical examination, monthly self-examination of the skin, and paying particular attention to moles, warts, and birthmarks.

Testicular cancer.   No prevention guidelines exist for testicular cancer. Cancer warning signs include swelling, a lump, or a heavy feeling in the testicle. Early detection includes an annual physical exam and monthly testicular self-examination.

Testicular Self-Examination

How to do testicular self-examination (TSE)

It is best to do TSE after a warm bath or shower, when the scrotal skin is loose and relaxed. Use both hands during the examination.

1. Lift your penis with your left hand. With the right hand, locate the epididymis, the cordlike structure at the back of your right testicle. Feel along it with your thumb and first two fingers. The epididymis extends upward into the spermatic cord. Squeeze along the length of this cord, feeling for lumps and masses as you progress upward.
2. To examine the right testicle, place your right thumb on the front of the testicle and your first two fingers behind it. Gently press your fingers and thumb together until they meet. Check the entire testicle in this manner.
3. Repeat steps 1 and 2 with the left testicle, using the left hand.

Normal testicles should feel firm to the touch, but you should be able to move them. They should feel smooth and rubbery and should be free of lumps. If you notice any lumps or masses or anything unusual, call your doctor.

From *Mosby's Patient Teaching Guides,* St Louis, 1996, Mosby.   *Continued*

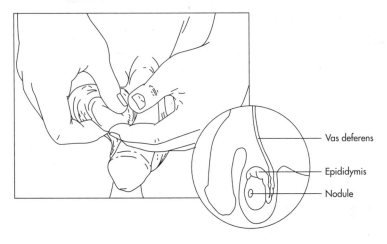

Testicular self-examination.

Breast Self-Examination

How to do breast self-examination

1. Undress and stand in front of a mirror with your arms at your sides. Look for any changes in the shape or size of your breasts or anything unusual, such as discharge from the nipples or puckering or dimpling of the skin (Figure 4-3, A).

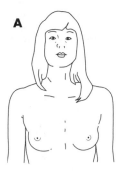

Figure 4-3, A

From *Mosby's Patient Teaching Guides,* St Louis, 1996, Mosby.

2. Raise your arms above and behind your head, and press your hands together. Look for the same things as in step 1 (Figure 4-3, B).

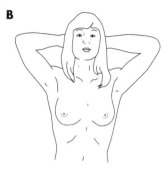

Figure 4-3, B

3. Place the palms of your hands firmly on your hips; look again for any changes (Figure 4-3, C).

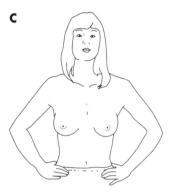

Figure 4-3, C

4. Raise your left arm over your head. Examine your left breast by firmly pressing the fingers of your right hand down and around in a circular motion until you have examined every part of the breast. You may use the wedge section, circular, or vertical strip examination method (see Figure 4-4). Be sure to include the area between your breast and armpit and the armpit itself. You are feeling for any lump or mass under the skin. If you find a lump, notify your doctor (Figure 4-3, D).

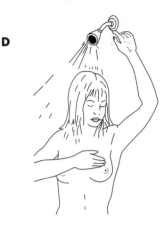

Figure 4-3, D

5. Gently squeeze the nipple, and look for any discharge (Figure 4-3, E). If there is any, see your doctor.

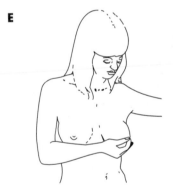

Figure 4-3, E

6. Repeat steps 4 and 5 on your right breast. (You may also perform steps 4 and 5 in the shower.)
7. Now, lie down on your back with a pillow under your right shoulder. Put your right arm over your head (Figure 4-3, F). This position flattens the breast and makes it easier to examine. Examine your right breast just as you did in steps 4 and 5. Repeat on your left breast.

F

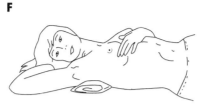

Figure 4-3, F

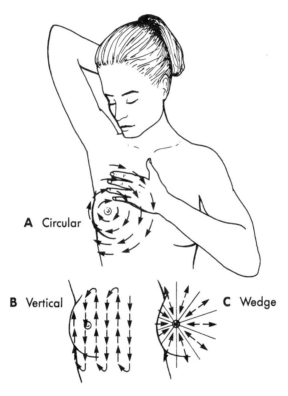

Figure 4-4 Three patterns of breast self-examination. **A,** Circular pattern. **B,** Vertical pattern. **C,** Wedge pattern.

Inform client that breast self-examination is important, but it is not a substitute for a doctor's examination and regular mammograms for women over age 40.

Skin Self-Examination

How to do skin self-examination

You will need a hand mirror and a full-length mirror to examine yourself.

1. Using a full-length mirror, examine the front and back of your body. Then raise your arms and examine the sides of your body (Figure 4-5, A).
2. Check the skin under your forearms and upper arms and on the palms of your hands.
3. Sit down and look at the backs of your legs. Examine your feet, including the soles and between your toes (Figure 4-5, B).
4. Examine the back of your neck and your scalp with a hand mirror (Figure 4-5, C).

From *Mosby's Patient Teaching Guides,* St Louis, 1996, Mosby.

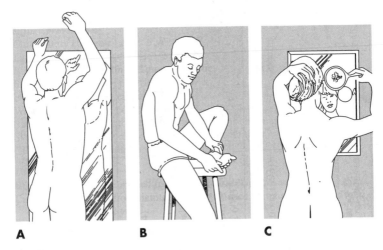

A   **B**   **C**

Figure 4-5

Vulvar Self-Examination

Cancer of the vulva is still a rare disease, but it is occurring more frequently. Women over age 50 are most susceptible to this cancer, but it can occur at any age. Examining your vulvar area once a month can help you discover the first symptoms of vulvar cancer, which can be cured if treated early. The vulvar area includes all the female external genital organs: the pubic mound, clitoris, urinary opening, vaginal opening, and anus (Figure 4-6, A).

How to do vulvar self-examination

Use a flashlight and a hand mirror to make viewing easier. You may do the examination while sitting on the edge of the toilet seat, your bed, or the bathtub. Sit with your legs spread apart, and check the entire vulvar region (Figure 4-6, B).

Examine both sides of the labia (the opening folds of the vulva) and see if they are similar.

With your fingers, separate the inner lips of the vulva, and check the clitoris, the urinary opening, the vagina, and the skin between the vagina and anus (Figure 4-6, C).

Press down on all areas of the vulva, feeling for any lumps or masses (Figure 4-6, D).

Gently squeeze the vaginal opening between your thumb and forefinger. It should feel soft and moist (not be tender or sore) (Figure 4-6, E).

If you see any of the following, see your doctor:

- Lumps, masses, or growths
- Any change in skin color
- Moles or birthmarks on the vulva that change color, bleed, or enlarge
- Burning in the vulva during urination
- Persistent itching
- Soreness or tenderness that does not go away
- Usually these signs do not indicate cancer, but check with your doctor to make sure.

From *Mosby's Patient Teaching Guides,* St Louis, 1996, Mosby.

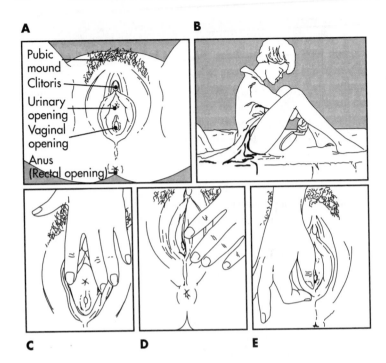

A

Pubic mound
Clitoris
Urinary opening
Vaginal opening
Anus (Rectal opening)

B

C   **D**   **E**

Figure 4-6

What causes vulvar cancer, and what can I do to prevent it?

It is unclear what causes cancer in the vulvar area, but certain conditions are thought to lead to the disease. These include poor hygiene, certain types of sexually transmitted diseases, cancer of other reproductive organs, and a condition called *dystrophy,* in which the skin of the vulva may thin or thicken, and red or white patches and sores may appear. You can help prevent some of these problems by seeing your gynecologist at least once a year, reporting any changes you find during your vulvar self-examination, and practicing good hygiene. Good hygiene of the vulva includes the following:

- Wiping from front to back after urination or a bowel movement
- Avoiding scented and perfumed products such as tampons, sanitary pads, feminine hygiene products, and scented soaps
- Using unscented, white toilet paper
- Wearing all-cotton underwear
- Avoiding tight clothing such as girdles, pantyhose, and form-fitting jeans

STROKE AND CARDIOVASCULAR DISEASE

Stroke—Signals and Actions

Know the common warning signs of stroke

- Sudden numbness or weakness of the face, arm or leg, especially on one side of the body.
- Sudden confusion, trouble speaking or understanding.
- Sudden trouble seeing in one or both eyes.
- Sudden trouble walking, dizziness, loss of balance or coordination.
- Sudden, severe headache with no known cause.

Be prepared for an emergency

- Keep a list of emergency rescue service numbers next to the telephone and in your pocket, wallet or purse.
- Find out which area hospitals have 24-hour emergency cardiovascular care.
- Know (in advance) which hospital or medical facility is nearest your home or office.

Take action in an emergency

- If you have one or more stroke symptoms that last more than a few minutes, don't delay! Immediately call 9-1-1 or the emergency medical service (EMS) number so an ambulance (ideally with advanced life support) can quickly be sent for you.
- If ambulance service isn't available in your area, immediately have someone drive you to the nearest hospital emergency room (or another facility with 24-hour life support).
- If you're with someone who may be having stroke symptoms, immediately call 9-1-1 or the EMS. Expect the person to protest—denial is common. Don't take "no" for an answer. Insist on taking prompt action.

Any of the above symptoms may be temporary and last only a few minutes. This may be due to a "little stroke" or "mini-stroke" called a **transient ischemic attack** (TIA).

Most strokes are not preceded by TIAs. However, of the people who've had one or more TIAs, more than a third will later have a stroke. In fact, a person who's had one or more TIAs is many times more likely to have a stroke than someone of the same age and sex who has not. **Thus TIAs are extremely important stroke warning signs.**

TIAs are more useful for predicting **if** a stroke will occur rather than **when** one will happen. They can occur days, weeks or even months before a major stroke. In about half of the cases the stroke occurs within one year of the TIA.

TIAs occur when a blood clot temporarily clogs an artery, and part of the brain doesn't get the blood it needs. The symptoms occur rapidly and last a relatively short time. Most TIAs last less than five minutes. The average is about a minute, although some last several hours. By definition, TIAs can last up to—but not over—24 hours, but this is very unusual. Unlike stroke, when a TIA is over, people return to normal.

From Heart and Stroke Facts, 2000, American Heart Association, Dallas, TX.

The usual TIA symptoms are the same as those of stroke, only temporary.
- Sudden numbness or weakness of the face, arm or leg, especially on one side of the body.
- Sudden confusion, trouble speaking or understanding.
- Sudden trouble seeing in one or both eyes.
- Sudden trouble walking, dizziness, loss of balance or coordination.
- Sudden, severe headache with no known cause.

The short duration of these symptoms and lack of permanent brain injury is the main distinction between TIA and stroke.

TIAs are very strong predictors of stroke risk. **Don't ignore them!** GET MEDICAL ATTENTION IMMEDIATELY. A doctor should determine if a TIA or stroke has occurred, or if it's another medical problem with similar symptoms (seizure, fainting, migraine, or general medical or cardiac condition). Prompt medical or surgical attention to these symptoms could prevent a fatal or disabling stroke from occurring.

Cerebrovascular Accident Conditions, Etiologies, Risk Factors, and Manifestations

Conditions Causing CVA
Thrombosis
Atherosclerosis in intracranial and extracranial arteries
Adjacency to intracerebral hemorrhage
Arteritis caused by collagen (autoimmune) disease or bacterial or arteritis
Hypercoagulability such as in polycythemia
Cerebral venous thromboses

Embolism
Valves damaged by rheumatic heart disease (RHD)
Myocardial infarction
Atrial fibrillation (this arrhythmia causes variable emptying of left ventricle; blood pools, and small clots form, and then at times the ventricle will be emptied completely with release of small emboli)
Bacterial endocarditis and nonbacterial endocarditis causing clots to form on endocardium

Hemorrhage
Hypertensive intracerebral hemorrhage
Subarachnoid hemorrhage
Rupture of aneurysm

From Long BC, Phipps WJ, Cassmeyer VL: *Medical-surgical nursing: a nursing process approach,* St Louis, 1993, Mosby.

Arteriovenous malformation

Hypocoagulation (as in patients with blood dyscrasias)

Generalized hypoxia

Severe hypotension, cardiopulmonary arrest, or severe depression in cardiac output caused by arrhythmias

Localized hypoxia

Cerebral artery spasms associated with subarachnoid hemorrhage

Cerebral artery vasoconstriction associated with migraine headaches

Etiologies of Ischemic Strokes

Atherosclerotic

Atherosclerosis affects both the large extracranial and intracranial arteries. The lumen of the vessel narrows and can be a target site for thrombus formation. Transient ischemic attacks occur in about half of patients before the stroke.

Small penetrating artery thrombosis/lacunar

Thrombosis of a small penetrating brain artery causes a small damaged area of tissue in the deep white matter structures of the brain, called a lacunae. Lacunae typically occur in the basal ganglia, internal capsule, pons, or thalamus.

Cardiogenic/embolic

Most of these strokes are the result of emboli, usually of cardiac origin, that break off and travel in the arterial circulation until they reach a vessel that is too narrow to allow further passage. Atrial fibrillation is the most common cause of the emboli.

Other

Ischemic strokes can also result from vasospasm, inflammation, coagulation disorders, and the effects of drug abuse, particularly cocaine.

Idiopathic

No identifiable cause is established in up to 30% of all ischemic strokes.

From Phipps WJ, Sands JK, Marek JF: *Medical-surgical nursing: concepts and clinical practice,* ed 6, St Louis, 1999, Mosby.

Factors to Consider When Assessing Coping in Stroke Clients

What losses has the client experienced as a result of the stroke?

Has the client experienced other recent losses in his life?

How do the client and family appraise their situation (primary, secondary)?

Does the client have deficits that interfere with appraisal of her situation?

What adaptive tasks does the client have to accomplish?

What goals do the client and family have?

Are goals of the client and family consistent with one another?

How did the client cope before the stroke?

How did the family cope before the stroke?

Are the client's coping strategies enabling him to manage his stressors effectively?

Are the family's coping strategies effective?

What are the sources of hope for the client and family?

Background/personal

What was the client's premorbid lifestyle?

What strengths do the client and family exhibit?

What weaknesses do the client and family exhibit?

What are the client's and family's values and beliefs?

What is the control orientation of the client and family?

What are the client's demographic characteristics (age, sex, cultural background, education level, employment status, socioeconomic status, and occupation)?

What is the likelihood that the client will resume prestroke roles in family, school, and employment?

Illness-related factors

Was the stroke onset sudden or gradual?

How recently did the stroke occur?

In what part of the brain is the lesion located?

How extensive is the stroke lesion?

What was the cause of the stroke?

Is the client at high risk for recurrence?

Does the client have concomitant acute or chronic illnesses?

From Bronstein KS, Popovich J, Stewart-Amidei CM: *Promoting stroke recovery: a research-based approach for nurses,* St Louis, 1991, Mosby.

What cognitive/perceptual deficits are present that may impair coping?

What are the type and severity of the client's functional limitations?

Environmental factors

Does/will the client receive rehabilitative care?

What is the extent and level of social support from family and friends?

What material resources are available (money, equipment, place for discharge)?

Will the client require a caregiver? If so, who?

Other Behavioral-Perceptual Consequences of Stroke

Clinical Manifestations

Transient ischemic attacks

Symptoms related to carotid involvement

Visual disturbances
   Temporary blindness in one eye
   Blurred vision
Motor disturbances
   Hemiparesis
   Localized motor deficits in face or extremities
Sensory disturbances
   Hemianesthesia
   Sensory deficits in face or extremities

Symptoms related to vertebral involvement

Motor disturbances
   Ataxia
   Dysarthria
   Dysphagia
   Unilateral or bilateral weakness
Visual disturbances
   Diplopia
   Bilateral blindness
Other
   Brief lapses in level of consciousness
   Sensory disturbance

From Phipps WJ, Sands JK, Marek JF: *Medical-surgical nursing: concepts and clinical practice,* ed 6, St Louis, 1999, Mosby.

Dizziness, vertigo
Tinnitus

Perceptual deficits caused by stroke

Unilateral neglect syndrome
A distortion in body image in which the patient ignores the affected side of the body

Anosognosia
Apparent unawareness or denial of any loss or deficit in physical functioning

Loss of proprioceptive skills
Lack of awareness of where various body parts are in relationship to each other and the environment

Agnosia
Inability to recognize a familiar object by use of the senses
Visual agnosia
Auditory agnosia
Tactile agnosia

Apraxia
Loss of ability to carry out a learned sequence of movements or use objects correctly when paralysis is not present
Constructional: may not be able to sequence a planned act necessary for activities of daily living (e.g., dressing, brushing teeth, combing hair)

Spatial relationships
Loss of ability to judge distance or size or localize objects in space
Impaired right-left discrimination

Left hemisphere vs. right hemisphere stroke

Left hemisphere stroke
(dominant hemisphere for most persons)
Motor deficits on right side
Language deficits
Fluent, nonfluent, or global aphasia
Agraphia or alexia
Right visual field deficits
Slow and cautious behavior
Severely anxious before attempting new skills

Visual Pathways

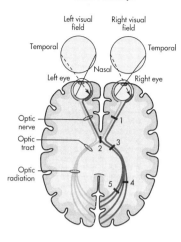

Visual field defects produced by selected lesions in the visual pathways. *From Phipps WJ, Sands JK, Marek JF: Medical-surgical nursing: concepts and clinical practice, ed 6, St Louis, 1999, Mosby.*

Visual Fields

Blackened Field Indicates Area of No Vision

Blind Right Eye (Right optic nerve)
A lesion of the optic nerve produces unilateral blindness.

1

Bitemporal Hemianopia (Optic chiasm)
A lesion at the optic chiasm may involve only those fibers that are crossing over to the opposite side. Because these fibers originate in the nasal half of each retina, visual loss involves the temporal half of each field.

2

Left Homonymous Hemianopia (Right optic tract)
A lesion of the optic tract interrupts fibers originating on the same side of both eyes. Visual loss in the eyes is therefore similar (homonymous) and involves half of each field (hemianopia).

3

Homonymous Left Upper Quadrantic Defect (Optic radiation, partial)
A partial lesion of the optic radiation may involve only a portion of the nerve fibers, producing, for example, a homonymous quadrantic defect.

4

5

Intellectual impairment
High level of frustration, depression over losses

Right hemisphere stroke
Motor deficits on left side
Left visual field deficits
Spatial perceptual deficits
Denial or unawareness of deficits
Poor judgment, overestimates abilities
Impulsive, highly distractible
Appears unconcerned over losses

Tests of Specific Disabilities That Commonly Follow Stroke

Hemianopia (loss of part of visual field)
Sitting opposite client, simultaneously hold up two pens of different colors 30 cm in front of patient and 30 cm apart; clients with hemianopia will be unable to see one of the pens or may turn head toward hemianopic side in an effort to see.

Proprioception (awareness of body in space)
The wrist of the affected arm is held between the thumb and forefinger of the examiner; client's hand is raised and lowered and client, with closed eyes, is asked the position of the hand; this exercise can also be done with fingers to determine even more specific loss of proprioception.

Sensation (feeling generated by sensory receptors)
With client's eyes closed, the examiner strokes the back of the unaffected hand and then the affected hand and in both cases asks the client to describe the sensation. The affected side may have varying degrees of loss of sensation or total loss of feeling.

Balance (bodily poise)
Client asked to sit on side of bed with feet off floor and maintain balance and sit unaided for 1 minute; it is usually readily apparent if individual has a problem maintaining balance.

Data summarized from Anderson R: *The aftermath of stroke: the experience of patients and their families,* Cambridge, 1992, Cambridge University Press. In Ebersole P, Hess P: *Toward healthy aging: human needs and nursing response,* ed 5, St Louis, 1998, Mosby.

Arm function (range of motion and control)

Client asked to lift affected arm to shoulder height and press against examiner's upheld hand:

Complete paralysis = inability to move arm

Severe weakness = can move arm but not lift up or push

Moderate weakness = able to lift arm but unable to push

Slight weakness = able to do task requested but cannot push as hard as with unaffected arm

No weakness = no difference in abilities of either arm

Cardiovascular Disease Risk Factors

Many deaths from cardiovascular disease are preventable. In addition, for people who already have been diagnosed with cardiovascular disease, the risk for death and further complications can be reduced. Research has uncovered several factors that contribute to heart attacks and strokes. The more risk factors a person has, the greater the chance of developing cardiovascular disease. Although some risk factors cannot be changed, you can modify others with your doctor's help, and still others can be eliminated altogether. The following checklists can help you determine your risk.

Major risk factors that cannot be changed

Heredity. A tendency toward heart disease runs in families. If one or both parents had cardiovascular disease, one's chances of developing it are higher.

Race. For reasons presently unknown, blacks have a much greater risk for developing high blood pressure than whites; twice as many have moderately high blood pressure, and three times as many have extremely high blood pressure. As a result, their risk for heart disease is greater.

Sex. Men have a higher risk for heart attack and stroke than women. During the childbearing years, women produce hormones that keep blood cholesterol levels low. Male hormones have the opposite effect—they raise blood cholesterol. However, women lose this protection after menopause or surgical removal of the ovaries, and women over age 55 have a 10 times greater risk than younger women. In recent years, however, more women under age 40 have developed coronary artery disease and high blood pressure. This probably results from the use of oral contraceptives and increased smoking.

Age. Fifty-five percent of heart attacks occur in people age 65 or older.

Major risk factors that can be changed

Smoking. Smokers have more than twice as many heart attacks as non-smokers. Sudden cardiac death occurs two to four times more frequently in smokers. Peripheral vascular disease (narrowing of the blood vessels in the arms and legs) is almost exclusively a disease of smokers. When people stop smoking, the risk for heart disease drops rapidly, and 10 years after quitting, their risk for death from cardiovascular disease is about the same as for people who never smoked.

High blood pressure. High blood pressure makes the heart work harder, causing it to enlarge and become weaker over time. This can lead to stroke, heart attack, kidney failure, and congestive heart failure. For some people, high blood pressure can be controlled by a low-salt diet, weight reduction, and regular exercise. Other people also require medication to lower their blood pressure.

Blood cholesterol levels. A cholesterol level between 200 and 240 mg/dL increases the risk for heart disease. A cholesterol level greater than 240 mg/dL doubles the risk for coronary artery disease. The American Heart Association Diet, which is low in cholesterol and other fats, is recommended for anyone with a level of 200 mg/dL or higher. Medication may also be necessary.

Other risk factors

Diabetes. Diabetes increases the risk for heart attack because it raises blood cholesterol levels. In addition, people who develop diabetes in midlife are often overweight, which is an additional risk factor.

Obesity. Excess weight forces the heart to work harder. People who are overweight are more prone to high blood pressure and high blood cholesterol levels. Obesity is defined as 30% or more over your ideal weight.

Physical inactivity. Researchers have found that people who seldom exercise do not recover as well from heart attacks. Although it is not clear if lack of exercise alone is a risk factor for developing heart disease, in combination with other risk factors, such as overweight, the risk is higher.

Stress. Excessive emotional stress over a prolonged period appears to increase the risk of heart disease. Stress can increase other existing risk factors, such as overeating, smoking, and high blood pressure.

Oral contraceptives. Birth control pills can worsen other risk factors. They raise blood cholesterol levels and increase blood pressure, so women who already have these problems should not take oral contraceptives. Smokers who take "the pill" run the risk of developing dangerous blood clots (thrombosis).

Alcohol. Heavy drinking can cause high blood pressure and lead to heart failure. Alcohol should be consumed only in moderate amounts—2 ounces of liquor a day or less.

Stroke Risk Factors

Age
Sixty to 75% of all strokes occur in persons over 65 years of age.

Sex
Men have a slightly increased incidence of stroke, possibly because of poorer control of hypertension and heart disease.

Race
African Americans are twice as likely to develop thrombotic strokes and three times more likely to develop hemorrhagic strokes. Whether this is truly a race-related risk is unknown.

Hypertension
Hypertension is a major risk factor for stroke, particularly in combination with atherosclerosis. The improved diagnosis and treatment of hypertension have decreased the incidence and mortality of stroke over the last two decades.

Heart disease
Heart disease is a major contributor to stroke both from atherosclerosis and as a common source of emboli.

Diabetes
Diabetes is associated with an accelerated rate of microvascular and macrovascular changes that contribute to atherosclerosis.

From Phipps WJ, Sands JK, Marek JF: *Medical-surgical nursing: concepts and clinical practice,* ed 6, St Louis, 1999, Mosby.

Other

Cigarette smoking

Oral contraceptive use (especially in smokers)

Alcohol use

Family history of transient ischemic attack or cerebrovascular accident

*Obesity

*Sedentary lifestyle

*Elevated serum cholesterol and triglycerides

---

*These factors are less well studied but are believed to contribute to stroke.

Clinical Manifestations of Stroke

NOTE: Specific symptoms will reflect the site and severity of ischemic damage. The following is a general listing of common deficits.

Motor

Hemiparesis or hemiplegia of the side of the body opposite the site of ischemia

Initially flaccid, progressing to spastic

Dysphagia

Swallowing reflex may also be impaired

Dysarthria

Bowel and bladder

Frequency, urgency, and urinary incontinence

Potential for bladder retraining is good if cognitively intact

Constipation

Related more to immobility than to the physical effects of stroke

Language

Nonfluent aphasia (also known as motor/expressive aphasia)—difficulty or inability to express self verbally

Fluent aphasia (also known as sensory/receptive aphasia)—difficulty or inability to comprehend speech

Alexia—inability to understand the written word

Agraphia—inability to express self in writing

Sensory-perceptual

Diminished response to superficial sensation

Touch, pain, pressure, heat, and cold

Diminished proprioception
   Knowledge of position of body parts in the environment
Visual deficits
   Decreased acuity
   Diplopia
   Homonymous hemianopia
Perceptual
   Unilateral neglect syndrome
   Distorted body image
   Apraxia—inability to carry out learned voluntary acts
   Agnosia—inability to recognize familiar objects through sight, sound, or touch
   Anosognosia—inability to recognize or denial of a physical deficit
   Possible deficits in
      Telling time
      Judging distance
      Right-left discrimination
      Memory of locations, objects

Cognitive-emotional

Emotional lability and unpredictability
   Behavior may be socially inappropriate (e.g., crying jags, swearing)
Depression
Memory loss
Short attention span, easy distractability
Loss of reasoning, judgment, and abstract thinking ability

Characteristics of Major Stroke Syndromes

Middle cerebral artery (MCA) syndrome (most common occlusion)

If blockage of the main stem of the MCA occurs, the infarction can affect most of the hemisphere, because the MCA accounts for about 80% of the blood supply to the cerebral hemispheres.

- Contralateral hemiparesis or hemiplegia—arm affected more severely than the leg
- Contralateral sensory impairment over same area affected by hemiplegia (proprioception, touch)
- Unilateral neglect or inattention (if nondominant hemisphere)

From Phipps WJ, Sands JK, Marek JF: *Medical-surgical nursing: concepts and clinical practice,* ed 6, St Louis, 1999, Mosby.

- Aphasia (if dominant hemisphere)
- Homonymous hemianopia

Internal carotid artery (ICA) syndrome
- Contralateral hemiparesis or hemiplegia
- Contralateral sensory losses
- Aphasia (if dominant hemisphere)

The symptoms of MCA and ICA strokes are almost identical, but if blockage of the main stem of the MCA occurs (see above), the deficits can be profound, because cerebral edema is usually extensive.

Vertebrobasilar artery syndromes
Occlusion of the vessels in this system creates unique symptoms that reflect the perfusion of the cerebellum and brain stem:

- Ataxia, clumsiness
- Dysphagia and dysarthria
- Dizziness and nystagmus
- Bilateral motor and sensory deficits
- Facial weakness and numbness

OTHER ILLNESSES

Fibrocystic Changes of the Breast

What are fibrocystic changes? Does this mean I have breast cancer?
Fibrocystic changes are the most common cause of breast lumps in women 30 to 50 years of age. These changes may also be referred to as fibrocystic disease, cystic disease, chronic cystic mastitis, or mammary dysplasia. This condition is not cancerous. At least 50% of women in their reproductive years have lumpy breasts as a result of this noncancerous condition.

How are breast changes diagnosed?
Usually fibrocystic changes can be diagnosed by physical examination or mammography, an x-ray of the breast. Fibrocystic changes may also be found with a biopsy, in which a small amount of tissue or fluid is removed from the breast and examined in the laboratory. Fortu-

nately, only about 5% of women who require biopsies for a fibrocystic condition have the type of changes that would be considered a risk factor for cancer.

What causes fibrocystic changes?

Fibrocystic changes occur because of the way breast tissue responds to monthly changes in the levels of estrogen and progesterone, two female hormones produced by the ovaries during a woman's reproductive years. Each month during the menstrual cycle, breast tissue alternately swells and returns to normal. Hormonal stimulation of breast tissue causes the blood vessels to swell, the milk glands and ducts to enlarge, and the breasts to retain water. The breasts frequently feel swollen, painful, tender, and lumpy at this time. After menstruation, the swelling decreases and the breasts feel less tender and lumpy; that's why the best time to examine your breasts for unusual or sudden changes is right after your menstrual period ends.

How do fibrocystic changes feel? What should I look for?

Repeated hormone stimulation from monthly changes causes breast tissue to become firmer, and pockets of fluid, called cysts, may form in obstructed or enlarged milk ducts. The breast tissue may feel like an irregularly shaped area of thicker tissue with a lumpy or ridgelike surface. Fibrocystic tissue may also feel like tiny beads scattered throughout the breast.

Fibrocystic changes usually are found in both breasts, most often in the upper outer quadrant and the underside of the breast, where a ridge may sometimes be felt. In premenopausal women with a fibrocystic condition, lumpy areas in the breast may increase in size, and the woman may feel discomfort ranging from a feeling of fullness or heaviness to a dull ache, extreme sensitivity to touch, or a burning sensation. For some women, the pain is so severe that it precludes exercise or even lying on the abdomen. The condition tends to subside after menopause (change of life).

How do I tell fibrocystic changes from a "lump" in my breast?

Confusion arises because not all women with lumps have fibrocystic changes. The breast is naturally a lumpy gland. The lumpy consistency arises from the milk glands and ducts and the fibrous tissue that separates and supports them. Practicing breast self-examination (BSE) regularly helps a woman distinguish between normal lumps and ones that must be evaluated by a physician.

How is a fibrocystic condition treated?

Treatment of a fibrocystic condition may require surgical removal (biopsy) of lumps that fail to disappear after brief observation or after attempts to remove fluid by a physician. For painful breasts, a physician may recommend aspirin or other pain relievers. Also, applying warmth to the breasts (such as with a heating pad), wearing a good support bra, and avoiding caffeine in coffee, tea, chocolate, and soft drinks may help decrease water retention. *Patients with cystic breasts should not have caffeine.* Occasionally a physician may prescribe medications such as vitamin E, danazol, or tamoxifen to help relieve the symptoms.

What is a mammogram?

A mammogram is a low-dose x-ray examination that can detect lumps infinitely smaller than fingers can feel, and with minimal risk. It is recommended that women between the ages of 35 and 39 who have no symptoms of breast cancer have a mammogram as a baseline for comparison; women ages 40 to 49 should have a mammogram every 1 or 2 years; and women age 50 or over should have a mammogram yearly.

Six Warning Signs of Kidney Disease

1. Burning or difficulty during urination
2. More frequent urination, particularly at night
3. Passage of bloody- or tea-colored urine
4. Puffiness around eyes, swelling of hands and feet, especially in children
5. Pain in small of back just below the ribs (not aggravated by movement)
6. High blood pressure

From National Kidney Foundation: *What everyone should know about kidneys and kidney disease,* New York, 1996, The Foundation.

Parkinson's Disease Manifestations and Teachings

Classic Clinical Manifestations of Parkinson's Disease

Tremor

- Most recognized and least disabling symptom
- Present in 75% of patients
- Nonintentional, present at rest but usually not during sleep
- Characterized by rhythmic movements of 4 or 5 cycles per second
  - Movement of the thumb across the palm gives a "pill-rolling" character
  - Tremor also seen in limbs, jaw, lips, lower facial muscles, and head

Rigidity

- Muscles feel stiff and require increased effort to move
- Discomfort or pain may be perceived in muscle when rigidity is severe
- "Cogwheel" rigidity refers to ratchetlike rhythmic contractions of the muscle that occur when the limbs are passively stretched

Bradykinesia/akinesia

- Slowness of active movement
- Difficulty initiating movement
- Often the most disabling symptom; interferes with activities of daily living (ADL) and predisposes patient to complications related to constipation, circulatory stasis, skin breakdown, and other related complications of immobility

Postural instability

- Changes in gait
  - Tendency to walk forward on the toes with small shuffling steps
  - Once initiated, movement may accelerate almost to a trot
  - Festination may occur, which propels the patient either forward or backward propulsively until falling is almost inevitable
- Changes in balance
  - Stooped-over posture when erect
  - Arms are semiflexed and do not swing with walking
  - Difficulty maintaining balance and sitting erect
  - Cannot "right" or brace self to prevent falling when balance is lost

From Phipps WJ, Sands JK, Marek JF: *Medical-surgical nursing: concepts and clinical practice,* ed 6, St Louis, 1999, Mosby.

Secondary Manifestations of Parkinson's Disease

Facial appearance
- Expressionless
- Eyes stare straight ahead
- Blinking is much less frequent than normal

Speech problems
- Low volume
- Slurred, muffled
- Monotone
- Difficulty with starting speech and word finding

Visual problems
- Blurred vision
- Impaired upward gaze
- Blepharospasm—involuntary prolonged closing of the eyelids

Fine motor function
- Micrographia—handwriting progressively decreases in size
- Decreased manual dexterity
- Clumsiness and decreased coordination
- Decreased capacity to complete ADL
- Freezing—sudden involuntary inability to initiate movement. Can occur during movement or inactivity

Autonomic disturbance
- Constipation (hypomotility and prolonged gastric emptying)
- Urinary frequency or hesitancy
- Orthostatic hypotension (dizziness, fainting, syncope)
- Dysphagia (neuromuscular incoordination)
- Drooling (results from decreased swallowing)
- Oily skin
- Excessive perspiration

Cognitive/behavioral
- Depression occurs in more than 50% of patients
- Slowed responsiveness
- Memory deficits
- Visual-spatial deficits
- Dementia

The Person with Parkinson's Disease

Activity and exercise

Perform range-of-motion exercise to all joints three times daily.

Massage and stretch muscles to reduce stiffness.

Use a broad base of support when ambulating. Consciously lift and place the feet when ambulating.

Pay attention to posture. Try walking with the hands clasped behind the back.

Explore the use of assistive devices.

Avoid staying in one position for prolonged periods. Alter position regularly.

Safety

Examine the home environment for risks of injury.

Modify the environment to improve lighting and remove hazards.

Consider installing devices such as raised toilet seats and grab bars.

Change positions slowly if orthostatic hypotension develops.

Be alert to the effects of heat, stress, and excitement on symptom severity.

Nutrition

Monitor weight once a week.

Evaluate dysphagia and modify diet to increase ease of chewing and swallowing if appropriate.

Practice swallowing and take small bites.

Provide an unhurried atmosphere and allow additional time for meals.

Follow a plan of small, frequent meals if fatigue is a problem during meals.

Avoid eating high-protein meals at times of medication administration.

Do not use vitamin supplements containing pyridoxine (vitamin B_6).

Ensure adequate fiber and fluid intake to prevent constipation.

Manage drooling problems with soft cloths.

Elimination

Monitor bowel elimination pattern.

Use diet, exercise, and fluids to ensure regularity if possible.

Use stool softeners if needed.

Keep a urinal or commode at the bedside.

Respond promptly to the urge to urinate, and be sure to empty the bladder at least every 2 to 4 hours. Bradykinesia can result in episodes of incontinence.

Cognitive/behavioral

Monitor for depression. Report its presence to healthcare provider.

Monitor for changes in sleep pattern, disordered thoughts, and the development of agitation, confusion, or hallucinations. Report these symptoms promptly.

Communication

Exercise the voice regularly by singing or reading aloud.

Attempt to project the voice and alter volume and pitch.

Consult a speech therapist if vocal problems are severe.

FAILURE TO THRIVE

Failure to Thrive—Nonorganic

Three general categories of failure to thrive are the following:

1. **Organic failure to thrive (OFTT)**—Result of a physical cause, such as congenital heart defects, neurologic lesions, microcephaly, chronic renal failure, gastroesophageal reflux, malabsorption syndrome, endocrine dysfunction, cystic fibrosis, or acquired immunodeficiency syndrome (AIDS).
2. **Nonorganic failure to thrive (NFTT)**—Has a definable cause that is unrelated to disease. NFTT is most often the result of psychosocial factors, such as inadequate nutritional information by the parent; deficiency in maternal care or a disturbance in maternal-child attachment; or a disturbance in the child's ability to separate from the parent, leading to food refusal to maintain attention.
3. **Idiopathic failure to thrive**—Unexplained by the usual organic and environmental etiologies but may also be classified as NFTT. Both categories of NFTT account for the majority of cases of FTT.

Traditionally the category of NFTT has implied a disturbance in the parent-child interaction. However, this is not always the case. Many other factors can lead to inadequate feeding of the infant, such as the following:

Poverty—Lack of funds to buy sufficient food; may dilute formula to extend available supply

---

From Wong DL, et al: *Whaley and Wong's nursing care of infants and children,* ed 6, St Louis, 1999, Mosby.

Health beliefs—Use of fad diets; excessive concern with preventing conditions such as obesity, hypercholesterolemia, or nursing caries

Inadequate nutritional knowledge—Cultural confusion of newly arrived immigrants who are unaware of appropriate food selections in American markets; parents with cognitive impairment

Family stress—Overwhelming involvement with another chronically ill child; any number of other stresses (financial, marital, excessive parenting and employment responsibilities, depression, chemical abuse, acute grief)

Feeding resistance—Result of nonoral nutritional therapy early in life

Insufficient breast milk—Result of a number of different causes (fatigue, illness, poor release of milk, insufficient glandular tissue, lack of maternal confidence)

Clinical Manifestations of Nonorganic Failure to Thrive

Growth failure—below fifth percentile in weight only or weight and height

Developmental retardation—social, motor, adaptive, language

Apathy

Poor hygiene

Withdrawn behavior

Feeding or eating disorders, such as vomiting, anorexia, pica, rumination

No fear of strangers (at age when stranger fear is normal)

Avoidance of eye contact

Wide-eyed gaze and continual scan of the environment ("radar gaze")

Stiff and unyielding or flaccid and unresponsive

Minimal smiling

From Wong DL, Perry SE: *Maternal child nursing care,* St Louis, 1998, Mosby.

Feeding Children With Nonorganic Failure to Thrive

Provide a primary core of staff to feed the child. The same nurses are able to learn the child's cues and respond consistently.

From Wong DL, et al: *Whaley and Wong's nursing care of infants and children,* ed 6, St Louis, 1999, Mosby.

Provide a quiet, unstimulating atmosphere. A number of these children are very distractible, and their attention is diverted with minimal stimuli. Older children do well at a feeding table; younger children should always be held.

Maintain a calm, even temperament throughout the meal. Negative outbursts may be commonplace in this child's habit formation. Limits on eating behavior definitely need to be provided, but they should be stated in a firm, calm tone. If the nurse is hurried or anxious, the feeding process will not be optimized.

Talk to the child by giving directions about eating. "Take a bite, Lisa" is appropriate and directive. The more distractible the child, the more directive the nurse should be to refocus attention on feeding. Positive comments about feeding are actively given.

Be persistent. This is perhaps one of the most important guidelines. Parents often give up when the child begins negative feeding behavior. Calm perseverance through 10 to 15 minutes of food refusal will eventually diminish negative behavior. Although forced feeding is avoided, "strictly encouraged" feeding is essential.

Maintain a face-to-face posture with the child when possible. Encourage eye contact and remain with the child throughout the meal.

Introduce new foods slowly. Often these children have been exclusively bottle-fed. If acceptance of solids is a problem, begin with puréed food and, once accepted, advance to junior and regular solid foods.

Follow the child's rhythm of feeding. The child will set a rhythm when the previous conditions are met.

Develop a structured routine. Disruption in their other activities of daily living has great impact on feeding responses, so bathing, sleeping, dressing, and playing, as well as feeding, are structured. The nurse should feed the child in the same way and place as often as possible. The length of the feeding should also be established (usually 30 minutes).

Characteristics of Failure-to-Thrive Family

Infant Characteristics

The most commonly identified physical and behavioral characteristics of failure-to-thrive infants include

- Failure to grow and gain weight
- Developmental slowness
- Gastrointestinal difficulties and feeding problems
- Unusual watchfulness
- Minimal smiling
- Decreased vocalizations
- Lack of cuddliness
- Position of tonic immobility
- Sleep disturbances
- Lack of interest in environmental stimuli or toys

Characteristics of the Failure-to-Thrive Family

Infant characteristics

Physical characteristics—failure to grow and gain weight
Behavioral characteristics—developmental slowness

Characteristics of mothers

Low self-esteem and feelings of inadequacy
Desire to be taken care of
Literal, concrete thinking patterns
Use of denial, isolation, and projection defense mechanisms
Predisposition to acting out, rather than thinking
Inaccessibility and suspicion of helping persons
Difficulty in accurately perceiving the infant's needs

Characteristics of fathers

Ineffectual in child-rearing behaviors
Often absent from home

Characteristics of siblings

Poor physical health

From Johnson S: *Nursing assessment and strategies for the family at risk: high-risk parenting,* ed 2, Philadelphia, 1986, JB Lippincott.

Family stability and socioeconomic characteristics
Marital problems
Low socioeconomic class

Other family difficulties
Guilt
Grief
Child abuse

NUTRITIONAL GUIDELINES

Form for Assessing Eating Habits and Nutritional State

Name _____ Date _____
　　　　　Height _____ Weight (lb) _____ (kg) _____ Age _____
　　　　　　　　　　　　　　　　　　　　　　　Ideal weight _____

Referral
Diagnosis
Diet order
Members of household
Occupation
Recreation, physical activity

Present food intake	Place	Hour	Frequency, form, and amount checklist
Morning			Milk
			Cheese
			Meat
			Fish
			Poultry
Noon			Eggs
			Cream
			Butter, margarine
			Other fats
Evening			Vegetables, green
			Vegetables, other
			Fruits (citrus)
			Legumes
			Potato
			Bread–kind
			Sugar
			Desserts
			Beverages
Summary			Alcohol
			Vitamins
			Candy

Nutrition history: activity-associated general day's food pattern. Also record general activity pattern throughout the day. *From Williams S:* Essentials of nutrition and diet therapy, *ed 7, St Louis, 1999, Mosby.*

Clinical Signs of Nutritional Status

Features	Good	Poor
General appearance	Alert, responsive	Listless, apathetic, cachexic
Hair	Shiny, lustrous, healthy scalp	Stringy, dull, brittle, depigmented
Neck glands	No enlargement	Thyroid enlarged
Skin, face, neck	Smooth, slightly moist, good color, reddish pink mucous membranes	Greasy, discolored, scaly
Eyes	Bright, clear, no fatigue circles	Dryness, signs of infection, increased vascularity, glassiness, thickened conjunctivae
Lips	Good color, moist	Dry, scaly, swollen, angular lesions (stomatitis)
Tongue	Good pink color, surface papillae present, no lesions	Papillary atrophy, smooth appearance, swollen, red, beefy (glossitis)
Gums	Good pink color, no swelling or bleeding, firm	Marginal redness or swelling, receding, spongy
Teeth	Straight, no crowding, well-shaped jaw, clean, no discoloration	Unfilled cavities, absent teeth, worn surface, mottled, malpositioned
Skin, general	Smooth, slightly moist, good color	Rough, dry, scaly, pale, pigmented, irritated; petechiae, bruises
Abdomen	Flat	Swollen
Legs, feet	No tenderness, weakness, swelling, good color	Edema, tender calf, tingling, weakness

Continued

From Williams S: *Nutrition and diet therapy*, ed 8, St Louis, 1997, Mosby.

Clinical Signs of Nutritional Status—cont'd

Features	Good	Poor
Skeleton	No malformations	Bowlegs, knock-knees, chest deformity at diaphragm, beaded ribs, prominent scapulas
Weight	Normal for height, age, body build	Overweight or underweight
Posture	Erect, arms and legs straight, abdomen in, chest out	Sagging shoulders, sunken chest, humped back
Muscles	Well-developed, firm	Flaccid, poor tone, undeveloped, tender
Nervous control	Good attention span for age, does not cry easily, not irritable or restless	Inattentive, irritable
Gastrointestinal function	Good appetite and digestion, normal, regular elimination	Anorexia, indigestion, constipation or diarrhea
General vitality	Endurance, energetic, sleeps well at night, vigorous	Easily fatigued, no energy, falls asleep in school, looks tired, apathetic

The Basic Food Groups

Food group	Servings	Major contributions	Foods and serving sizes*
Bread, cereals, rice, pasta	6-11	Starch Thiamin Riboflavin† Iron Niacin Folate Magnesium‡ Fiber‡ Zinc	1 slice of bread 1 oz ready-to-eat cereal ½-¾ cup cooked cereal, rice, pasta
Vegetables	3-5	Vitamin A Vitamin C Folate Magnesium Fiber	½ cup raw or cooked vegetables 1 cup raw leafy vegetables
Fruits	2-4	Vitamin C Fiber	¼ cup dried fruit ½ cup cooked fruit ¾ cup juice 1 whole piece of fruit 1 melon wedge

*May be reduced for child servings.
†If enriched.
‡Whole grains especially.
From the US Department of Agriculture, revised edition of former *Basic Four Food Groups Guide.*

Continued

The Basic Food Groups—cont'd

Food group	Servings	Major contributions	Foods and serving sizes*
Milk, yogurt, cheese	2 (adults§) 3 (children, teens, young adults, pregnant or lactating women)	Calcium Riboflavin Protein Potassium Zinc	1 cup milk 1½ oz cheese 2 oz processed cheese 1 cup yogurt 2 cups cottage cheese 1 cup custard/pudding 1½ cups ice cream
Meat, poultry, fish, dry beans, eggs, nuts	2-3	Protein Niacin Iron Vitamin B_6 Zinc Thiamin Vitamin B_{12}‖	2-3 oz cooked meat, poultry, fish 1-1½ cups cooked dry beans 4 tbsp peanut butter 2 eggs ½-1 cup nuts
Fats, oils, sweets	Foods from this group should not replace any from the other groups. Amounts consumed should be determined by individual energy needs.		

§≥25 years of age.
‖Present only in animal food choices.

Promotion of Good Dietary Habits: Food for Everyday Use

Sample Menus for Children and Adolescents Based on Food Guide Pyramid

YOUNG CHILD (AGE 4-6)*

Breakfast	1 oz dry, unsweetened cereal
	¼ cup orange juice
	4 oz low-fat milk
	1 slice toast
Snack	½ banana
Lunch	2 tbsp peanut butter
	2 tsp all-fruit preserves
	1 slice whole wheat bread
	½ cup peas
	4 oz low-fat milk
Snack	2 graham crackers
	4 oz low-fat milk
	½ cup carrots, raw
Dinner	1 chicken leg, roasted without skin
	½ cup macaroni and cheese
	½ cup green beans, cooked
	1 whole wheat roll
	4 oz low-fat milk
Snack	½ cup canned peaches
Total Servings	
Grain group	6
Vegetable group	3
Fruit group	2
Milk group	2
Meat group	2
school-age children	

Serving sizes are minimums for nutritional adequacy. Many children eat more.

*Use fats, oils, and sweets sparingly. Increase fluids with servings of water.

†Adolescents require increased portions in the milk, yogurt, and cheese group to meet the recommended 1200 mg calcium required for bone growth.

This section may be photocopied and distributed to families.

From Wong DL, Hess CS: *Wong and Whaley's clinical manual of pediatric nursing,* ed 5, 2000, Mosby, St Louis.

SCHOOL-AGE CHILD*

Breakfast	2 four-inch waffles
	2 tbsp syrup
	½ cup orange juice
Lunch	4 oz lean hamburger and bun
	½ cup raw carrot sticks
	¾ cup apple juice
Snack	1 cup frozen yogurt *or*
	1 cup unsweetened cereal with low-fat milk
Dinner	1 cup spaghetti with tomato sauce
	1 piece garlic bread
	Green salad with romaine lettuce and dressing
	½ cup broccoli
	1 banana
	1 cup low-fat milk
Snack	2 cups plain popcorn
	½ cup grape juice

Total Servings

Grain group	6-7
Vegetable group	3
Fruit group	3-4
Milk group	2
Meat group	2

ADOLESCENT*

Breakfast	8 oz of 1% milk†
	½ cup orange juice
	2 oz dry, unsweetened cereal
	1 banana
Lunch	1 cheeseburger with lettuce, tomato, and onion
	1 small order French fries
	1 medium low-fat milk shake
Snack	1 peanut butter sandwich
	8 oz of 1% milk
	1 cup yogurt

Dinner	½ cup canned mixed fruit
	12 oz baked chicken breast
	1 slice whole wheat bread
	½ cup cooked rice
	1 serving corn on the cob
	1½ cup tossed green salad with low-fat dressing
	8 oz Snapple fruit drink
Snack	¾ cup vegetable juice (e.g., V8)
	2-3 graham crackers

Total Servings

Grain group	7
Vegetable group	5
Fruit group	4
Milk group	5
Meat group	2

Recommended Nutritional Intake for Pregnant Adolescents

Food	No. servings*
Dairy products: one serving equals 1 cup milk, 1 oz hard cheese, 1¼ cups cottage cheese, ⅓ cup dry milk, or 1¾ cup ice cream (use low-fat milk)	4
Meat and meat alternatives: one serving equals 2 eggs, 2 oz lean meat, 1 cup beans or split peas, 4 tablespoons peanut butter, 2 oz cheddar cheese, or ½ cup cottage cheese	3
Fruits, vegetables, or juices: one serving equals ½ cup or 1 medium fresh fruit or vegetable	At least 5
Breads and cereals: one serving equals 1 slice of bread, ½ cup cooked cereal, ¾ cup ready-to-eat cereal, or ½ to ¾ cup cooked macaroni, spaghetti, rice, or grits, pasta	6-11
Fats, oils, sweets	Use sparingly

*Suggested amounts should support adequate weight gain

Modified from Murray RB, Zentner JP: *Health assessment and promotion strategies throughout the lifespan,* ed 6, Stamford, CT, 1997, Appleton & Lange.

Recommended Nutritional Intake for Young Adults

Foods	Young adult	Pregnant woman	Lactating woman
Traditional basic four			
Milk and milk products	2 or more cups	3 or 4 cups	4 or more cups
Meat, fish, or protein equivalent	2 (2- or 3-ounce) servings	3 (2- or 3-ounce) servings	3 or 4 (2- or 3-ounce) servings
Fruits and vegetables (including a high vitamin C source)	4 (½-cup) servings	4 or 5 (½-cup) servings	4 or 5 (½-cup) servings
Grain, bread, and cereals	4 servings	4 or more servings	4 or more servings
Suggested change			
Milk and milk products	2 or 3 cups	3 or 4 cups	4 or more cups
Meat, fish, poultry, dry beans, eggs, nuts	2 or 3 (2- or 3-ounce) servings	3 (2- or 3-ounce) servings	3 or 4 (2- or 3-ounce) servings
Fruits	2-4 (½-cup) servings	2-4 (½-cup) servings	2-4 (½-cup) servings
Vegetables	3-5 (½-cup) servings	3-5 (½-cup) servings	3-5 (½-cup) servings
Breads, cereal, rice, pastas	6-11 servings	6-11 servings	6-11 servings
Fats, oils, sweets	Use sparingly for all age groups		

From Murray RB, Zentner JP: *Health assessment and promotion strategies through the lifespan*, ed 6, Stamford, CT, 1997, Appleton & Lange.

Recommended Nutritional Intake for Elderly People

	Milk and milk products	Protein foods	Breads, cereals, and whole grains	Vitamin C-rich fruits/vegetables	Dark green and yellow fruits and vegetables	Other fruits and vegetables
Number of servings	2	3	4	2	2	2

Have small, frequent meals. Liquids are important even if not thirsty. Use whole grains to avoid constipation. Socializing with groups will help to increase activity and increase motivation to eat with company. May need vitamin and mineral supplements, especially calcium in the order of 1200 mg per day. Avoid alcohol. Nutrient-drug interactions can be minimized by eating a balanced diet and carefully following the instructions for use.

Modified from Gutierrez Y, May K: Nutrition and the family. In Gilliss C, et al: *Toward a science of family nursing*, Reading, Mass, 1989, Addison-Wesley.

Single-Room Occupant Foods

Milk products
Box of dry skim or whole milk
Small can evaporated milk
Instant cocoa
Instant pudding to use with dry milk
Small pieces of cheese (if wrapped airtight and kept in cool place)

Meat products
Small can of tuna fish, sardines, salmon
Canned potted meat
Peanut butter
Cottage cheese
Hard cooked eggs

Fruits and vegetables
Small cans of any fruits and vegetables
Dried fruit (raisins, apricots, dates)
Fresh apples, oranges, seasonal fruits

Miscellaneous foods
Instant coffee
Tea
Sugar
Condiments of choice

From Ebersole P, Hess P: *Toward healthy aging: human needs and nursing response,* ed 5, St Louis, 1998, Mosby.

Developmental Milestones Associated With Feeding

Age (months)	Development
Birth	Has sucking, rooting, and swallowing reflexes
	Feels hunger and indicates desire for food by crying; expresses satiety by falling asleep
1	Has strong extrusion reflex
3-4	Extrusion reflex is fading
	Begins to develop hand-eye coordination

From Wong D, Whaley L: *Clinical manual of pediatric nursing,* ed 4, St Louis, 1996, Mosby.

Age (months)	Development
4-5	Can approximate lips to the rim of a cup
5-6	Can use fingers to feed self a cracker
6-7	Chews and bites
	May hold own bottle, but may not drink from it (prefers for it to be held)
7-9	Refuses food by keeping lips closed; has taste preferences
	Holds a spoon and plays with it during feeding
	May drink from a straw
	Drinks from a cup with assistance
9-12	Picks up small morsels of food (finger foods) and feeds self
	Holds own bottle and drinks from it
	Drinks from a household cup without assistance but spills some
	Uses a spoon with much spilling
12-18	Drools less
	Drinks well from a household cup, but may drop it when finished
	Holds cup with both hands
24	Can use a straw
	Chews food with mouth closed and shifts food in mouth
	Distinguishes between finger and spoon foods
	Holds small glass in one hand; replaces glass without dropping
36	Spills small amount from spoon
	Begins to use fork; holds it in fist
	Uses adult pattern of chewing, which involves rotary action of jaw
48	Rarely spills when using spoon
	Serves self finger foods
	Eats with fork held with fingers
54	Uses fork in preference to spoon
72	Spreads with knife
84	Cuts tender food with knife

Nutrition Education and Counseling Screening Alerts

If older individuals indicate that the following questions listed on the Checklist, Level I and II screen alerts are descriptive of their condition or life situation, nutrition education interventions may help them solve their nutritional problems and improve their nutritional status.

From American Academy of Family Physicians, American Dietetic Association, National Council on the Aging, Nutritional Screening Initiative: *Nutrition interventions manual for professional caring for older americans,* Washington, DC, 1992, The Academy.

Determine Your Nutritional Health

The warning signs of poor nutritional health are often overlooked. Use this checklist to find out if you or someone you know is at nutritional risk.

Read the statements below. Circle the number in the *yes* column for those that apply to you or someone you know. For each *yes* answer, score the number in the box. Total your nutritional score.

	YES
I have an illness or condition that made me change the kind and/or amount of food I eat.	2
I eat fewer than 2 meals per day.	3
I eat few fruits or vegetables or milk products.	2
I have 3 or more drinks of beer, liquor, or wine almost every day.	2
I have tooth or mouth problems that make it hard for me to eat.	2
I don't always have enough money to buy the food I need.	4
I eat alone most of the time.	1
I take 3 or more different prescribed or over-the-counter drugs per day.	1
Without wanting to, I have lost or gained 10 pounds in the last 6 months.	2
I am not always physically able to shop, cook, and/or feed myself.	2
TOTAL	

Total Your Nutritional Score. If it's—

0-2   *Good!* Recheck your nutritional score in 6 months.

3-5   *You are at moderate nutritional risk.* See what can be done to improve your eating habits and lifestyle. Your office on aging, senior nutrition program, senior citizens center, or health department can help. Recheck your nutritional score in 3 months.

6 or more   *You are at a high nutritional risk.* Bring this checklist the next time you see your doctor, dietitian, or other qualified health or social service professional. Talk with them about any problems you may have. Ask for help to improve your nutritional health.

Checklist for the "warning signs" of poor nutritional health. *Reprinted with the permission of the Nutritional Screening Initiative, a project of American Academy of Family Physicians, American Dietetic Association, and National Council on Aging, and funded in part by a grant from Ross Laboratories, a division of Abbott Laboratories.*

Level I screen alerts

Has lost or gained 10 lbs or more in the past 6 months.
Body mass index <22.
Body mass index >27.
Has poor appetite.
Is on a special diet.
Eats vegetables two or fewer times daily.

Eats milk or milk products once or not at all daily.

Eats fruit or drinks fruit juice once or not at all daily.

Eats breads, cereals, pasta, rice, or other grains five or fewer times daily.

Has difficulty chewing or swallowing.

Has more than one alcoholic drink per day (if woman); more than two drinks per day (if man).

Has pain in mouth, teeth, or gums.

Lives on an income of less than $6000 per year (per individual in the household).

Is unable or prefers not to spend money on food (<$25-$30 per person spent on food each week).

Usually or always needs assistance with preparing food, shopping for food or other necessities.

Level II screen alerts

Has lost or gained 10 lbs or more in the past 6 months.

Body mass index <22.

Body mass index >27.

Has poor appetite.

Is on a special diet.

Eats vegetables two or fewer times daily.

Eats milk or milk products once or not at all daily.

Eats fruit or drinks fruit juice once or not at all daily.

Eats breads, cereals, pasta, rice, or other grains five or fewer times daily.

Has difficulty chewing or swallowing.

Has more than one alcoholic drink per day (if woman); more than two drinks per day (if man).

Has pain in mouth, teeth, or gums.

Lives on an income of less than $6000 per year (per individual in the household).

Is unable or prefers not to spend money on food (<$25-$30 per person spent on food each week).

Usually or always needs assistance with preparing food, shopping for food or other necessities.

Three or more prescription drugs, over-the-counter (OTC) medications, or vitamin/mineral supplements daily.

Skin changes (dry, loose nonspecific lesions, edema).

Nutrition Education and Counseling Interventions

Screening alerts	Older adults, family, friends	Social service professionals	Dietitians, health professionals/nurses	Physicians
Doesn't eat enough (skips meals, eats few meals daily, doesn't spend enough money on food)	✔ Eat at least 3 meals daily ✔ Eat in social settings ✔ Eat small, frequent meals and snacks ✔ Cook large meals in advance and freeze leftovers ✔ Buy ready-to-eat foods ✔ Eat out at senior centers, inexpensive restaurants (ask about discount)	✔ All prior interventions ✔ Bring easily prepared foods (soups, mixes) ✔ Call older adults to encourage eating ✔ Identify social isolation and encourage socialization ✔ Eat with the person	✔ All prior interventions ✔ Arrange eating clubs ✔ Give large print/colorful schedules with times for meals and snacks and suggested foods to eat ✔ Rearrange kitchen to simplify cooking	✔ All prior interventions ✔ Screen for protein-energy malnutrition, deficiency diseases ✔ Make referral to dietitian
Doesn't eat food from all groups (vegetables, fruits, grains, dairy, meat)	✔ Use milk and cheese in soups and casseroles ✔ Chop vegetables in blender and add to soups and casseroles ✔ Eat canned fruits for desserts and snacks ✔ Eat puddings made with milk, ice cream, frozen yogurt, cocoa with milk	✔ All prior interventions ✔ Encourage older adults to attend adult education classes on nutrition, cooking, dining out ✔ Determine if money is an issue	✔ All prior interventions ✔ Identify reason for avoiding food group(s) (afraid of adverse gastrointestinal (GI) problems, dislike taste, hard to prepare, etc.) and recommend diet modifications/substitutions accordingly	✔ All prior interventions ✔ Screen for deficiency diseases ✔ Advise if eating habits could make existing health conditions worse ✔ Make referral to dietitian

Inadequate/ unbalanced diet	✔ Eat well-balanced diet: • 3-5 servings vegetables • 2-4 servings fruits • 6-11 servings breads, cereals, rice, pasta • 2-3 servings milk • 2-3 servings poultry, fish, meats, eggs ✔ Consume sugars, salt, and fat in moderation	✔ All prior interventions ✔ Determine whether older adult has difficulty understanding/ reading English so that recommendations can be made in appropriate language	✔ Adjust therapeutic diet ✔ Suggest alternatives or use food/nutritional supplements ✔ All prior interventions ✔ Do complete nutrition assessment ✔ Check functional status ✔ Determine if food texture/consistency should be modified ✔ Consider vitamin/ mineral supplements	✔ All prior interventions ✔ Screen for deficiency diseases ✔ To encourage compliance, reinforce recommendations of dietitian ✔ Seek nutrition support interventions
Special diet (due to illness or self-imposed)	✔ Ask doctor or dietitian before eating any special diet that hasn't been prescribed ✔ Ask doctor or dietitian if special diet is needed due to change in health	✔ All prior interventions ✔ Weigh older adults weekly and monitor for other changes in health ✔ Assist in selecting, preparing, and eating	✔ All prior interventions ✔ Review diet/disease status to identify deficiencies/excesses and to prescribe appropriate diet, medical nutritionals	✔ All prior interventions ✔ Screen for deficiency diseases ✔ Advise if eating habits could make existing health conditions worse

Continued

From American Academy of Family Physicians, American Dietetic Association, National Council on the Aging. Nutritional Screening Initiative: *Nutrition interventions manual for professional caring for older Americans,* Washington, DC, 1992, The Academy.

Nutrition Education and Counseling Interventions—cont'd

Screening alerts	Older adults, family, friends	Social service professionals	Dietitians, health professionals/nurses	Physicians
			✔Recommended that food texture/consistency be modified as needed ✔Adjust therapeutic diet	✔Make referral to dietitian ✔See medications use and nutrition support interventions
			special or modified foods (pureed, thickened)	
Overweight or underweight	✔Ask doctor whether current body weight is healthy ✔Contact dietitian to modify diet to achieve healthy body weight ✔Eat more protein foods if underweight and fewer fatty foods (especially sweets) if overweight	✔All prior interventions ✔Weigh older adults weekly ✔Encourage appropriate eating patterns and food selection	✔All prior interventions ✔Screen for nutrient deficiencies/excesses ✔Recommend nutritional supplements, hypercaloric diet for weight gain ✔Recommend low-fat/hypocaloric diet for weight loss ✔Encourage physical activity	✔All prior interventions ✔Screen for protein-energy malnutrition, physical (cancer, diabetes, HIV, etc.) and psychiatric (depression, dementia, etc.) causes for weight change ✔See nutrition support interventions ✔Make referral to dietitian
Consumes alcohol regularly	✔Complete questionnaire on alcohol use (CAGE, HEAT, MAST)	✔All prior interventions ✔Monitor alcohol take for pattern of	✔All prior interventions ✔Monitor diet of home and hospitalized older	✔All prior interventions ✔Screen for blood alcohol levels, anemia,

✔Limit number of daily drinks to one or none if woman, two or fewer if man ✔Contact counseling center if concerned about alcohol use/abuse	alcohol use	adults with alcohol-related problems for adequate protein, complex carbohydrates, micronutrients, and fluids ✔Provide alcohol counseling ✔Make referral to dietitian	malnutrition, weight loss, cardiac arrhythmias, GI bleeding, trauma, hypertension, heart failure, edema, mental changes, chronic fatigue, seizures, etc.

Food Sources of Calcium (RDAs for Adults: 800 mg)

	Quantity	Calcium (mg)
Bread, cereal, rice, pasta		
Bran muffin, homemade	1 muffin	54
Bread, whole wheat	1 slice	18
Corn muffin, from mix	1 muffin	96
Cream of wheat (cooked)	3/4 cup	38
Pasta, enriched (cooked)	1 cup	16
Rice, enriched	1 cup	21
Wheat flakes	1 cup	43
Vegetables		
Artichoke (boiled)	1 med	47
Asparagus (boiled)	½ cup (6 spears)	22
Avocado (raw)	1 med	19
Broccoli (raw)	½ cup	21
Brussels sprouts (boiled)	½ cup (4 sprouts)	28
Carrots (raw)	1 med	19
Collards (boiled)	1 cup	148
Corn, yellow (boiled)	½ cup	2
Kale (chopped)	½ cup	47
Peas, green (boiled)	½ cup	19
Potato (baked, with skin)	1 med	115
Tomato (raw)	1 med	8
Fruits		
Apricots (raw)	3 med	15
Banana (raw)	1 med	7
Cantaloupe (raw)	½ cup	8
Figs (dried)	10 figs	269
Orange juice (fresh)	8 fl oz	27
Orange, navel (raw)	1 med	56
Papaya (raw)	1 med	72
Raspberries (raw)	½ cup	14
Strawberries (raw)	½ cup	11
Tangerine (raw)	1 med	12
Meat, poultry, fish, dry beans, eggs, nuts		
Almonds (roasted)	1 oz	148
Beef liver (fried)	3.5 oz	11
Cashews (roasted)	1 oz	13
Chicken, dark (roasted, without skin)	3.5 oz	179
Chicken, light (roasted, without skin)	3.5 oz	216
Egg, whole	1 large	90
Ham (canned)	3.5 oz	6
Kidney beans (boiled)	1 cup	50
Lentils (boiled)	1 cup	37

From Williams SR: *Nutrition and diet therapy,* ed 8, St Louis, 1997, Mosby.

	Quantity	Calcium (mg)
Lima beans (boiled)	1 cup	32
Peanuts (roasted)	1 oz	15
Soybeans (boiled)	1 cup	175
Milk, dairy products		
Milk, skim	8 fl oz	302
Milk, whole	8 fl oz	290
Yogurt, whole	8 fl oz	355
Fats, oils		
This food group is not an important source of calcium.		
Sugar		
Brown sugar	1 cup	123
Molasses, Barbados	1 tbsp	49

Optimal Calcium Requirements

Group	Optimal daily calcium intake (mg)
Infant	
Birth-6 months	400
6 months-1 year	600
Children	
1-5 years	800
6-10 years	800-1200
Adolescents/young adults	
11-24 years	1200-1500
Men	
25-65 years	1000
Over 65 years	1500
Women	
25-50 years	1000
Over 50 years (postmenopausal)	
On estrogen replacement therapy	1000
Not on estrogen replacement therapy	1500
Over 65 years	1500
Pregnant and nursing	1200-1500

From NIH Consensus Development Conference, 1994.

Food Sources of Potassium (Estimated Safe and Adequate Daily Intake for Adults: 1875-5625 mg)

	Quantity	Potassium (mg)
Bread, cereal, rice, pasta		
Bran flakes	¾ cup	184
Bran muffin, homemade	1 muffin	99
Bread, whole wheat	1 slice	44
Oatmeal (cooked)	¾ cup	99
Pasta, enriched (cooked)	1 cup	85
Rice, white, enriched	1 cup	57
Wheat flakes	1 cup	110
Wheat germ, toasted	¼ cup (1 oz)	268
Vegetables		
Artichoke (boiled)	1 med	316
Asparagus (boiled)	½ cup (6 spears)	279
Avocado (raw)	1 med	1097
Broccoli (raw)	½ cup, chopped	143
Brussels sprouts (boiled)	½ cup (4 sprouts)	247
Carrot (raw)	1 med	233
Corn, yellow (boiled)	½ cup	204
Mushrooms (boiled)	½ cup, pieces	277
Potato (baked, with skin)	1 med	844
Spinach (boiled)	1 med	397
Sweet potato (baked)	½ cup	419
Tomato (raw)	1 med	254
Fruits		
Apple (raw, with skin)	1 med	159
Banana	1 med	451
Cantaloupe	1 cup, pieces	494
Dates (dried)	10 dates	541
Figs (dried)	10 figs	1332
Orange juice (fresh)	8 fl oz	486
Orange, navel	1 med	250
Prunes (dried)	10 prunes	626
Prune juice (canned)	8 fl oz	706
Raisins, seedless	⅔ cup	751
Meat, poultry, fish, dry beans, eggs, nuts		
Almonds (dry roasted)	1 oz (22 nuts)	219
Beef liver (fried)	3.5 oz	364
Beef, top round, lean (broiled)	3.5 oz	442
Black-eyed peas (boiled)	1 cup	476
Chicken, dark (roasted, without skin)	3.5 oz	240

From Williams SR: *Nutrition and diet therapy,* ed 8, St Louis, 1997, Mosby.

	Quantity	Potassium (mg)
Chicken, light (roasted, without skin)	3.5 oz	247
Clams (steamed)	3 oz (9 small)	534
Crab, blue (steamed)	3 oz	275
Egg, whole	1 large	65
Ground beef, regular (broiled)	3.5 oz	292
Halibut (baked)	3 oz	490
Ham, canned (lean)	3.5 oz	364
Lentils (boiled)	1 cup	731
Lima beans (boiled)	1 cup	955
Lobster (steamed)	3 oz	299
Mackerel (baked)	3 oz	341
Oysters (steamed)	3 oz (12 med)	389
Peanut butter, creamy	1 tbsp	110
Peanuts (dry roasted)	1 oz	184
Pinto beans (boiled)	1 cup	800
Salmon (baked)	3 oz	319
Sirloin steak, lean (broiled)	3.5 oz	403
Soybeans (boiled)	1 cup	886
Trout, rainbow (baked)	3 oz	539
Tuna, light, canned in water (with salt)	3 oz	267

Milk, dairy products

	Quantity	Potassium (mg)
Cottage cheese, creamed	1 cup	177
Milk, skim	8 fl oz	406
Milk, whole	8 fl oz	368
Yogurt, whole	8 fl oz	351

Fats, oils

This food group is not an important source of potassium.

Sugar

	Quantity	Potassium (mg)
Molasses, black	1 tbsp	585
Sugar, brown	1 cup	499

High-Fiber Foods

Dietary fiber (g per serving)	Food			
	Grain products	Fruits	Dried beans and peas	Vegetables
10 or more	All Bran (⅓ c) Fiber One (½ c) Wheat bran (½ c)	Figs, dried (10) Peaches, dried (10 halves) Prunes, dried (10) Prunes, dried, cooked (½ c)		
5 to 9	Bran Buds (⅓ c) Bran flakes (¾ c) Raisin Bran (¾ c)		Beans, cooked: great northern, kidney, lima, red, or refried (½ c) Bean soup (1 c)	
3 to 5	English muffin, whole grain or bran (1) Crackling Oat Bran (⅓ c) Fruit & Fibre (½ c) Mueslix (⅔ c) Muffin, bran (1) Nutri-Grain (⅔ c) Ry-Krisp (2) Waffle, frozen (2) Wheat Chex (⅔ c) Wheat germ (¼ c)	Apple with skin (1 med) Apricots, dried (10 halves) Avocado (1 med) Blackberries (½ c) Dates, dried (10) Orange (1 med) Papaya (1 med) Pear, raw (1)	Beans, baked (½ c) Beans or peas, cooked: garbanzos, lentils, navy, pinto, white, blackeye (½ c) Pea soup (1 c)	Brussels sprouts, cooked (½ c) Corn, cooked (½ c) Peas, green, canned or frozen (½ c)

1 to 2

Bread: cracked wheat, whole-wheat, mixed grain, rye, oat bran, oatmeal (1 slice)
Brown rice, cooked (1 c)
Cornbread (1 piece)
Cornflakes (1 c)
Cheerios (1¼ c)
French toast (2 slices)
Granola (¼ c)
Grape-Nuts (¼ c)
Muffin, all except bran (1)
Pancakes (2)
Ry-Krisp (1)
Shredded wheat (1 large biscuit)

Applesauce (½ c)
Apricots (3 med)
Blueberries, raw (½ c)
Cantaloupe (1 c)
Cherries, sweet, raw (10)
Grapes (1 c)
Kiwifruit (1 med)
Mango (1 med)
Nectarine (1 med)
Peaches, canned (1 c)
Peach, raw (1 med)
Pear, canned (½ c)
Pineapple, raw or canned (1 c)
Raisins (2 tbsp)
Strawberries, raw or frozen (½ c)
Watermelon (1½ c)

Broccoli, raw or cooked (½ c)
Carrot, cooked (½ c)
Carrot, raw (1 med)
Cauliflower, raw or cooked (½ c)
Green beans, frozen, canned, or fresh (½ c)
Mushrooms, raw or canned (1 c)
Olives (10)
Onions, raw (½ c)
Peppers, sweet, raw (½ c)
Potato, baked or boiled without skin (1 med)
Potato salad (½ c)
Soups: minestrone or vegetable (1 c)
Spinach, cooked (½ c)
Squash, summer or winter, cooked (½ c)
Sweet potatoes, cooked, (½ c)
Tomato, raw (1 med)
Turnip, cooked (½ c)

Moore MC: *Pocket guide to nutritional care*, ed 3, St Louis, 1997, Mosby.

Relationship Between Fiber and Various Health Problems

Problem	Effect of fiber	Possible mode of action	Future research needs
Diabetes mellitus	Reduces fasting blood glucose levels Reduces glycosuria Reduces insulin requirements Increases insulin sensitivity	Slows carbohydrate absorption by: Delaying gastric emptying time Forming gels with pectin or guar gum in the intestine, thus impeding carbohydrate absorption "Protecting" carbohydrates from enzymatic activity with a fibrous coat Allows "protected" carbohydrates to escape into large colon where they are digested by bacteria	Influence of short-chain fatty acid production or metabolism of glucose and fats in the liver Exact mechanisms by which fiber influences glucose metabolism
	Inhibits postprandial (after meals) hyperglycemia	Alters gut hormones (for example, glucagon) to enhance glucose metabolism in the liver	
Obesity	Increases satiety rate	Prolongs chewing and swallowing movements	Cause of increased satiety rate reported by subjects
	Reduces nutrient bioavailability	Increases fecal fat content	Effect of nutrient binding on nutritional status

	Reduces energy density	Inhibits absorption of carbohydrates in high-fiber foods	Studies based on food composition and kcal density instead of fiber content alone
		Decreases transit time	Effects of different types of fiber on gastric, small intestine, and colonic emptying time
	Alters hormonal response	Alters action of insulin, gut glucagon, and other intestinal hormones	
	Alters thermogenesis		
Coronary heart disease	Inhibits recirculation of bile acids	Alters bacterial metabolism of bile acids	Influence of fiber on cholesterol content of specific lipoprotein fractions
		Alters bacterial flora, resulting in a change in metabolic activity	Influence on production of short-chain fatty acids
		Forms gels that bind bile acids	Role of dietary fiber as an independent variable in reducing risk of heart disease
		Alters the function of pancreatic and intestinal enzymes	
	Reduces triglyceride and cholesterol levels*	Reduces insulin levels†	Relationship between lipoprotein turnover and glucose turnover/sensitivity to insulin
		Binds cholesterol, preventing absorption	Effect of higher concentration of bile salts on colon function
		Slows fat absorption by forming gel matrices in the intestine	

From Williams SR: *Nutrition and Diet Therapy*, ed 8, St Louis, 1999, Mosby.

*This effect is based on epidemiologic studies, usually observed in combination with reduced fat intake.

†Insulin is required for fat synthesis.

Continued

Relationship Between Fiber and Various Health Problems—cont'd

Problem	Effect of fiber	Possible mode of action	Future research needs
Colon cancer	Reduces incidence of disease‡	Bile acids or their bacterial metabolites may affect the structure of the colon, its cell turnover rate, and function	Testing of current hypotheses regarding the effects of dietary factors on the structure of the colon and cell turnover rate
Other gastrointestinal disorders	Reduces pressure from within the intestinal lumen	Decreases transit time	
Diverticular disease	Increases diameter of the intestinal lumen, thus allowing intestinal tract to contract more, propelling contents more rapidly and inhibiting segmentation§	Increases water absorption resulting in a larger, softer stool	
Constipation			
Hiatal hernia			
Hemorrhoids			

‡Preventive effect of fiber is assumed from epidemiologic studies that associate low-fiber, high-fat diets with an *increased* incidence of disease.
§Segmentation increases pressure and weakness along the walls of the intestinal tract.

Tips for a Low-Sodium Diet

Restrictions for a Mild Low-Sodium Diet (2 to 3 g/day)
Do not use
1. Salt at the table (use salt lightly in cooking)
2. Salt-preserved foods such as salted or smoked meat (bacon and bacon fat, bologna, dried or chipped beef, corned beef, frankfurters, ham, kosher meats, luncheon meats, salt pork, sausage, smoked tongue), salted or smoked fish (anchovies, caviar, salted and dried cod, herring, sardines) sauerkraut, olives
3. Highly salted foods such as crackers, pretzels, potato chips, corn chips, salted nuts, salted popcorn
4. Spices and condiments such as bouillon cubes,* catsup,* chili sauce,* celery salt, garlic salt, onion salt, monosodium glutamate, meat sauces, meat tenderizers,* pickles, prepared mustard, relishes, Worcestershire sauce, soy sauce
5. Cheese,* peanut butter*

Restrictions for a Moderate Low-Sodium Diet (1000 mg/day)
Do not use
1. Salt in cooking or at the table
2. Salt-preserved foods such as salted or smoked meat (bacon and bacon fat, bologna, dried or chipped beef, brains, corned beef, frankfurters, ham, kosher meats, luncheon meats, salt pork, sausage, smoked tongue, kidneys), salted or smoked fish (anchovies, caviar, salted and dried cod, herring, sardines, frozen fish fillets, canned salmon,* tuna*), sauerkraut, olives
3. Highly salted foods such as crackers, pretzels, potato chips, corn chips, salted nuts, salted popcorn
4. Spices and condiments such as bouillon cubes,* catsup,* chili sauce,* celery salt, garlic salt, onion salt, monosodium glutamate, meat sauces, meat tenderizers,* pickles, prepared mustard, relishes, Worcestershire sauce, soy sauce
5. Cheese,* peanut butter*
6. Buttermilk (unsalted buttermilk may be used) instead of skimmed milk
7. Canned vegetables,* canned vegetable juices*

---

*Dietetic low-sodium kind may be used.

From Williams SR: *Basic nutrition and diet therapy,* ed 10, St Louis, 1995, Mosby.

8. Frozen peas, frozen lima beans, frozen mixed vegetables, any frozen vegetables to which salt has been added
9. More than 1 serving of any of these vegetables in 1 day: artichokes, beet greens, beets, carrots, celery, dandelion greens, kale, mustard greens, spinach, Swiss chard, turnips (white)
10. Regular bread, rolls,* crackers*
11. Dry cereals,* except puffed rice, puffed wheat, and shredded wheat
12. Quick-cooking Cream of Wheat
13. Shellfish: clams, crab, lobster, shrimp (oysters may be used)
14. Salted butter, salted margarine, commercial French dressings,* mayonnaise,* other salad dressings*
15. Regular baking powder,* baking soda, or anything containing them; self-rising flour
16. Prepared mixes: pudding,* gelatin,* cake, biscuit
17. Commercial candies

Restrictions for a Strict Low-Sodium Diet (500 mg/day)

Do not use

1. Salt in cooking or at the table
2. Salt-preserved foods such as salted or smoked meat (bacon and bacon fat, bologna, dried or chipped beef, brains, corned beef, frankfurters, ham, kosher meats, luncheon meats, salt pork, sausage, smoked tongue, kidneys), salted or smoked fish (anchovies, caviar, salted and dried cod, herring, sardines, frozen fish fillets, canned salmon,* tuna*), sauerkraut, olives
3. Highly salted foods such as crackers, pretzels, potato chips, corn chips, salted nuts, salted popcorn
4. Spices and condiments such as bouillon cubes,* catsup,* chili sauce,* celery salt, garlic salt, onion salt, monosodium glutamate, meat sauces, meat tenderizers,* pickles, prepared mustard, relishes, Worcestershire sauce, soy sauce
5. Cheese,* peanut butter*
6. Buttermilk (unsalted buttermilk may be used) instead of skimmed milk
7. More than 2 cups skimmed milk per day, including that used on cereal
8. Any commercial foods made of milk (ice cream, ice milk, milkshakes)

---

*Dietetic low-sodium kind may be used.

9. Canned vegetables,* canned vegetable juices*
10. Frozen peas, frozen lima beans, frozen mixed vegetables, any frozen vegetables to which salt has been added
11. These vegetables: artichokes, beet greens, beets, carrots, celery, dandelion greens, kale, mustard greens, spinach, Swiss chard, turnips (white)
12. Regular bread,* rolls,* crackers
13. Dry cereals,* except puffed rice, puffed wheat, and shredded wheat
14. Quick-cooking Cream of Wheat
15. Shellfish: clams, crab, lobster, shrimp (oysters may be used)
16. Salted butter, salted margarine, commercial French dressings,* mayonnaise,* other salad dressings*
17. Regular baking powder,* baking soda, or anything containing them; self-rising flour
18. Prepared mixes: pudding,* gelatin,* cake, biscuit
19. Commercial candies

General Guidelines for Over-the-Counter (OTC) Drugs

- If asked about OTC remedies, first assess the patient. What symptoms or problems require treatment? What has the patient used successfully in the past?
- Remember that many patients do not consider drugs purchased without a prescription as true drugs; that is, if questioned about medications they are taking, they may not think to include OTC preparations.
- As a part of assessment, ask specifically about medicine purchased at the drugstore or health food store. It may be helpful to include some leading questions such as: "Do you take any cold medicines, cough syrups, vitamins, or other medicines that you can buy without a prescription?" It may also help to know of local health problems or habits. For example, in an area where there are frequent high pollen counts, causing frequent allergy problems, ask questions about allergies and what the patient uses to relieve allergy symptoms.
- In asking how a patient uses OTC drugs, try to frame questions in a nonjudgmental way to learn about actual use patterns. Most patients

From Freeman JB, Queener SF, Karb VB: *Pharmacologic basis of nursing practice,* ed 5, St Louis, 1997, Mosby.

want to use medications correctly and will welcome instruction about drug use but not if they feel defensive about their current practices.

Patient and family education

- Point out to the patient that many OTC preparations contain multiple drugs. Encourage the patient to consider purchasing products that contain only the drug needed. This may be difficult since the ingredients for a product may be listed in generic names, which are not usually familiar to the patient.

- Ideally, the nurse would accompany the patient to the drugstore and review product labeling during the instruction. In the absence of this possibility, suggest that the patient talk over the medication needs with the pharmacist. In addition, the pharmacist can help the patient choose the least expensive but most effective product available at that store.

- Talking about OTC drug use may provide the ideal opportunity to review general safe practices regarding drug use.

- Suggest that the patient periodically look over all the medications in the house and discard those that look discolored or crumbled or that have passed the expiration date. Emphasize to patients the need to discard medications in a way that children or animals cannot find them and take them. Small amounts of liquids can be poured down the sink or toilet, and a few remaining tablets or capsules can be flushed also. If there is a large quantity of medication, consider checking with a local pharmacy or poison control center for guidance about proper disposal.

- Encourage patients who are not obtaining relief from appropriate OTC medications to seek medical care for the problem.

Food Sources of Sodium (Estimated Safe and Adequate Daily Intakes for Adults: 1100-3300 mg)

	Quantity	Sodium (mg)
Bread, cereal, rice, pasta		
Bran flakes	¾ cup	264
Bran muffin, homemade	1 muffin	168
Bread, whole wheat	1 slice	159
Corn flakes	1 cup	310
Wheat flakes	1 cup	270

From Williams SR: *Nutrition and diet therapy,* ed 8, St Louis, 1999, Mosby.

	Quantity	Sodium (mg)
Vegetables		
Artichoke (boiled)	1 med	79
Broccoli (boiled)	½ cup	12
Brussels sprouts (boiled)	½ cup	17
Carrot (raw)	1 med	25
Potato (baked, with skin)	1 med	16
Spinach (boiled)	½ cup	63
Tomato (raw)	1 med	10
Fruits		
This food group is not an important source of sodium.		
Meat, poultry, fish, dry beans, eggs, nuts		
Almonds (roasted, unsalted)	1 oz (22 nuts)	3
Bacon (broiled/fried)	3 med pieces	303
Beef liver (fried)	3.5 oz	106
Beef, top round, lean (broiled)	3.5 oz	61
Black-eyed peas (boiled)	1 cup	6
Chicken, dark (roasted, without skin)	3.5 oz	93
Chicken, light (roasted, without skin)	3.5 oz	77
Clams (steamed)	3 oz	237
Crab, blue (steamed)	3 oz (9 small)	95
Egg, whole	1 large	69
Ground beef, regular (broiled)	3.5 oz	83
Halibut (baked)	3 oz	59
Ham, canned (lean)	3.5 oz	1255
Lentils (boiled)	1 cup	4
Lobster (steamed)	3 oz	323
Mackerel (baked)	3 oz	71
Oysters (steamed)	3 oz (12 med)	190
Peanut butter, creamy (unsalted)	1 tbsp	3
Peanut butter, creamy (with salt)	1 tbsp	131
Shrimp (steamed)	3 oz (15 large)	190
Sirloin steak, lean (broiled)	3.5 oz	66
Soybeans (boiled)	1 cup	1
Tuna, light, canned in water (with salt)	3 oz	303
Milk, dairy products		
Cheddar cheese	1 oz	176
Cottage cheese, creamed	1 cup	850
Milk, skim	8 fl oz	126
Milk, whole	8 fl oz	119
Swiss cheese	1 oz	74
Yogurt, whole	8 fl oz	105

Continued

Food Sources of Sodium (Estimated Safe and Adequate Daily Intakes for Adults: 1100-3300 mg)—cont'd

	Quantity	Sodium (mg)
Fats, oils, sugar		
Butter (salted)	1 tbsp	123
Butter (unsalted)	1 tbsp	2
Margarine, stick, corn oil (salted)	1 tbsp	132
Margarine, stick, corn oil (unsalted)	1 tbsp	3
Molasses, black	1 tbsp	19
Sugar, brown	1 cup	44

Salt-Free Seasoning Guide

Fish	Beef	Poultry and veal	Gravies and sauces
Breaded, battered fillets Dry mustard and onion; oregano, basil, and garlic; thyme Broiled steaks or fillets Chili or curry powder; tarragon Fillets in butter sauce Thyme and chervil; dill; fennel Fish soup Italian seasoning; bay leaf, thyme, and tarragon Fish cakes Tarragon and savory; dry mustard and white pepper; red pepper and oregano	Swiss steak Rosemary and black pepper; bay leaf and thyme; clove Roast beef Basil and oregano; bay leaf; nutmeg; tarragon and marjoram Beef stew Chili powder; bay leaf and tarragon; caraway; marjoram Meatballs Garlic and thyme; basil, oregano, and onion; thyme and garlic; black pepper and dry mustard Beef stroganoff Red pepper, onion, and garlic; nutmeg and onion; curry powder	Fried chicken Basil, oregano, and garlic; onion and dill; sesame seed and nutmeg Roast chicken or turkey Ginger and garlic; onion, thyme, and tarragon Chicken croquettes Dill; curry; chili and cumin; tarragon and oregano Veal patties Italian seasoning; tarragon; dill, onion, and sesame seed Barbecue chicken Garlic and dry mustard; clove, allspice, and dry mustard; basil, garlic, and oregano	Barbecue Bay leaf, thyme, and red pepper; cinnamon, ginger, allspice, dry mustard, and red pepper; chili powder Brown Chervil and onion; onion, bay leaf, and thyme; onion and nutmeg; tarragon Chicken Dry mustard; ginger and garlic; marjoram, thyme, and bay leaf Cream White pepper and dry mustard; curry powder; dill, onion, and paprika; tarragon and thyme

Continued

From Williams SR: *Nutrition and diet therapy*, ed 8, St Louis, 1997, Mosby.

Salt-Free Seasoning Guide—cont'd

Soups	Salads	Pasta, beans, and rice	Vegetables
Chicken Thyme and savory; ginger; clove, white pepper, and allspice	**Chicken** Curry or chili powder; Italian seasoning; thyme and tarragon	**Baked beans** Dry mustard; chili powder; clove and onion; ginger and dry mustard	**Asparagus** Ginger; sesame seed; basil and onion
Clam chowder Basil and oregano; nutmeg and white pepper; thyme and garlic powder	**Coleslaw** Dill; caraway; poppy; dry mustard and ginger	**Rice and vegetables** Curry; thyme, onion, and paprika; rosemary and garlic; ginger, onion, and garlic	**Broccoli** Italian seasoning; marjoram and basil; nutmeg and onion; sesame seed
Mushroom Ginger; oregano; thyme and tarragon; bay leaf and black pepper; chili powder	**Fish or seafood** Dill; tarragon, ginger, dry mustard, and red pepper; ginger, onion, and garlic	**Spanish rice** Cumin, oregano, and basil; Italian seasoning	**Cabbage** Caraway; onion and nutmeg; allspice and clove
Onion Curry and caraway; marjoram and garlic; cloves	**Macaroni** Dill; basil, thyme, and oregano; dry mustard and garlic	**Spaghetti** Italian seasoning and nutmeg; oregano, basil, and nutmeg; red pepper and tarragon	**Carrots** Ginger; nutmeg; onion and dill
Tomato Bay leaf and thyme; Italian seasoning; oregano and onion; nutmeg	**Potato** Chili powder; curry; dry mustard and onion	**Rice pilaf** Dill; thyme; savory and black pepper	**Cauliflower** Dry mustard; basil; paprika and onion
Vegetable Italian seasoning; paprika and caraway; rosemary and thyme; fennel and thyme			**Tomatoes** Oregano; chili powder; dill and onion
			Spinach Savory and thyme; nutmeg; garlic and onion

Food Sources High in Iron

If your blood iron levels are low, eat the foods listed below. (Try to eat two of these foods every day.)

- Liver
- Meats
- Eggs
- Whole and enriched grains
- Legumes
- Dark green leafy vegetables

Cooking in cast iron pots increases the iron in your food.

To increase iron absorption, drink orange juice or another food high in vitamin C along with these high-iron foods.

Food Sources of Iron*

	Quantity	Iron (mg)
Bread, cereal, rice, pasta		
Bran flakes	¾ cup	4.50
Bran muffin, homemade	1 muffin	1.26
Bread, whole wheat	1 slice	0.86
Cream of wheat, regular (cooked)	¾ cup	7.70
Oatmeal (cooked)	¾ cup	1.19
Pasta, enriched (cooked)	1 cup	2.40
Rice, white, enriched	1 cup	1.80
Wheat flakes	1 cup	4.45
Vegetables		
Artichoke (boiled)	1 med	1.62
Avocado (raw)	1 med	2.04
Broccoli (raw)	½ cup	0.89
Brussels sprouts (boiled)	½ cup	0.94
Peas, green (boiled)	½ cup	1.24
Potato (baked, with skin)	1 med	2.75
Spinach (boiled)	½ cup	3.21
Fruits		
Dates (dried)	10 dates	0.96
Figs (dried)	10 figs	4.18
Prune juice (canned)	8 fl oz	3.03
Prunes (dried)	10 prunes	2.08
Raisins, seedless	⅔ cup	2.08

From Williams SR: *Nutrition and diet therapy,* ed 8, St Louis, 1997, Mosby.

Continued

Food Sources High in Iron—cont'd

	Quantity	Iron (mg)
Meat, poultry, fish, dry beans, eggs, nuts		
Almonds (roasted)	1 oz (22 nuts)	1.08
Beef liver (fried)	3.5 oz	6.28
Beef, top round, lean (broiled)	3.5 oz	2.88
Black-eyed peas (boiled)	1 cup	4.29
Cashews (roasted)	1 oz	1.70
Chicken, dark (roasted, without skin)	3.5 oz	1.33
Chicken, light (roasted, without skin)	3.5 oz	1.06
Chick-peas (boiled)	1 cup	4.74
Clams (steamed)	3 oz (9 small)	23.76
Crab, blue (steamed)	3 oz	0.77
Egg, whole	1 large	1.04
Ground beef, regular (broiled)	3.5 oz	2.44
Halibut (baked)	3 oz	0.91
Ham, canned (lean)	3.5 oz	0.94
Lentils (boiled)	1 cup	6.59
Lima beans (boiled)	1 cup	4.50
Mackerel (baked)	3 oz	1.33
Oysters (steamed)	3 oz (12 med)	11.39
Pinto beans (boiled)	1 cup	4.47
Shrimp (steamed)	3 oz (15 large)	2.62
Sirloin steak, lean (broiled)	3.5 oz	3.36
Sole (baked)	3.5 oz	1.40
Soybeans (boiled)	1 cup	8.84
Trout, rainbow (baked)	3 oz	2.07
Tuna, light, canned in water	3 oz	2.72
Milk, dairy products		
Cheddar cheese	1 oz	0.19
Cottage cheese, creamed	1 cup	0.29
Milk, skim	8 fl oz	0.10
Milk, whole	8 fl oz	0.12
Yogurt, whole	8 fl oz	0.11

Fats, oils

This food group is not an important source of iron.

Sugar		
Molasses, black	1 tbsp	3.20
Sugar, brown	1 cup	4.90

*RDAs for adult women, 15 mg; for adult men, 10 mg.

Low-Gluten Diet for Children With Celiac Disease

Dietary principles

- Kcalories—high, usually about 20% above normal requirement, to compensate for fecal loss
- Protein—high, usually 6 to 8 g/kg body weight
- Fat—low, but not fat-free, because of impaired absorption
- Carbohydrates—simple, easily digested sugars (fruits, vegetables) should provide about one half of the kcalories
- Feedings—small, frequent feedings during ill periods; afternoon snack for older children
- Texture—smooth, soft, avoiding irritating roughage initially, using strained foods longer than usual for age, adding whole foods as tolerated and according to age of child
- Vitamins—supplements of B vitamins, vitamins A and B in water-miscible forms, and vitamin C
- Minerals—iron supplements if anemia is present

Food groups	Foods included—low gluten	Foods excluded—high gluten
Milk	Milk (plain or flavored with chocolate or cocoa) Buttermilk	Malted milk; preparations such as Cocomalt, Hemo, Postum, Nestles chocolate
Meat or substitute	Lean meat, trimmed well of fat Eggs, cheese Poultry, fish Creamy peanut butter (if tolerated)	Fat meats (sausage, pork) Luncheon meats, corned beef, frankfurters, all common prepared meat products with any possible wheat filler

From Williams, SR: *Nutrition and diet therapy,* ed 8. St Louis, 1999, Mosby.

Continued

Low-Gluten Diet for Children With Celiac Disease—cont'd

Food groups	Foods included—low gluten	Foods excluded—high gluten
		Duck, goose Smoked salmon Meat prepared with bread, crackers, or flour
Fruits and juices	All cooked and canned fruits and juices Frozen or fresh fruits as tolerated, avoiding skins and seeds	Prunes, plums (unless tolerated)
Vegetables	All cooked, frozen, canned as tolerated (prepared *without* wheat, rye, oat, or barley products); raw as tolerated	Any causing individual discomfort All prepared with wheat, rye, oat, or barley products
Cereals	Corn or rice	Wheat, rye, oat, barley; any product containing these cereals
Breads, flours, cereal products	Breads, pancakes, or waffles made with suggested flours (cornmeal, cornstarch; rice, soybean, lima bean, potato, buckwheat)	All bread or cracker products made with gluten: wheat, rye, oat, barley, macaroni, noodles, spaghetti; any sauces, soups, or gravies prepared with gluten flour, wheat, rye, oat, or barley
Soups	Broth, bouillon (no fat or cream; no thickening with wheat, rye, oat, or barley products); soups and sauces may be thickened with cornstarch	All soups containing wheat, rye, oat, or barley products

Caffeine Content of Beverages and Foods*

Food or beverage	Caffeine (mg)
Coffee, drip, 5 fl oz	137
Coffee, percolated, 5 fl oz	117
Coffee, instant, 5 fl oz	60
Coffee, decaffeinated, 5 fl oz	3
Tea, black, 5 min brew, 5 fl oz	46
Tea, instant, 6 fl oz	33
Cola, diet or regular, 12 fl oz	30-46
Baking chocolate, 1 oz	25-35
Milk chocolate candy, 1 oz	6
Cocoa (beverage), 6 fl oz	5

*Many over-the-counter and some prescription drugs contain higher levels of caffeine than these foods and beverages. Consult the package label or a pharmacist for information about the caffeine content of drugs.

From Moore MC: *Pocket guide to nutritional care,* ed 3, St Louis, 1997, Mosby.

Caffeine Content of Soft Drinks

12-ounce beverage	Caffeine (mg)
Jolt	71.2
Sugar-Free Mr. Pibb	58.8
Pepsi One	55.5
Mountain Dew	55.0 (none in Canada)
Diet Mountain Dew	55.0
Kick citrus	54
Mellow Yellow	52.8
Surge	51.0
Tab	46.8
Coca-Cola	45.6
Diet Coke	45.6
Shasta Cola	44.4
Shasta Cherry Cola	44.4
Shasta Diet Cola	44.4
Mr. Pibb	40.8
Sunkist orange	40
Dr. Pepper	39.6

Based on data from National Soft Drink Association, US Food and Drug Administration, Bunker and McWilliams, Pepsi.   *Continued*

Caffeine Content of Soft Drinks—cont'd

12-ounce beverage	Caffeine (mg)
Storm	38
Big Red	38
Pepsi-Cola	37.2
Diet Pepsi	37
Aspen	36.0
RC Cola	36.0
Diet RC	36.0
Canada Dry Cola	30.0
Barq's Root Beer	23
Canada Dry Diet Cola	1.2
Diet Rite Cola	0
Sprite	0
7-Up	0
Mug Root Beer	0
Sundrop Orange	0
Minute Maid Orange	0
A & W Root Beer	0

Facts About Cholesterol

Types of cholesterol

LDL "bad cholesterol"	HDL "good cholesterol"
Clogs blood vessels	Cleans blood vessels
<200 mg/dL (<5.17 mmol/L*)	<130 mg/dL (<3.36 mmol/L)
Desirable blood cholesterol	Desirable LDL cholesterol
200 mg/dL to 239 mg/dL (5.17 mmol/L to 6.18 mmol/L)	130 mg/dL to 159 mg/dL (3.36 mmol/L to 4.11 mmol/L)
Borderline-high blood cholesterol	Borderline-high-risk LDL cholesterol
≥240 mg/dL (≥6.21 mmol/L)	≥160 mg/dL (≥4.13 mmol/L)
High blood cholesterol	High-risk LDL cholesterol

*To convert mg/dL cholesterol to mmol/L, divide cholesterol by 38.7 or multiply by 0.02586.

Source: National Cholesterol Education Program, National Heart, Lung, and Blood Institute: *Blood cholesterol,* National Institutes of Health, Public Health Service, US Department of Health and Human Services, 1996, NIH Pub #94-2686. Available: http://www.nhlbi.nih.gov/health/public/heart/chol/fabc/index.htm.

What is cholesterol and why should it be of concern?

Cholesterol is a soft, fatlike substance found in the bloodstream. It comes from the *animal source* foods you eat and the cholesterol your body makes. Too much cholesterol can clog the blood vessels and lead to strokes and heart attacks.

To prevent or decrease high cholesterol in the blood, what can one eat?

Increase fiber:

1. Whole wheat bread
2. Hot cereals (oatmeal)

Increase exercise:

1. Walking three times per week if doctor approves

Follow these suggestions:

1. Limit intake of meats, poultry, and seafood to no more than 5-7 oz per day.
2. Use fish, chicken, or turkey in most of your main meals, limiting "red" meats to 3-4 servings per week.
3. Use "low-meat" dishes or vegetable protein dishes such as dried beans or peas for regular entrees.
4. Use low-fat dairy products—2 cups skim milk daily.
5. Limit egg yolks to 2 per week including those in cooking. (1 egg = 274 mg cholesterol)
6. Limit added fat to 5-8 teaspoons daily. Use soft margarines, vegetable oils (olive oil, too) in cooking.

For cholesterol control

Foods to eat	Foods to limit
Egg whites	Egg yolks
Skim milk and low-fat cheeses mozzarella, gouda, ricotta, farmer's and low-fat cottage cheese	Liver
	Heart
	Kidney and other organ meats
	Whole milk
Liquid vegetable oil	Cheese
Olive oil	Oysters
Fish, chicken, turkey (no skin)	Shrimp
Fruits, vegetables, and whole grain foods	Crabs
	Lobster
	Butter
	Cream
	Red meat

Continued

Facts About Cholesterol—cont'd

	Low cholesterol		High cholesterol
Substitute:	Skim milk	for	Whole milk
	Liquid corn oil Margarine	for	Butter
	Safflower oil Corn oil	for	Vegetable shortening

Other tips

Use smaller portions of red meats!

Use less animal food, more plant food.

Switch to whole grains (i.e., whole wheat bread, wheat or oats cereals, brown rice.)

Cholesterol: The Numbers

- For total cholesterol levels, you do not need to fast.
- For triglycerides, you do need to fast.

Cholesterol level	Classification (adults over age 20)
Total cholesterol level	
Less than 200 mg/dL	Desirable
200-239 mg/dL	Borderline-high
Greater than 240 mg/dL	High
LDL ("bad") cholesterol level	
Less than 130 mg/dL	Desirable
130-159 mg/dL	Borderline-high
Greater than 160 mg/dL	High
HDL ("good") cholesterol level	
Average for men is 45 mg/dL	
Average for women is 55 mg/dL	
Below 35 mg/dL is a cause for concern	
Triglyceride levels	
Less than 250 mg/dL	Desirable
250-500 mg/dL	Borderline-high
Greater than 500 mg/dL	High

From Quinnipiack Valley Health Department, Conn.

Total cholesterol = LDL + HDL + (Triglycerides ÷ 5)
(formula for calculating VLDL)

LDL/HDL ratio—less than 3:1 is desirable
(mg/dL = milligrams per deciliter of blood)

Diet and Cancer

- Reduce intake of dietary fat from 40% to 30% of total calories.
- Increase the intake of fresh fruits and vegetables.
- Increase the intake of whole grain breads and cereals.
- Drink alcoholic beverages in moderation, if at all.
- Avoid obesity by regulating total caloric intake.
- Increase intake of foods rich in vitamins A and C.
- Increase intake of cabbage family (cruciferous) vegetables.
- Choose lean meats or legumes as protein sources.
- Trim off excess fat from meats.
- Limit intake of butter, cream, margarine, shortening, and coconut oil, and foods made with such products.
- Broil, bake, or boil rather than fry foods.
- Moderate intake of eggs and organ meats.
- Substitute skim or low-fat milk for whole milk.

Modified from Cancer Information Services, National Institutes of Health. Available: http://www.cis.nci.nih.gov/contact/cancer.html.

Diet Guidelines for a Healthy Heart

These guidelines offer a brief summary of three diets for a healthy heart. If your doctor has prescribed one of these diets for you, you need more complete information. The American Heart Association has free pamphlets available that explain the low-cholesterol and low-sodium diets in detail.

Reading labels

Labels on packaged foods make it easier to select healthier products, but you must understand how to interpret them. If the product makes any nutritional claim, the label lists two categories of information. **"Nutritional Information per Serving"** lists the amount of calories, protein, carbohydrates, fat, and sodium (salt) in one serving. It also tells you how much is considered *one* serving, which can be confusing. For example, one normal serving of milk is 1 cup, or 8 ounces. If you pour milk into a tall drinking glass, however, you may have 10 to 16 ounces.

The second category is **"Percentage of US Recommended Dietary Allowances (U.S. RDA)"** for protein, vitamins, and minerals in each serving. Remember that these numbers are percentages, so if the label on a milk carton says "Protein 20," this means that 1 cup provides 20% of the protein you need each day.

Packaged foods that don't claim to provide nutrition don't have these labels, but they do list the ingredients. The largest quantity is listed first and the smallest amount last. For example, a jar of sweet pickles lists the ingredients as "Cucumbers, water, corn syrup, vinegar, peppers, salt, natural and artificial flavors, preservatives, and artificial coloring." This tells you cucumbers are the main ingredient, water the next highest ingredient, and so forth.

Of course, fresh meats, fish and seafood, fruits, and vegetables do not carry labels. You need to learn which ones are the best for your diet and which ones to avoid.

Low-cholesterol diet

The average American consumes a large amount of cholesterol every day: men about 500 milligrams (mg) and women about 320 mg. A low-cholesterol diet limits cholesterol intake to less than 300 mg per day. To manage this, only 30% (or less) of the total calories you eat every day should come from fat. In addition, most of this fat should come from **polyunsaturated fat,** the "good" fat that helps lower blood cholesterol.

How can you tell the difference between "good" and "bad" fat? Polyunsaturated oil is usually liquid and comes from vegetables such as corn, cottonseed, soybean, sunflower, and safflower. Peanut, canola, and olive oil are **monounsaturated fats** that are neutral and do not add cholesterol. The "bad" fats are **saturated fats,** which harden at room temperature and are found in meat, dairy products made from whole milk or cream, solid and hydrogenated shortening, coconut oil, palm oil, and cocoa butter.

Here are some tips for avoiding too much saturated fat:

1. Eat less meat. Adults need about 5-7 ounces of meat, poultry, fish, or seafood per day.

2. Avoid "prime grade" or heavily marbled meats, corned beef, pastrami, regular ground beef, frankfurters, sausage, bacon, lunch meat, goose, duck, or organ meats. Select very lean cuts of meat. Trim skin off chicken and turkey.

3. Avoid fried meat, chicken, fish, or seafood. Use a rack to drain off fat when broiling, baking, or roasting.

4. Eat no more than two whole eggs (yolks and whites) per week. (Egg whites are allowed because they contain little cholesterol.)

5. Avoid dairy products containing more than 1% milk fat, such as butter, sour cream, cream cheese, creamed cottage cheese, and most natural and processed cheeses. Select milk products that contain only up to 1% milk fat. Use polyunsaturated margarine.

6. Avoid packaged foods or bakery items that contain egg yolks, whole milk, saturated fats, cream sauces, or butter. Select only those that have a low-cholesterol rating.

7. Avoid cashews, coconut, pistachios, and macadamia nuts. Most other types of vegetables, fruits, nuts, and seeds are low in cholesterol.

Low-sodium diet

The average American consumes about 1 to 2 teaspoons of salt every day (6 to 18 grams), and most of this salt is added at the table. Your body needs only about 0.5 gram of salt per day. Since most foods that come from animals (meat, poultry, fish, eggs, milk) are naturally high in sodium, your body's requirements are easily met without adding salt to your food.

What is the difference between salt and sodium? Sodium keeps the right amount of water in your body, so some is necessary for good health. However, too much sodium causes water retention, which raises your blood pressure.

It may take a little time to get used to a low-sodium diet, particularly if you are accustomed to eating highly salted foods. Start by eliminating salt from the table. Use spices and herbs that contain no sodium to add flavor, and try some of the new salt substitutes that contain no sodium.

Many packaged and processed foods are now marketed as low-sodium, including cheeses, luncheon meats, canned and packaged food, and even snacks such as potato chips. However, beware if the package reads "reduced sodium"; the sodium content may still be too high. If you are not sure of a product, read the ingredients carefully and look for the words "salt, sodium, soda, baking powder, monosodium glutamate (MSG), and disodium phosphate." If you are still in doubt, don't eat it.

Here are some tips for eliminating the "hidden" sodium from your diet:

1. Avoid cured or smoked meat, poultry, or fish. These include ham, bacon, corned beef, regular luncheon meats, sausage, commercially frozen fish, canned fish packed in oil or brine, and canned shellfish.
2. Avoid frozen, canned, and dehydrated main-dish foods such as pizza, TV dinners, spaghetti, chili, stews, and soups.
3. Avoid canned vegetables and vegetable juices.
4. Avoid cheese, buttermilk, and cocoa mixes.
5. Avoid commercial sauces (catsup, chili sauce, steak sauce, soy sauce), mayonnaise, salad dressing, olives, pickles, meat tenderizers, and seasoning salts.

Low-calorie diet

Losing weight (or keeping weight off) is an important part of controlling blood pressure and reducing blood cholesterol levels. Your doctor, a dietitian, or a nutritionist can advise you about calories, because this depends on how active you are, your height, and your physical condition.

The low-cholesterol diet is an excellent basis for a weight loss program. Fats are high in calories, and the low-cholesterol diet is essentially a low-fat diet. For example, 1 cup of whole milk contains 150 calories, but the same amount of skim milk has only 86 calories. Also, because it emphasizes fresh fruits and vegetables and discourages processed foods, the low-cholesterol diet is nutritionally well balanced.

Weight loss should be gradual. Remember: it probably took you several years to put the pounds on, so expect it to take several months to lose them.

Here are some other tips for helping you lose weight:

1. Divide your daily calorie allowance into several small meals a day, instead of eating one or two large meals.
2. For between-meal snacks, choose high-fiber, low-calorie foods such as apples or celery. High-fiber foods make your stomach feel full quicker.
3. For between-meal hunger pangs, fool your stomach with a glass of ice water, hot tea, or calorie-free soda.

4. If you eat when you're bored, busy yourself to take your mind off food. Change your activity—do something you enjoy, take a walk, or take a shower.

5. If you eat when you are "blue," try the "buddy system" with a dieting friend. Agree to call each other for help whenever you're tempted to indulge.

6. Regular exercise that burns calories (walking, jogging, swimming, etc.) is the magic ingredient in many people's exercise programs. Check with your doctor first about the safest program for you.

7. "Too good to be true" weight loss programs are just that—they are either worthless or dangerous. Follow a diet that has been medically recommended and skip the fad diets.

Cultural and Regional Foods

Name of food	Culture/region	Type of food	Description
Adobo	Filipino	Meat	Meat with soy sauce
Ajinomoto	Japanese	Grain	Wheat germ
Anadama	New England	Grain	Cornmeal-molasses yeast bread
Arroz blanco	Puerto Rican	Grain	Enriched white rice
Bacalao	Puerto Rican	Meat	Salted codfish
Bagels	Jewish	Grain	Bread dough, doughnut-shaped, boiled in water and baked
Baklava	Greek	Dessert	Layered pastry made with honey
Bok choy	Asian	Vegetable	Green leafy, stalk-like vegetable
Brioche	French	Grain	Egg-rich cake bread, used as sweet roll or shell for entrees
Bulgur	Middle Eastern	Grain	Granular wheat product with nut-like flavor
Burrito	Mexican	Combination	Sandwich; tortilla filled with beef-bean mixture and fried or baked
Café con leche	Latin American	Beverage	Coffee with milk
Cape Cod turkey	New England	Meat	Codfish balls
Challah	Jewish	Grain	Sabbath or holiday twisted egg-bread
Chayote	Mexican	Vegetable	Squash-like vegetable
Chitterlings	Southern US	Meat	Intestine of young pigs, soaked, boiled, and fried
Chorizo	Mexican	Meat	Sausage
Cilantro	Mexican	Seasoning	Coriander, similar to parsley
Crackling	Southern US	Snack	Crispy pieces of fried pork fat
Croissant	French	Grain	Buttery, flaky, crescent-shaped roll
Crumpets	English	Grain	Muffin-like product cooked on griddle then toasted
Cush	Montana	Grain	Cornbread mixed with butter and water and fried
Dandelion greens	Southern US	Vegetable	Leaves from dandelion plant

Continued

Dolmathes	Greek	Grape leaves stuffed with beef
Enchiladas	Mexican	Tortilla filled with meat and cheese
Escargots	French	Snails
Falafel	Middle Eastern	Vegetarian-type meatball
Fatback	Southern US	Fat from loin of pig
Feijoada	Brazilian	Black beans with meat
Feta	Greek	Soft, salty white cheese from sheep or goat milk
Finnan haddie	Scottish	Salted, smoked haddock
Frijoles fritos	Mexican	Refried pinto beans
Gazpacho	Spanish	Cold soup with chopped tomatoes, green peppers, and cucumbers
Gefilte fish	Jewish	Seasoned fish ground and shaped into balls
Goulash	Hungarian	Stew seasoned with paprika
Grits	Southern US	Hulled and coarsely ground corn
Guava	Cuban	Small, yellow or red sweet tropical fruit
Gumbo	Creole	Well-seasoned okra stew with meat or seafood
Hangtown fry	California	Fried oysters and eggs
Hoe cake	Southeast US	Thin corn cake
Hog maw	Southern US	Stomach of pig
Hoppin' John	Southern US	Blackeyed peas and rice
Hushpuppies	Southern US	Fried cornbread
Jalapeños	Latin American	Hot peppers
Jambalaya	Creole	Well-seasoned combination of seafoods, tomatoes, and rice
Kale	Southern US	Dark green leafy vegetable, similar to spinach
Kasha	Jewish	Coarsely ground buckwheat, toasted before cooking in liquid

From Davis JR, Sherer K: *Applied nutrition and diet therapy for nurses,* ed 2, Philadelphia, 1994, WB Saunders.

Cultural and Regional Foods—cont'd

Name of food	Culture/region	Type of food	Description
Kelp	Asian	Vegetable	Seaweed
Kibbeh	Middle Eastern	Meat	Fresh raw lamb, ground and seasoned, similar to meat loaf
Kielbasa	Polish	Meat	Sausage
Kimchi	Korean	Vegetable	Peppery fermented combination of pickled cabbage, turnips, radishes, and other vegetables
Kuchen	German	Dessert	Yeast cake
Latkes	Jewish	Grain	Pancakes, sometimes from potatoes
Lard	—	Fat	Shortening-like product from pork
Limpa	Swedish	Grain	Rye bread
Lox	Jewish	Meat	Smoked salmon
Matzo	Jewish	Grain	Unleavened bread
Menudo	Mexican	Meat	Stew made with tripe (cow's stomach)
Minestrone	Italian	Soup	Vegetable soup
Miso	Asian	"Meat"	Fermented soybean paste
Moussaka	Greek	Combination	Meat and eggplant casserole
Mush	Southwest US	Grain	Cooked cereal, usually cornmeal
Pan Dowdy	New England	Dessert	Dumplings and fruit
Papaya	—	Fruit	Large, yellow melon-like tropical fruit
Pasta	Italian	Grain	Macaroni, spaghetti, and noodles in various shapes made from wheat
Pepperoni	Italian	Meat	Hot sausage
Phyllo	Greek	Grain	Paper-thin pastry for making meat, vegetables, cheese and egg dishes, and sweet pastries
Pilaf	Middle Eastern	Grain	Rice enriched with fat and sometimes vegetables, bits of meat, and spices

Continued

Poi	Polynesian	Vegetable	Root vegetable, especially taro, cooked and pounded, mixed with water, and sometimes fermented
Polenta	Italian	Grain	Cornmeal or cornmeal mush
Poke	Southern US	Vegetable	Dark green leafy vegetable
Potato latkes	Jewish	Vegetable	Potato pancakes
Pot liquor (likker)	Southern US	Vegetable	Liquid from cooking green vegetables or bones
Prosciutto	Italian	Meat	Ready-to-eat, cured, smoked ham
Prickly pear	Native American	Fruit	Fruit of cactus
Pumpernickel	—	Grain	Yeast bread with wheat, corn, rye, and potatoes
Ratatouille	French	Vegetable	Well-seasoned casserole of eggplant, zucchini, tomato, and green pepper
Red-eye gravy	Southern US	Gravy	Fried ham gravy
Safrito	Puerto Rican	Seasoning	Specially seasoned tomato sauce
Sake	Asian	Beverage	Rice wine
Salt pork	Southern US	Fat	Salted pork fat from the belly
Sancocho	Puerto Rican	Combination	Soup with meat and viandas
Sashimi	Japanese	Meat	Raw fish
Sauerbrauten	German	Meat	Pot roast in spicy, aromatic, sweet-and-sour marinade
Scone	English	Grain	Round, flat, unleavened sweetened bread
Scrapple	Pennsylvania Dutch	Combination	Solid mush from cornmeal and the by-products of hog butchering
Shoofly pie	Pennsylvania Dutch	Dessert	Molasses pie
Shoyu	Japanese	Seasoning	Soy sauce
Sopapillas	Mexican	Grain	Rich fried bread
Spaetzle	German	Grain	Small dumplings
Spoonbread	Virginia	Grain	Baked dish with cornmeal
Spumoni	Italian	Dessert	Fruited ice cream
Stollen	German	Dessert	Christmas fruitcake

Cultural and Regional Foods—cont'd

Name of food	Culture/region	Type of food	Description
Strickle sheets	Pennsylvania Dutch	Dessert	Coffee cake
Strudel	German	Dessert	Light pastry, filled with fruit or cheese
Tacos	Mexican	Combination	Fried tortillas, filled with meat, vegetables, and hot sauce
Tempura	Japanese	Combination	Deep-fried seafood or vegetables
Teriyaki sauce	Hawaiian	Seasoning	Sweetened soy sauce
Tofu	Asian	"Meat"	Soybean curd
Tortillas	Mexican	Grain	Pancake-like leathery bread
Trotters	Southern US	Meat	Pig's feet
Viandas	Puerto Rican	Vegetable	Starchy tropical vegetables, including plantain, green bananas, and sweet potatoes

Food Restrictions of Various Religions

Jewish dietary laws

Food selected and prepared according to these rules are called *kosher.* Present Jewish dietary laws govern the slaughter, preparation, and serving of meat; to the combining of meat and milk; to fish; and to eggs. Various food restrictions exist.

1. *Meat.* No pork is used. Forequarters of other meats are allowed, as well as all commonly used forms of poultry. All forms of meat used are strictly cleansed of all blood.
2. *Meat and milk.* No combining of meat and milk is allowed. Orthodox homes maintain two sets of dishes, one for serving meat and the other for meals using dairy products.
3. *Fish.* Only fish with fins and scales are allowed. These may be eaten with either meat or dairy meals. No shellfish or eels may be used.
4. *Eggs.* No egg with a blood spot may be eaten. Eggs may be used with either meat or dairy meals.

From Williams SR: *Nutrition and diet therapy,* ed 8, St Louis, 1997, Mosby.

Other religious dietary restrictions

RELIGIOUS GROUP AND FOOD RESTRICTIONS	CLINICAL IMPLICATIONS WITH INSTITUTIONAL SITUATIONS OR WITH MODIFIED DIETS
Catholic Abstinence from meat, meat soups, or gravy on Ash Wednesday and Fridays during Lent	Fish or other meat substitutes are generally offered on these days
Mormon No alcoholic beverages No stimulants	Substitutes should be given to clients for regular coffee, tea, and most carbonated beverages, specially if the client is on a liquid diet

From Davis JR, Sherer K: *Applied nutrition and diet therapy for nurses,* ed 2, Philadelphia, 1994, WB Saunders.

Continued

RELIGIOUS GROUP AND FOOD RESTRICTIONS	CLINICAL IMPLICATIONS WITH INSTITUTIONAL SITUATIONS OR WITH MODIFIED DIETS
Muslim	
No pork or pork products; no animal shortenings	Hospitalized clients may need assistance in selecting from hospital menus to see that vegetables are not cooked with any animal shortenings or pork seasonings
Only kosher meats allowed	Although institutional meats are not normally kosher, they may be purchased
Regular gelatin made with pork, marshmallow, and other confections made with pork are not allowed	Nurses should assist the client in selecting from the hospital menu to be certain he or she receives adequate food considering these restrictions
No alcoholic products or beverages (including extracts such as vanilla or lemon)	
Fasting is common (mandatory for 1 mo each year)	Fasting can be precarious with some medical problems, especially diabetes and hypoglycemia
Recommended foods: honey, milk, dates, meat, seafood, and vegetable and olive oil	Some of these foods may be contraindicated on a special diet (honey on a diabetic diet) and should be noted
Seventh-Day Adventist	
Optional vegetarianism: (1) strict vegetarianism, (2) ovolactovegetarianism, (3) no pork or pork products, shellfish, or blood	If sodium is restricted, the use of soy-based meat analogues should be noted because they are high in sodium. Strict vegetarians need assistance to select a well-balanced menu from the regular hospital diet. Assist clients in choosing from hospital menu to receive foods not seasoned with pork
No alcoholic beverages No beverages containing caffeine	Substitutes should be made for the regular coffee, tea, and some carbonated beverages ordinarily given, especially if the client is on a liquid diet
Snacking between meals is discouraged (mealtimes are are at intervals of 5 to 6 hr)	Some diabetic, hypoglycemia, and ulcer-type diets require more frequent feedings

Nutritional Analysis of Fast Foods

Food name	Amount	Unit	Grams	kCalories	Carbohydrates (g)	Protein (g)	Fat (g)	Saturated fat (g)	Monounsaturated fat (g)	Polyunsaturated fat (g)	Fiber (g)	Cholesterol (mg)	Folate (µg)	Vitamin A (RE)	Vitamin B6 (mg)	Vitamin B12 (µg)	Vitamin C (mg)	Vitamin E (mg)	Thiamin (mg)	Riboflavin (mg)	Calcium (mg)	Iron (mg)	Magnesium (mg)	Niacin (mg)	Phosphorus (mg)	Potassium (mg)	Sodium (mg)	Zinc (mg)
Arby's-Beef'N Cheddar Sandwich	1	Each	194.0	443	30	35	20	10	4	1	—	85	45	64	.4	2.3	1	.4	.5	.4	202	5.6	44	6.5	442	380	1801	6
Arby's-Chicken Breast Fillet Sandwich	1	Each	204.0	547	53	26	28	11	11	2	—	101	35	17	.7	.4	0	2.9	.4	.5	123	3.9	51	16.4	322	366	1130	1.9
Arby's-Curly Fries	1	Each	99.2	337	43	4	18	—	—	—	—	0	—	—	—	—	16	.8	.1	.1	16	1.9	—	1.9	724	—	167	—
Arby's-Regular Roast Beef	1	Each	155.9	388	38	25	16	8	4	2	1	58	45	71	.3	1.4	2	.2	.3	.4	61	4.7	35	6.6	268	354	888	3.8
Burger King-Bacon Double Cheeseburger	1	Each	202.0	613	29	34	40	17	6	1	—	115	32	74	.4	3.4	8	.4	.3	.4	162	4.1	39	8.4	386	480	833	6.6
Burger King-Double Cheeseburger	1	Each	191.4	537	32	33	30	14	12	2	—	111	34	111	.3	2	7	2	.3	.2	210	3.3	34	5.5	339	383	947	4.5
Burger King-Hamburger	1	Each	122.9	310	35	16	12	—	—	—	—	—	—	—	—	—	—	—	—	—	—	—	—	—	—	—	560	—
Burger King-Salad w/House Dressing	1	Each	176.0	159	8	3	13	—	—	—	—	11	—	25	—	—	0	—	—	—	352	.1	95	.2	592	402	293	.1
Burger King-Salad w/Reduced-Calorie Italian	1	Each	176.0	42	7	2	1	—	—	—	—	0	—	—	—	—	0	—	—	—	320	.1	105	.2	472	390	430	.1
Burger King-Whopper	1	Each	283.5	684	54	28	39	18	15	3	—	113	34	209	.3	3.1	14	4.2	0	—	113	6.5	54	5.6	339	565	1075	5.8
Dunkin' Donuts-Banana Nut Muffin	1	Each	103.0	310	49	7	10	—	—	3	—	30	—	—	—	—	—	—	—	—	—	—	—	—	—	—	410	—
Dunkin' Donuts-Bran Muffin w/Raisins	1	Each	104.0	310	51	6	9	—	—	4	—	15	—	—	—	—	—	—	—	—	—	—	—	—	—	—	560	—

Continued

From Williams SR: *Nutrition and diet therapy,* ed 8, St Louis, 1997, Mosby.

Nutritional Analysis of Fast Foods—cont'd

Food name	Amount	Unit	Grams	kCalories	Carbohydrates (g)	Protein (g)	Fat (g)	Saturated fat (g)	Monounsaturated fat (g)	Polyunsaturated fat (g)	Fiber (g)	Cholesterol (mg)	Folate (µg)	Vitamin A (RE)	Vitamin B6 (mg)	Vitamin B12 (µg)	Vitamin C (mg)	Vitamin E (mg)	Riboflavin (mg)	Thiamin (mg)	Calcium (mg)	Iron (mg)	Magnesium (mg)	Niacin (mg)	Phosphorus (mg)	Potassium (mg)	Sodium (mg)	Zinc (mg)
Dunkin' Donuts-Cake Ring, Plain	1	Each	62.0	270	25	4	17	—	—	1	—	0	—	—	—	—	—	—	—	—	—	—	—	—	—	—	330	—
Dunkin' Donuts-Chocolate Frosted Yeast Ring	1	Each	55.0	200	25	4	10	—	—	1	—	0	—	—	—	—	—	—	—	—	—	—	—	—	—	—	190	—
Dunkin' Donuts-Croissant, Plain	1	Each	72.0	310	27	7	19	—	—	2	—	0	—	—	—	—	—	—	—	—	—	—	—	—	—	—	240	—
Dunkin' Donuts-Glazed Chocolate Rings	1	Each	71.0	324	34	4	21	—	—	2	—	0	—	—	—	—	—	—	—	—	—	—	—	—	—	—	383	—
Dunkin' Donuts-Jelly Filled	1	Each	67.0	220	31	4	9	—	1	—	2	0	—	—	—	—	—	—	—	—	—	—	—	—	—	—	230	—
Fast Food-Biscuit w/Egg	1	Each	136.0	316	24	11	20	8	6	4	—	233	30	178	.1	.7	0	—	.3	.3	154	3.1	20	—	185	160	654	1.1
Fast Food-Biscuit w/Egg and Sausage	1	Each	180.0	581	41	19	39	15	16	4	—	302	40	164	.2	1.4	0	—	.5	.4	155	3.6	25	—	490	320	1141	2.2
Fast Food-Biscuit w/Egg, Cheese, and Bacon	1	Each	144.0	477	33	16	31	14	11	3	—	261	37	166	.1	1.1	2	—	.4	.3	164	2.5	20	—	459	230	1260	1.5
Fast Food-Burrito w/Beans	1	Each	108.5	224	36	7	7	2	3	1	—	2	59	16	.2	.5	1	—	.3	.3	56	2.3	43	—	49	327	493	.8
Fast Food-Burrito w/Beans, Cheese, and Beef	1	Each	101.5	165	20	7	7	2	1	—	—	62	30	75	.1	.5	.3	—	.1	.2	65	1.9	25	—	70	205	495	1.2
Fast Food-Burrito w/Beef	1	Each	110.0	262	29	13	10	4	5	0	—	32	20	14	.2	1	.1	—	.5	.3	42	3.2	41	—	87	370	746	2.4
Fast Food-Cheeseburger, Large, Double Patty	1	Each	258.0	704	40	38	44	18	17	5	—	142	49	54	.4	3.4	1	—	.4	.5	240	5.9	52	—	395	596	1148	6.7
Fast Food-Cheeseburger, Large, Single Patty	1	Each	219.0	563	38	28	33	13	15	2	—	88	28	129	.3	2.6	8	1.2	.5	.4	206	4.7	44	—	311	445	1108	4.6

Food	Amt	Measure																								
Fast Food-Cheeseburger, Triple Patty, Plain	1	Each	304.0	796	27	56	51	22	22	3	—	161	52	85	.6	5.9	3	—	.6	.6	283	8.3	61	11.5	541	821	1213	10.9
Fast Food-Chicken Fillet Sandwich, Plain	1	Each	182.0	515	39	24	29	9	10	8	—	60	29	31	.2	.4	9	—	.2	.3	60	4.7	35	6.8	233	353	957	1.9
Fast Food-Chicken Nuggets, w/Barb. Sauce	1	Each	17.0	43	3	2	2	1	1	0	—	8	4	6	0	0	0	—	0	0	3	.2	3	.9	28	42	108	.1
Fast Food-Chicken Nuggets, w/Sweet and Sour	1	Each	17.0	45	4	2	2	1	1	0	—	8	2	10	0	0	0	—	0	0	3	.2	3	.9	28	36	89	.1
Fast Food-Chili Con Carne	1	Cup	253.0	256	22	25	8	3	3	1	—	134	30	167	.3	1.1	2	—	1.1	.1	68	5.2	46	2.5	197	691	1007	3.6
Fast Food-Chimichanga, w/Beef	1	Each	174.0	425	43	20	20	9	8	1	—	9	31	16	.3	1.5	5	—	.6	.5	63	4.5	63	5.8	124	586	910	5
Fast Food-Clams, Breaded and Fried	3	Ounce	85.1	333	29	9	20	5	8	5	—	65	7	27	0	.8	0	—	.2	.5	63	2.3	23	2.1	176	196	617	1.2
Fast Food-Corn on the Cob w/Butter	1	Each	146.0	155	32	4	3	2	1	1	—	6	44	96	.3	0	7	—	.1	.2	4	.9	41	2.2	108	359	29	.9
Fast Food-Croissant w/Egg and Cheese	1	Each	127.0	368	24	13	25	14	8	1	—	216	37	255	.1	.8	0	—	.4	.2	244	2.2	22	1.5	348	174	551	1.8
Fast Food-Croissant w/Egg, Cheese, and Ham	1	Each	152.0	474	24	19	34	17	11	2	—	213	36	117	.2	1	11	—	.3	.5	144	2.1	26	3.2	336	272	1081	2.2
Fast Food-Danish Pastry, Fruit	1	Each	94.0	335	45	16	5	3	10	2	—	19	15	24	.1	.2	2	—	.2	.3	22	1.4	14	1.8	69	110	333	.5
Fast Food-Enchilada w/Cheese	1	Each	163.0	319	29	29	19	11	6	1	—	44	34	186	.4	.7	1	—	.4	.1	324	1.3	51	1.9	134	240	784	2.5
Fast Food-Enchirito w/Cheese, Beef, and Beans	1	Each	193.0	344	34	18	16	8	7	0	—	50	253	133	.2	1.6	5	—	.7	.2	218	2.4	71	3	224	560	1251	2.8
Fast Food-Eng. Muffin w/Egg, Cheese, and Can. Bacon	1	Each	146.0	383	31	20	20	9	7	2	—	234	44	158	.2	.8	1	.6	.5	207	3.3	34	3.9	320	213	784	1.8
Fast Food-Fish Fillet, Battered and Fried	1	Each	91.0	211	15	13	11	3	2	6	—	31	51	11	.1	.1	1	—	.1	.1	16	1.9	22	1.9	156	291	484	.4
Fast Food-Fried Pie, Fruit (Apple, Cherry, or Lemon)	1	Each	85.0	266	33	2	14	7	6	1	—	13	4	33	0	.1	1	1.4	.1	.1	13	.9	8	1	37	51	325	.2
Fast Food-Frijoles w/Cheese	3	Ounce	85.1	115	15	6	4	2	2	0	—	19	57	36	.1	.3	1	—	.2	.1	96	1.1	43	.8	89	308	449	.9

Continued

Nutritional Analysis of Fast Foods—cont'd

Food name	Amount Unit	Grams	kCalories	Protein (g)	Carbohydrates (g)	Fat (g)	Saturated fat (g)	Monounsaturated fat (g)	Polyunsaturated fat (g)	Fiber (g)	Cholesterol (mg)	Folate (µg)	Vitamin A (RE)	Vitamin B6 (mg)	Vitamin B12 (µg)	Vitamin C (mg)	Vitamin E (mg)	Riboflavin (mg)	Thiamin (mg)	Calcium (mg)	Iron (mg)	Magnesium (mg)	Niacin (mg)	Phosphorus (mg)	Potassium (mg)	Sodium (mg)	Zinc (mg)
Fast Food-Hamburger, Double Patty w/Cond and Veg	1 Each	226.0	540	34	40	27	11	10	3	—	122	27	11	.5	4.1	1	—	.4	.4	102	5.9	50	7.6	314	570	791	5.7
Fast Food-Hamburger, Large, Single Patty w/Cond and Veg	1 Each	218.0	512	26	40	27	10	11	2	—	87	37	33	.3	2.4	3	—	.4	.4	96	4.9	44	7.3	233	480	824	4.9
Fast Food-Hamburger, Single Patty, Plain	1 Each	90.0	275	12	31	12	4	5	1	—	35	25	0	.1	.9	0	—	.3	.3	63	2.4	19	3.7	103	145	387	2
Fast Food-Hot Dog w/Chili	1 Each	114.0	296	14	31	13	5	7	1	—	51	50	6	0	.3	3	—	.2	.3	19	3.3	10	3.7	192	166	480	.8
Fast Food-Hot Dog w/Corn Flour Coating (Corndog)	1 Each	175.0	460	17	56	19	5	9	3	—	79	60	37	.1	.4	0	—	.7	.3	102	6.2	18	4.2	166	263	973	1.3
Fast Food-Hot Dog, Plain	1 Each	98.0	242	10	18	15	5	7	2	—	44	29	0	.1	.5	0	—	.2	.2	24	2.3	13	3.6	97	143	670	2
Fast Food-Ice Milk, Vanilla, Soft-serve w/Cone	1 Each	103.0	164	4	24	6	4	2	0	—	28	5	52	.1	.2	.4	.1	.2	.1	153	.2	15	.3	139	169	92	.6
Fast Food-Nachos w/Cheese	3 Ounce	85.1	260	7	27	14	6	6	2	—	14	8	69	.2	.6	1	—	.2	.1	205	1	42	1.2	208	129	614	1.3
Fast Food-Nachos w/Cheese, Beans, Ground Beef	3 Ounce	85.1	190	7	19	10	4	4	2	—	7	13	156	.1	.3	2	—	.1	.1	128	.9	32	1.1	129	151	600	1.2
Fast Food-Onion Rings, Breaded and Fried	1 Each	10.0	33	0	4	2	1	1	0	—	2	1	0	0	0	0	0	.1	.1	9	.1	2	.1	10	16	52	0
Fast Food-Pancakes w/Butter and Syrup	1 Each	74.0	166	3	29	4	2	2	1	—	19	11	22	0	.1	1	—	.4	.1	41	.8	16	1.1	152	80	352	.3
Fast Food-Pizza w/Cheese, Sausage, and Vegetables	1 Slice	79.0	184	13	21	5	2	3	1	—	21	27	101	.1	.4	2	—	.2	.2	101	1.5	18	2	131	179	382	1.1
Fast Food-Pizza w/Pepperoni	1 Slice	71.0	181	10	20	7	2	3	1	—	14	53	55	.1	.2	2	—	.2	.1	65	.9	9	3	75	153	267	.5

Food	Portion	Weight	Cal																								
Fast Food-Potato, Baked w/Cheese Sauce and Broccoli	1 Each	339.0	403	47	14	21	9	8	4	—	20	61	278	.8	.3	48	—	.3	.3	336	3.3	78	3.6	346	1441	485	2
Fast Food-Potato, French Fried in Beef Tallow	1 Large	115.0	359	44	5	19	9	8	1	—	21	38	3	.3	.1	6	—	0	.2	18	1.6	38	2.6	153	819	187	.6
Fast Food-Potato, French Fried in Vegetable Oil	1 Large	115.0	355	44	5	19	6	9	3	—	0	38	3	.3	.1	6	—	0	.2	18	1.6	38	2.6	153	819	187	.6
Fast Food-Potatoes, Hashed Brown	1/2 Cup	72.0	151	16	2	9	4	4	0	—	9	8	3	.2	0	5	.1	0	.1	7	.5	16	1.1	69	267	290	.2
Fast Food-Salad, w/o Dressing, w/Chicken	1/2 Cup	72.7	35	1	6	1	0	0	0	—	24	23	32	.1	.1	6	—	0	0	12	.4	11	2	57	149	70	.3
Fast Food-Shrimp, Breaded and Fried	1 Ounce	28.4	79	7	3	4	1	3	0	—	35	8	6	0	0	0	—	.2	0	14	.5	7	0	60	32	250	.2
Fast Food-Submarine Sandwich w/Cold Cuts	1 Each	228.0	456	51	22	19	7	8	2	—	36	55	80	.1	1.1	12	—	.8	1	189	2.5	68	5.5	287	394	1651	2.6
Fast Food-Submarine Sandwich w/Tuna Salad	1 Each	256.0	584	55	30	28	5	13	7	—	49	56	41	.2	1.6	4	—	.3	.5	74	2.6	79	11.3	220	335	1293	1.9
Fast Food-Sundae, Hot Fudge	1 Each	158.0	284	48	6	9	5	2	1	0	21	9	57	.1	.6	2	.7	.3	.1	207	.6	33	1.1	228	395	182	.9
Fast Food-Sundae, Strawberry	1 Each	153.0	268	45	6	8	4	3	1	0	21	18	58	.1	.6	2	.8	.3	.1	161	.3	24	.9	155	271	92	.7
Fast Food-Taco	1 Large	263.0	568	41	32	32	17	10	1	—	87	37	226	.4	1.6	3	—	.7	.2	339	3.7	108	4.9	313	729	1233	6
Fast Food-Tostada w/Guacamole	1 Ounce	28.4	39	3	1	3	1	1	0	—	4	12	24	0	.1	0	—	.1	0	46	.2	8	.2	25	71	87	.4
Fast Food-Tostada, w/Beans and Cheese	1 Each	144.0	223	27	10	10	5	3	1	—	30	75	85	.2	.7	1	—	.3	.1	210	1.9	59	1.3	117	403	543	1.9
Hardee's-Big Deluxe	1 Each	248.1	675	—	—	—	—	—	—	—	—	—	—	—	—	—	—	—	—	—	—	—	—	—	—	1063	—
Hardee's-Big Fish Sandwich	1 Each	191.4	514	49	20	26	—	—	—	—	—	—	—	—	—	—	—	—	—	—	—	—	—	—	—	314	—
Hardee's-Cheeseburger	1 Each	100.6	335	29	17	17	—	—	—	—	—	—	—	—	—	—	—	.3	—	—	—	—	—	—	—	789	—
Hardee's-Chicken Fillet	1 Each	191.4	510	42	27	26	—	—	—	—	—	—	—	—	—	2	—	—	—	—	—	—	5.5	—	—	360	—
Hardee's-Hot Dog	1 Each	50.0	346	26	11	22	—	—	—	—	—	—	—	—	—	—	—	—	—	—	—	—	—	—	—	744	—
Jack in the Box-Bacon Cheeseburger	1 Each	242.0	705	41	35	45	15	16	9	—	113	70	—	—	—	8	—	.5	.2	200	2.8	—	8.4	—	—	1240	—

Continued

Nutritional Analysis of Fast Foods—cont'd

Food name	Amount	Unit	Grams	kCalories	Carbohydrates (g)	Protein (g)	Fat (g)	Saturated fat (g)	Monounsaturated fat (g)	Polyunsaturated fat (g)	Fiber (g)	Cholesterol (mg)	Folate (µg)	Vitamin A (RE)	Vitamin B6 (mg)	Vitamin B12 (µg)	Vitamin C (mg)	Vitamin E (mg)	Riboflavin (mg)	Thiamin (mg)	Calcium (mg)	Iron (mg)	Magnesium (mg)	Niacin (mg)	Phosphorus (mg)	Potassium (mg)	Sodium (mg)	Zinc (mg)
Jack in the Box-Jumbo Jack	1	Each	222.0	497	41	25	26	10	11	2	—	72	67	.3	2.4	4	—	.3	—	.4	121	4.1	40	10.5	236	444	1023	3.8
K.F.C.-Colonel's Chicken Sandwich	1	Each	166.0	482	39	21	27	6	4	9	1	47	29	14	.6	.3	0	2.3	.3	.4	100	3.1	41	10.6	261	297	1060	1.5
K.F.C.-Mashed Potatoes and Gravy	1	Each	98.0	71	12	2	2	1	0	0	—	—	—	—	—	0	—	—	—	—	16	.2	—	—	—	—	339	—
K.F.C.-Original Recipe Center Breast	1	Each	103.0	261	9	25	15	4	2	0	—	87	4	15	.6	.4	0	.5	.1	.1	—	1.2	31	14	238	265	603	1.1
K.F.C.-Original Recipe Thigh	1	Each	95.0	324	11	16	24	6	3	0	—	103	8	28	.3	.3	.5	.2	.1	.1	13	1.4	23	6.5	176	224	549	2.4
McDonald's-Apple Danish	1	Each	115.0	390	51	6	17	11	2	2	—	25	3	35	0	0	—	—	.1	.1	14	1.4	8	2.2	31	69	370	.2
McDonald's-Big Mac	1	Each	215.0	560	43	25	32	10	20	2	—	103	21	106	.3	1.8	2	—	.3	.5	256	4	38	6.8	314	237	950	4.7
McDonald's-Chef Salad	1	Each	265.0	215	7	20	12	6	3	1	—	120	—	385	.3	—	13	—	.3	—	240	1.4	—	3.4	—	—	459	—
McDonald's-Chicken McNuggets	1	Each	18.5	45	3	3	3	1	1	—	—	9	—	—	—	0	—	—	—	.1	—	—	—	1.3	—	—	97	—
McDonald's-Egg McMuffin	1	Each	135.0	284	27	18	11	4	4	1	—	221	43	147	.2	.8	1	1.8	.3	.5	250	2.7	32	3.6	312	208	724	1.8
McDonald's-Filet O' Fish	1	Each	141.0	437	38	14	26	5	10	11	1	50	20	44	.1	.8	—	.1	.3	.3	164	1.8	27	2.7	227	149	1023	.9
McDonald's-Hotcakes w/Margarine and Syrup	1	Each	174.0	440	74	8	12	2	5	5	—	8	50	40	—	—	—	—	.3	.3	80	1	—	2.9	—	—	685	—
McDonald's-McChicken	1	Each	187.0	415	39	19	20	5	9	7	—	50	20	—	—	.2	—	—	.9	—	120	1.5	—	8.6	—	—	830	—
McDonald's-Quarter Pounder	1	Each	166.0	410	34	23	20	8	—	1	—	85	40	—	—	—	—	—	.3	.4	120	2	—	6.7	—	—	645	—
McDonald's-Sausage McMuffin	1	Each	135.0	345	27	15	20	7	11	2	—	57	40	—	—	—	—	—	.5	—	160	1.5	—	4.8	—	—	770	—

Continued

Food	Amt	Unit	Wt	Cal																							
McDonald's-Side Salad	1	Each	106.0	30	4	2	1	0	0	1	0	33	—	800	—	—	.1	.1	16	.4	—	—	35	—			
McDonald's-Strawberry Lowfat Milk Shake	1	Each	294.1	320	67	11	1	1	0	1	0	10	—	60	—	—	.5	.1	280	—	—	.4	170	—			
Pizza Hut-Cheese Pizza, Pan	1	Slice	70.0	246	29	15	9	5	—	5	—	17	—	45	—	.3	4	.3	.3	252	1.5	26	2.5	188	160	470	2
Pizza Hut-Cheese Pizza, Thin 'n Crispy	1	Slice	70.0	199	19	14	9	5	—	3	—	17	—	35	—	.3	2	.2	.2	264	.9	21	2.3	188	131	434	1.8
Pizza Hut-Pepperoni Personal Pan Pizza	1	Each	250.0	675	76	37	29	13	17	—	—	53	—	120	—	.4	10	.7	.6	584	3.2	53	7.8	360	408	1335	3.8
Pizza Hut-Pepperoni Pizza, Hand Tossed	1	Slice	70.0	250	25	14	12	6	5	—	—	25	—	50	—	.3	4	.3	.3	176	1.4	26	2.7	156	208	634	1.9
Pizza Hut-Super Supreme Pizza, Thin 'n Crispy	1	Slice	70.0	232	22	15	11	5	5	—	—	28	—	50	—	.4	4	.2	.3	184	1.4	26	2.6	168	232	668	2.3
Pizza Hut-Supreme Personal Pan Pizza	1	Each	250.0	647	76	33	28	11	17	—	—	49	—	120	—	.5	11	.7	.6	416	3.7	53	7.6	320	487	1313	3.8
Pizza Hut-Supreme Pizza, Hand Tossed	1	Slice	70.0	270	25	16	13	6	7	—	—	28	—	55	—	.4	6	.3	.3	192	2.3	35	3.4	184	289	735	2.9
Red Lobster-Atlantic Ocean Perch, Lunch	1	Each	141.8	130	1	24	4	1	—	1	—	75	—	55	—	.3	—	.1	.1	—	—	21	1.5	160	—	190	.3
Red Lobster-Calamari, Breaded and Fried, Lunch	1	Each	141.8	360	30	13	21	6	2	—	2	140	—	—	—	2	—	.1	.2	—	.6	21	1.5	360	—	1150	.9
Red Lobster-Chicken Breast, Skinless, Lunch	1	Each	113.4	140	0	26	3	1	1	—	1	70	—	—	—	—	—	.1	.1	—	.4	21	11.4	160	—	60	.9
Red Lobster-Halibut, Lunch Portion	1	Each	141.8	110	1	25	1	0	1	—	1	60	—	—	—	.3	—	.3	.2	—	—	28	2.9	240	—	105	—
Red Lobster-Norwegian Salmon, Lunch	1	Each	141.8	230	3	27	12	3	5	—	5	80	—	—	—	.2	—	.1	.2	16	—	35	6.7	240	—	60	.3
Red Lobster-Shrimp, Lunch Portion	1	Each	198.5	120	0	25	2	1	1	—	1	230	—	—	—	.5	—	—	0	32	—	35	1.9	120	—	110	1.5
Subway-BMT, on Honey Wheat Bread	1	12 in.	220.0	1011	88	45	57	20	25	7	6	133	63	67	.5									—	1002	3199	—
Subway-BMT, on Italian Roll	1	12 in.	213.0	982	83	44	55	20	24	7	5	133	63	67	.5	2.3	5	5.1	.3	.3	64000	4.3	66	5.1	308	917	3139	6.1

Nutritional Analysis of Fast Foods—cont'd

Food name	Amount	Unit	Grams	kCalories	Carbohydrates (g)	Protein (g)	Fat (g)	Saturated fat (g)	Monounsaturated fat (g)	Polyunsaturated fat (g)	Fiber (g)	Cholesterol (mg)	Folate (µg)	Vitamin A (RE)	Vitamin B6 (mg)	Vitamin B12 (µg)	Vitamin C (mg)	Vitamin E (mg)	Thiamin (mg)	Riboflavin (mg)	Calcium (mg)	Iron (mg)	Magnesium (mg)	Niacin (mg)	Phosphorus (mg)	Potassium (mg)	Sodium (mg)	Zinc (mg)
Subway-Cold Cut Combo, on Italian Roll	1	12 in.	184.0	853	83	46	40	12	15	10	5	166	39	87	.2	1.2	17	.9	.3	.4	227000	2.9	28	3.8	315	876	2218	2.7
Subway-Ham and Cheese, on Wheat	1	12 in.	194.0	673	86	39	22	7	8	—	6	73	—	—	—	—	—	—	—	—	—	—	—	—	—	918	2508	—
Subway-Meat Ball Sandwich, on Italian Roll	1	12 in.	215.0	918	96	42	44	17	17	4	3	88	35	72	.4	3.2	19	1	.4	.3	78000	5	47	9.4	263	1210	2022	6.2
Subway-Seafood, on Wheat Roll	1	12 in.	219.0	1015	100	31	58	16	11	28	3	56	—	—	—	—	—	—	—	—	—	—	—	—	—	557	1967	—
Subway-Turkey Breast, on Wheat Roll	1	12 in.	192.0	674	88	20	20	7	7	—	3	67	—	—	—	—	—	—	—	—	—	—	—	—	—	605	2520	—
Taco Bell-Bean Burrito	1	Each	206.0	387	63	15	14	7	3	2	—	9	—	53	—	2	—	—	—	.4	190	4	—	2.8	—	495	1148	—
Taco Bell-Burrito Supreme	1	Each	198.0	440	55	20	22	—	8	2	3	33	—	26	—	2.1	—	—	—	.4	190	4	—	3.6	—	501	1181	—
Taco Bell-Light Bean Burrito	1	Each	198.0	330	55	14	6	—	—	—	—	5	—	300	—	—	2	—	—	—	120	2	—	—	—	—	1340	—
Taco Bell-Light Burrito Supreme	1	Each	248.0	350	50	20	8	—	1	2	—	25	—	600	—	—	9	—	.2	.4	96	1.5	—	—	—	—	1160	—
Taco Bell-Light Soft Taco	1	Each	99.0	180	19	13	5	—	4	—	—	25	—	40	—	—	0	—	—	—	48	.6	—	2.8	—	196	554	—
Taco Bell-Light Taco Salad	1	Each	464.0	330	35	30	9	—	1	2	—	50	—	1200	—	—	27	—	—	1.5	120	1.5	—	—	—	—	1610	—
Taco Bell-Nachos	1	Each	106.0	346	37	7	18	—	6	—	—	9	—	2	—	—	—	—	—	.2	191	1	—	.6	—	159	399	—
Taco Bell-Nachos Bell Grande	1	Each	287.0	649	61	22	35	12	3	4	—	36	—	58	—	—	—	—	.3	.1	297	3	—	2.2	—	674	997	—
Taco Bell-Taco	1	Each	78.0	183	11	10	11	5	1	1	—	32	—	1	—	—	—	—	.1	.1	84	1	—	1.2	—	159	276	—
Wendy's-Big Classic	1	Each	251.0	480	44	27	23	8	7	—	—	75	—	60	—	—	12	—	.3	.5	120	3.5	—	6.7	—	500	850	—

Food																										
Wendy's-Bkd Potato w/Bacon and Cheese	1	Each	380.0	510	75	17	17	4	3	8	—	15	—	100	—	36	—	.2	—	.5	80	2.5	—	6.7	—	1370	1170	—
Wendy's-Bkd Potato w/Broccoli and Cheese	1	Each	411.0	450	77	9	14	2	3	7	—	0	—	200	—	60	—	.1	—	.3	80	2.5	—	4.8	—	1310	450	—
Wendy's-Chili, Large	1	Each	340.0	290	31	28	9	4	2	1	—	60	—	150	—	12	—	.2	—	.2	80	4.5	—	2.9	—	660	1000	—
Wendy's-French Fries, Biggie	1	Each	170.0	450	62	6	22	5	15	1	—	0	—	—	—	12	—	.1	—	.3	16	.8	—	3.8	—	950	280	—
White Castle-Cheeseburger Sandwich	1	Each	64.8	200	16	8	11	—	—	3	—	—	—	—	—	—	—	—	—	—	—	—	—	—	—	—	361	—
White Castle-Hamburger Sandwich	1	Each	58.5	161	15	6	8	—	—	2	—	—	—	—	—	—	—	—	—	—	—	—	—	—	—	—	266	—
White Castle-Onion Rings	1	Each	60.2	245	27	3	13	—	—	3	—	—	—	—	—	—	—	—	—	—	—	—	—	—	—	—	566	—
White Castle-Sausage and Egg Sandwich	1	Each	96.3	322	16	13	22	—	—	3	—	—	—	—	—	—	—	—	—	—	—	—	—	—	—	—	698	—

Labeling: What's Old and What's New

To improve communication between producers and consumers, we must all use the same "dictionary"—supplied by the Food and Drug Administration (FDA). Whether these terms are used in the common format of nutrition information in the box titled "Nutrition Facts" (see opposite) or elsewhere as part of the manufacturer's product description, everyone must work from the same FDA "dictionary." Here is a sample:

Daily values (DV)

A label reference value that relates the nutrition information to a total daily diet of 2000 kcalories, which is appropriate for most women, teenage girls, and some sedentary men. The footnote indicates daily values for a 2500-kcaloric diet, which meets needs of most men, teenage boys, and active women. To help consumers determine how a food fits into a healthy diet, the following nutrients in the order given must be listed as percent of the daily value (DV%):

- Total fat
- Saturated fat
- Cholesterol
- Sodium
- Total carbohydrate
- Dietary fiber
- Vitamins A and C
- Calcium and iron

Daily reference value (DRV)

A part of the Daily Value (DV) above; a set of dietary standards for eight nutrients: total fat, saturated fat, cholesterol, total carbohydrate, dietary fiber, protein, potassium, and sodium. It does not appear on the label, since it is part of the food's Daily Value (DV).

Reference daily intake (RDI)

Part of the Daily Value (DV) above; a set of dietary standards for essential vitamins and minerals, and in some cases protein. It is based on the actual current (edition 10, 1989) Recommended Dietary Allowances (RDAs), thus replacing the old, confusing term "US RDA", which was developed by food manufacturers as an estimate based on

---

Williams SR: *Basic nutrition and diet therapy,* ed 10, St Louis, 1995, Mosby.

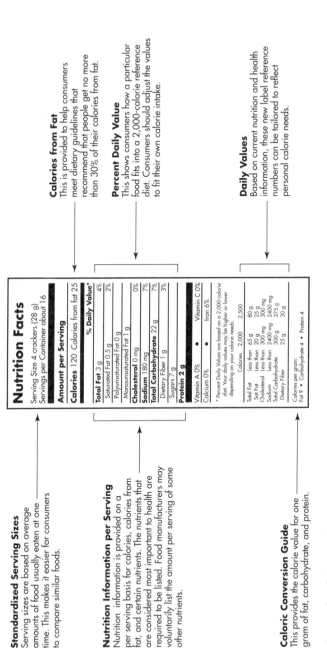

Standardized Serving Sizes
Serving sizes are based on average amounts of food usually eaten at one time. This makes it easier for consumers to compare similar foods.

Nutrition Information per Serving
Nutrition information is provided on a per serving basis for calories, calories from fat, and certain nutrients. The nutrients that are considered most important to health are required to be listed. Food manufacturers may voluntarily list the amount per serving of some other nutrients.

Caloric Conversion Guide
This provides the calorie value for one gram of fat, carbohydrate, and protein.

Calories from Fat
This is provided to help consumers meet dietary guidelines that recommend that people get no more than 30% of their calories from fat.

Percent Daily Value
This shows consumers how a particular food fits into a 2,000-calorie reference diet. Consumers should adjust the values to fit their own calorie intake.

Daily Values
Based on current nutrition and health information, these new label reference numbers can be tailored to reflect personal calorie needs.

A sample of the new food label. Most packaged food is required to carry the information presented in this example. These labels help consumers plan healthy diets. *From Food and Drug Administration: FDA backgrounder: the new food label, Dec. 10, 1992.*

old RDAs. The RDI does not appear on the label, since it is part of the Daily Value (DV).

Descriptive terms on products

The FDA has specifically defined many terms that manufacturers must follow if they wish to use the term on their product. The following are some examples:

- **Fat free.** Less than 0.5 g of fat per serving.
- **Low cholesterol.** 20 mg of cholesterol or less per serving and per 100 g; 2 g saturated fat or less per serving. Any label claim about low cholesterol is prohibited for all foods that contain more than 2 g of saturated fat per serving.
- **Light** or **Lite.** At least a one-third reduction in kcalories (40 kcal with minimum fat reduction of 3 g; if fat contributes 50% or more of total kcalories, fat content must be reduced by 50% compared with the reference food).
- **Less sodium.** At least a 25% reduction; 140 mg or less per reference amount per serving.
- **High.** 20% or more of the Daily Value (DV) per serving.
- **Reduced saturated fat.** At least 25% less saturated fat per reference amount than an appropriate reference food.
- **Lean.** Applied to meat, poultry, and seafood; less than 10 g fat, 4 g saturated fat, and 95 mg cholesterol per reference amount and 100 g for individual foods.
- **Extra lean.** Applied to meat, poultry, and seafood; less than 5 g fat, 2 g saturated fat, and 95 mg cholesterol per reference amounts and 100 g for individual foods.

Health claims

The FDA guidelines indicate that any label health claim must be supported by substantial scientific evidence and has found that several meet this test and can be used:

- Sodium and hypertension
- Calcium and osteoporosis
- Dietary fat and cancer
- Dietary cholesterol and saturated fat and coronary heart disease
- Fiber-containing grain products, fruits and vegetables and cancer
- Grain products, fruits and vegetables that contain fiber, especially soluble fiber, and coronary heart disease.
- Fruits and vegetables rich in vitamins A or C and cancer.

Definitions of FDA Food Labeling Terms

High (rich in, excellent source): contains ≥20% of recommended daily intake for the nutrient

Good source: contains 10%-19% of the daily value/serving for a desirable nutrient

More (fortified, enriched, added): contains ≥10% of daily value for protein, vitamins, minerals, dietary fiber, or dietary potassium than the reference food; may not be used as a claim on meat or poultry items

Low (little, few, low source): foods that can be eaten in reasonable amount without exceeding dietary guidelines

Low calorie: ≤40 kcal/serving

Low fat: ≤3 g/serving; low saturated fat: ≤1 g/serving and <15% of calories from saturated fat

Low cholesterol: ≤20 mg/serving

Low sodium: ≤140 mg/serving; very low sodium: ≤35 mg/serving

Free (without, no, zero): contains very small or insignificant amounts of one or more of the following: fat, saturated fat, cholesterol, sodium, sodium/salt, sugars, or calories

Light/lite: one-third fewer calories or 50% less fat; also may be used to describe texture or color (must be specified on label)

Reduced, less, fewer: food has been changed to contain at least 25% less of a nutrient or calories than the reference food

Lean: <10 g fat, <4 g saturated fat, <95 mg cholesterol/serving per 100 g of meats, poultry, seafood, or game meats

Extra lean: <5 g fat, <2 g saturated fat, <95 mg cholesterol per 100 g of meats, poultry, seafood, or game meats

Fresh: raw or unprocessed food never frozen, heated, or preserved (milk and bread excepted)

Fresh frozen: allowed on foods that have been quickly frozen while fresh

Modified from American Dietetic Association: *Understanding food labels* [pamphlet], Chicago, 1993, The Association. In Phipps WJ, et al: *Medical-surgical nursing: concepts and clinical practice,* ed 5, St Louis, 1995, Mosby.

Selected Examples of Bacterial Foodborne Disease

Foodborne disease	Causative organisms (genus and species)	Food source	Symptoms and course
Bacterial food infections			
Escherichia coli O157:H7 infection	*Escherichia* E. coli O157:H7	Undercooked meat, mainly ground beef	Severe cramps, nausea, vomiting; bloody and nonbloody diarrhea; acute renal failure. Appears 1-8 days after eating, typically lasts 3-4 days; sometimes fatal.
Salmonellosis	*Salmonella* S. typhi S. paratyphi	Milk, custards, egg dishes, salad dressings, sandwich fillings, polluted shellfish	Mild to severe diarrhea, cramps, vomiting. Appears 12-24 hours or more after eating; lasts 1-7 days.
Shigellosis	*Shigella* S. dysenteriae	Milk and milk products, seafood, salads	Mild diarrhea to fatal dysentery (especially in young children). Appears 7-36 hours after eating; lasts 3-14 days.
Listeriosis	*Listeria* L. monocytogenes	Soft cheese, poultry, seafood, raw milk, meat products (paté)	Severe diarrhea, fever, headache, pneumonia, meningitis, endocarditis. Symptoms begin after 3-21 days.

Bacterial food poisoning

	Organism	Food involved	Symptoms
Staphylococcal	*Staphylococcus S. aureus*	Custards, cream fillings, processed meats, ham, cheese, ice cream, potato salad, sauces, casseroles	Severe abdominal pain, cramps, vomiting, diarrhea, perspiration, headache, fever, prostration. Appears suddenly 1-6 hours after eating; symptoms subside generally within 24 hours.
Clostridial Perfringens enteritis	*Clostridium C. perfringens*	Cooked meats, meat dishes held at warm or room temperature	Mild diarrhea, vomiting. Appears 8-24 hours after eating; lasts a day or less.
Botulism	*C. botulinum*	Improperly home-canned foods; smoked and salted fish, ham, sausage, shellfish	Symptoms range from mild discomfort to death within 24 hours; initial nausea, vomiting, weakness, dizziness, progressing to motor and sometimes fatal breathing paralysis.

Williams SR: *Nutrition and diet therapy*, ed 8, St Louis, 1997, Mosby.

Food Safety

Food contaminated with bacteria, viruses, or parasites can cause illness. The following tips are designed to help you guard against contaminated food. **Wash hands with soap before and after handling food.** Most food contamination happens at home.

Commercially packaged food

The US government has strict standards aimed at protecting the consumer from improperly canned and packaged foods. Even so, contaminated foods occasionally find their way to the grocery shelves. Observe the following guidelines and remember: **If in doubt, throw it out! Do not even taste a small amount.**

- Do not buy containers that appear to have been opened or have broken seals on jar lids.
- Do not buy or use cans that have bulging ends, leaks, or rust.
- Do not use food that shows spoilage, such as mold, an off-color, or an off-odor. A can that spurts liquid when opened is unsafe.
- Be sure to refrigerate a jar after opening it if the label so instructs.

Home-canned foods

Home canning requires following very precise methods of preparing the food, using the proper kind of jars, and sealing the jars carefully. Nonacid foods are especially susceptible to the bacteria responsible for botulism. (Note: Nonacid foods include all vegetables, tomatoes, meat, poultry, and fish.) Pressure canning using 10 pounds of pressure at 240° F is the only method recommended for nonacid foods. The botulism bacteria does not cause an odor, a change in color or texture, or the formation of gas. **Never taste home-canned nonacid food before first cooking!** To cook nonacid home-canned foods, vigorously boil in an uncovered pot (vegetables for 3 to 5 minutes; meat, poultry, and fish for 10 minutes).

Meat and poultry

Salmonella and other bacteria may be present in raw meat and poultry. Any kitchen equipment that comes in contact with raw meat or poultry should be washed thoroughly before it is used with other foods.

- Use hot water and detergent to wash utensils that have touched raw meat or poultry before using the equipment with other food.

- When cutting raw meat or poultry, use a nonporous cutting board (plastic, marble, or glass) and wash it immediately.
- Keep meat refrigerated at 35° F to 40° F. Ground meats are very perishable and should be cooked (or frozen) within 24 hours after purchase. Roasts will keep for 3 or 4 days without freezing. Poultry should be eaten within 2 days. Before cooking, check the odor of meats and poultry. Do not risk it if there is an unpleasant smell. Wash hands between handling raw meat and other foods, and **cook** all meat.

Pork

Pork may contain a parasite that causes trichinosis. The only way to destroy the parasite is to cook pork thoroughly until the meat is white or grayish all the way through or registers 137° F on a meat thermometer.

Eggs

Eggs may be infected with *Salmonella* or other bacteria. Never use an egg that has an unpleasant odor or that has a cracked shell. Eat only eggs that have been cooked. Refrigerate eggs and prepared food that contain eggs (mayonnaise and other salad dressings) until ready to serve.

Milk and dairy products

Milk and other dairy products made from raw (unpasteurized) milk have caused tuberculosis. Buy only pasteurized dairy products.

Fish and shellfish

Because of environmental pollution, hepatitis has been caused by eating raw oysters, and several types of bacterial food poisoning can occur from eating raw shellfish or fish. Avoid eating any uncooked fish and shellfish.

Travel outside the United States

Travelers to developing countries should not drink local water or eat uncooked vegetables. Fruits that require peeling are safe, but peel them yourself. Do not eat food from street vendors.

ACQUIRED IMMUNE DEFICIENCY SYNDROME (AIDS)

Risk of Exposure to Human Immunodeficiency Virus (HIV) Related to Behaviors and Practice

Risk/levels of safety	Sexual contact	Injecting drug use	Perinatal exposure
Absolutely safe	Abstinence Mutually monogamous with noninfected partner	Not using injection drugs	Abstinence Sterilization
Safe	Noninsertive sexual practices Dry kissing Masturbation on intact skin Oral sex with a condom External "water sports" Touching Fantasy	Exchanging needles and syringes for sterile supplies Using sterilized injection paraphernalia	Abortion
Possibly safe	Insertive sexual practices with the use of condoms	Not sharing equipment Cleaning injection paraphernalia with full-strength bleach	Use of hormonal contraceptives, intrauterine devices Use of condoms Pregnancy
Risky	Wet kissing Fellatio, cunnilingus without a latex barrier Masturbation on broken skin	Cleaning equipment with other disinfectants, water	
Dangerous	Intercourse without a condom Internal "water sports" Fisting Rimming	Sharing equipment Use of "shooting galleries" Sex under the influence of drugs or alcohol	Pregnancy Breast-feeding

From Ungvarski PJ, Flaskerud JH: *HIV/AIDS: a guide to primary care management,* ed 4, Philadelphia, 1999, WB Saunders.

Clinical Categories for Children With HIV Infection

Category N: not symptomatic

Children who have no signs or symptoms considered to be the result of HIV infection or who have only *one* of the conditions listed in Category A

Category A: mildly symptomatic

Children with *two* or more of the following conditions but none of the conditions listed in Category B or C:

Lymphadenopathy	Dermatitis
Hepatomegaly	Parotitis
Splenomegaly	Recurrent or persistent upper respiratory infection, sinusitis, or otitis media

Category B: moderately symptomatic

Children who have symptomatic conditions other than those listed for Category A or C that are attributed to HIV infection. Examples of conditions in Category B include but are not limited to:

Anemia ($<$8 g/dL, neutropenia ($<$1000/mm^3), or thrombocytopenia ($<$100,000/mm^3) persisting $\geq$30 days

Bacterial meningitis, pneumonia, or sepsis (single episode)

Candidiasis, oropharyngeal (thrush), persisting $>$2 months in children $>$6 months of age

Cardiomyopathy

Cytomegalovirus infection, with onset before 1 month of age

Diarrhea, recurrent or chronic

Hepatitis

Herpes simplex virus (HSV) stomatitis, recurrent (more than two episodes within 1 year)

HSV bronchitis, pneumonitis, or esophagitis with onset before 1 month of age

Herpes zoster (shingles) involving at least two distinct episodes or more than one dermatome

Leiomyosarcoma

Lymphoid interstitial pneumonia (LIP) or pulmonary lymphoid hyperplasia complex

Data from Centers for Disease Control and Prevention: 1994 revised classification system for human immunodeficiency virus infection in children less than 13 years of age, *MMWR*, 43(RR-12): 1-19, 1994.

Nephropathy
Nocardiosis
Persistent fever (lasting >1 month)
Toxoplasmosis, onset before 1 month of age
Varicella, disseminated (complicated chickenpox)

Category C: severely symptomatic
Children who have any condition listed in the 1987 surveillance case definition for acquired immunodeficiency syndrome, with the exception of LIP (which is a Category B condition)

What are the Symptoms of HIV?

The only way to determine for sure whether one is infected is to be tested for HIV infection. You cannot rely on symptoms to know whether or not someone is infected with HIV. Many people who are infected with HIV do not have any symptoms at all for many years.

The following **may be** warning signs of infection with HIV:

- Rapid weight loss
- Dry cough
- Recurring fever or profuse night sweats
- Profound and unexplained fatigue
- Swollen lymph glands in the armpits, groin, or neck
- Diarrhea that lasts for more than a week
- White spots or unusual blemishes on the tongue, in the mouth, or in the throat
- Pneumonia
- Red, brown, pink, or purplish blotches on or under the skin or inside the mouth, nose, or eyelids
- Memory loss, depression, and other neurologic disorders

Similarly, you cannot rely on symptoms to establish that a person has AIDS. **The symptoms of AIDS are similar to the symptoms of many other illnesses.** AIDS is a medical diagnosis made by a doctor based on specific criteria established by the Centers for Disease Control and Prevention (CDC).

From Centers for Disease Control and Prevention; National Center for HIV, STD, and TB Prevention. Available: http://www.cdc.gov/nchstp/hiv_aids/pubs/faq/faq5.htm.

How is HIV Passed From One Person to Another?

HIV transmission can occur when blood, semen (including pre-seminal fluid, or "pre-cum"), vaginal fluid, or breast milk from an infected person enters the body of an uninfected person.

HIV can enter the body through a vein (e.g., injection drug use), the anus or rectum, the vagina, the penis, the mouth, other mucous membranes (e.g., eyes or inside of the nose), or cuts and sores. Intact, healthy skin is an excellent barrier against HIV and other viruses and bacteria.

These are the most common ways that HIV is transmitted from one person to another:

- by having sexual intercourse (anal, vaginal, or oral sex) with an HIV-infected person
- by sharing needles or injection equipment with an injection drug user who is infected with HIV
- from HIV-infected women to babies before or during birth, or through breastfeeding after birth

HIV also can be transmitted through transfusions of infected blood or blood clotting factors. However, since 1985, all donated blood in the United States has been tested for HIV. Therefore, the risk of infection through transfusion of blood or blood products is extremely low. The US blood supply is considered to be among the safest in the world.

From Centers for Disease Control and Prevention; National Center for HIV, STD, and TB Prevention. Available: http://www.cdc.gov/nchstp/hiv_aids/pubs/faq/faq16.htm.

Lifestyle Recommendations

In 1985, the Public Health Service published several lifestyle recommendations designed to reduce the risk of contracting AIDS. The recommendations were as follows:

1. Do not have sexual contact with persons known to have or suspected of having AIDS.
2. Do not have sex with multiple partners.
3. Do not use intravenous (IV) drugs.

From U.S. Public Health Service, 1985.

4. Do not have sex with people who are known to inject drugs.
5. Do not use inhalant nitrites. They may play a role in regard to Kaposi's sarcoma.
6. Avoid anal intercourse.
7. Protect yourself and your partner during sexual intercourse by using condoms, avoiding oral-genital contact and open mouth kissing, and avoiding contact with body fluids (semen, blood, urine, and feces).

Guidelines for Safer Sex

Five steps to a healthier and safer sex life

1. *Use a condom every time.*

   - Condoms offer the best protection against sexually transmitted diseases (STDs) for people having sexual intercourse.

> **Condoms Work!** In a 1987-1991 study of couples in which one partner had HIV, all 123 couples who used condoms every time for 4 years prevented transmission of HIV. In 122 couples who did not use condoms every time, 12 partners became infected.
>
> A similar 1993 study showed that using condoms every time prevented HIV transmission for all but two of 171 women with male partners with HIV. However, eight out of 55 women whose partners didn't use condoms every time became infected.

2. Talk with your partners before the heat of passion, *and use a condom every time.*

   - Partners should care about each other and be interested in one another's pleasure, comfort, and health.
   - Be open. Let your partner know your health concerns and sexual health history, and encourage your partner to be open, too.
   - Be direct. Talk about your sexual needs and expectations.
   - Be persistent. Don't let your partner remain silent on these issues.

3. Keep medically fit *and use a condom every time.*

   - Have a checkup for STDs every year.

---

*From Planned Parenthood Federation of America, Inc: *Sex—safer and satisfying: a guide for the sexually active,* New York, 1996, The Federation.

- Protect your immune system. Eat well, get enough rest, and limit your use of alcohol, tobacco, and other drugs.

4. If you think you or your partner has an STD, do the following:

   - See a clinician for testing, diagnosis, and treatment.
   - Find out if your partner(s) needs to be examined and treated too.
   - Use all the medication that is prescribed since symptoms often disappear before an infection is cured.
   - Do not take anyone else's medicine, and do not share your own.
   - Do not have sex until your infection is under control, *then use a condom every time.*

5. Stay in charge, *and use a condom every time.*

   - Alcohol and other drugs weaken good judgment and self-control. Don't let them jeopardize your self-control.

How to use condoms

Don't tear the condom while unwrapping it. Don't use one that's brittle, stiff, or sticky.

Use plenty of water-based lubricant. It helps prevent rips and tears, and it increases sensitivity. Oil-based lubricants destroy latex condoms.

Use a condom only once. Have a good supply on hand.
Practice makes perfect.

- Put a drop or two of lubricant inside the condom.
- Place the rolled condom over the tip of the hard penis.
- Leave a half-inch space at the tip to collect semen.
- If uncircumcised, pull back the foreskin before rolling on the condom.
- Pinch the air out of the tip with one hand. Friction against air bubbles causes most condom breaks.
- Unroll the condom over the penis with the other hand.
- Unroll it all the way down to the base of the penis.
- Smooth out any air bubbles.
- Lubricate the outside of the condom.

Enjoy.

- Pull out before the penis softens.
- Don't spill the semen. Hold the condom against the base of the penis while pulling out.

HIV Risk Comparisons

Here are some common sexual behaviors grouped according to relative risk for the transmission of HIV:

Very low risk
No reported cases due to the following behaviors:

- Masturbation/mutual masturbation
- Touching/massage
- Erotic massage/body rubbing
- Kissing/deep kissing
- Oral sex on a man with a condom
- Oral sex on a woman with a dental dam, plastic wrap, or cut-open condom

(Don't worry about getting vaginal secretions, menstrual flow, urine, or semen on unbroken skin away from the vulva.)

Low risk
Rare reported cases due to the following behaviors:

- Oral sex
- Vaginal intercourse with a condom or vaginal pouch
- Anal intercourse with a condom or vaginal pouch

(Try not to get semen or blood into the mouth or on broken skin.)

High risk
Millions of reported cases due to the following behaviors:

- Vaginal intercourse without a condom
- Anal intercourse without a condom

Some of the drugs that encourage taking risks with sex
- Alcohol
- Poppers
- Cocaine
- Ecstasy
- Speed
- Marijuana
- Crack cocaine

From Planned Parenthood Federation of America, Inc: *The condom,* New York, 1995, The Federation.

Some of the feelings that encourage taking risks with sex

- Desire to be swept away
- Fear of losing a partner
- Insecurity
- Embarrassment
- Anger
- Shame
- Low self-esteem
- Need to be loved

Practicing Safer Sex

What does it mean to practice "safer sex"?

The term "safer sex" refers to the practice of protecting yourself against sexually transmitted diseases (STDs), sometimes referred to as venereal disease (VD). There are at least 50 different kinds of STDs, some of them even life-threatening. You can catch an STD by having sex with someone who is infected.

What if I have sex without actually having intercourse?

You can still get an STD without having vaginal intercourse or penetration. STDs are spread by having vaginal, oral, or anal sex with an infected person. STD-causing germs can pass from one person to another through body fluids, such as semen, vaginal fluid, saliva, and blood; genital warts and herpes are STDs that are spread by direct contact with a wart or blister.

No one I date looks to me as if they could have an STD. They look really healthy.

You can't tell if a person has an STD just by appearance. In fact, some people with STDs have no signs at all and may not even know they are infected. Still, some signs to look for in your partner are a heavy discharge, rash, sore, or redness near your partner's sex organs. If you see any of these, don't have sex or be sure to use a condom.

How can I tell if I might have an STD?

You may have an STD if you experience the following: burning or pain when urinating; sores, bumps, or blisters near the genitals or mouth; swelling around the genitals; fever, chills, night sweats, or swollen

---

glands; or tiredness, vomiting, diarrhea, or sore muscles. In addition, you may have any of the following: an unusual discharge or smell from the vagina; burning and itching around the vagina; pain in the lower abdomen; vaginal pain during sex; or vaginal bleeding between periods. *But don't forget, you may not have any warning signs at all. Regular medical checkups are essential to your health. If you have sex with more than one partner, routine cultures and blood tests may be needed.*

I think I have an STD! What should I do?
Get help right away. If you don't you may pass the STD to your partner or, if you're pregnant, to your baby. In fact, without treatment an STD may make it impossible for you to have a baby at all. You may also develop brain damage, blindness, cancer, heart disease, or arthritis. In some cases you can even die. So go to a doctor or clinic right away.

If your healthcare provider determines that you do have an STD, tell your partner or partners to get tested too. Take all of your medication; don't stop just because all your symptoms go away. Do not have sex until you have received full treatment. The disease could still be present in your body. Finally, keep all your appointments, and always use a condom and spermicide when you have sex.

What are the signs of STDs?
There are many different kinds of STDs, and some of them have similar symptoms. You should never attempt to make a diagnosis on your own. The nurse can give you a list with general descriptions of a few of the most common STDs.

How can I reduce my chances of contracting an STD?
Remember, the more sexual partners you have, the greater your risk. Naturally, the best way to reduce your risk is by not having sex or by having sex with one mutually faithful, uninfected partner, or by using a latex condom and spermicide with nonoxynol 9 during sex. Some STDs may be avoided by placing spermicide in the vagina before having sex, because it kills sperm and some STD germs. It helps to urinate and wash after sex (but do not douche, because douching may actually force germs higher up into the body). Avoid having sex with someone who uses intravenous drugs or engages in anal sex. Don't engage in oral, anal, or vaginal sex with an infected person. If you think you may be at risk for AIDS or an STD, seek medical help immediately. Use a new condom each time you have sexual intercourse. *Recent research indicates that the prevention of HIV transmission and developing AIDS is not 100% effective when using condoms as a barrier against this infection.*

What if the condom breaks? What should we do?

If a condom breaks, do not douche. Insert more spermicide into the vagina right away. Men should wash their genitals immediately. Go to a doctor or clinic for an STD examination as soon as possible.

Centers for Disease Control and Prevention Classification System for HIV-Infected Clients

Group	Classification and description
I	Acute HIV infection: Clients with transient signs and symptoms of HIV infection.
II	Asymptomatic HIV infection: Clients without previous signs or symptoms leading to classification in Group III or IV.
III	Persistent generalized lymphadenopathy (PGL): Clients with lymph nodes >1 cm in diameter that persisted for longer than 3 months at two or more extrainguinal sites.
IV	Other HIV disease: *Subgroup A (constitutional disease):* clients with one or more of the following: fever for longer than 1 month, involuntary weight loss >10%, diarrhea for longer than 1 month. *Subgroup B (neurologic disease):* clients with dementia, myelopathy, or peripheral neuropathy. *Subgroup C (secondary infectious disease):* clients diagnosed with infectious disease from the following categories: *Category C-1:* 1 of 12 specified diseases listed in the CDC surveillance definition of AIDS: *Pneumocystis carinii* pneumonia, chronic cryptosporidiosis, toxoplasmosis, extraintestinal strongyloidiasis, isosporiasis, candidiasis (esophageal, bronchial, or pulmonary), cryptococcosis, histoplasmosis, mycobacterial infection with *Mycobacterium avium* complex or *M. kansasii,* cytomegalovirus infection, chronic mucocutaneous or disseminated herpes simplex virus infection, and progressive multifocal leukoencephalopathy. *Category C-2:* symptomatic or invasive disease with oral, hairy leukoplakia, multidermatomal herpes zoster, recurrennt *Salmonella* bacteremia, nocardiosis, tuberculosis, or oral candidiasis.

Adapted from Centers for Disease Control and Prevention: Classification system for human T-lymphotropic virus type III/lymphadenopathy-associated virus infections, *MMWR* 35:334, 1986, and Raiten DJ: Nutrition and HIV infection: a review and evaluation of the extant knowledge of the relationship between nutrition and HIV infection, *Nutr Clin Prac* 6(3):1S, 1992. In Williams SR: *Nutrition and diet therapy,* ed 8, St Louis, 1997, Mosby. *Continued*

Centers for Disease Control and Prevention Classification System for HIV-Infected Clients—cont'd

Group	Classification and description
	Subgroup D (secondary cancers): clients diagnosed with cancers known to be associated with HIV infection: Kaposi's sarcoma, non-Hodgkin's lymphoma (small, noncleaved lymphoma or immunoblastic sarcoma), or primary lymphoma of the brain.
	Subgroup E (other conditions in HIV infection): clients exhibiting clinical findings which may be due to HIV disease: chronic lymphoid interstitial pneumonitis, constitutional symptoms not meeting Subgroup IV-A, clients with infectious diseases not meeting Subgroup IV-C, and clients with neoplasms not meeting subgroup IV-D.

Medical Treatment of HIV-Infected Clients

Evaluation for antiretroviral therapy and prophylaxis for *Pneumocystis carinii* pneumonia (PCP) by monitoring T-helper lymphocyte count and clinical status.

T-cell count <500 is an indication for zidovudine

T-cell count <200 is an indication for PCP prophylaxis

History of tuberculin reactivity, tuberculosis (TB) exposure, or chest x-ray compatible with old TB should lead to evaluation for prophylaxis

Education to improve general health knowledge and to avoid possible sources of infection.

Discussion of applicable research protocols.

Regular follow-ups to alert physician to earliest signs of AIDS-related complications.

Consideration of antiretroviral therapy failure in client on prolonged treatment who develops new or recurrent symptoms and to rule out AIDS-related complications.

Adapted from Gold JWM: HIV-1 infection: diagnosis and management, *Med Clin North Am* 76(1):1, 1992. In Williams SR: *Nutrition and diet therapy,* ed 7, St Louis, 1993, Mosby.

Toxicities of Dideoxynucleoside Drugs

AZT (azidothymidine, zidovudine, 3′-azido-2′,3′-dideoxythymidline)

Bone marrow suppression; anemia with increased mean corpuscular volume; leukopenia and thrombocytopenia often dose-limiting
Nausea and vomiting
Headache
Malaise, fatigue, fever
Myalgias
Seizures (rare, but reported to be fatal)
Confusion, tremulousness
Encephalopathy resembling Wernicke's encephalopathy
Bluish pigmentation of finger and toenails
Hepatic transaminase elevation
Stevens-Johnson syndrome

ddI (dideoxyinosine, 2′,3′-dideoxyinosine)

Painful peripheral neuropathy
Sporadic pancreatitis (may be fatal)
Hyperamylasemia, hypertriglyceridemia
Headache
Insomnia, restlessness
Hepatic transaminase elevations (occasional hepatitis)
Hyperuricemia (with high doses)

ddC (dideoxycytidine, 2′,3′-dideoxycytidine)

Painful peripheral neuropathy
Aphthous stomatitis
Maculopapular rash (occasionally pseudovesicular)
Fevers
Arthralgias, edema
Thrombocytopenia

d4T (2′,3′-dideoxythymidinene, 2′,3′-dideoxy-2′,3′-didehydrothymidine)

Painful peripheral neuropathy
Anemia
Hepatic transaminase elevations

Adapted from Pluda JM, et al: Hematologic effects of AIDS therapies, *Hematol Oncol Clin North Am* 5(2):229, 1991. In Williams SR: *Nutrition and diet therapy,* ed 7, St Louis, 1993, Mosby.

The ABCDs of Nutrition Assessment in AIDS

Biochemical indices
- Serum proteins: albumin, prealbumin, transferrin
- Liver function test (evaluate liver function)
- Blood urea nitrogen, serum electrolytes (evaluate renal function)
- Urinary urea nitrogen excretion over 24 hours (nitrogen balance)
- Creatinine height index
- Complete blood cell count (evaluate for anemia)
- Fasting glucose (evaluate for hyperglycemia or hypoglycemia)

Clinical observations
- General signs of nutritional status
- Drug effects

Diet evaluation
- Usual intake, current intake, restrictions, modifications (use both 24-hour recall and food diaries)
- Nutrition supplements, vitamin-mineral supplements
- Food allergies, intolerances
- Activity level (general kcal expended per day)
- Support system (caregivers to help with nutrition care plan)

Environmental, behavioral, and psychologic assessment
- Living situation, personal support
- Food environment, types of meals, eating assistance needed

Financial assessment
- Medical insurance
- Income, financial support through care givers
- Current medical and other expenses
- Ability to afford food, enteral supplements, added vitamins-minerals

From Williams SR: *Nutrition and diet therapy,* ed 7, St Louis, 1993, Mosby.

Planning Nutrition Care for Clients with AIDS

Type of problem	Possible causes	Patient care plan considerations
Food intake	Anorexia Drug, food interaction HIV, other infection Taste alteration Food intolerances, allergies Lack of access or ability to prepare food Depression	Patient, caregiver roles Motivation, patient decision-making Education, counseling Resource materials Nutrition supplements Vitamin-mineral supplements Drug or food reactions Special enteral or parenteral nutrition support Monitoring, adjustments as needed
Nutrient absorption	HIV-related infections or cancers Diminished gastric HCL secretion Altered mucosal absorbing surface Organ involvement: liver, pancreas, gallbladder, kidney Drug or nutrient interaction	Treatment of underlying disease or disorder Pancreatic enzymes supplement Drug or nutrient reactions Special enteral-parenteral nutrition support, appropriate formula design Monitoring, adjustments as needed
Altered metabolism, excretion	HIV infection Associated infections, diseases Drug or nutrient interactions Altered hormonal function Organ dysfunction	Review of drug dose, schedule Modification of diet, meal pattern Treatment of infection, symptoms Review of diet nutrients, increase or decrease Special enteral-parenteral nutrition support, appropriate formula design Monitoring, adjustments as needed

Adapted from Newman CF: *Practical guide for improving nutritional status in HIV-related disease,* University of California, Davis Medical School Fifth Annual Conference on Clinical Nutrition, Nutrition in the Treatment of Serious Medical Problems, Feb 28-29, 1992. In Williams SR: *Nutrition and diet therapy,* ed 7, St Louis, 1993, Mosby.

PREGNANCY THROUGH CHILDHOOD CARE

Prenatal, postnatal, and maternal-child care are important components of public/community health nursing. Through education, the nurse can promote and improve the health of pregnant women and infants. The tools on the following pages will assist in this endeavor.

PREGNANCY

Normal Discomforts Experienced during Pregnancy

Discomfort	Known or probable cause	Nursing suggestions for relief
Backache	Changes in posture, such as increased lumbar curve Excessive bending and lifting	Practice good posture Perform pelvic rocking Wear comfortable, low-heeled shoes Squat to lift Avoid prolonged sitting Sleep on firm mattress
Constipation	Pressure of enlarged uterus Slowed peristalsis caused by progesterone Side effect of iron supplement	Increase fluid intake, especially juices Eat high-fiber foods Exercise Drink warm liquids in morning Only if other methods fail, use mild laxative, stool softener, or glycerine suppository
Fatigue	Decreased metabolic rate in early pregnancy	Get full night's sleep Nap or rest during day Share work load when possible "Usually better after first trimester"
Hemorrhoids	Constipation Pressure of enlarged uterus	Relieve constipation with measures just listed Take sitz baths

From Edelman CL, Mandle CL: *Health promotion throughout the lifespan,* ed 4, St Louis, 1998, Mosby.

Discomfort	Known or probable cause	Nursing suggestions for relief
		Use ice pack or witch hazel for local relief
		Reinsert hemorrhoid; do perineal tightening exercises
		Local preparation for analgesia
Leg cramps	Pressure of large uterus on blood vessels	Take calcium supplement
	Fatigue or chilling	Practice gentle, steady stretch to relieve cramp
	Lack of calcium	Never massage cramping muscle
	Sudden stretching or over-extension of the foot	Avoid toe-pointing when exercising
	Excessive phosphorus in diet	
Leukorrhea (increased vaginal discharge)	Increased vascularity of cervix and vagina	Wear cotton-crotched panties
		Wash genital area more frequently
		If infection develops, have physician treat
		Do not douche
Nausea and vomiting (may occur any time of day)	Increase in estrogen and progesterone levels	Eat small, frequent meals
	Change (especially lowering) of blood glucose levels	Eat dry cracker before getting up in morning
		Snack at bedtime
		Usually stops after first trimester
Urinary frequency (day and night)	Pressure of uterus on bladder in first and third trimesters	(Explanation of why frequency is occurring)
	Nocturia caused by increased venous return from extremities when lying down	If interfering with sleep, reduce fluids in evening
		Rest during day
Varicosities	Increased vascularity of pelvic organs	Avoid knee socks and tight elastic on underwear
	Venous return slowed by pressure of uterus	Elevate feet for 10 to 15 minutes several times a day
	Familial tendency	Avoid long periods of standing
	Progesterone effect in smooth muscles	Avoid crossing legs when sitting
		Wear support stockings

Prenatal High-Risk Factors

Specific Pregnancy Problems/Related Risk Factors

Preterm labor
Age less than 16 or more than 35 years
Low socioeconomic status
Maternal weight below 50 kg (110 lb)
Poor nutrition
Previous preterm birth
Incompetent cervix
Uterine anomalies
Smoking
Drug addiction and alcohol abuse
Pyelonephritis, pneumonia
Multiple gestation
Anemia
Abnormal fetal presentation
Premature rupture of membranes
Placental abnormalities
Infection

Polyhydramnios
Diabetes mellitus
Multiple gestation
Fetal congenital anomalies
Isoimmunization (Rh or ABO)
Nonimmune hydrops
Abnormal fetal presentation

Intrauterine growth restriction (IUGR)
Multiple gestation
Poor nutrition
Maternal cyanotic heart disease
Chronic hypertension
Pregnancy-induced hypertension
Recurrent antepartum hemorrhage
Smoking
Maternal diabetes with vascular problems
Fetal infections
Fetal cardiovascular anomalies

From DeCherney A, Pernol M, editors: *Current obstetric and gynecologic diagnosis and treatment,* ed 8, Norwalk, Conn, 1994, Appleton & Lange.

Drug addiction and alcohol abuse
Fetal congenital anomalies
Hemoglobinopathies

Oligohydramnios
Renal agenesis (Potter's syndrome)
Prolonged rupture of membranes
Intrauterine growth retardation
Intrauterine fetal death

Postterm pregnancy
Anencephaly
Placental sulfatase deficiency
Perinatal hypoxia, acidosis
Placental insufficiency

Chromosomal abnormalities
Maternal age 35 years or more
Balanced translocation (maternal and paternal)

Factors that Place the Postpartum Woman and Neonate at High Risk

The mother
Hemorrhage
Infection
Abnormal vital signs
Traumatic labor or birth
Psychosocial factors

The infant (for admission to NICU)
High-risk category
Infants who continue with or develop signs of RDS or other respiratory distress
Asphyxiated infants (Apgar score <6 at 5 min), resuscitation required at birth
Preterm infants, dysmature infants
Infants with cyanosis or suspected cardiovascular disease, persistent cyanosis
Infants with major congenital malformations requiring surgery, chromosomal anomalies

---

Lowdermilk DL, Perry SE, Boback IM: *Maternity nursing,* ed 5, St Louis, 1999, Mosby.

Infants with convulsions, sepsis, hemorrhagic diathesis, or shock
Meconium aspiration syndrome
CNS depression for more than 24 hr
Hypoglycemia
Hypocalcemia
Hyperbilirubinemia

Moderate risk

Dysmaturity
Prematurity (weight between 2,000 and 2,500 g)
Apgar score <5 at 1 min
Feeding problems
Multifetal birth
Transient tachypnea
Hypomagnesemia or hypermagnesemia
Hypoparathyroidism
Failure to gain weight
Jitteriness or hyperactivity
Cardiac anomalies not requiring immediate catheterization
Heart murmur
Anemia
CNS depression for less than 24 hr

CNS, Central nervous system; *NICU*, neonatal intensive care unit; *RDS*, respiratory distress syndrome.

Categories of High-Risk Factors

Biophysical factors

1. *Genetic considerations.* Genetic factors may interfere with normal fetal or neonatal development, result in congenital anomalies, or create difficulties for the mother. These factors include defective genes, transmissible inherited disorders and chromosome anomalies, multiple pregnancy, large fetal size, and ABO incompatibility.

2. *Nutritional status.* Adequate nutrition, without which fetal growth and development cannot proceed normally, is one of the most important determinants of pregnancy outcome. Conditions that influence nutritional status include young age; three pregnancies in the previous 2 years; tobacco, alcohol, or drug use; inadequate dietary intake because of chronic illness or food fads; inadequate or excessive weight gain; and hematocrit value less than 33%.

3. *Medical and obstetric disorders.* Complications of current and past pregnancies, obstetric-related illnesses, and pregnancy losses put the patient at risk.

Psychosocial factors

1. *Smoking.* A strong, consistent, causal relationship has been established between maternal smoking and reduced birth weight. Risks include low–birth-weight infants, higher neonatal mortality rates, increased spontaneous abortions, and increased incidence of premature rupture of membranes. These risks are aggravated by low socioeconomic status, poor nutritional status, and concurrent use of alcohol.

2. *Caffeine.* Birth defects in humans have not been related to caffeine consumption. High intake (three or more cups of coffee per day) has been related to a slight decrease in birth weight.

3. *Alcohol.* Although its exact effects in pregnancy have not been quantified and its mode of action is largely unexplained, alcohol exerts adverse effects on the fetus, resulting in fetal alcohol syndrome, fetal alcohol effects, learning disabilities, and hyperactivity.

4. *Drugs.* The developing fetus may be adversely affected by drugs through several mechanisms. They can be teratogenic, cause metabolic disturbances, produce chemical effects, or cause depression or alteration of central nervous system function. This category includes medications prescribed by a healthcare provider or bought over the counter, as well as commonly abused drugs such as heroin, cocaine, and marijuana.

5. *Psychologic status.* Childbearing triggers profound and complex physiologic, psychologic, and social changes, with evidence to suggest a relationship between emotional distress and birth complications. This risk factor includes conditions such as specific intrapsychic disturbances and addictive lifestyles; a history of child or spouse abuse; inadequate support systems; family disruption or dissolution; maternal role changes or conflicts; noncompliance with cultural norms; unsafe cultural, ethnic, or religious practices; and situational crises.

Sociodemographic factors

1. *Low income.* Poverty underlies many other risk factors and leads to inadequate financial resources for food and prenatal care, poor general health, increased risk of medical complications of pregnancy, and greater prevalence of adverse environmental influences.

2. *Lack of prenatal care.* Failure to diagnose and treat complications early is a major risk factor arising from financial barriers or lack of access to care; depersonalization of the system, resulting in long

waits, routine visits, variability in healthcare personnel, and unpleasant physical surroundings; lack of understanding of the need for early and continued care or cultural beliefs that do not support this need; and fear of the healthcare system and its providers.

3. *Age.* Women at both ends of the childbearing age spectrum have a higher incidence of poor outcomes; however, age may not be a risk factor in all cases. Both physiologic and psychologic risks should be evaluated.

   Adolescents—More complications are seen in young mothers (less than 15 years old), who have a 60% higher mortality rate than those over age 20, and in pregnancies occurring less than 3 years after menarche. Complications include anemia, pregnancy-induced hypertension (PIH), prolonged labor, and contracted pelvis and cephalopelvic disproportion. Long-term social implications of early motherhood are lower educational status, lower income, increased dependence on government support programs, higher divorce rates, and higher parity.

   Mature mothers—The risks to older mothers are not from age alone but from other considerations such as number and spacing of previous pregnancies; genetic disposition of the parents; and medical history, lifestyle, nutrition, and prenatal care. The increased likelihood of chronic diseases and complications that arise from more invasive medical management of a pregnancy and labor combined with demographic characteristics put an older woman at risk. Medical conditions more likely to be experienced by mature women include hypertension and PIH, diabetes, extended labor, cesarean birth, placenta previa, abruptio placentae, and mortality. Her fetus is at greater risk for low birth weight and macrosomia, chromosomal abnormalities, congenital malformations, and neonatal mortality.

4. *Parity.* The number of previous pregnancies is a risk factor that is associated with age and includes all first pregnancies, especially a first pregnancy at either end of the childbearing-age continuum. The incidence of PIH and dystocia is higher with a first birth.

5. *Marital status.* The increased mortality and morbidity rates for nonmarried women, including a greater risk for PIH, are often related to inadequate prenatal care and a younger childbearing age.

6. *Residence.* The availability and quality of prenatal care varies widely with geographic residence. Women in metropolitan areas have more prenatal visits than those in rural areas, who have fewer opportunities for specialized care and consequently a higher incidence of maternal mortality. Healthcare in the inner city, where residents are usually poorer and begin childbearing earlier and con-

tinue longer, may be of lower quality than in a more affluent neighborhood.

7. *Ethnicity.* Although ethnicity itself is not a major risk factor, race is an indicator of other sociodemographic risk factors. Nonwhite women are more than three times as likely as white women to die of pregnancy-related causes. African-American babies have the highest rates of prematurity and low birth weight, with the infant mortality rate among African-Americans being more than double than that for whites.

Environmental factors

Various environmental substances can affect fertility and fetal development, the chance of a live birth, and the child's subsequent mental and physical development. Environmental influences include infections; radiation; chemicals such as pesticides, therapeutic drugs, illicit drugs, industrial pollutants, cigarette smoke; stress; and diet. Paternal exposure to mutagenic agents in the workplace has been associated with an increased risk of spontaneous abortion.

Risk Factors Affecting Pregnancy

1. Low socioeconomic, educational status (influencing especially nutrition, prenatal care supervision, and compliance)
2. Little or no prenatal care
3. Maternal age younger than 18 or older than 35 years
4. More than four pregnancies (especially if older than 35)
5. Conception within 2 months of last delivery
6. Living at high altitude
7. The presence of coincidental maternal disease or significant health problems involving the following:
   a. Cardiovascular disease
   b. Renal disease
   c. Diabetes mellitus
   d. Tuberculosis or other pulmonary disease
   e. Herpes simplex, syphilis, viral infections
   f. Hereditary anomaly or possible carrier state (e.g., sickle cell anemia, myelomeningocele, cystic fibrosis, osteogenesis imperfecta)

From Novak JC, Broom BL: *Ingalls and Salerno's maternal and child health nursing,* ed 9, St Louis, 1999, Mosby.

g. Use of drugs: alcohol, nicotine, and street drugs

h. Ingestion of fetotoxic medication, exposure to radiation or toxic chemicals

i. Obesity (more than 20% greater than standard weight for height)

8. Previous obstetric complications that may recur, such as the following:

a. Preeclampsia-eclampsia (pregnancy-induced hypertension)

b. Severe anemia, clotting problems, intrapartum or postpartum hemorrhage

c. Cephalopelvic disproportion

9. Previous poor fetal outcome (repetitive fetal loss, stillbirth)

10. Deviations in the current pregnancy such as the following:

a. Twinning or other multiple pregnancies

b. Premature or small-for-date fetus

c. Postmature fetus (more than 42 weeks)

d. Breech presentation

e. Polyhydramnios or oligohydramnios

f. Preterm or prolonged rupture of membranes

g. Any of the complications noted in No. 8

h. Obstetric complications (e.g., placenta previa, abruptio placentae, abnormal presentation, Rh or blood group sensitization)

Assessment Focus at First Prenatal Visit and Return Visits

Focus during first prenatal visit

Existence of pregnancy

Past and present maternal health status through health history, physical examination, and laboratory data

Risk factors for childbearing and early parenting, including physical, psychologic, and sociologic factors

Signs and symptoms of pregnancy

Well-being of embryo or fetus

Psychosocial adaptation to pregnancy

From Sherwen L, Scoloveno M, Weingarten C: *Nursing care of the childbearing family,* ed 2, Norwalk, Conn., 1995, Appleton & Lange.

Cultural, socioeconomic, or other factors that influence healthcare practices
Client/family strengths and resources
Client/family educational needs

Focus during return visits
Maternal health status through updated health history, physical examination, and laboratory testing as indicated
Risk factors (new or ongoing)
Progress of pregnancy
Fetal well-being
Progression of psychosocial adaptation to pregnancy
Cultural, socioeconomic, or other factors that influence healthcare practices as pregnancy progresses
Client/family strengths and resources
Client/family educational needs

Nursing Strategies for Working With Childbearing Clients Experiencing Crisis and Grief

- Anticipate the potential for crisis and grief. For example, clients who receive news of a high-risk condition, particularly a condition requiring a change in lifestyle or having long-term implications, may be expected to experience crisis.
- Assess the event itself and its implications for the client's health and well-being.
- Assess the responses of the client and family in light of their religious and cultural backgrounds.
- Provide an atmosphere of privacy and confidentiality to encourage the client to express her feelings.
- Allow adequate time to discuss the high-risk condition and the family's feelings. Listen carefully, but do not make unrealistic promises, such as "Everything will turn out fine." Having another nurse temporarily "cover" other clients can allow the staff nurse the opportunity to talk uninterrupted with a client in crisis.
- Help clients identify physical, emotional, and behavioral responses related to crisis and grief. Reassure clients when responses are

From Sherwen L, Scoloveno M, Weingarten C: *Nursing care of the childbearing family,* ed 2, Norwalk, Conn., 1995, Appleton & Lange.

normal. Promptly enlist the assistance of mental health resources if a client's responses pose a threat to the health or safety of herself or others.

- Ensure that the client receives support in coping with crisis and grief. Assist the client in identifying sources of support within her own network of family and friends. Offer to speak with significant others if the client so desires. Provide the client with referrals, for example, for appropriate support groups, for telephone hotline assistance, for relevant counseling, or for appropriate financial aid services. Make certain that a plan for follow-up of the client experiencing crisis and grief is implemented (e.g., telephone contact at intervals or home visits if appropriate).

- Communicate with other health care providers directly involved in the family's care so that a consistent and supportive approach may be implemented.

- Provide a mechanism to deal with tension on the part of health care providers, such as interdisciplinary staff conferences, so that staff members can discuss their own feelings related to working with clients in crisis and grief.

Family System Changes During the Childbearing Cycle

Family system component	Change during childbearing
Structure	First pregnancy involves shift from a stable dyad to a volatile triangle. Subsequent pregnancies involve development of several complex, shifting triangular structures. Family members must occasionally cope with being the "isolate" in a triangle. Stress and tension may increase. Additional subsystems must be established: mother–child; father–child; sibling; grandparent–grandchild
Power	Patterns often alter; egalitarian power patterns often become more "traditional," with father as decision maker. Fetus and newborn may become very powerful in family system, producing major changes in parents' behavior and family patterns.
Boundaries	Mother's boundary incorporates another human within, the embryo/fetus. Becomes a "protective container" for fetus, progressively closing in and focusing her attention inward.

From Sherwen L, Scoloveno M, Weingarten C: *Nursing care of the childbearing family,* ed 2, Norwalk, Conn., 1995, Appleton & Lange.

Family system component	Change during childbearing
	Father's boundary must expand to give support and become empathetic with mother.
	Family boundary must become permeable to selected input, for example, healthcare and education.
Affect or feelings	Stress arising from structural change may alter feeling tone in family system. Danger signs are perception of hidden anger and hostility; pervasive depression; and apathy, unresponsiveness, or "flat" emotion.
Intergenerational patterns and roles	Parents' parents must "move up" a generation to become grandparents.
	Each member of the family system (both nuclear and extended) must assume new roles, whether it is a first or subsequent pregnancy.
Communication patterns	Family members must learn to communicate as a triangle. One member needs to learn to be a temporary outsider or "isolate" left out of communications, because only two people can communicate at one time.
Cultural background and rituals	Family members from different cultural backgrounds may have different values concerning pregnancy and childbearing, may perceive new roles differently, and may have different practices and rituals for this event. Differences can produce family conflict and stress.

INFANCY

Parenting Tasks for Developmental Landmarks in Infancy

Age (months)	Landmark	Parenting task
1	Lifts head when prone	Place infant in prone position and dangle colorful object above head
2	Social smile	Promote by talking to infant and allowing opportunity to smile
4	Squeals	Encourage and praise for doing
5	Rolls from back to front	Place infant in protected area (crib, playpen) and encourage to move by placing toy out of reach
8-9	Uses pincer grasp to feed self cracker	Make finger foods available

From Edelman CL, Mandle CL: *Health promotion throughout the lifespan,* ed 4, St Louis, 1998, Mosby.

Parenting Tasks for Developmental Landmarks in Infancy—cont'd

Age (months)	Landmark	Parenting task
10	Pulls self to standing position	Provide safe environment: place chair or object of appropriate height in reach
11-12	Initiates vocalization	Talk to infant frequently and include in family gatherings
12-15	Walks	Encourage and provide clutter-free, safe walkway; praise for attempts
15	Drinks from cup	Supply cup with appropriate drink; do not scold for clumsiness in handling cup or spills
18	Mimics household chores	Give rag to help with dusting, allow to fold clothes, and so on

Normal Sleep Patterns for Infants

Age (months)	Hours in 24-hour period
2-3	Low: 10 Average: 16½ High: 23 (Two to four naps)
3-4	Low: 8-10 nightly High: 11-12 nightly (Two or three naps daily)
6-12	11-12 nightly (Two or three naps daily)
12-18	8-12 nightly (One or two naps daily)

From Edelman CL, Mandle CL: *Health promotion throughout the lifespan,* ed 4, St Louis, 1998, Mosby.

Visual Development Milestones During Infancy

Age (months)	Milestones
1-3	Stares at objects
	Follows light with eyes
	Looks toward sound
3-5	Fixates on objects 3 feet away
	Accommodation begins to develop
	Follows moving objects well
	Looks at and grabs objects
	Visual acuity is 20/200
5-7	Developing hand-eye coordination
	Ultimate color of iris is established
	Eye movements coordinated and mature
	Searches for fallen objects
7-12	Depth perception begins to develop
	Demonstrates interest in small objects
	Reaches for unseen object
	Visual acuity is 20/100
12-18	Looks at pictures with interest
	Able to identify forms
	Convergence becomes well established

Modified from Chinn PL: *Child health maintenance: concepts in family-centered care,* ed 2, St Louis, 1979, Mosby. In Edelman CL, Mandle CL: *Health promotion throughout the lifespan,* ed 4, St Louis, 1998, Mosby.

Progressive Auditory Development of Infants During Infancy

Age (months)	Development
1-2	Startled by sounds (Moro reflex)
	Quiets when hears voice
	Turns head toward familiar sound
3-5	Searches for sound in room
	Stops sucking to listen
	Locates sound below ear
6-8	Reacts to changes in music volume
	Recognizes familiar sounds
9-12	Listens to talking
	Responds to simple commands
	Begins to differentiate between words
12-18	Begins to show voluntary control over responses to sound
	Begins to develop gross discrimination by learning to distinguish between sounds

Modified from Chinn PL: *Child health maintenance: concepts in family-centered care,* ed 2, St Louis, 1979, Mosby. In Edelman CL, Mandle CL: *Health promotion throughout the lifespan,* ed 4, St Louis, 1998, Mosby.

Clinical Assessment of Nutritional Status

Evidence of adequate nutrition	Evidence of deficient or excess nutrition	Deficiency/excess*
General growth		
Within 5th and 95th percentiles for height, weight, and head circumference	Below 5th or above 95th percentiles for growth	Protein, calories, fats, and other essential nutrients, especially A, pyridoxine, niacin, calcium, iodine, manganese, zinc
Steady gain with expected growth spurts during infancy and adolescence	Absence of or delayed growth spurts; poor weight gain	
Sexual development appropriate for age	Delayed sexual development	Excess vitamin A, D
Skin		
Smooth, slightly dry to touch	Hardening and scaling	Vitamin A
Elastic and firm	Seborrheic dermatitis	Excess niacin
Absence of lesions	Dry, rough, petechiae	Riboflavin
Color appropriate to genetic background	Delayed wound healing	Vitamin C
	Scaly dermatitis on exposed surfaces	Riboflavin, vitamin C, zinc
	Wrinkled, flabby	Niacin
	Crusted lesions around orifices, especially nares	Protein and calories
	Pruritus	Zinc
	Poor turgor	Excess vitamin A, riboflavin, niacin
	Edema	Water, sodium
		Protein, thiamin
		Excess sodium
	Yellow tinge (jaundice)	Vitamin B$_{12}$
		Excess vitamin A, niacin

	Signs associated with deficiency or excess*	Nutrient
	Depigmentation	Protein, calories
	Pallor (anemia)	Pyridoxine, folic acid, vitamin B$_{12}$, C, E (in premature infants), iron
		Excess vitamin C, zinc
		Excess riboflavin
	Paresthesia	
Hair		
Lustrous, silky, strong, elastic	Stringy, friable, dull, dry, thin	Protein, calories
	Alopecia	Protein, calories, zinc
	Depigmentation	Protein, calories, copper
	Raised areas around hair follicles	Vitamin C
Head		
Even molding, occipital prominence, symmetric facial features	Softening of cranial bones, prominence of frontal bones, skull flat and depressed toward middle	Vitamin D
Fused sutures after 18 months	Delayed fusion of sutures	Vitamin D
	Hard tender lumps in occiput	Excess vitamin A
	Headache	Excess thiamin
Neck		
Thyroid not visible, palpable in midline	Thyroid enlarged; may be grossly visible	Iodine

*Nutrients listed are deficient unless specified as excess.

From Wong DL: *Whaley and Wong's essentials of pediatric nursing*, ed 5, St Louis, 1997, Mosby.

Continued

Clinical Assessment of Nutritional Status—cont'd

Evidence of adequate nutrition	Evidence of deficient or excess nutrition	Deficiency/excess*
Eyes		
Clear, bright	Hardening and scaling of cornea and conjunctiva	Vitamin A
Good night vision	Night blindness	Riboflavin
Conjunctiva—pink, glossy	Burning, itching, photophobia, cataracts, corneal vascularization	
Ears		
Tympanic membrane—pliable	Calcified (hearing loss)	Excess vitamin D
Nose		
Smooth, intact nasal angle	Irritation and cracks at nasal angle	Riboflavin, Excess vitamin A
Mouth		
Lips—smooth, moist, darker color than skin	Fissures and inflammation at corners	Riboflavin, Excess vitamin A
Gums—firm, coral pink color, stippled	Spongy, friable, swollen, bluish red or black color, bleed easily	Vitamin C
Mucous membranes—bright pink, smooth, moist	Stomatitis	Niacin

Tongue—rough texture, no lesions, taste sensation	Glossitis	Niacin, riboflavin, folic acid
	Diminished taste sensation	Zinc
Teeth—uniform white color, smooth, intact	Brown mottling, pits, fissures	Excess fluoride
	Defective enamel	Vitamin A, C, D, calcium, phosphorus
	Caries	Excess carbohydrates
Chest		
In infants, shape is almost circular	Depressed lower portion of rib cage	Vitamin D
In children, lateral diameter increases in proportion to anteroposterior diameter	Sharp protrusion of sternum	
Smooth costochondral junctions	Enlarged costochondral junctions	Vitamin C, D
Breast development—normal for age	Delayed development	See "General growth," especially zinc
Cardiovascular system		
Pulse and blood pressure (BP) within normal limits	Palpitations	Thiamin
	Rapid pulse	Potassium
		Excess thiamin
	Arrhythmias	Magnesium, potassium
		Excess niacin, potassium
	Increased blood pressure (BP)	Excess sodium
	Decreased BP	Thiamin; excess niacin
Abdomen		
In young children, cylindric and prominent	Distended, flabby, poor musculature	Protein, calories
	Prominent, large	Excess calories
Older children, flat	Potbelly, constipation	Vitamin D

Continued

*Nutrients listed are deficient unless specified as excess.

Clinical Assessment of Nutritional Status—cont'd

Evidence of adequate nutrition	Evidence of deficient or excess nutrition	Deficiency/excess*
Abdomen—cont'd		
Normal bowel habits	Diarrhea	Niacin
		Excess vitamin C
	Constipation	Excess calcium, potassium
Musculoskeletal system		
Muscles—firm, well-developed, equal strength bilaterally	Flabby, weak, generalized wasting	Protein, calories
	Weakness, pain, cramps	Thiamin, sodium, chloride, potassium, phosphorus, magnesium
		Excess thiamin
	Muscle twitching, tremors	Magnesium
	Muscular paralysis	Excess potassium
	Kyphosis, lordosis, scoliosis	Vitamin D
Spine—cervical and lumbar curves (double S curve)		
Extremities—symmetric; legs straight with minimum bowing	Bowing of extremities, knock-knees	Vitamin D, calcium, phosphorus
	Epiphyseal enlargement	Vitamin A, D
	Bleeding into joints and muscles, joint swelling, pain	Vitamin C
	Thickening of cortex of long bones with pain and fragility, hard tender lumps in extremities	Excess vitamin A
Joints—flexible, full range of motion, no pain or stiffness	Osteoporosis of long bones	Calcium; excess vitamin D

Neurologic system

Behavior—alert, responsive, emotionally stable	Listless, irritable, lethargic, apathetic (sometimes apprehensive, anxious, drowsy, mentally slow, confused)	Thiamin, niacin, pyridoxine, vitamin C, potassium, magnesium, iron, protein, calories Excess vitamin A, D, thiamin, folic acid, calcium Excess manganese
	Masklike facial expression, blurred speech, involuntary laughing	
Absence of tetany, convulsions	Convulsions	Thiamin, pyridoxine, vitamin D, calcium, magnesium Excess phosphorus (in relation to calcium)
Intact peripheral nervous system	Peripheral nervous system toxicity (unsteady gait, numb feet and hands, fine motor clumsiness)	Excess pyridoxine
Intact reflexes	Diminished or absent tendon reflexes	Thiamin, vitamin E

Development of Feeding Skills

Age	Oral and neuromuscular development	Feeding behavior
Birth	Rooting reflex Swallowing reflex	Turns mouth toward nipple or any object brushing cheek Initial swallowing involves the posterior of the tongue; by 9-12 weeks anterior portion is increasingly involved, which facilitates ingestion of semisolid food
	Extrusion reflex	Pushes food out when placed on tongue; strong the first 9 weeks
	Sucking reflex	By 6-10 weeks recognizes the feeding position and begins mouthing and sucking when placed in this position
3-6 months	Beginning coordination between eyes and body movements	Explores world with eyes, fingers, hands, and mouth; starts reaching for objects at 4 months but overshoots; hands get in the way during feeding
	Learning to reach mouth with hands at 4 months	Finger sucking; by 6 months all objects go into the mouth Sucking reflex becomes voluntary, and lateral motions of the jaw begin
	Extrusion reflex present until 4 months	May continue to push out food placed on tongue
	Able to grasp objects voluntarily at 5 months	Grasps objects in mitten-like fashion
6-12 months	Eyes and hands working together	Can approximate lips to rim of cup by 5 months; chewing action begins; by 6 months begins drinking from cup Brings hand to mouth; at 7 months able to feed self biscuit Bangs cup and objects on table at 7 months
	Sits erect with support at 6 months Sits erect without support at 9 months	

Development of grasp (finger-to-thumb opposition)	Holds own bottle at 9-12 months
	Pincer approach to food
Relates to objects at 10 months	Pokes at food with index finger at 10 months
	Reaches for food and utensils, including those beyond reach; pushes plate around with spoon
	Insists on holding spoon, not to put in mouth, but to return to plate or cup
	Increased desire to feed self
1-3 years Development of manual dexterity	*15 months*: begins to use spoon but turns it before reaching mouth; may hold cup, likely to tilt cup rather than head, causing spilling
	18 months: eats with spoon, spills frequently, turns spoon in mouth; holds glass with both hands
	2 years: inserts spoon correctly, occasionally with one hand; holds glass; plays with food; distinguishes between food and inedible materials
	2-3 years: self-feeding complete with occasional spilling; uses fork; pours from pitcher; obtains drink of water from faucet

Adapted from Wong DL: *Whaley and Wong's essentials of pediatric nursing*, ed 5, St Louis, 1997, Mosby; Lowdermilk D, Perry S, Bobak I: *Maternity nursing*, ed 5, St Louis, 1999, Mosby.

Feeding for the First 12 Months of Life

1	2	3	4	5	6	7	8	9	10	11	12
Breast milk: nutritionally sound; believed to provide immunity; facilitates a close mother-baby relationship; decreases incidence of dental caries and malocclusion											
Formula: 24-32 oz/24 hr; well tolerated when breast milk is not available											
				Iron-fortified rice cereal: source of calories, iron, and fiber; avoid wheat products first 12 months of life							
						Strained vegetables: source of calories, fiber, iron, vitamins A and B, and minerals; introduce yellow vegetables before green					
							Strained fruits: source of calories, iron, fiber, vitamin C, and minerals; will offset constipating effect of cereals				
								Plain lowfat yogurt: excellent source of calcium, phosphorus, vitamin B, and protein			
								Meats: source of protein, calories, iron, and vitamins			
								Finger foods: assist in teething and fine motor coordination			

From Ingalls JA, Salerno MC: *Ingalls and Salerno's maternal and child health nursing*, ed 9, St Louis, 1999, Mosby.

Infant State-Related Behavior Chart

Behavior/description of behavior	Infant state consideration	Implications for caregiving
Alertness		
Widening and brightening of the eyes. Infants focus attention on stimuli, whether visual, auditory, or objects to be sucked	From drowsy or active alert to quiet alert	Infant state and timing are important. When trying to alert infants, try to do the following: 1. Unwrap infant (arms out at least). 2. Place infant in upright position. 3. Talk to infant, putting variation in your pitch and tempo. 4. Show your face to infant. 5. Elicit the rooting, sucking, or grasp reflexes.
Visual response		
Newborns have pupillary responses to differences in brightness. Infants can focus on objects or faces about 7-8 inches away. Newborns have preferences for more complex patterns, human faces, and moving objects.	Quiet alert	Newborn's visual alertness provides opportunities for eye-to-eye contact with caregivers, an important source of beginning caregiver–infant interaction.
Auditory response		
Reaction to a variety of sounds, especially in the human voice range. Infants can hear sounds and locate the general direction of the sound (if the source is constant).	Drowsy, quiet alert, active alert	Enhances communication between infants and caregivers. Crying infants can often be consoled by voice.

Continued

Modified from Bobak IM, Lowermilk DL, Jensen MD: *Maternity nursing*, ed 5, St Louis, 1999, Mosby.

Infant State-Related Behavior Chart—cont'd

Behavior/description of behavior	Infant state consideration	Implications for caregiving
Irritability How easily infants are upset by loud noises, handling by caregivers, temperature changes, removal of blankets or clothes, etc.	From deep sleep, light sleep, drowsy, quiet alert, or active alert to fussing or crying	Irritable infants need more frequent consoling and more subdued external environments. Parents can be helped to cope with more irritable infants.
Readability The cues infants give through motor behavior and activity, looking, listening, and behavior patterns.	All states	Parents need to learn that newborns' behaviors are part of their individual temperaments and not reflections on their parenting abilities. By observing and understanding an infant's characteristic pattern, parents can respond more appropriately.
Smile Ranging from a faint grimace to a full-fledged smile; reflexive.	Drowsy, active alert, quiet alert, light sleep	Initial smile in the neonatal period is the forerunner of the social smile at 3 to 4 weeks of age. Important for caregivers to respond to it.
Habituation The ability to lessen one's response to repeated stimuli, seen where the Moro response is repeatedly elicited. If a noise is continually repeated, infants will usually cease to respond.	Deep sleep, light sleep, also seen in drowsy	Because of this ability, families can carry out normal activities without disturbing infants. Infants who have more difficulty with this will probably not sleep well in active environments.

Cuddliness

Infants' response to being held. Infants nestle and work themselves into the contours of caregivers' bodies.

Primarily in awake states

Cuddliness is usually rewarding behavior for the caregivers. If infants do not nestle and mold, show the caregivers how to position infants to maximize this response.

Consolability

Measured when infants have been crying for at least 15 seconds. The ability of infants to bring themselves or to be brought by others to a lower state.

From crying to active alert, quiet alert, drowsy, or sleep states

Crying is the infant behavior that presents the greatest challenge to caregivers. Parents' success or failure in consoling their infants has a significant impact on their feelings of competence as parents.

Self-consoling

Maneuvers used by infants to console themselves and move to a lower state:
1. Hand-to-mouth movement
2. Sucking on fingers, fist, or tongue
3. Paying attention to voices or faces
4. Changes in position

From crying to active alert, quiet alert, drowsy, or sleep states

If caregivers are aware of these behaviors, they may allow infants the opportunity to gain control of themselves. This does not imply that newborns should be left to cry. Once newborns are crying and do not initiate self-consoling activities, they may need attention from caregivers.

Consoling by caregivers

After crying for longer than 15 seconds, the caregivers may try to:
1. Show face to infant.
2. Talk to infant in a steady, soft voice.
3. Hold both infant's arms close to body.
4. Swaddle infant.

From crying to active alert, quiet alert, drowsy, or sleep states

Often parental initial reaction is to pick up infants or feed them when they cry. Parents could be taught to try other soothing maneuvers, after ascertaining that the diaper is clean and dry.

Continued

Infant State-Related Behavior Chart—cont'd

Behavior/description of behavior	Infant state consideration	Implications for caregiving
Consoling by caregivers—cont'd 5. Pick up infant. 6. Rock infant. 7. Give infant a pacifier or feed.		
Motor behavior and activity Spontaneous movements of extremities and body when stimulated vs. when left alone. Smooth, rhythmical movements vs. jerky ones.	Quiet alert, active alert	Smooth, nonjerky movements with periods of inactivity seem most natural. Some parents see jerky movements and startles as negative response to their caregiving and are frightened.

Common Concerns and Problems of the First Year

Problem or concern	Assessment	Nursing intervention
Burping	Swallowed air bubbles trapped in stomach; occurs more frequently in bottle-fed infants who cry during feeding.	Burp frequently during feeding (i.e., before, during, and after, or after every 1 ounce of formula or every 4-5 minutes at breast). Use upright position to burp (gently rub infant's back while baby sits on parent's knee and rests forward against parent's arm). Try to burp every 10-15 minutes while awake if not successful burping during and after feeding. Sit upright in infant seat for 30-45 minutes after feeding if awake or position with head elevated and on right side if sleeping.
Colic	Unexplained bouts of crying frequently occurring at same time of day (usually busiest) and often accompanied by abdominal distention, spasms, drawing up legs to stomach and/or passing gas. May be caused by feeding problems, maternal anxiety, or allergy, and is aggravated by tension in household. Can last 3 months. Also see Crying (below).	Review basic infant needs with parents (i.e., is infant hungry, wet, does infant have air bubble, is infant in uncomfortable position). Review feeding method, technique and burping, review maternal diet for offending foods if breast-fed. Record time when colic episodes occur. Soothe and comfort before "attack." Swaddle infant (i.e., wrap warmly and in an encompassing manner). Walk, rock, and hold infant over shoulder.

Adapted from Kenner C, Lott J, Flondermeyer A: *Comprehensive neonatal nursing,* ed 2, Philadelphia, 1998, WB Saunders; Lowdermilk D, Perry S, Bobak I: *Maternity nursing,* ed 5, St Louis, 1999, Mosby; Novak J, Broom B: *Ingalls and Salerno's maternal and child health nursing,* ed 9, St Louis, 1999, Mosby; Wong D: *Whaley and Wong's nursing care of infants and children,* ed 5, St Louis, 1995, Mosby.

Continued

Common Concerns and Problems of the First Year—cont'd

Problem or concern	Assessment	Nursing intervention
Colic—cont'd		Try a monotonous soothing noise (music, ticking clock) or activity (ride in a car).
		Change infant position from stomach to side to back to sitting position.
		Rest infant on abdomen on warm hard surface (e.g., parent knee, warmed crib surface).
		Change household routine if indicated, create a quiet environment.
		Try pacifier or sugar water; if bottle fed, try soy formula.
		Reassure parents that infant is not ill, that they are providing good care, and that colic will definitely go away.
		Provide support to parents, giving them an opportunity to discuss feelings.
		Explain theories about origin and cycle of colic.
Crying	Periodic crying for unexplained reason; ascertain if a pattern exists for crying spells; may be related to colic; obtain a detailed history of time and length of spell; feeding frequency, method, technique and burping; stool patterns; meeting contact and sucking needs; parental handling of crying and feelings regarding crying; other	See previous section on colic.
		Reinforce that babies cry for a reason. Best to respond to cry vs. letting baby cry it out. Crying is a release and/or exercise for infant. One or two periods a day of 5-10 minutes is normal for most infants.
		Assist parents to develop positive, relaxed approach.
		Reassure and support parents in this time of stress.

	household factors (e.g., siblings, relative advice, parental support of each other, presence of other symptoms and/or allergies).	Suggest parents alternate infant care and meeting infant demands.
Constipation	Consistency of stool that is hard, pebbly, rocklike. Not related to frequency, straining, grunting or number of days between stools. Ascertain color, consistency, frequency, and presence of blood or mucus. Review infant diet and verify parent perception of constipation and expectation of normal stool patterns.	Discuss normal elimination/stool patterns for type of feeding method (i.e., breast-fed stools vs. bottle-fed stools). Reassure that straining, grunting, and infrequent number are normal. Reinforce that each infant has individual stool pattern and educate parents regarding what constipation actually is (i.e., consistency). Discuss parents attitude regarding toilet habits and expectations about stool patterns. If constipated, increase liquids in diet; may offer water between meals. If introduced to solids too early or in too large a quantity, discontinue use until constipation clears, then begin again with smaller amounts. Karo syrup, 1 tsp/3 oz of water may be given several times a day. If appropriate for feeding stage, add prunes (up to 3 tbsp) or prune juice to diet.
Flatus	Air in stomach or intestines causing abdominal distress, distension, and discomfort; frequently expelled through anus. May be caused by excess swallowing of air, overfeeding, underfeeding, or allergy. Ascertain details regarding feeding (e.g., frequency and size of nipple, type of bottle	Burp frequently during and after feedings (see Burping). Calm infant when crying and burp after crying. Place on left side to ease expelling of gas. If allergies are suspected, try soy formula or elimination diet. Reassure parents.

Continued

Common Concerns and Problems of the First Year—cont'd

Problem or concern	Assessment	Nursing intervention
Flatus—cont'd	used, breast-feeding technique, maternal diet, use of pacifier, propping of bottle, burping).	
Hiccoughs	Sudden sharp involuntary spasms of diaphragm usually occur following a meal.	Reassure parents that infant will cry if truly distressed. Offer infant something to suck (e.g., pacifier, breast, bottle with warm water).
Pacifier	Infants demonstrate a need for non-nutritional sucking.	Assist parents to understand aspects of positive and negative use of pacifier. Positive use: indicated immediately after birth before newborn can manipulate thumb into mouth; assists in developing sucking function; contributes to establishment of breast-feeding; good means of satisfying sucking need especially for bottle-fed infants who need extra sucking time; does not usually become a habit unless child sucks beyond infancy; most infants substitute thumb for pacifier around 3-4 months. Parents should look for clues to eliminate pacifier use at this time and provide stimulation suitable for the age. Negative use: pacifiers do not replace parent holding the baby; stimulation, or needs satisfaction; pacifiers should not be used constantly, especially before tending to infants needs; parents should be encouraged to discontinue use by age 5 months since continued use may become hard to overcome.

If thumb is substituted, it generally is used less frequently than pacifier.

Concern	Description	Management
Spoiling	Ascertain parent definition of spoiling. Generally it is the result of basic needs not being met in early infancy leading to a demanding, undisciplined child because the need for gratification continues beyond normal time; overgratification usually occurs then. It generally is believed that infants cannot be spoiled under 6 months of age.	Parents require counseling and education that reinforces the following: Early infant needs must be gratified. A child cannot handle frustrations well until the age of 8-9 months, and is unable to delay gratification of needs until this age. A gradual and gentle approach to limits and delaying gratification is best. A relaxed, positive approach is helpful. Parents often find support groups helpful in dealing with this problem.
Biting	In first year, it is frequently related to teething. It is particularly a problem for breast-feeding mothers. In toddlers it is related to normal aggressive impulses.	If related to teething, see Teething (below) for alleviation of discomfort. Breast-feeding mothers should remove infant from breast at every occurrence and may accompany with a "no"; should also allow time to lapse before finishing feeding.
Separation anxiety	Occurs at 9-10 months as infant is learning to differentiate self from mother. Can occur again in toddlerhood as child is learning to distance and separate self from mother in attempt to establish autonomy.	Reassure mother that this is a normal developmental process. Advise parents, especially mother, to do the following: • Play "peek-a-boo" games. • Allow sufficient time (30-45 minutes) for child to acquaint himself or herself with new person (e.g., visitor, babysitter).

Continued

Common Concerns and Problems of the First Year—cont'd

Problem or concern	Assessment	Nursing intervention
Separation anxiety—cont'd		• Avoid "sneaking out." Tell child firmly that "mommy leaves, mommy comes back." Reinforce this with "peek-a-boo" or "hide and seek" games. • Avoid making major changes in child's or household routines during this period (e.g., mother returning to work; changing child's room, changing regular babysitter or day care situation).
Stranger anxiety	Begins at 6-8 months and gradually diminishes by 18 months. Process of child development.	See preceding section on separation anxiety. Advise parents, particularly mother, to hold infant in presence of strangers. If infant is to be left, mother should spend a short time with stranger.
Infant sleep patterns	Some infants have difficulty releasing into sleep or awaken easily. Separation anxiety, teething, and illness are among the common causes. Ascertain history of problem to include how long infant sleeps, what the feeding schedule is, bedtime and household routines, the presence of illness or teething, and how the problem is handled.	Counseling should be directed toward education of the parents; infants need gratification and normal sleep patterns, emphasizing the following: • Differences in temperament and incidence of sleep problems can be related. • Infants generally sleep through the night by age 3 months. • Infant may need help getting to sleep by rocking, holding, pacifier, walking, etc. • Environment and atmosphere conducive to sleep (e.g., quiet and dim) should be provided.

		• If sleep problem is related to a physical problem, measures to remedy this should be implemented.
Teething	Eruption of primary or deciduous teeth starting at about 6 months, usually with lower incisors; will continue every 2 months for first 2 years. Signs which may be included, but are not always present: red, swollen gums, irritability, crying and rubbing gums. Since other events in infant development are occurring simultaneously, nurse must help parents distinguish between these and teething as follows: • Drooling, which normally occurs at 3 to 4 months and has little to do with teething, although it may persist throughout teething. • Fever does not usually accompany teething; must be assessed separately because maternal antibody protection is diminishing and presence of fever is suspect for infectious process. • Separation anxiety, sleep disturbances, or fussiness from other causes are all common development symptoms associated with the infant age group, as is reaching for and mouthing objects.	Recommend to parents hard, clean objects for baby to chew on (e.g., rubber teething rings, beads, hard rubber toys, a cool spoon, teething biscuits, or pretzels). Parents should avoid use of teething toys or rings filled with liquid because plastic covers are easily broken and liquid can be ingested.
Diaper rashes	Rashes of various types occurring in diaper area. Persistent rashes which do not respond to home management, or which continue to occur despite	Preventive measures to keep the diaper area clean, dry, and aerated including the following: • Diapers should be changed frequently.

Continued

Common Concerns and Problems of the First Year—cont'd

Problem or concern	Assessment	Nursing intervention
Diaper rashes—cont'd	preventive measures, should be referred to the appropriate care provider for medical evaluation.	• Cleanse with water (and mild soap after bowel movement) at each changing; dry area well. • Thick diapers and/or absorbent pads are recommended; plastic or rubber pants are not. • A *thin* film of lubrication, such as A and D ointment or petroleum jelly, may be used. • Remove diapers for short periods every day. Wash diapers well as follows: 1. Soak soiled diapers in Borateen or borax solution (½ cup to 1 gallon of water). 2. Prerinse before washing. 3. Wash in full cycle with mild soap, such as Ivory, Dreft, or Lux. 4. Avoid softeners and strong detergents. 5. Rinse diapers 2 to 3 times, and ¼ to ½ cup vinegar may be added to final rinse. 6. Dry in sun if possible. Home management of diaper rash includes the following: • Follow preventive measures with an emphasis on leaving diaper off more frequently, changing when wet, and cleaning area thoroughly during changes.

		• Zinc oxide ointment often is helpful in checking early nonfungal rashes.
		• Cornstarch is never recommended for rashes or their prevention.
		• Seek medical help if rash worsens or does not improve.
Cradle cap	Form of seborrheic dermatitis in neonate characterized by scalping, flaking of scalp skin especially over anterior fontanelle. May persist beyond neonatal age into infancy.	Preventive measures include the following:
		• Teach parents how to shampoo infant head and recommend shampooing every other day.
		• Reassure that vigorous scrubbing will not injure fontanelle or skull.
		Home management for mild cases:
		• Shampoo head daily with warm water and soap, using firm pressure on scalp.
		• Loosen cap by applying mineral or baby oil to scalp 15 to 20 minutes before shampooing. Remove with shampoo.
		• Comb scalp with fine comb to loosen and dislodge scaly cap.
		• Severe cases will require medical attention, and are generally managed with antiseborrheic shampoos.
Problems related to feeding		
Parental concerns about overfeeding or underfeeding	Some parents find it difficult to determine the appropriate amount of milk and/or solid food to give an infant. Ascertain parents' understanding, knowledge, and perceptions through the following:	Assist parents in constructing a workable feeding schedule.
		Discuss normal feeding pattern for breast- and bottle-fed infants.
		Discuss infants needs for non–nutrient sucking.

Continued

Common Concerns and Problems of the First Year—cont'd

Problem or concern	Assessment	Nursing intervention
Problems related to feeding—cont'd		
Parental concerns about overfeeding or underfeeding—cont'd	• Diet history • Height and weight measurement and charting on growth curve • Elimination habits and description	Convey that infants will eat more than they need or require if food is offered at each cry. Offer water between feedings to postpone next feeding to a reasonable time. Suggest a schedule of solid food introduction. Reassure parents that if infant is gaining weight, he or she is not underfed. Explain growth and appetite spurts.
Refusal of solids	Infant may refuse new foods for a number of reasons (e.g., temperature, texture, manner presented by person feeding, or too-early introduction). Ascertain through diet history which foods accepted, and likes and dislikes and parental feelings and perception regarding solid foods.	Discuss normal feeding patterns for age. Review the following indications for starting or not starting solid foods: • No need for solid foods before 4 to 6 months. • Digestion begins with salivation around 4 months. • Feeding of solid foods is not necessarily related to sleeping through the night. • Tongue thrusting of solid food is normal and not a refusal. Discuss ways to encourage solid food acceptance. Some examples follow: • Allow infant to feed self.

Refusal of food and variations in appetite	Once solid foods have been introduced and established, infants and especially toddlers will go through periods of refusal, pickiness, and preference. Obtain a diet history as reviewed in Refusal of solids.

- Avoid forcing infant to eat since this will only increase resistance.
- Solids may be stopped for a while, offering only ones that infant likes.
- Offer solid foods before milk when infant is hungriest.
- Offer food in a calm, positive manner.

See Refusal of solids.

Discuss the following with parents:

- Refusal may be due to loss of interest in food when more active or due to a form of negativism and a means to control.
- Avoid use of food as a substitute for attention or stimulation.
- Some degree of refusal and variation in appetite is normal for age.

Try the following approaches:

- Offer small amounts of food frequently.
- Emphasize favorite foods as much as possible.
- Use as few non–nutritive foods as possible.
- Allow the child to feed self if he desires and provide finger foods.
- Be patient as child tries to master use of utensils.
- Eating should be an enjoyable and sociable time. If hunger does not permit infant to wait until family dinner time, feed before and offer nibbles during family meal.
- Give older infant and toddler a place, chair, utensils, and plate at the table.

Continued

Common Concerns and Problems of the First Year—cont'd

Problem or concern	Assessment	Nursing intervention
Spitting up	Regurgitation commonly following a feeding; usually related to air swallowed with food, inability to relax esophageal sphincter, possible overfeeding, or allergy to milk. Ascertain nature of regurgitation (e.g., frequency, amount, color, consistency) as well as diet history and data regarding weight gain. Regurgitation is frequently outgrown by the time the infant is sitting well in upright position.	Reinforce the following with parents: • Correct preparation of formula. • Use of appropriate size nipple and nipple hole. • Regular and frequent burping is needed. • Place infant in an upright position for 30 minutes after feeding. • Correct position of infant during feeding. Determine the need to change the method of feeding or formula.
Weaning	A transition of feeding methods. May be from bottle to cup or from breast to bottle and/or cup. Weaning from breast is difficult if parents (especially mother) have ambivalent feelings or if infant refuses alternative methods. Ascertain who wants baby weaned and why, as well as schedule of feedings. Weaning from bottle should be attempted gradually when child is ready, usually around 1 year. Ascertain who wants child weaned, what has been tried, feeding schedule and number of bottles, and ability to use cup.	Assist parents to make decision to wean. The criteria include the following: • Should be discussed and decided by both parents. • If breast-feeding, it is helpful to mother to assess every 3 months whether or not to continue nursing. • Positive attitude toward weaning is essential, especially for breast-feeding mothers. • Weaning at times of separation anxiety is not advised, especially in breast-fed infants. • If possible, an infant should be weaned from breast to cup. This avoids having to wean from bottle later on.

Weaning—cont'd

Active weaning for breast-feeding mothers includes:

- Start by substituting a bottle or cup for the breast at one feeding and allow 5-6 days before substituting second breast-feeding.
- If resistance is encountered, try giving water or juice in a bottle or cup before weaning starts, using nipple similar to breast or pacifier if one is used, heating milk before offering, and having someone other than mother offer the bottle or cup. Keep to a schedule and be firm, positive, and patient.

Active weaning to cup—continue preceding steps with the following additions:

- Reinforce idea of accomplishment in using a cup to child.
- May give child one bottle a day, but should contain only water to avoid incidence of dental caries.
- Avoid forcing child to wean; forcing the use of a cup may increase the need to suck.
- A calm, relaxed, positive approach is essential.

Infant Stimulation Guide

Age (months)	Visual stimulation	Auditory stimulation	Tactile stimulation	Kinetic stimulation
Suggested activities				
Birth-1	Look at infant at close range Hang bright, shiny object within 20-25 cm (8-10 inches) of infant's face and in midline Hang mobiles with black-and-white contrast designs	Talk to infant, sing in soft voice Play music box, radio, television Have ticking clock or metronome nearby	Hold, caress, cuddle Keep infant warm May like to be swaddled	Rock infant, place in cradle Use carriage for walks
2-3	Provide bright objects Make room bright with pictures or mirrors on walls Take infant to various rooms while doing chores Place infant in infant seat for vertical view of environment	Talk to infant Include in family gather-ings Expose to various envi-ronmental noises other than those of home Use rattles, wind chimes	Caress infant while bath-ing, at diaper change Comb hair with a soft brush	Use infant swing Take in car for rides Exercise body by moving extremities in swim-ming motion Use cradle gym
4-6	Place infant in front of unbreakable mirror	Talk to infant, repeat sounds infant makes	Give infant soft squeeze toys of various textures	Use swing or stroller Bounce infant in lap

Continued

Age	Visual stimulation	Auditory stimulation	Tactile stimulation	Kinetic/Motor stimulation
	Give brightly colored toys to hold (small enough to grasp)	Laugh when infant laughs Call infant by name Crinkle different papers by infant's ear Place rattle or bell in hand	Allow to splash in bath Place nude on soft furry rug and move extremities	while holding in standing position Support infant in sitting position, let infant lean forward to balance self Place infant on floor to crawl, roll over, sit Hold upright to bear weight and bounce Pick up, say "up" Put down, say "down" Place toys out of reach; encourage infant to get them Play pat-a-cake
6-9	Give infant large toys with bright colors, movable parts, and noisemakers Place unbreakable mirror where infant can see self Play peekaboo, especially hiding face in a towel Make funny faces to encourage imitation Give ball of yarn or string to pull apart	Call infant by name Repeat simple words such as "dada," "mama," "bye-bye" Speak clearly Name parts of body, people, and foods Tell infant what you are doing Use "no" only when necessary Give simple commands Show how to clap hands, bang a drum	Let infant play with fabrics of various textures Have bowl with foods of different size and textures to feel Let infant "catch" running water Encourage "swimming" in large bathtub or shallow pool Give wad of sticky tape to manipulate	
6-12	Show infant large pictures in books Take infant to places where there are animals, many people, different objects	Read infant simple nursery rhymes Point to body parts and name each one Imitate sounds of animals	Give infant finger foods of different textures Let infant mess and squash food Let infant feel cold (ice cube) or warm objects;	Give large push-pull toys Place furniture in a circle to encourage cruising Turn in different positions

From Wong DL: *Whaley and Wong's essentials of pediatric nursing*, ed 5, St Louis, 1997, Mosby.

Infant Stimulation Guide—cont'd

Age (months)	Visual stimulation	Auditory stimulation	Tactile stimulation	Kinetic stimulation
Suggested activities—cont'd	(shopping center) Play ball by rolling it to child, demonstrate "throwing" it back Demonstrate building a two-block tower		say what temperature each is Let infant feel a breeze (fan blowing)	
Suggested toys Birth-6	Nursery mobiles Unbreakable mirrors See-through crib bumpers Contrasting colored sheets	Music boxes Musical mobiles Crib dangle bells Small-handled clear rattle	Stuffed animals Soft clothes Soft or furry quilt Soft mobiles	Rocking crib/cradle Weighted or suction toy Infant swing (wind-up)
6-12	Various colored blocks Nested boxes or cups Books with rhymes and bright pictures Strings of big beads Simple take-apart toys Large ball Cup and spoon Large puzzles Jack-in-the box	Rattles of different sizes, shapes, tones, and bright colors Squeaky animals and dolls Records with light, rhyth-mic music	Soft, different-textured animals and dolls Sponge toys, floating toys Squeeze toys Teething toys Books with textures and objects, such as fur and zipper	Push-pull toys Baby swing (wind-up) Activity box for crib

Tips for a Baby's Safety

Back carriers
	YES	NO
1. Carrier has restraining strap to secure child.	____	____
2. Leg openings are small enough to prevent child from slipping out.	____	____
3. Leg openings are large enough to prevent chafing.	____	____
4. Frames have no pinch points in the folding mechanism.	____	____
5. Carrier has padded covering over metal frame near baby's face.	____	____

THE COMMISSION RECOMMENDS: Do not use until baby is 4 or 5 months old. By then baby's neck is able to withstand jolts and not sustain an injury.

Bassinets and cradles
	YES	NO
1. Bassinet/Cradle has a sturdy bottom and a wide base for stability.	____	____
2. Bassinet/Cradle has smooth surfaces, no protruding staples or other hardware that injure the baby.	____	____
3. Legs have strong, effective locks to prevent folding while in use.	____	____
4. Mattress is firm and fits snugly.	____	____

THE COMMISSION RECOMMENDS: Follow manufacturer's guidelines on weight and size of baby who can safely use these products.

Baby bath rings or seats
	YES	NO
1. Suction cups securely fastened to product.	____	____
2. Suction cups securely attached to SMOOTH SURFACE of tub.	____	____
3. Tub filled only with enough water to cover baby's legs.	____	____
4. Baby should NEVER be left alone or with a sibling while in bath ring, even for a moment!	____	____

From Consumer Product Safety Commission: *Tips for your baby's safety,* CPSC Document A200. Available: http://www.cpsc.gov/cpscpub/pubs/200.html.

THE COMMISSION RECOMMENDS: NEVER leave a baby unattended or with a sibling in a tub of water. Do not rely on a bath ring to keep your baby safe.

Carrier seats

	YES	NO
1. Carrier seat has a wide sturdy base for stability.	——	——
2. Carrier has non-skid feet to prevent slipping.	——	——
3. Supporting devices lock securely.	——	——
4. Carrier seat has crotch and waist strap.	——	——
5. Buckle or strap is easy to use.	——	——

THE COMMISSION RECOMMENDS: Never use the carrier as a car seat.

Changing tables

	YES	NO
1. Table has safety straps to prevent falls.	——	——
2. Table has drawer or shelves that are easily accessible without leaving the baby unattended.	——	——

THE COMMISSION RECOMMENDS: Do not leave baby on the table unattended. Always use the straps to prevent the baby from falling.

Cribs

	YES	NO
1. Slats are spaced no more than 2⅜ inches (60 mm) apart.	——	——
2. No slats are missing or cracked.	——	——
3. Mattress fits snugly–less than two finger's width between edge of mattress and crib side.	——	——
4. Mattress support is securely attached to the head and footboards.	——	——
5. Corner posts are no higher than ¹⁄₁₆ inch (1.5 mm) to prevent entanglement of clothing or other objects worn by child.	——	——
6. No cutouts in the head and footboards which allow head entrapment.	——	——
7. Drop-side latches cannot be easily released by baby.	——	——
8. Drop-side latches securely hold sides in raised position.	——	——
9. All screws or bolts that secure components of crib are present and tight.	——	——

THE COMMISSION RECOMMENDS: Do not place crib near draperies or blinds where child could become entangled and strangle on the cords. When the child reaches 35 inches in height or can climb and/or fall over the sides, the crib should be replaced with a bed.

Crib toys	YES	NO
1. No strings with loops or openings having perimeters greater than 14 inches (356 mm).	____	____
2. No strings or cords longer than 7 inches (178 mm) should dangle into the crib.	____	____
3. Crib gym has label warning to remove from crib when child can push up on hands and knees or reaches 5 months of age, whichever comes first.	____	____
4. Components of toys are not small enough to be a choking hazard.	____	____

THE COMMISSION RECOMMENDS: Avoid hanging toys across the crib or on crib corner posts with strings long enough to result in strangulation. Remove crib gyms when child is able to pull or push up on hands and knees.

Gates and enclosures	YES	NO
1. Openings in gate are too small to entrap a child's head.	____	____
2. Gate has a pressure bar or other fastener that will resist forces exerted by a child.	____	____

THE COMMISSION RECOMMENDS: To avoid head entrapment, do not use accordion-style gates or expandable enclosures with large v-shaped openings along the top edge, or diamond-shaped openings within.

High chairs	YES	NO
1. High chair has waist and crotch restraining straps that are independent of the tray.	____	____
2. Tray locks securely.	____	____
3. Buckle on waist strap is easy to use.	____	____
4. High chair has a wide stable base.	____	____
5. Caps or plugs on tubing are firmly attached and cannot be pulled off and choke a child.	____	____
6. If it is a folding high chair, it has an effective locking device to keep the chair from collapsing.	____	____

THE COMMISSION RECOMMENDS: Always use restraining straps; otherwise child can slide under the tray and strangle.

Hook-on chairs	YES	NO
1. Chair has a restraining strap to secure the child.	___	___
2. Chair has a clamp that locks onto the table for added security.	___	___
3. Caps or plugs on tubing are firmly attached and cannot be pulled off and choke a child.	___	___
4. Hook-on chair has a warning never to place the chair where the child can push off with feet.	___	___

THE COMMISSION RECOMMENDS: Don't leave a child unattended in a hook-on chair.

Pacifiers	YES	NO
1. No ribbon, string, cord or yarn attached to pacifier.	___	___
2. Shield is large enough and firm enough to not fit in child's mouth.	___	___
3. Guard or shield has ventilation holes so the baby can breath if the shield does get into the mouth.	___	___
4. Pacifier nipple has no holes or tears that might cause it to break off in baby's mouth.	___	___

THE COMMISSION RECOMMENDS: To prevent strangulation, never hang pacifier or other items on a string around a baby's neck.

Playpens	YES	NO
1. Drop-side mesh playpen or crib has label warning never to leave side in the down position.	___	___
2. Mesh has small weave (less than ¼ inch openings).	___	___
3. Mesh has no tears, holes or loose threads.	___	___
4. Mesh is securely attached to top rail and floorplate.	___	___
5. Top rail cover has no tears or holes.	___	___
6. Wooden playpen has slats spaced no more than 2 inches (60 mm) apart.	___	___
7. If staples are used in construction, they are firmly installed and none are missing or loose.	___	___

THE COMMISSION RECOMMENDS: Never leave an infant in a mesh playpen or crib with the drop-side down. Even a very young infant can roll into the space between the mattress and loose mesh side and suffocate.

Rattles, squeeze toys, teethers   YES   NO

1. Rattles, squeeze toys and teethers are too large to lodge in a baby's throat.   _____   _____
2. Rattles are of sturdy construction that will not break apart in use.   _____   _____
3. Squeeze toys do not contain a squeaker that could detach and choke a baby.   _____   _____

THE COMMISSION RECOMMENDS: Take rattles, squeeze toys, teethers and other toys out of the crib or playpen when the baby sleeps to prevent suffocation.

Strollers and carriages   YES   NO

1. Wide base to prevent tipping.   _____   _____
2. Seat belt and crotch strap securely attached to frame.   _____   _____
3. Seat belt buckle is easy to use.   _____   _____
4. Brakes securely lock the wheel(s).   _____   _____
5. Shopping basket is low on the back and directly over or in front of rear wheels for stability.   _____   _____
6. When used in carriage position, leg hold openings can be closed.   _____   _____

THE COMMISSION RECOMMENDS: Always secure the seat belts. Never leave a child unattended in a stroller. Keep child's hands away from pinching areas when stroller is being folded or unfolded or the seat back is being reclined.

Toy chests   YES   NO

1. No lid latch which could entrap child within the chest.   _____   _____
2. Hinged lid has a spring-loaded lid support that will support the lid in any position and will not require periodic adjustment.   _____   _____
3. Chest has ventilation holes or spaces in front or sides, or under the lid should a child get inside.   _____   _____

THE COMMISSION RECOMMENDS: If you already own a toy chest or trunk with a freely falling lid, remove the lid to avoid a head injury to a small child or install a spring-loaded lid support.

Walkers   YES   NO

1. Wide wheel base for stability.   _____   _____
2. Covers over coil springs to avoid finger pinching.   _____   _____

3. Seat is securely attached to frame or walker.   ____ ____

4. No x-frames that could pinch or amputate
  fingers.   ____ ____

THE COMMISSION RECOMMENDS: Place gates or guards at top
of all stairways or keep stairway doors closed to prevent falls. Do not
use walker as baby sitters.

_____

For more nursery equipment information write for a free copy of *The safe nursery, a
buyer's guide,* Office of Information and Public Affairs, Washington, D.C., 20207.

Protocol for Postpartum Home Visit

Previsit interventions

1. Contact family to arrange details for home visit.
  a. Identify self, credentials, and agency role.
  b. Review purpose of home visit follow-up.
  c. Schedule convenient time for visit.
  d. Confirm address and route to family home.
2. Review and clarify appropriate data.
  a. All available assessment data for mother and infant (i.e., referral
    forms, hospital discharge summaries, family identified learning
    needs).
  b. Review records of any previous nursing contacts.
  c. Contact other professional caregivers as necessary to clarify
    data (i.e., obstetrician, nurse-midwife, pediatrician, referring
    nurse).
3. Identify community resources and teaching materials appropriate
  to meet needs already identified.
4. Plan the visit and prepare bag with equipment, supplies, and materials necessary for the assessments of mother and infant, actual
  care anticipated for mother and infant, and teaching.

In-home interventions: establishing a relationship

1. Reintroduce self and establish purpose of postpartum follow-up
  visit for mother, infant, and family; offer family opportunity to
  clarify their expectations of contact.

_____

From Bobak IM, Lowdermilk DL, Jensen MD: *Maternity nursing,* ed 4, St Louis, 1995,
Mosby.

2. Spend brief time socially interacting with family to become acquainted and establish trusting relationship.

In-home interventions: working with family

1. Conduct systematic assessment of mother and newborn to determine physiologic adjustment and any existing complications.
2. Throughout visit, collect data to assess the emotional adjustment of individual family members to newborn and lifestyle changes. Note evidence of family-newborn bonding and sibling rivalry; note relationships among mother, father, children, and grandparents.
3. Determine adequacy of support system.
   a. To what extent does someone help with cooking, cleaning, and other home management tasks?
   b. To what extent is help being provided in caring for the newborn and any other children?
   c. Are support persons encouraging the new mother to care for herself and get adequate rest?
   d. Who is providing helpful information? Emotional support?
4. Throughout the visit, observe home environment for adequacy of resources.
   a. Space: privacy, safe play of children, sleeping.
   b. Overall cleanliness and state of repair.
   c. Number of steps new mother must climb.
   d. Adequacy of cooking arrangements.
   e. Adequacy of refrigeration and other food storage areas.
   f. Adequacy of bathing, toileting, and laundry facilities.
   g. Arrangements in home for newborn: sleeping, bathing, formula preparation (if needed), layette items, and diapers.
5. Throughout the visit, observe home environment for overall state of repair and existence of safety hazards.
   a. Storage of medications, household cleaners, and other substances hazardous to children.
   b. Presence of peeling paint on furniture, walls, or pipes.
   c. Factors that contribute to falls, such as dim lighting, broken steps, scatter rugs.
   d. Presence of vermin.
   e. Use of crib or playpen that fails to meet safety guidelines.
   f. Existence of emergency plan in case of fire; fire alarm or extinguisher.
6. Provide care to mother and/or newborn as prescribed by their respective primary care provider or in accord with agency protocol.
7. Provide teaching on basis of previously identified needs.

8. Refer family to appropriate community agencies or resources, such as warm lines and support groups.
9. Ascertain that woman knows potential problems to watch for and whom to call if they occur.
10. Ensure that used disposable items have been handled appropriately and that reusable items are cleaned and repacked appropriately in the nurse's bag.

In-home interventions: ending the visit*
1. Summarize the activities and main points of the visit.
2. Clarify future expectations, including schedule of next visit.
3. Review teaching plan, and provide major points in writing.
4. Provide information about reaching the nurse or agency if needed before the next scheduled visit.

Postvisit interventions
1. Document the visit thoroughly, using the necessary agency forms to serve as a legal record of the visit and to allow third-party reimbursement, as possible.
2. Initiate the plan of care on which the next encounter with the client/family will be based.
3. Communicate appropriately (by telephone, letter, progress notes, or referral form) with primary care provider, other health professionals, or referral agencies on behalf of client/family.

---

*If this is the nurse's final planned encounter with the woman/family, it is important to recognize that both the woman and nurse may have feelings evoked by ending a meaningful relationship and by saying goodbye. Such feelings as anger, denial, and sadness are normal in this situation. Freely expressing these feelings at the end of the relationship is encouraged. Often patients are encouraged to do so if the nurse shares such feelings first.

Index